D0019728

HURST'S
THE HEART
MANUAL OF CARDIOLOGY

NOTICE

Medicine is an ever-changing science. As new research and clinical experience broaden our knowledge, changes in treatment and drug therapy are required. The editors and the publisher of this work have checked with sources believed to be reliable in their efforts to provide information that is complete and generally in accord with the standards accepted at the time of publication. However, in view of the possibility of human error or changes in medical sciences, neither the editors nor the publisher nor any other party who has been involved in the preparation or publication of this work warrants that the information contained herein is in every respect accurate or complete, and they disclaim all responsibility for any errors or omissions or for the results obtained from use of the information contained in this work. Readers are encouraged to confirm the information contained herein with other sources. For example and in particular, readers are advised to check the product information sheet included in the package of each drug they plan to administer to be certain that the information contained in this work is accurate and that changes have not been made in the recommended dose or in the contraindications for administration. This recommendation is of particular importance in connection with new or infrequently used drugs.

TWELFTH EDITION

HURST'S
THE HEART
MANUAL OF CARDIOLOGY

EDITORS

Robert A. O'Rourke, MD, MACC, MACP, FAHA
Distinguished Professor of Medicine, Emeritus
University of Texas Health Sciences Center at San Antonio
San Antonio, Texas

Richard A. Walsh, MD, FACC, FAHA
John H. Hord Professor
Chair, Department of Medicine
Case Western Reserve University
Physician-in-Chief
University Hospitals Health System
Cleveland, Ohio

Valentin Fuster, MD, PhD, FACC, FAHA
Professor of Cardiology
Director, Mount Sinai Heart
Director, the Zena and Michael A. Wiener Cardiovascular Institute and
the Marie-Josée and Henry R. Kravis Center for Cardiovascular Health
The Mount Sinai Medical Center
New York, New York

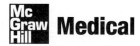

New York   Chicago   San Francisco   Lisbon   London   Madrid
Mexico City   Milan   New Delhi   San Juan   Seoul   Singapore   Sydney   Toronto

The **McGraw·Hill** Companies

HURST'S THE HEART, Twelfth Edition
MANUAL OF CARDIOLOGY

Copyright © 2009, 2005, 2001, by The McGraw-Hill Companies, Inc. All rights
reserved. Printed in the United States of America. Except as permitted under the
United States Copyright Act of 1976, no part of this publication may be reproduced
or distributed in any form or by any means, or stored in a data base or retrieval
system, without the prior written permission of the publisher.

4 5 6 7 8 9 0   DOC/DOC   12 11 10

ISBN 978-0-07-159298-7
MHID 0-07-159298-9

This book was set in Adobe Garamond by International Typesetting and Composition.
The editors were Ruth Weinberg and Christie Naglieri.
The production supervisor was Catherine Saggese.
Project management was provided by Vasundhara Sawhney, International Typesetting
and Composition.
The text designer was Alan Barnett.
The art director was Margaret Webster-Shapiro.
Cover photograph: Illustration of a healthy human heart.
Credit: Brian Evans / Photo Researchers Inc.
The indexer was Robert Swanson.
RR Donnelley was printer and binder.

This book is printed on acid-free paper.

Library of Congress Cataloging-in-Publication Data

Hurst's the heart manual of cardiology / editors, Robert A. O'Rourke,
    Richard A. Walsh, Valentin Fuster. — 12th ed.
        p. ; cm.
    Companion handbook to: Hurst's the heart. 12th ed. ©2008.
    Includes bibliographical references and index.
    ISBN-13: 978-0-07-159298-7 (pbk. : alk. paper)
    ISBN-10: 0-07-159298-9 (pbk. : alk. paper)   1. Heart—Diseases—Handbooks,
manuals, etc. 2.
Cardiology—Handbooks, manuals, etc.   I. Hurst, J. Willis (John Willis),
    1920-   II. O'Rourke, Robert A.   III. Walsh, Richard A., 1946-   IV. Fuster,
Valentin. V. Title: Heart manual of cardiology.
    [DNLM: 1. Cardiovascular Diseases—Handbooks. WG 39 H966 2009]
    RC669.15.H87 2009
    616.1'2—dc22

                                                        2008027734

CONTENTS

CONTRIBUTORS

Jamil A. Aboulhosn, MD
Professor of Medicine, Division of Cardiology, David Geffen School of
Medicine at UCLA, Los Angeles, California
Chapter 46, Congenital Heart Disease in Adults

Masood Akhtar, MD
Clinical Professor of Medicine, Cardiovascular Disease Section, Department
of Medicine, University of Wisconsin School of Medicine and Public Health,
Milwaukee, Wisconsin
Chapter 14, Techniques of Electrophysiologic Evaluation

Suhail Allaqaband, MD
Clinical Associate Professor of Medicine, University of Wisconsin School of
Medicine and Public Health, Milwaukee, Wisconsin
Chapter 58, Endovascular Treatment of Peripheral Vascular Disease

Charles Antzelevitch, PhD
Director of Research, Gordon K. Moe Scholar, Masonic Medical Research
Library, Utica, New York
Chapter 8, Mechanisms of Cardiac Arrhythmias and Conduction Disturbances

Faisal A. Arian, MD
Vascular Medical Fellow, Mayo Clinic College of Medicine, Rochester,
Minnesota
*Chapter 57, Diagnosis and Management of Diseases of the Peripheral Arteries
and Veins*

Tanvir Bajwa, MD
Clinical Professor of Medicine, University of Wisconsin School of Medicine
and Public Health, Milwaukee, Wisconsin
Chapter 58, Endovascular Treatment of Peripheral Vascular Disease

Julio A. Barcena, MD
Cardiology Fellow, University Hospitals Case Medical Center, Cleveland,
Ohio
Chapter 60, Adverse Cardiovascular Drug Interactions and Complications

Jeroen J. Bax, MD
Professor, Department of Cardiology, Leiden University Medical Center,
Leiden, Netherlands
Chapter 4, Noninvasive Testing for Myocardial Ischemia

Daniel S. Berman, MD
Professor of Medicine, David Geffen School of Medicine at UCLA, Los Angeles, California
Chapter 4, Noninvasive Testing for Myocardial Ischemia

William E. Boden, MD, FACC
Professor of Medicine and Preventive Medicine, University at Buffalo Schools of Medicine and Public Health, Buffalo, New York
Chapter 27, Mechanical Intervention in Acute Myocardial Infarction

Michael R. Bristow, MD, PhD
Professor of Medicine, University of Colorado Health Sciences Center, Denver, Colorado
Chapter 39, Dilated Cardiomyopathies

Craig S. Broberg, MD
Assistant Professor of Cardiovascular Medicine, Oregon Health and Science University, Portland, Oregon
Chapter 52, Heart Disease and Pregnancy

Alexander Burashnikov, PhD
Research Scientist, Masonic Medical Research Library, Utica, New York
Chapter 8, Mechanisms of Cardiac Arrhythmias and Conduction Disturbances

Louis R. Caplan, MD
Professor of Neurology, Harvard Medical School, Boston, Massachusetts
Chapter 55, Cerebrovascular Disease and Neurovascular Manifestations of Heart Disease

Mark D. Carlson, MD, MA
Adjunct Professor of Medicine, University Hospitals Case Medical Center, Cleveland, Ohio
Chapter 17, Diagnosis and Management of Syncope

Agustin Castellanos, MD
Professor of Medicine, University of Miami, Miller School of Medicine, Miami, Florida
Chapter 2, The Resting Electrocardiogram
Chapter 12, Brady Arrhythmias and Pacing

Pamela Charney, MD
Clinical Professor of Medicine, Albert Einstein College of Medicine, Nyack, New York
Chapter 51, Women and Coronary Heart Disease

Paul T. L. Chiam, MBBS, MRCP
Consultant, Department of Cardiology, National Heart Centre, Singapore
Chapter 56, The Nonsurgical Approach to Carotid Disease

John S. Child, MD
Professor of Medicine and Cardiology, David Geffen School of Medicine at UCLA, Los Angeles, California
Chapter 46, Congenital Heart Disease in Adults

Marco A. Costa, MD, PhH, FACC, FSCAI
Professor of Medicine, Division of Cardiovascular Medicine, University Hospitals Case Medical Center, Cleveland, Ohio
Chapter 7, Cardiac Catheterization and Coronary Angiography

Rebecca B. Costello, MD
Nutrition Scientist, Office of Dietary Supplements, National Institutes of Health, Bethesda, Maryland
Chapter 62, Complementary Medicine in Relation to Cardiovascular Disease

Freddy Del-Carpio Munoz, MD
Fellow in Clinical Cardiac Electrophysiology, Mayo Clinic College of Medicine, Rochester, New York
Chapter 2, The Resting Electrocardiogram

James A. deLemos, MD
Associate Professor of Medicine, University of Texas Southwestern Medical Center, Dallas, Texas
Chapter 25, Diagnosis and Management of Patients with Unstable Angina and Non–ST-Segment Elevation Myocardial Infarction

John S. Douglas, Jr, MD
Professor of Medicine, Emory University School of Medicine, Atlanta, Georgia
Chapter 26, Percutaneous Coronary Intervention

Kim A. Eagle, MD
Albion Walter Hewlett Professor of Internal Medicine, University of Michigan Health System, Ann Arbor, Michigan
Chapter 47, Perioperative Evaluation of Patients with Known or Suspected Cardiovascular Disease Who Undergo Noncardiac Surgery

John A. Elefteriades, MD
William W.L. Glenn Professor and Chief, Cardiothoracic Surgery, Yale University School of Medicine, New Haven, Connecticut
Chapter 54, Diseases of the Aorta

Sammy Elmariah, MD
Fellow, Cardiovascular Disease, The Zena and Michael A. Wiener Cardiovascular Institute, The Mount Sinai Medical Center, New York, New York
Chapter 49, Diabetes and Cardiovascular Disease

Gordon A. Ewy, MD
Professor and Chief of Cardiology, University of Arizona College of Medicine, Tucson, Arizona
Chapter 19, CPR and Post-Resuscitation Management

Emily A. Farkas, MD
Assistant Professor of Surgery, Division of Cardiothoracic Surgery, Saint Louis
University School of Medicine, Saint Louis, Missouri
Chapter 54, Diseases of the Aorta

Peter F. Fedullo, MD
Professor of Medicine, University of California San Diego, San Diego, California
Chapter 31, Pulmonary Embolism

Gary S. Francis, MD
Professor, University of Minnesota, Minneapolis, Minnesota
Chapter 20, Diagnosis and Management of Heart Failure

Michael Froeschl, MD, FRCP
Assistant Professor of Medicine, University of Ottawa Heart Institute, Ottawa,
Ontario
Chapter 45, Cardiovascular Diseases Caused by Genetic Abnormalities

Valentin Fuster, MD
Professor of Cardiology, The Mount Sinai Medical Center, New York, New York
Chapter 6, Cardiac CT and MRI
Chapter 23, Definitions and Pathogenesis of Acute Coronary Syndromes
Chapter 49, Diabetes and Cardiovascular Disease

Jon C. George, MD
Cardiology Fellow, Division of Cardiology, University Hospitals Case
Medical Center, Cleveland, Ohio
Chapter 5, Noninvasive Testing for Cardiac Dysfunction

Bernard J. Gersh, MD
Professor of Medicine, Mayo Clinic College of Medicine, Rochester, Minnesota
*Chapter 24, Diagnosis and Management of Patients with ST-Segment Elevation
Myocardial Infarction*

Edward M. Gilbert, MD
Professor, Department of Cardiology, University of Utah Health Sciences
Center, Salt Lake City, Utah
Chapter 39, Dilated Cardiomyopathies

Joey P. Granger, MD
Professor of Physiology and Medicine, Department of Physiology and
Biophysics, University of Mississippi Medical Center, Jackson, Mississippi
Chapter 28, Systemic Hypertension: Pathogenesis and Etiology

Scott M. Grundy, MD, PhD
Professor of Internal Medicine, UT Southwestern Medical Center at Dallas,
Dallas, Texas
Chapter 21, Dyslipidemia and Other Cardiac Risk Factors
Chapter 48, Metabolic Syndrome, Obesity, and Diet

Gary L. Grunkemeier, PhD
Professor, Providence Health System, Providence, Rhode Island
Chapter 36, Prosthetic Heart Valves: Choice of Valve and Management of the Patient

Anjan Gupta, MD
Clinical Associate Professor of Medicine, University of Wisconsin School of Medicine and Public Health, Milwaukee, Wisconsin
Chapter 58, Endovascular Treatment of Peripheral Vascular Disease

Saptsari Haldar, MD
Assistant Professor of Medicine, University Hospitals Case Medical Center, Cleveland, Ohio
Chapter 38, Infective Endocarditis

John E. Hall, MD
Arthur C. Guyton Chair and Professor, Department of Physiology and Biophysics, University of Mississippi Medical Center, Jackson, Mississippi
Chapter 28, Systemic Hypertension: Pathogenesis and Etiology

Michael E. Hall, MD
Professor, Department of Physiology and Biophysics, University of Mississippi Medical Center, Jackson, Mississippi
Chapter 28, Systemic Hypertension: Pathogenesis and Etiology

Brian D. Hoit, MD
Professor of Medicine, Physiology, and Biophysics, University Hospitals Case Medical Center, Cleveland, Ohio
Chapter 5, Noninvasive Testing for Cardiac Dysfunction
Chapter 41, Restrictive, Obliterative, and Infiltrative Cardiomyopathies
Chapter 44, Diseases of the Pericardium

Robert L. Huang, MD, MPH
Clinical Fellow, Division of Cardiovascular Medicine, Vanderbilt University School of Medicine, Nashville, Tennessee
Chapter 21, Dyslipidemia and Other Cardiac Risk Factors

Sriram S. Iyer, MD
Professor, Lenox Hill Heart and Vascular Institute of New York, New York, New York
Chapter 56, The Nonsurgical Approach to Carotid Disease

Jooby John, MD
Fellow, Cardiology, Sarver Heart Center, Tucson, Arizona
Chapter 19, CPR and Post-Resuscitation Management

Daniel W. Jones, MD
Professor of Medicine, University of Mississippi Medical Center, Jackson, Mississippi
Chapter 28, Systemic Hypertension: Pathogenesis and Etiology

Mark E. Josephson, MD
Professor of Medicine, Harvard Medical School, Boston, Massachusetts
Chapter 18, Sudden Cardiac Death

Joseph Jozic, MD
Interventional Cardiology Fellow, Division of Cardiovascular Medicine,
University Hospitals Case Medical Center, Cleveland, Ohio
Chapter 7, Cardiac Catheterization and Coronary Angiography

Prashant Kaul, MD
Fellow in Cardiovascular Disease, Division of Cardiology, Duke University
Medical Center, Durham, North Carolina
Chapter 62, Complementary Medicine in Relation to Cardiovascular Disease

Richard E. Kerber, MD
Professor of Medicine, University of Iowa College of Medicine,
Iowa City, Iowa
*Chapter 16, Indications and Techniques of Electrical Defibrillation and
Cardioversion*

Spencer B. King III, MD, MACC
Professor of Medicine Emeritus, Emory University School of Medicine,
Atlanta, Georgia
Chapter 26, Percutaneous Coronary Intervention

Mitchell W. Krucoff, MD
Professor Medicine/Cardiology, Duke University Medical Center, Durham,
North Carolina
Chapter 62, Complementary Medicine in Relation to Cardiovascular Disease

Megan C. Leary, MD
Instructor in Neurology, Harvard Medical School, Boston, Massachusetts
*Chapter 55, Cerebrovascular Disease and Neurovascular Manifestations of Heart
Disease*

Steve L. Liao, MD
Instructor of Medicine, Mount Sinai School of Medicine, New York, New York
Chapter 6, Cardiac CT and MRI

Michael J. Lim, MD
Associate Professor of Internal Medicine, Saint Louis University School of
Medicine, Saint Louis, Missouri
*Chapter 47, Perioperative Evaluation of Patients with Known or Suspectd
Cardiovascular Disease Who Undergo Noncardiac Surgery*

Brian D. Lowes, MD
Associate of Medicine, University of Colorado Health Sciences Center,
Denver, Colorado
Chapter 39, Dilated Cardiomyopathies

Judith A. Mackall, MD
Associate Professor of Medicine, University Hospitals Case Medical Center, Cleveland, Ohio
Chapter 17, Diagnosis and Management of Syncope

Donna M. Mancini, MD
Professor of Medicine, New York-Presbyterian/Columbia, New York, New York
Chapter 42, Myocarditis and Specific Cardiomyopathies

Daniel B. Mark, MD, MPH
Professor of Medicine, Duke University Medical Center, Durham, North Carolina
Chapter 62, Complementary Medicine in Relation to Cardiovascular Disease

David J. Maron, MD
Associate Professor of Medicine and Emergency Medicine, Vanderbilt University School of Medicine, Nashville, Tennessee
Chapter 21, Dyslipidemia and Other Cardiac Risk Factors

Thomas H. Marwick, MBBS, PhD, FRACP, FESC, FACC
Professor of Medicine, University of Queensland, Brisbane, Australia
Chapter 4, Noninvasive Testing for Myocardial Ischemia

Susan A. Matulevicius, MD
Cardiology Fellow, University of Texas Southwestern Medical Center, Dallas, Texas
Chapter 25, Diagnosis and Management of Patients with Unstable Angina and Non–St-Segment Elevation Myocardial Infarction

John H. McAnulty, MD
Professor Emeritus, Oregon Health and Science University, Portland, Oregon
Chapter 37, Antithrombotic Therapy for Valvular Heart Disease
Chapter 52, Heart Disease and Pregnancy

Christopher D. McCoy, MD
Cardiology Fellow, University Hospitals Case Medical Center, Cleveland, Ohio
Chapter 41, Restrictive, Obliterative, and Infiltrative Cardiomyopathies

Robert McCray, MD
Cardiology Fellow, Department of Cardiology, Heart and Vascular Institute at the Cleveland Clinic, Cleveland, Ohio
Chapter 20, Diagnosis and Management of Heart Failure

Luisa Mestroni, MD
Professor of Medicine/Cardiology, University of Colorado Health Sciences Center, Denver, Colorado
Chapter 39, Dilated Cardiomyopathies

Marc A. Miller, MD
Fellow, Cardiovascular Disease, The Zena and Michael A. Wiener Cardiovascular
Institute, The Mount Sinai Medical Center, New York, New York
Chapter 49, Diabetes and Cardiovascular Disease

Raul D. Mitrani, MD
Voluntary Associate Professor of Medicine, University of Miami, Miller
School of Medicine, Miami, Florida
Chapter 12, Brady Arrhythmias and Pacing

M. Eyman Mortada, MD
Clinical Assistant Professor, Department of Medicine, Cardiovascular Disease
Section, University of Wisconsin School of Medicine and Public Health,
Milwaukee, Wisconsin
Chapter 14, Techniques of Electrophysiologic Evaluation

Robert J. Myerburg, MD
Professor of Medicine and Physiology, Division of Cardiology, University
of Miami, Miller School of Medicine, Miami, Florida
Chapter 2, The Resting Electrocardiogram
Chapter 12, Brady Arrhythmias and Pacing

Ajith P. Nair, MD
Clinical Instructor, Mount Sinai School of Medicine, New York, New York
Chapter 42, Myocarditis and Specific Cardiomyopathies

Vidya Narayan, MD
Fellow in Cardiology, Keck School of Medicine, University of Southern
California, Los Angeles, California
Chapter 32, Aortic Valve Disease

Ira S. Nash, MD, FACC, FAHA, FACP
Associate Professor, Mount Sinai School of Medicine, New York, New York
Chapter 59, Practice Guidelines and Cardiovascular Care

Patrick T. O'Gara, MD
Associate Professor of Medicine, Harvard Medical School, Boston,
Massachusetts
Chapter 38, Infective Endocarditis

Robert A. O'Rourke, MD, MACC, MACP, FAHA
Distinguished Professor of Medicine, Emeritus, University of Texas Health
Science Center at San Antonio, San Antonio, Texas
Chapter 1, The History, Physical Examination, and Cardiac Auscultation
Chapter 3, Cardiac Roentgenography
Chapter 9, Approach to the Patient with Cardiac Arrhythmias
Chapter 10, Atrial Fibrillation, Atrial Flutter, and Supraventricular Tachycardia
Chapter 13, Long-Term Continuous Electrocardiographic Recording
Chapter 22, Management of Patients with Chronic Ischemic Heart Disease

Chapter 34, Mitral Regurgitation (Including Mitral Valve Prolapse)
Chapter 40, Hypertrophic Cardiomyopathy
Chapter 50, Autoimmune Disorders and the Cardiovascular System
Chapter 61, Treatment Consideration in Elderly Patients with Cardiovascular Diseases

Richard L. Page, MD, FACC, FAHA, FHRS
Robert A. Bruce Professor of Medicine/Cardiology, Division of Cardiology, University of Washington School of Medicine, Washington DC
Chapter 11, Ventricular Arrhythmias

Thomas A. Pearson, MD
Albert D. Kaiser Professor, Senior Associate Dean for Clinical Research, University of Rochester, Rochester, New York
Chapter 21, Dyslipidemia and Other Cardiac Risk Factors

Lakshmana K. Pendyala, MD
Cardiology Fellow, Saint Joseph's Translational Research Institute, Atlanta, Georgia
Chapter 53, The Heart and Obesity

Illeana A. Piña, MD
Professor of Medicine, Cardiology, University Hospitals Case Medical Center, Cleveland, Ohio
Chapter 60, Adverse Cardiovascular Drug Interactions and Complications

Sean P. Pinney, MD
Assistant Professor of Medicine, Mount Sinai School of Medicine, New York, New York
Chapter 42, Myocarditis and Specific Cardiomyopathies

Duane S. Pinto, MD
Assistant Professor of Medicine, Harvard Medical School, Boston, Massachusetts
Chapter 18, Sudden Cardiac Death

Aly Rahimtoola, MD
Partner, Division of Cardiovascular Medicine, The Oregon Clinic, Portland, Oregon
Chapter 32, Aortic Valve Disease

Shahbudin H. Rahimtoola, MD
Distinguished Professor, Keck School of Medicine, University of Southern California, Los Angeles, California
Chapter 32, Aortic Valve Disease
Chapter 33, Mitral Valve Stenosis
Chapter 36, Prosthetic Heart Valves: Choice of Valve and Management of the Patient
Chapter 37, Antithrombotic Therapy for Valvular Heart Disease

Mahboob Rahman, MD
Associate Professor of Medicine, University Hospitals Case Medical Center, Cleveland, Ohio
Chapter 29, Diagnosis and Treatment of Hypertension

Matthew R. Reynolds, MD
Assistant Professor of Medicine, Harvard Medical School, Boston, Massachusetts
Chapter 18, Sudden Cardiac Death

Robert W. Rho, MD, FACC
Associate Professor of Medicine, University of Washington School of Medicine, Washington DC
Chapter 11, Ventricular Arrhythmias

Paul M. Ridker, MD
Eugene Braunwald Professor of Medicine, Harvard Medical School, Boston, Massachusetts
Chapter 21, Dyslipidemia and Other Cardiac Risk Factors

Robert Roberts, MD, FRCP, MACE
Professor of Medicine, University of Ottawa Heart Institute, Ottawa, Ontario
Chapter 45, Cardiovascular Diseases Caused by Genetic Abnormalities

Sharon L. Roble, MD
Cardiology Fellow, University Hospitals Case Medical Center, Cleveland, Ohio
Chapter 44, Diseases of the Pericardium

Anand Rohatgi, MD
Assistant Professor, University of Texas Southwestern Medical Center, Dallas, Texas
Chapter 25, Diagnosis and Management of Patients with Unstable Angina and Non–St-Segment Elevation Myocardial Infarction

Jose F. Roldan, MD
Assistant Professor of Medicine, Department of Medicine, University of Texas Health Science Center at San Antonio, San Antonio, Texas
Chapter 50, Autoimmune Disorders and the Cardiovascular System

Gary S. Roubin, MD, PhD
Professor, Lenox Hill Heart and Vascular Institute of New York, New York, New York
Chapter 56, The Nonsurgical Approach to Carotid Disease

Darrell C. Rubin, MD, PhD
Resident, Internal Medicine, University Hospitals Case Medical Center, Cleveland, Ohio
Chapter 29, Diagnosis and Treatment of Hypertension

Lewis J. Rubin, MD
Professor of Medicine, University of California, School of Medicine, La Jolla, California
Chapter 30, Pulmonary Hypertension

Christian T. Ruff, MD
Professor, Cardiovascular Division, Harvard Medical School, Boston, Massachusetts
Chapter 38, Infective Endocarditis

Habib Samady, MD, FACC, FSCAI
Associate Professor of Medicine, Interventional Cardiology, Andreas Gruentzig
Cardiovascular Center, Emory University School of Medicine, Atlanta, Georgia
Chapter 26, Percutaneous Coronary Intervention

Chirag M. Sandesara, MD
Electrophysiology Fellow, University of Iowa College of Medicine, Iowa City, Iowa
Chapter 16, Indications and Techniques of Electrical Defibrillation and Cardioversion

John T. Schindler, MD
Assistant Professor of Medicine, University of Pittsburgh Medical Center, Pittsburgh, Pennsylvania
Chapter 35, Tricuspid Valve and Pulmonic Valve Disease

James A. Shaver, MD
Professor of Medicine, University of Pittsburgh Medical Center, Pittsburgh, Pennsylvania
Chapter 35, Tricuspid Valve and Pulmonic Valve Disease

Leslee J. Shaw, MD
Professor of Medicine, Department of Medicine, Emory University School of Medicine, Atlanta, Georgia
Chapter 4, Noninvasive Testing for Myocardial Ischemia

Lian R. Shaw, MD
Cascade Heart Clinic, Vancouver, Washington
Chapter 40, Hypertrophic Cardiomyopathy

Amardeep K. Singh, MD
Cardiology Fellow, University of Southern California, Los Angeles, California
Chapter 33, Mitral Valve Stenosis

Andrew L. Smith, MD
Associate Professor of Medicine, Emory University School of Medicine, Atlanta, Georgia
Chapter 43, The Heart and Noncardiac Drugs, Electricity, Poisons, and Radiation

Sidney C. Smith, Jr, MD
Professor of Medicine, Division of Cardiology, Department of Internal Medicine, University of North Carolina at Chapel Hill, Chapel Hill, North Carolina
Chapter 48, Metabolic Syndrome, Obesity, and Diet

Albert Starr, MD
Professor, Providence Health System, Providence, Rhode Island
Chapter 36, Prosthetic Heart Valves: Choice of Valve and Management of the Patient

Eric C. Stecker, MD, MPH
Professor, Division of Cardiology, Legacy Good Samaritan Hospital, Portland, Oregon
Chapter 37, Antithrombotic Therapy for Valvular Heart Disease

William G. Stevenson, MD
Professor of Medicine, Harvard Medical School, Boston, Massachusetts
Chapter 15, Treatment of Cardiac Arrhythmias with Ablation Therapy

H. Robert Superko, MD
Executive Director, Center for Genomics and Human Health, Saint Joseph's Translational Research Institute, Atlanta, Georgia
Chapter 53, The Heart and Obesity

Joseph M. Sweeny, MD
Fellow, Cardiovascular Disease, Mount Sinai School of Medicine, New York, New York
Chapter 23, Definitions and Pathogenesis of Acute Coronary Syndromes

Anwar Tandar, MD
Assistant Professor of Medicine, State University of New York at Buffalo, Buffalo, New York
Chapter 27, Mechanical Intervention in Acute Myocardial Infarction

Usha B. Tedrow, MD, MSc
Instructor of Medicine, Harvard Medical School, Boston, Massachusetts
Chapter 15, Treatment of Cardiac Arrhythmias with Ablation Therapy

Mintu Turakhia, MD
Instructor, Stanford University, Palo Alto, California
Chapter 18, Sudden Cardiac Death

Rajesh Vedanthan, MD, MPH
Fellow in Cardiovascular Medicine, Mount Sinai School of Medicine, New York, New York
Chapter 59, Practice Guidelines and Cardiovascular Care

Mohan N. Viswanathan, MD
Assistant Professor of Medicine/Cardiology, Division of Cardiology, University of Washington School of Medicine, Washington DC
Chapter 11, Ventricular Arrhythmias

Jiri J. Vitek, MD
Professor, Lenox Hill Heart and Vascular Institute of New York, New York,
New York
Chapter 56, The Nonsurgical Approach to Carotid Disease

John H. K. Vogel, MD
Chairman, Department of Cardiology, Santa Barbara Cottage Hospital,
Santa Barbara, California
Chapter 62, Complementary Medicine in Relation to Cardiovascular Disease

Stanley S. Wang, MD
Professor, University of Texas Southwestern Medical Center at Dallas, Dallas,
Texas
Chapter 48, Metabolic Syndrome, Obesity, and Diet

Paul W. Wennberg, MD
Assistant Professor of Medicine, Mayo Clinic College of Medicine,
Rochester, Minnesota
*Chapter 57, Diagnosis and Management of Diseases of the Peripheral Arteries
and Veins*

Arie Wolak, MD
Lecturer, Ben Gurion University of the Negev, School of Medicine, Faculty
of Health Sciences, Beer Sheva, Israel
Chapter 4, Noninvasive Testing for Myocardial Ischemia

Jackson T. Wright, Jr, MD, PhD
Program Director, W.T. Dahms MD Clinical Research Unit, University
Hospitals Case Medical Center, Cleveland, Ohio
Chapter 29, Diagnosis and Treatment of Hypertension

YingXing Wu, MD
Professor, Providence Health System, Providence, Rhode Island
*Chapter 36, Prosthetic Heart Valves: Choice of Valve and Management
of the Patient*

Eric H. Yang, MD, FACC
Assistant Professor of Medicine, University of North Carolina at Chapel
Hill, Chapel Hill, North Carolina
*Chapter 24, Diagnosis and Management of Patients with ST-Segment Elevation
Myocardial Infarction*

Gordon L. Yung, MD
Associate Clinical Professor of Medicine, University of California San Diego,
San Diego, California
Chapter 31, Pulmonary Embolism

PREFACE

This manual of cardiology provides an up-to-date compendium for the diagnosis and management of a wide spectrum of patients with cardiovascular disease. It contains useful clinical information relating to heart disease patients for all health care providers, and meets the needs of physicians and students for a concise, portable handbook that can be used any time, day or night, when there is no access to larger reference material (such as the recently published 12th edition of *Hurst's the Heart*).

Written by many of the same experts who contributed to the larger textbook, the manual has been considerably revised including additional material such as myocardial imaging and genetic causes of cardiovascular disease. The manual also can be used as a stand-alone source for quick information concerning the presentation, natural history, and treatment of various cardiovascular disorders. Important information from the ACC/AHA *Clinical Practice Guidelines* is included in many chapters, and this book contains tables and algorithms not available in the larger text, in order to provide the reader with appropriate, easily accessible indications for specific therapy.

We express our gratitude to the authors of the individual chapters of this practical concise resource for cardiovascular diagnostics and therapeutics.

Finally we wish to thank our families for their support and the many sacrifices they made to make this manual possible.

The Editors
Robert A. O'Rourke
Richard A. Walsh
Valentin Fuster

CHAPTER (1)

History, Physical Examination, and Cardiac Auscultation

Robert A. O'Rourke

In assessing patients with definite or suspected heart disease, the history and physical examination, along with various noninvasive studies, can provide relevant information. Integration of these data often results in accurate diagnoses and appropriate decisions regarding further diagnostic studies, therapeutic options, or both. The history and physical examination should be the foundation for evaluating any patient with known or suspected heart disease.

This chapter is composed of three sections, covering the salient features of the history, physical examination, and particularly cardiac auscultation.

HISTORY

The history is the first step in the assessment of the patient. The most common complaint among patients with heart disease is chest pain; however, particular attention should be paid to the chief complaint, with clarification of all relevant symptoms. These may include exercise intolerance, shortness of breath (particularly with exertion), orthopnea, and paroxysmal nocturnal dyspnea. Symptoms of edema, ascites, cough, hemoptysis, palpitation, fatigue, and peripheral embolization can be consistent with heart disease. Chest discomfort is the foremost manifestation of myocardial ischemia and the most commonly encountered symptom. The differential diagnosis of chest pain is extensive and is given in Table 1-1.

Angina pectoris is defined as chest pain or discomfort of cardiac origin that usually results from a temporary imbalance between myocardial oxygen supply and demand. The important characteristics of angina include the quality of the pain, precipitating factors, mode of onset, duration, location, and pattern of disappearance.

The quality of the pain is typically described as "tightness," "pressure," "burning," "heaviness," "aching," "strangling," or "compression." The description of the quality may be influenced by the patient's intelligence, social background, and education.

The most common precipitating factor is physical exertion. Angina also can be provoked by emotional distress, cold weather, or eating. It typically has a crescendo pattern, but it can occur acutely, as with the acute coronary syndromes. An episode may last up to 20 minutes. Most patients have relief of symptoms within 5 minutes after cessation of physical activity or by nitroglycerin lingual spray or sublingual tablets. Failure of rest or nitroglycerin to relieve symptoms suggests another cause of the pain or impending myocardial infarction. Localizing the site of chest discomfort is also helpful in determining the cause. Angina pectoris is usually retrosternal or slightly to the left of midline. Pain tends to radiate into the arms, neck, and jaw. In the arms, the pain radiates down the ulnar aspect and the volar surface to the wrist and the ulnar fingers. Patients with angina pectoris are classified functionally from classes I to IV (Table 1-2).

TABLE 1-1

Differential Diagnosis of Chest Pain

1. Angina pectoris/myocardial infarction
2. Other cardiovascular causes
   a. Likely ischemic in origin
      (1) Aortic stenosis
      (2) Hypertrophic cardiomyopathy
      (3) Severe systemic hypertension
      (4) Severe right ventricular hypertension
      (5) Aortic regurgitation
      (6) Severe anemia/hypoxia
   b. Nonischemic in origin
      (1) Aortic dissection
      (2) Pericarditis
      (3) Mitral valve prolapse
3. Gastrointestinal
   a. Esophageal spasm
   b. Esophageal reflux
   c. Esophageal rupture
   d. Peptic ulcer disease
4. Psychogenic
   a. Anxiety
   b. Depression
   c. Cardiac psychosis
   d. Self-gain
5. Neuromusculoskeletal
   a. Thoracic outlet syndrome
   b. Degenerative joint disease of cervical/thoracic spine
   c. Costochondritis (Tietze's syndrome)
   d. Herpes zoster
   e. Chest wall pain and tenderness
6. Pulmonary
   a. Pulmonary embolus with or without pulmonary infarction
   b. Pneumothorax
   c. Pneumonia with pleural involvement
7. Pleurisy

TABLE 1-2

Canadian Cardiovascular Society Functional Classification of Angina Pectoris

I. Ordinary physical activity, such as walking and climbing stairs, does not cause angina. Angina results from strenuous or rapid or prolonged exertion at work or recreation.
II. Slight limitation of ordinary activity. Walking or climbing stairs rapidly, walking uphill, walking or stair climbing after meals, in cold, in wind, or when under emotional stress, or only during the few hours after awakening. Walking more than two blocks on the level and climbing more than one flight of ordinary stairs at a normal pace and under normal conditions.
III. Marked limitations of ordinary physical activity. Walking one to two blocks on the level and climbing more than one flight under normal conditions.
IV. Inability to carry on any physical activity without discomfort—anginal syndrome may be present at rest.

Modified from Campeau L. Letter: Grading of angina pectoris. *Circulation.*19;54:522. Reproduced with permission from the American Heart Association, Inc., and the author.

TABLE 1-3

The Old New York Heart Association Functional Classification

Class 1. No symptoms with ordinary physical activity.
Class 2. Symptoms with ordinary activity. Slight limitation of activity.
Class 3. Symptoms with less than ordinary activity. Marked limitation of activity.
Class 4. Symptoms with any physical activity or even at rest.

Data compiled from the Criteria Committee of the New York Heart Association. *Diseases of the Heart and Blood Vessels: Nomenclature and Criteria for Diagnosis of the Heart and Great Vessels.* 6th ed. New York: New York Heart Association/Little Brown; 1964.

Other cardiovascular diseases can also precipitate chest pain in the absence of coronary atherosclerosis. Increased oxygen demand resulting in chest pain can occur with aortic stenosis, hypertrophic cardiomyopathy, and systemic arterial hypertension. In addition, chest discomfort resulting from myocardial ischemia can be caused by aortic valve regurgitation. Chest pain that is not related to myocardial ischemia can be caused by pericarditis, aortic dissection, and mitral valve prolapse.

A separate New York Heart Association functional classification exists for assessing cardiac disability for patients with heart failure (Table 1-3). Patients should be asked sufficient questions to allow proper assessment according to this classification. The classification based on symptoms is used frequently in medical literature, multicenter research trials, and clinical practice.

PHYSICAL EXAMINATION

Important information concerning the patient with definite or suspected heart disease is often obtained by a careful and deliberate physical examination, which includes a general inspection of the patient, an indirect measurement of the arterial blood pressure in both arms and one or both lower extremities, an examination of central and peripheral arterial pulses, an evaluation of the jugular venous pressure and pulsations, palpation of the precordium, and cardiac auscultation. Based on this rather inexpensive evaluation, a definite diagnosis is often made and noninvasive and invasive testing may be unnecessary.

【 】 ARTERIAL PRESSURE PULSE

The arterial pulse wave begins with aortic valve opening and the onset of left ventricular ejection (Fig. 1-1). The rapid-rising portion of the arterial pressure curve is often termed the *anacrotic limb* (from the Greek, meaning "upbeat"). During isovolumic relaxation, a transient reversal of flow from the central arteries toward the ventricle just prior to aortic valve closure is associated with an incisura on the descending limb of the aortic pressure pulse.

A small weak pulse, *pulsus parvus*, is common in conditions with a diminished left ventricular stroke volume, narrow pulse pressure, and increased peripheral vascular resistance. A hypokinetic pulse may be due to hypovolemia, left ventricular failure, restrictive pericardial disease, or mitral stenosis. In aortic valve stenosis, the delayed systolic peak, *pulsus tardus*, results from obstruction to left ventricular ejection. In contrast, a large, bounding (hyperkinetic) pulse is usually associated with an increased left ventricular

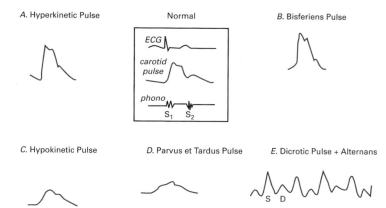

A. Hyperkinetic Pulse   Normal   *B.* Bisferiens Pulse

ECG

carotid
pulse

phono
          S₁ S₂

C. Hypokinetic Pulse   *D.* Parvus et Tardus Pulse   *E.* Dicrotic Pulse + Alternans

S D

FIGURE 1-1. Schematic representation of the normal carotid arterial pulse, five types of abnormal pulses, and pulsus alternans. (ECG, electrocardiogram; phono, phonocardiogram; S₁, S₂, first and second heart sounds; S, systole; D, diastole.)

stroke volume, a wide pulse pressure, and a decrease in peripheral vascular resistance. This pattern occurs characteristically in patients with an elevated stroke volume, with hyperkinetic circulation, or with a rapid runoff of blood from the arterial system—such as with an arteriovenous (AV) fistula. Patients with mitral regurgitation or a ventricular septal defect also may have a bounding pulse. In aortic regurgitation, the rapidly rising, bounding arterial pulse results from an increased left ventricular volume and an increased rate of ventricular ejection. The *bisferiens* pulse, which has two systolic peaks, is characteristic of aortic regurgitation (with or without accompanying stenosis) and of hypertrophic cardiomyopathy. The *dicrotic* pulse has two palpable waves, the second in diastole. It occurs most frequently in patients with a very low stroke volume, including those with dilated cardiomyopathy.

Pulsus alternans is a pattern in which there is regular alteration of the pressure pulse amplitude, despite a regular rhythm. It denotes severe impairment of left ventricular function and commonly occurs in patients who also have a loud third heart sound. In *pulsus paradoxus*, the decrease in systolic arterial pressure that normally accompanies the reduction in arterial pulse amplitude during inspiration is accentuated. In patients with pericardial tamponade, airway obstruction (asthma), or superior vena cava obstruction, the decrease in systolic arterial pressure frequently exceeds the normal decrease of 10 mm Hg, and the peripheral pulse may disappear completely during inspiration.

【 】 JUGULAR VENOUS PULSE

The two main objectives of the examination of the neck veins are inspection of their waveforms and estimation of the central venous pressure (CVP). In most patients, the right internal jugular vein is best for both purposes. Usually, the pulsation of the internal jugular vein is optimal when the trunk is inclined less than 30 degrees. In patients with elevated venous pressure, it may be necessary to elevate the trunk further, sometimes to as much as 90 degrees. Simultaneous palpation of the left carotid artery aids the examiner in determining which pulsations are venous and in relating the venous pulsations to their timing in the cardiac cycle.

The normal jugular venous pulse (JVP) consists of two to three positive waves and two negative troughs (Fig. 1-2). The positive, presystolic *a* wave is produced by venous distention due to right atrial contraction and is the dominant wave in the JVP. Large *a* waves indicate that the right atrium is contracting against increased resistance, as occurs

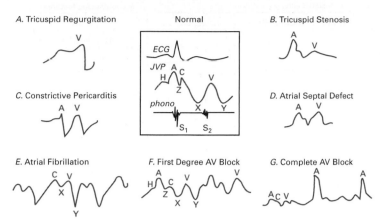

FIGURE 1-2. Schematic representation of the normal jugular venous pulse (JVP), four types of abnormal JVPs, and the JVPs in three arrhythmias. See text under "Jugular Venous Pulse" for definitions of h, a, z, c, x, v, and y.

with tricuspid stenosis or more commonly with increased resistance to right ventricular filling. Large a waves ("cannon"*a* waves) also occur during arrhythmias whenever the right atrium contracts while the tricuspid valve is still closed. The *a* wave is absent in patients with atrial fibrillation, and there is an increased delay between the *a* wave and the carotid arterial pulse in patients with first-degree atrioventricular block.

The *c* wave is a positive wave produced by the bulging of the tricuspid valve into the right atrium during right ventricular isovolumetric systole and by the distention of the carotid artery located adjacent to the jugular vein. The *x* descent is due both to atrial relaxation and to the downward displacement of the tricuspid valve during ventricular systole. The *x* descent is reversed in tricuspid regurgitation. The positive late systolic *v* wave results from right atrial filling during ventricular systole, when the tricuspid valve is closed. Tricuspid regurgitation causes the *v* wave to become more prominent; when tricuspid regurgitation becomes severe, the combination of a prominent *v* wave and the obliteration of the *x* descent results in a single large, positive systolic wave (i.e., "ventricularization"—a pattern similar to the right ventricular pressure tracing). The negative descending limb, the *y* descent of the JVP, is produced by the opening of the tricuspid valve and the rapid inflow of blood into the right ventricle. A venous pulse characterized by a sharp *y* descent, a deep *y* trough, and a rapid ascent to the baseline is seen in patients with constrictive pericarditis or with severe right heart failure and a high venous pressure.

The right internal jugular vein is the best vein to use for accurate estimation of the CVP. The sternal angle is used as the reference point, because the center of the right atrium lies approximately 5 cm below the sternal angle. The patient is best examined at the optimal degree of trunk elevation for visualization of the jugular venous pulsations. The vertical distance between the top of the oscillating venous column and the level of the sternal angle is determined; generally it is less than 3 cm (3 cm + 5 cm = 8 cm blood or water; multiply by 0.8 to convert to mm Hg). In patients suspected of having right ventricular failure who have a normal CVP at rest, the abdominojugular reflux test may be helpful. The palm of the examiner's hand is placed over the abdomen, and firm pressure is applied for 10 seconds or more. When right heart function is impaired, the upper level of venous pulsations usually increases. A positive abdominojugular reflux test is best defined as an increase in the JVP during 10 seconds of firm midabdominal compression followed by a rapid drop in pressure by 4 cm blood on release of the compression.

Graphic Representation
(Palpable features in heavy line)

Type of movement and associated clinical condition	Graphic Representation	Location and accompanying features
NORMAL ADULT APEX IMPULSE	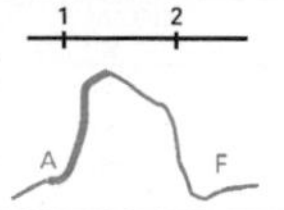	Cardiac apex; moderate systolic thrust; A and F waves usually imperceptible
HYPERKINETIC APEX IMPULSE Normal Child Hyperdynamic states Ventricular septal defect Patent ductus arteriosus Mitral regurgitation Aortic regurgitation	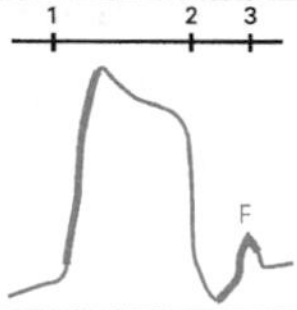	Exaggerated thrust at cardiac apex; F wave may be palpable, coincident with third heart sound
HYPERKINETIC RIGHT VENTRICULAR IMPULSE Atrial septal defect Pulmonary regurgitation	Same as above	Maximal at left sternal edge in third and fourth intercostal spaces
SUSTAINED APEX IMPULSE Left ventricular hypertrophy, as in: Aortic stenosis Hypertension Insert: a variation that may occur in hypertrophic cardiomyopathy	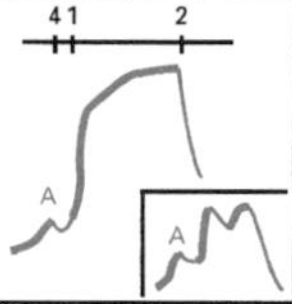	Maximal at cardiac apex; A wave may be visible and palpable coincident with fourth heart sound
SUSTAINED RIGHT VENTRICULAR IMPULSE Right ventricular hypertrophy, as in: Pulmonary hypertension Pulmonary stenosis	Same impulse as in Sustained above	Maximal at left sternal edge in third and fourth intercostal spaces
ECTOPIC LEFT VENTRICULAR IMPULSE Ventricular aneurysm	Same impulse as in Sustained above	Maximal over mid-precordium rather than at apex
LEFT ATRIAL EXPANSION Severe mitral regurgitation	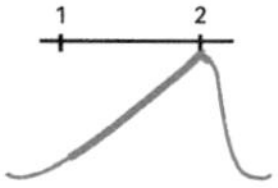	Left sternal edge or entire precordium; hyperkinetic apex impulse due to left ventricular volume overload
PULMONARY ARTERY PULSATION Pulmonary hypertension	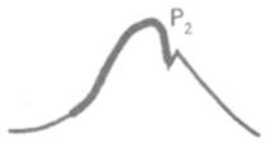	Second left intercostal space; palpable P_2
INWARD MOVEMENT DURING SYSTOLE Constrictive pericarditis Tricuspid regurgitation; primary	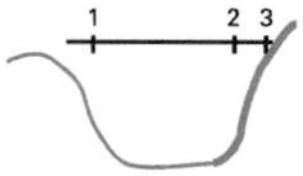	Cardiac apex or entire precordium; reversal of direction during systole as compared with preceding examples
DIASTOLIC MOVEMENTS Cardiomyopathy	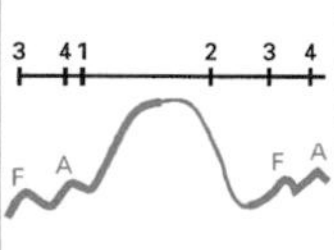	Cardiac apex; systolic movement may be inconspicuous; diastolic movements F and A correspond to 3rd and 4th heart sounds which may merge in tachycardia to form a summation gallop

FIGURE 1-3. Graphic representation of apical movements in health and disease. Heavy line indicates palpable features. (P_2, pulmonary component of second heart sound; A, atrial wave, corresponding to a fourth heart sound (S_4) or atrial gallop; F, filling wave, corresponding to third heart sound (S_3) or ventricular gallop. (Reproduced with permission from O'Rourke RA, Shaver JA, Silverman ME: The History, Physical Examination, and Cardiac Auscultation. In: Fuster V, Alexander W, O'Rourke RA: The Heart 10th edition, New York: McGraw-Hill;2001.)

Kussmaul's sign—an increase rather than the normal decrease in the CVP during inspiration—is most often caused by severe right-sided heart failure; it is also a frequent finding in patients with constrictive pericarditis or right ventricular infarction.

【 】 PRECORDIAL PALPATION

The location, amplitude, duration, and direction of the cardiac impulse usually can be best appreciated with the fingertips. Left ventricular hypertrophy (LVH) results in exaggeration of the amplitude, duration, and often size (normal diameter is < 3 cm) of the left ventricular thrust. The impulse may be displaced laterally and downward into the sixth or seventh interspace, particularly in patients with an LV volume load, as in the case of aortic regurgitation or dilated cardiomyopathy (Fig. 1-3).

Additional abnormal features detectable at the left ventricular apex include marked presystolic distention of the LV, which is often accompanied by a fourth heart sound (S_4) in patients with an excessive LV pressure load or myocardial ischemia or infarction, and a prominent early diastolic rapid-filling wave, which is often accompanied by a third heart sound (S_3) in patients with left LV failure or mitral valve regurgitation.

Right ventricular hypertrophy often results in a sustained systolic lift at the lower left parasternal area that starts in early systole and is synchronous with the LV apical impulse.

A left parasternal lift is frequently present in patients with severe mitral regurgitation. This pulsation occurs distinctly later than the LV apical impulse, is synchronous with the *v* wave in the left atrial pressure curve, and is due to anterior displacement of the right ventricle by an enlarged, expanding left atrium. Pulmonary artery pulsation is often visible and palpable in the second left intercostal space. Although this pulsation may be normal in children or in thin young adults, in others, it usually denotes pulmonary hypertension, increased pulmonary blood flow, or poststenotic pulmonary artery dilation.

CARDIAC AUSCULTATION

To obtain the most information from cardiac auscultation, the observer should keep several principles in mind:

1. Auscultation should be performed in a quiet room.

2. Attention must be focused on the phase of the cardiac cycle during which the auscultory event is expected to occur.

3. The timing of a heart sound or murmur can be determined accurately from its relation to other observable events in the cardiac cycle.

4. It is often necessary to observe alterations in the timing or intensity of a heart sound during various physiologic and/or pharmacologic interventions (dynamic auscultation).

【 】 HEART SOUNDS

The intensity of the first heart sound (S_1) is influenced by (1) the position of the mitral valve leaflets at the onset of ventricular systole, (2) the rate of rise of the LV pressure pulse, (3) the presence or absence of structural disease of the mitral valve, and (4) the amount of tissue, air, or fluid between the heart and the stethoscope. The S_1 sound is louder if diastole is shortened (tachycardia) or if atrial contraction precedes ventricular contraction by an unusually short interval, reflected in a short PR interval. The loud S_1 in mitral stenosis usually signifies that the valve is pliable (Fig. 1-4).

A reduction in the intensity of S_1 may be due to poor conduction of sound through the chest wall, a long PR interval, or imperfect closure, as in mitral regurgitation.

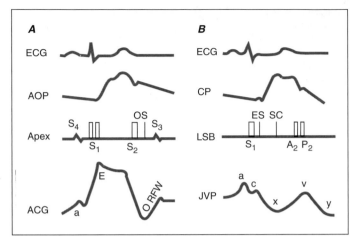

FIGURE 1-4. A. Schematic representation of ECG, aortic pressure pulse (AOP), phonocardiogram recorded at the apex, and apex cardiogram (ACG). On the phonocardiogram, S_1, S_2, S_3, and S_4 represent the first through fourth heart sounds; OS represents the opening snap of the mitral valve, which occurs coincident with the O point of the apex cardiogram. S_3 occurs coincident with the termination of the rapid-filling wave (RFW) of the ACG, while S_4 occurs coincident with the a wave of the ACG. **B.** Simultaneous recording of ECG, indirect carotid pulse (CP), phonocardiogram along the left sternal border (LSB), and indirect jugular venous pulse (JVP). (ES, ejection sound; SC, systolic click.)

Splitting of the two high-pitched components of S_1 is a normal phenomenon. The first component of S_1 is attributed to mitral valve closure and the second to tricuspid valve closure. Widening of S_1 is due most often to complete right bundle branch block.

Splitting of S_2 into aortic (A_2) and pulmonic (P_2) components occurs normally during inspiration. Physiologic splitting of S_2 is accentuated in conditions associated with right ventricular volume overload and a distensible pulmonary vascular bed. However, in patients with an increase in pulmonary vascular resistance, narrow splitting of S_2 is present. Splitting that persists with expiration (heard best at the pulmonic or left sternal border) when the patient is in the upright position is usually abnormal. Such splitting may be due to delayed activation of the right ventricle (right bundle branch block), left ventricular ectopic beats, a LV pacemaker, pulmonary embolism or pulmonic stenosis, or atrial septal defect.

In pulmonary hypertension, P_2 is increased in intensity, and the splitting of the second heart sound may be diminished, normal, or accentuated. Early aortic valve closure, which occurs with mitral regurgitation or a ventricular septal defect, also may produce splitting that persists during expiration. In patients with an atrial septal defect, the volume and duration of right ventricular ejection are not significantly increased by inspiration, and there is little inspiratory exaggeration of the splitting of S_2. This phenomenon, termed *fixed splitting* of the second heart sound, is of considerable diagnostic value.

A delay in aortic valve closure, causing P_2 to precede A_2, results in reversed (*paradoxic*) splitting of S_2. Splitting is then maximal during expiration and decreases during inspiration. The most common causes of reversed splitting of S_2 are left bundle branch block and delayed excitation of the LV from a right ventricular ectopic beat. Mechanical prolongation of LV systole, resulting in reversed splitting of S_2, also may be caused by severe aortic outflow obstruction, a large aorta-to-pulmonary artery shunt, systolic hypertension, and ischemic heart disease or cardiomyopathy with left ventricular failure.

A P$_2$ that is greater than A$_2$ suggests pulmonary hypertension, except in patients with atrial septal defect.

The third heart sound (S$_3$) is a low-pitched sound produced in the ventricle after A$_2$. In patients over 40 years old, an S$_3$ usually indicates impairment of ventricular function, AV valve regurgitation, or some other condition that increases the rate or volume of ventricular filling. The left-sided S$_3$ is best heard with the bell of the stethoscope at the left ventricular apex during expiration and with the patient in the left lateral position. The right-sided S$_3$ is best heard at the left sternal border or just beneath the xiphoid and usually is louder with inspiration.

Third heart sounds often disappear with the treatment of heart failure. The *opening snap* (OS) is a brief, high-pitched, early diastolic sound that is usually due to stenosis of an AV valve, most often the mitral valve. It is generally heard best at the lower left sternal border and radiates well to the base of the heart. The A$_2$–OS interval is inversely related to the mean left atrial pressure. The OS of tricuspid stenosis occurs later in diastole than the mitral OS and is often overlooked in patients with more prominent mitral valve disease.

The fourth heart sound (S$_4$) is a low-pitched, presystolic sound produced in the ventricle during ventricular filling; it is associated with an effective atrial contraction (and thus is absent in atrial fibrillation) and is heard best with the bell of the stethoscope. The S$_4$ is present frequently in patients with systemic hypertension, aortic stenosis, hypertrophic cardiomyopathy, ischemic heart disease, and acute mitral regurgitation. Most patients with an acute myocardial infarction and sinus rhythm have an audible S$_4$. It is heard best at the LV apex when the patient is in the left lateral position, and is accentuated by mild isotonic or isometric exercise in the supine position. In patients with chronic obstructive pulmonary disease (COPD) and increased anteroposterior (AP) diameter of the chest, the fourth heart sound (and often a third heart sound) may be heard best at the base of the neck or in the infra or supraclavicular areas.

The *ejection sound* is a sharp, high-pitched sound occurring in early systole and closely following the first heart sound. Ejection sounds occur in the presence of semilunar valve stenosis and in conditions associated with dilatation of the aorta or pulmonary artery. The aortic ejection sound is usually heard best at the LV apex and the second right intercostal space; the pulmonary ejection sound is strongest at the upper left sternal border. The latter, unlike most other right-sided acoustical events, is heard better during expiration. *Nonejection* or *midsystolic clicks*, occurring with or without a late systolic murmur, often denote prolapse of one or both leaflets of the mitral valve.

【 】 HEART MURMURS

The intensity of murmurs may be graded from I to VI. A grade I murmur is so faint that it can be heard only with special effort; a grade VI murmur is audible with the stethoscope removed from contact with the chest. The configuration of a murmur may be crescendo, decrescendo, crescendo-decrescendo (diamond-shaped), or plateau. The precise time of onset and time of cessation of a murmur depend on the instant in the cardiac cycle at which an adequate pressure difference between two chambers arises and disappears (Fig. 1-5).

The location on the chest wall where the murmur is best heard and the areas to which it radiates can be helpful in identifying the cardiac structure from which the murmur originates.

In addition, by noting changes in the characteristics of the murmur during maneuvers that alter cardiac hemodynamics (dynamic auscultation), the auscultator often can identify its correct origin and significance.

Accentuation of a murmur during inspiration implies that the murmur originates on the right side of the circulation. The Valsalva maneuver reduces the intensity of most murmurs by diminishing both right and left ventricular filling. The systolic murmur associated with hypertrophic cardiomyopathy and the late systolic murmur due to mitral valve prolapse are exceptions and may be paradoxically accentuated during the Valsalva

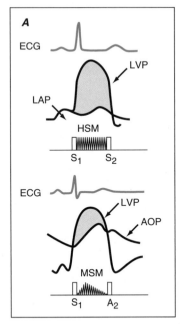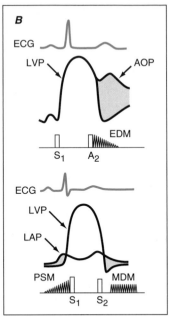

FIGURE 1-5. A. Schematic representation of ECG, aortic pressure (AOP), left ventricular pressure (LVP), and left atrial pressure (LAP). The shaded areas indicate a transvalvular pressure difference during systole. (HSM, holosystolic murmur; MSM, midsystolic murmur). **B.** Graphic representation of ECG, aortic pressure (AOP), left ventricular pressure (LVP), and left atrial pressure (LAP), with shaded areas indicating transvalvular diastolic pressure difference. (EDM, early diastolic murmur; PSM, presystolic murmur; MDM, mid-diastolic murmur.)

maneuver. Murmurs due to flow across a normal or obstructed semilunar valve increase in intensity in the cycle following a premature ventricular beat or a long RR interval in atrial fibrillation. In contrast, murmurs due to AV valve regurgitation or a ventricular septal defect do not change appreciably during the beat following a prolonged diastole. Standing accentuates the murmur of hypertrophic cardiomyopathy and occasionally the murmur due to mitral valve prolapse. Squatting increases most murmurs, except those caused by hypertrophic cardiomyopathy and mitral regurgitation due to a prolapsed mitral valve. Sustained hand-grip exercise often accentuates the murmurs of mitral regurgitation, aortic regurgitation, and mitral stenosis, but usually diminishes those due to aortic stenosis or hypertrophic cardiomyopathy. Transient arterial occlusion by the inflation of bilateral arm cuffs to 20 mm Hg above the systolic pressure for 5 seconds usually intensifies murmurs due to left-sided regurgitant lesions.

【 】 SYSTOLIC MURMURS

Holosystolic (pansystolic) murmurs are generated when there is flow between two chambers that have high pressure gradients throughout systole. Therefore, holosystolic murmurs accompany mitral or tricuspid regurgitation and ventricular septal defect. Although the typical high-pitched murmur of mitral regurgitation usually continues throughout systole (Fig. 1-6), the shape of the murmur may vary considerably. The holosystolic murmurs of mitral regurgitation and ventricular septal defect are augmented by transient exercise and are diminished by inhalation of amyl nitrate. The murmur of

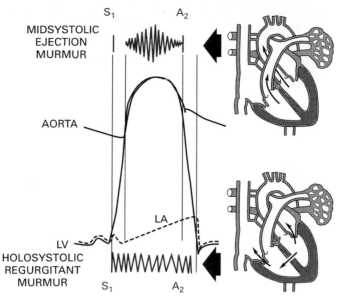

FIGURE 1-6. Midsystolic ejection murmurs are caused by forward flow across the left ventricular (LV) or right ventricular (RV) outflow tract, whereas pansystolic regurgitant murmurs are caused by retrograde flow from a high-pressure cardiac chamber to a low-pressure one. *Left.* Diagrammatic representation of the midsystolic ejection murmur and the pansystolic regurgitant murmur, as related to LV, aortic, and left atrial (LA) pressures. The systolic ejection murmur occurs during the period of LV ejection; the onset of the murmur is separated from S_1 by the period of isovolumic contraction, and the crescendo-decrescendo murmur terminates before A_2. The pansystolic regurgitant murmur begins with, or may replace, S_1, and the murmur continues up to and through A_2 as LV pressure exceeds left atrial pressure during the period of isovolumic relaxation. The murmur has a plateau configuration and varies little with respiration. *Right.* Flow diagram. (Left panel reproduced from Reddy PS, Shaver JA, Leonard JJ. Cardiac systolic murmurs: pathophysiology and differential diagnosis. *Prog Cardiovasc Dis.* 1971;14:19. Entire figure reproduced with permission from Shaver JA. Systolic murmurs. *Heart Dis Stroke.* 1993;2:10.)

tricuspid regurgitation associated with pulmonary hypertension is holosystolic and frequently increases during inspiration. Midsystolic murmurs, also called *systolic ejection murmurs*, which are often crescendo-decrescendo in shape, occur when blood is ejected across the aortic or pulmonic outflow tracts (Fig. 1-6). When the semilunar valves are normal, an increased flow rate, ejection into a dilated vessel beyond the valve, or increased transmission of sound through a thin chest wall may be responsible for this murmur. Most benign functional murmurs are midsystolic and originate from the pulmonary outflow tract. Valvular or subvalvular obstruction of either ventricle also may cause such a midsystolic murmur.

The murmur of aortic stenosis (AS) is the prototype of the left-sided midsystolic murmur. In valvular aortic stenosis, the murmur is usually maximal in the second right intercostal space, with radiation into the neck. In supravalvular aortic stenosis, the murmur is occasionally loudest above the second intercostal space, with disproportionate radiation into the right carotid artery. In hypertrophic cardiomyopathy, the midsystolic murmur originates in the LV cavity and is usually maximal at the lower left sternal edge and apex, with relatively little radiation to the carotids. When the aortic valve is immobile (calcified), the aortic closure sound (A_2) may be soft and inaudible, so that the length and configuration of the murmur are difficult to determine. Midsystolic murmurs also occur in patients with mitral regurgitation resulting from papillary muscle dysfunction.

Midsystolic aortic and pulmonic murmurs are intensified after amyl nitrate inhalation and during the cardiac cycle following a premature ventricular beat, while those due to mitral regurgitation are unchanged or softer.

Early systolic murmurs begin with the first heart sound and end in midsystole. An early systolic murmur is a feature of tricuspid regurgitation occurring in the absence of pulmonary hypertension. Patients with acute mitral regurgitation into a noncompliant left atrium and a large v wave often have a loud early systolic murmur that diminishes as the pressure gradient between the left ventricle and the left atrium decreases in late systole.

Late systolic murmurs are faint or moderately loud, high-pitched apical murmurs that start well after ejection and do not mask either heart sound. They are probably related to papillary muscle dysfunction and may appear only during angina, but they are common in patients with myocardial infarction or diffuse myocardial disease. Late systolic murmurs following midsystolic clicks are often due to late systolic mitral regurgitation caused by prolapse of the mitral valve into the left atrium. The timing of the murmur does not necessarily correlate with its severity.

【 】 DIASTOLIC MURMURS

Early diastolic murmurs begin with or shortly after S_2 (Fig. 1-7). The high-pitched murmurs of aortic regurgitation or of pulmonic regurgitation due to pulmonary hypertension are generally decrescendo. The faint, high-pitched murmurs of aortic regurgitation are difficult to hear unless they are specifically sought by applying firm pressure on the diaphragm over the left midsternal border while the patient sits, leaning forward, and holds a breath in full expiration. The diastolic murmur of aortic regurgitation is enhanced by hand-grip exercise and diminishes with amyl nitrate inhalation.

Mid-diastolic murmurs, usually arising from the AV valves, occur during early ventricular filling. Such murmurs may be quite loud (grade III) despite only slight AV valve stenosis. Conversely, the murmurs may be soft or even absent despite severe obstruction if the cardiac output is markedly reduced. When the stenosis is marked, the diastolic murmur is prolonged, and so the duration of the murmur is more reliable than its intensity as an index of the severity of valve obstruction.

The low-pitched, mid-diastolic murmur of mitral stenosis characteristically follows the OS. It should be specifically sought by placing the bell of the stethoscope at the site of the left ventricular impulse, which is best localized with the patient in the left lateral position. Frequently, the murmur of mitral stenosis is present only at the left ventricular apex, and it may be increased in intensity by mild supine exercise or by inhalation of amyl nitrate. In tricuspid stenosis, the mid-diastolic murmur is localized to a relatively limited area along the left sternal border and may be stronger during inspiration.

A soft, mid-diastolic murmur may sometimes be heard in patients with acute rheumatic fever (Carey Coombs murmur). In acute, severe aortic regurgitation, the left ventricular diastolic pressure may exceed the left atrial pressure, resulting in a mid-diastolic murmur due to "diastolic mitral regurgitation." In severe, chronic aortic regurgitation, a murmur is frequently present that may be either mid-diastolic or presystolic (Austin Flint murmur).

Presystolic murmurs begin during the period of ventricular filling that follows atrial contraction, and therefore occur in sinus rhythm. They are usually due to stenosis of the AV valve and have the same quality as the mid-diastolic filling rumble, but they are usually crescendo, reaching peak intensity at the time of a loud S_1. It is the presystolic murmur that is most characteristic of tricuspid stenosis and sinus rhythm.

【 】 CONTINUOUS MURMURS

Continuous murmurs begin in systole, peak near S_2, and continue into all or part of diastole. A patent ductus arteriosus causes a continuous murmur as long as the pressure

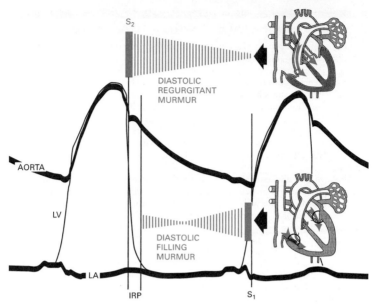

FIGURE 1-7. Diastolic filling murmurs or rumbles are caused by forward flow across the AV valves, whereas diastolic regurgitant murmurs are caused by retrograde flow across incompetent semilunar valves. *Left.* Diagrammatic representation of the diastolic filling murmur and the diastolic regurgitant murmur as related to left ventricular (LV), aortic, and left atrial (LA) pressures. The diastolic filling murmur occurs during the diastolic filling period and is separated from S_2 by the isovolumic relaxation period. The rumbling murmur is most prominent during rapid, early ventricular filling and presystole, terminating with S_1. The diastolic regurgitant murmur begins immediately after S_2 and continues in a decrescendo fashion up to S_1, closely paralleling the aortic LV diastolic pressure gradient. *Right.* Flow diagram. (*From* Shaver JA: Diastolic murmurs. *Heart Dis Stroke.* 1993;1:98–103. Reproduced with permission from the American Heart Association.)

in the pulmonary artery is much lower than that in the aorta. The murmur is intensified by elevation of the systemic arterial pressure and reduced by amyl nitrate inhalation. When pulmonary hypertension is present, the diastolic portion may disappear, leaving the murmur confined to systole.

Continuous murmurs may result from congenital or acquired systemic arteriovenous fistulas, coronary arteriovenous fistula, anomalous origin of the left coronary artery from the pulmonary artery, and communications between the sinus of Valsalva and the right side of the heart.

In nonconstricted arteries, continuous murmurs may be due to rapid flow through a tortuous bed. Such murmurs typically occur within the bronchial arterial collateral circulation in cyanotic patients with severe pulmonary outflow obstruction.

【 】 PERICARDIAL FRICTION RUB

These adventitious sounds may have presystolic, systolic, and early diastolic scratchy components; they may be confused with a murmur or extracardiac sound when they are heard only in systole. A pericardial friction rub is best appreciated with the patient upright and leaning forward and may be accentuated during inspiration.

APPROACH TO THE PATIENT WITH A HEART MURMUR

The evaluation of a patient with a heart murmur may vary greatly, depending on many of the considerations discussed earlier, including the intensity of the cardiac murmur, its timing in the cardiac cycle, its location and radiation, and its response to various physiologic maneuvers. Also of importance are the presence or absence of cardiac and noncardiac symptoms and whether other cardiac or noncardiac physical findings suggest that the cardiac murmur is clinically significant. The skill and confidence of the cardiac auscultator, the relative cost of various diagnostic approaches, and the accuracy and reliability of additional tests in the laboratory where they are performed are likewise important factors. One systematic approach to patients with a heart murmur is depicted in Fig. 1-8. This algorithm is particularly applicable to children and adults younger than 40 years.

Although two-dimensional echocardiography and color Doppler flow imaging can provide important information about patients with cardiac murmurs, they are not necessary tests for all patients with cardiac murmurs, and they usually add little but expense to the evaluation of asymptomatic patients with short grade I to grade II midsystolic murmurs, otherwise normal physical findings, and no history suggestive of cardiac disease.

It is important to consider that many recent studies indicate that with the improved sensitivity of Doppler ultrasound devices, valvular regurgitation may be detected through the tricuspid and pulmonic valves in a very high percentage of young, healthy subjects and through left-sided valves in a variable but lower percentage. In a recent study of 200 healthy Japanese subjects, mitral regurgitation could be detected by Doppler in up to 45% of individuals, tricuspid regurgitation in up to 70%, and pulmonic regurgitation in up to 88%, even though these patients were healthy, had no cardiac auscultation evidence of heart disease, and had normal ECGs. "Normal" aortic regurgitation is encountered much less frequently, and its incidence increases with increasing age (Fig. 1-9). Thus, echocardiographic interpretations of mild or trivial (physiologic) valvular regurgitation may lead to the echocardiographic diagnosis of cardiac disease in patients with no clinical heart disease.

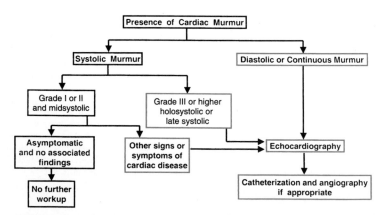

FIGURE 1-8. A schematic approach to the workup of a patient with a cardiac murmur according to whether the murmur is probably innocent or secondary to cardiac pathology. This algorithm is particularly relevant to children and adults younger than 40 years, and echocardiography is recommended before cardiac consultation.

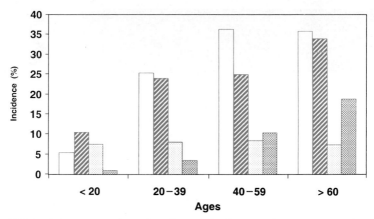

FIGURE 1-9. Percent incidence of mitral, tricuspid, pulmonic, and aortic regurgitation by Doppler echocardiography in clinically normal subjects according to age, from younger than 20 to older than 60 years. (Modified from Choong CY, Abascal VM, Weyman J. Prevalence of valvular regurgitation by Doppler echocardiography in patients with structurally normal hearts by 2-dimensional echocardiography. *Am Heart J.* 1989;117:636–642.)

SUGGESTED READING

Ewy GA. Venous and arterial pulsations: bedside insights into hemodynamics. In: Chizner M, ed. *Classic Teachings in Clinical Cardiology: A Tribute to W. Proctor Harvey.* Cedar Grove, NJ: Laennec; 1996.

Leon DF, Shaver JA, eds. *Physiologic Principles of Heart Sounds and Murmurs.* Monograph 46. New York: American Heart Association; 1975.

O'Rourke RA. Approach to the patient with a murmur. In: Goldman L, Braunwald E, eds. *Primary Cardiology.* 2nd ed. Philadelphia, PA: Saunders; 2003.

O'Rourke RA, Braunwald E. Physical examination of the cardiovascular system. In: Fauci AS, Braunwald E, Isselbacher KJ, et al., eds. *Harrison's Principles of Internal Medicine.* 15th ed. New York, NY: McGraw-Hill; 2007.

O'Rourke RA, Silverman ME, Shaver JA. The history, physical examination, and cardiac auscultation. In: Fuster V, O'Rourke RA, Walsh RA, et al., eds. *Hurst's The Heart.* 12th ed. New York, NY: McGraw-Hill; 2008.

CHAPTER (2)

The Resting Electrocardiogram

Freddy Del-Carpio Munoz, Robert J. Myerburg,
and Agustin Castellanos

The electrocardiogram (ECG) has many uses. It may function as an independent marker of myocardial disease; it may reflect anatomic, hemodynamic, molecular, ionic, and drug-induced cardiac abnormalities; and it may provide essential information for the proper diagnosis and therapy of many cardiac problems. In fact, it is the most commonly used laboratory procedure for the diagnosis of heart disease. All physicians who interpret ECGs as well as those learning electrocardiographic interpretation should read the *Guidelines for Electrocardiography of the American College of Cardiology, American Heart Association Task Force.* (See also Chapter 59.)

VENTRICULAR DEPOLARIZATION AND REPOLARIZATION

In the resting or polarized state, the charges are at rest. A unipolar electrode facing the epicardial side of a left ventricular strip, such as V_6, registers an isoelectric line. Depolarization occurs with an endocardium-to-epicardium *sequence*. Depolarization has been described as a moving wave *with the positive charges in front* of the negative charges. The unipolar lead will record a positivity because it consistently faces positive charges throughout the entire depolarization sequence. On the other hand, the *sequence* of ventricular repolarization is from epicardium to endocardium, but with the negative charges in front. Thus, V_6 will record a positive deflection because it constantly faces positive charges. The earlier-occurring epicardial end of repolarization has been attributed to the shorter duration of repolarization that epicardial cells have in comparison to endocardial cells. Therefore, when repolarization finishes at the epicardium, it still has not been completed at the endocardium. This simplistic view is of didactic value only, since it fails to consider the role played by the M cells described by Antzelevitch and coworkers. M cells play a determining role in the inscription of the T wave, since currents flowing down voltage gradients on either side of the usual (but not necessarily) mid-myocardial cells determine both the height and the width of the T wave as well as the degree to which the ascending or descending limbs of the T wave are interrupted. A transmural dispersion of repolarization is created by differences in repolarization time among the three myocardial layers, with the M cells having the longest repolarization time. The greater the transmural dispersion of repolarization (the difference between repolarization times between mid-myocardium and endo/epicardium), the greater the risk for arrhythmic events.

ELECTROCARDIOGRAPHIC LEADS

【 】 STANDARD AND EXTREMITY LEADS

An ECG lead can be defined as a pair of terminals with designated polarity, each of which is connected either directly or by way of a passive-active network to recording electrodes. Einthoven and associates first developed a method of studying the electrical activity of the heart by representing it graphically in a *two-dimensional* geometric figure—namely, an equilateral triangle. Although there are three bipolar leads and three unipolar extremity leads, the information contained in limb leads is redundant. If any two of the six are recorded, the other four can be derived using Einthoven's equation (III = II − I) and the relationship between bipolar and unipolar limb leads (I = VL − VR, II = VF − VR, and III = VF − VL). When the electrodes are placed proximally to the roots of the extremities, they lose their relatively "far" distance from the heart. Hence, Einthoven's equilateral theory does not hold. This explains why leads placed proximally to the roots of the extremities—such as those used for exercise testing, monitoring in the coronary care unit, and ambulatory ECG recordings—by being only "equivalent" to the corresponding bipolar leads, are in some cases markedly different from the "true" standard bipolar leads.

【 】 UNIPOLAR PRECORDIAL LEADS

Unipolar precordial leads should be viewed in a slightly different context. Precordial (V) leads yield a positive deflection when facing positive charges and a negative deflection when facing negative charges. Wilson called this the *solid angle*, which is an imaginary cone extending from the site in the chest through the heart. The precordial electrode is at its apex, and its base is at the opposite epicardial surface. According to Wilson's scalar concept of electrocardiography, this occurs because the solid angle subtended by the corresponding lead records the electrical activity from the regions of the heart over which it is placed as well as from distant regions. Thus, if V_2 is placed over (and thereby faces) the right ventricle, part of the initial positive ventricular deflection reflects right ventricular activation, with the corresponding electrical forces moving toward the electrode. Most portions of the terminal S wave represent activation of muscle other than the right ventricle (the septum and free left ventricular wall), reflecting electrical forces moving away from the electrode. Acceptance that the amount of muscle activity recorded by various unipolar leads is not the same implies different "real" durations of depolarization and repolarization, even though the one supposedly results from the projections of a vector on an idealized horizontal plane of a "corrected" spatial vectorcardiographic (such as the Frank) system.

NORMAL ACTIVATION OF THE HEART: VENTRICULAR DEPOLARIZATION

After emerging from the sinus node, the cardiac impulse propagates throughout the atria toward the atrioventricular (AV) node. The sequence of atrial depolarization occurs in an inferior, leftward, and somewhat posterior direction. The PR interval (used to estimate AV conduction time) includes conduction through the "true" AV structures (AV node, His bundle, bundle branches, and main divisions of the left bundle branch) as well as through those parts of the atria located between the sinus and AV nodes. The onset of ventricular depolarization (defined as the beginning of the normal Q wave) reflects activation of the left side of the interventricular septum. Hence, the normal initial depolarization is oriented from left to right, explaining the small Q wave in lead V_6 and the small R wave in V_1. Thereafter, the interventricular septum is activated in both directions.

Septal activation is encompassed within or neutralized by subsequent free-wall activation. The greater mass of the left ventricular (LV) free wall explains why LV free-wall events overpower those of the interventricular septum and right ventricular free wall.

ELECTRICAL AXIS

The electrical axis (EA) may be defined as a vector originating in the center of Einthoven's equilateral triangle. When applied to the EA of the QRS complexes, the vector that represents it also gives the direction of the activation process as projected in the plane of the limb leads. The classical approach recommends calculating the net *areas* enclosed by the QRS complex in leads I to III. A simpler, though less precise, method of calculating the quadrant (or part of a quadrant) in which the EA is located consists of using the maximal QRS deflection in leads I and aVF and, when necessary, lead II. A normal QRS axis orientation in the frontal plane lies between +90 degrees and −30 degrees.

CARDIAC MEMORY

Rosenbaum and associates studied the prolonged depolarization occurring during long periods of ventricular stimulation and found two types of altered ventricular repolarization. One, corresponding to Wilson's classic theory, was primary and proportional in magnitude to the QRS complex, but of opposite polarity. The other, concealed by (and during) the former, required a longer time (even days) both to reach maximal effect and to disappear, becoming apparent *only when* normal activation recurred. The latter type was attributed to modulated electrotonic interactions occurring during cardiac activation in such a way that repolarization was accelerated at ventricular sites where depolarization begins and delayed in areas where depolarization terminates. Abnormal T-wave changes occurring after the disappearance of prolonged periods of abnormal repolarization induced by abnormal depolarization showed accumulation and (fading) *long-term* memory for a variable period of time. The occurrence of *short-term* affects memory, after periods of altered ventricular depolarization (and repolarization) as short as 1 minute in duration, has recently been reported. The term *memory* has also been applied to gradual adjustments of action potential duration (roughly corresponding to QT intervals) after abrupt changes in cycle lengths (events influenced by past history), without necessarily requiring previous abnormal ventricular repolarization. Cardiac memory can be seen in the surface electrocardiogram as persistent abnormal repolarization (T waves), for example, after disappearance of preexcitation, resolution of bundle branch block, RV pacing, and wide QRS complex tachycardias.

ABNORMAL ST-SEGMENT CHANGES

In orthodox ECG language, *injury* implies *abnormal ST-segment changes*; *necrosis* or *fibrosis* implies *abnormal Q waves; and ischemia* implies *symmetrical T-wave inversion* (or elevation). Various hypotheses have been postulated to explain how the injury-related diastolic hypopolarization is manifested as abnormal ST-segment shifts. One hypothesis is based on the existence of a *diastolic* current of "injury," and the other presupposes a true, active, *systolic* displacement. Most likely, injury reflects both the disappearance of diastolic baseline shifts and active ST-segment elevation. In addition, loss or depression of the action potential dome in epicardium but not endocardium underlies the development of prominent ST-segment elevation. Some authors consider ST-segment changes in ventricular aneurysms to be a result of the earlier repolarization of a ring of persistently viable tissue surrounding the aneurysm; however, others believe that they reflect functional (echocardiographic) dyskinesia. ST-segment elevation from epicardial injury

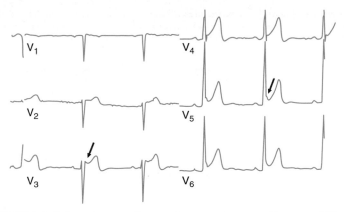

FIGURE 2-1. Early repolarization. This normal variant is characterized by narrow QRS complexes with J-point and ST-segment elevation in the chest leads. Left chest leads often show tall R waves with a distinct notch or slur in their downstroke (arrow in V_5), while the right chest leads may display ST segments having a "saddleback" or "humpback" shape (arrow in V_3).

due to pericarditis should be differentiated from the benign "early repolarization" pattern (Fig. 2-1), a normal variant characterized by J-point elevation with an upwardly concave ST segment and tall R waves with a distinct notch on the downstroke commonly seen in the precordial leads and affected by exercise and hyperventilation. Although the mechanism of early repolarization has not been fully elucidated, it has been related to enhanced activity of the right sympathetic nerves.

【 】 SELECTIVE NON-ISCHEMIC ST-SEGMENT ELEVATION IN THE RIGHT PRECORDIAL LEADS

High-takeoff ST segments of either the caved or saddleback type localized to the right chest leads, associated with different degrees of right bundle branch block (RBBB) with or without T-wave inversion, are seen in the Brugada syndrome (see Chapters 8, 11, and 16). Strong sodium channel–blocking drugs can produce ST-segment elevations even in patients without any evidence of syncope or ventricular fibrillation. Slight ST-segment elevation with an incomplete RBBB pattern showing an epsilon wave has been described in some patients with arrhythmogenic right ventricular dysplasia. Hyperkalemic "injury" can produce an anteroseptal myocardial infarction (MI) pattern (dialyzable current of injury).

ABNORMAL Q WAVES

Abnormal Q waves appearing several hours after total occlusion of a coronary artery result from the necrosis secondary to the decreased blood supply. The number of affected cells has to be large enough to produce changes that are reflected at the body surface, and abnormal Q waves can occur in MIs that are not completely transmural. The following changes have been said to be equivalent to Q waves in non–Q-wave MIs: R/S ratio changes, acute frontal- plane right-axis deviation, new left-axis deviation or left bundle branch block (LBBB), initial and terminal QRS notching, and some types of "poor R-wave progression" not related to precordial lead misplacement.

The concept of non–Q-wave MI as a discrete clinicopathologic entity that differs from Q-wave MI has gained almost universal acceptance, but is still controversial to some electrocardiographers.

ISCHEMIC T-WAVE CHANGES

Symmetrical T waves, inverted or upright (as in "hyperacute" T waves), characteristic of ECG "ischemia" have been considered to reflect a type or degree of cellular affection resulting in action potentials of increased and different duration with regional alterations of the duration of the depolarized state. T-wave inversions do not always reflect "physiologic" ischemia (due to decreased blood supply), since they can also be seen in evolving pericarditis, myocardial contusion, and increased intracranial pressure, and in the right chest leads of young patients (persistent juvenile pattern).

SECONDARY ST-T-WAVE CHANGES

Alterations in the sequence of (and sometimes delay in) ventricular depolarization (as produced by BBBs, ventricular pacing, ectopic ventricular impulse formation, pre-excitation syndromes, and ventricular hypertrophy) result in an obligatory change in the sequence of ventricular repolarization. This causes nonischemic T-wave inversions (secondary T-wave changes) in leads showing predominantly positive QRS deflections. Disappearance of these alterations of ventricular depolarization may be followed by narrow QRS complexes with negative T waves due to cardiac memory, as previously stated.

NONSPECIFIC ST-T-WAVE CHANGES

Nonspecific (or rather, nondiagnostic) ST-T-wave changes are the most commonly diagnosed ECG abnormalities. They have not been adequately categorized and represent different findings for various interpreters. When ECGs were analyzed without clinical information, this diagnosis was made in 40% of 410 abnormal ECGs, with the number reduced to 10% when clinical data became available. In the absence of structural heart disease, these changes can be due to a variety of physiologic, pharmacologic, and extracardiac factors.

ACUTE MYOCARDIAL INFARCTION

Myocardial infarctions are classified as non–ST-segment elevation and ST-segment elevation. The former in most cases does not lead to Q-wave formation, while the latter in most cases does lead to Q-wave formation if no reperfusion is established. In the thrombolytic era, the prevalence of non–ST-segment elevation MI seems to be greater (see Chapter 25). The prethrombolytic "classic" evolution of acute ST-segment elevation MI has been transformed by pharmacologic therapy and interventional techniques. The succession of events in the course of a classic ST-segment elevation MI is from hyperacute positive T waves (on occasion) to ST segment elevation to abnormal Q waves to T-wave inversion. Acceleration of these phases can occur with effective reperfusion. The time course of ST-segment elevation is a good predictor of reperfusion. Because prethrombolytic 12-lead ECG studies of ST-segment evolutions were based on static recordings obtained at fixed time intervals, it became clear that continuous monitoring in the coronary care unit was essential to adequately record the dynamics of ST-segment trends

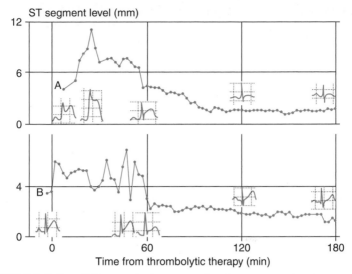

FIGURE 2-2. Plots of ST segment levels versus time from therapy in two selected patients with patency of the infarct-related vessel at 60 minutes. Note that a 50% decrease in ST segment levels within 60 minutes occurred only when measurements were made from the peak ST segment level (highest ST segment level measurement within the last 60 minutes).

(Fig. 2-2). Sensitivity increases as frequency of monitoring increases. Continuous monitoring is thus essential to evaluate the occurrence of reperfusion. Resolution of ST-segment elevation has been defined as a progressive decrease within 40 to 60 minutes to less than 50% of its maximally elevated value. It has been suggested that in patients treated with thrombolytics, the dichotomization for Q-wave and non–Q-wave MI should be made by the predischarge rather than the 24-hour ECG because of possible crossover from one group to another (see also Chapter 23).

【 】 DETERMINING THE SITE OF OCCLUSION IN THE CORONARY ARTERY IN ST-SEGMENT ELEVATION MYOCARDIAL INFARCTION

Right Coronary Artery Occlusion
- ST depression in lead I.
- ST elevation in lead III greater than in lead II.

PROXIMAL
- ST elevation more than 1 mm with positive T wave in lead V_4R.

DISTAL
- ST isolectric with a positive T wave in lead V_4R

Left Circumflex Artery Occlusion

- ST elevation in lead II greater than lead III.
- ST isoelectric or elevated in lead I.
- ST isoelectric or depressed with negative T wave in V_4R.

Extension to Posterior Wall

- ST depression in precordial leads.

Extension to Lateral Wall

- ST elevation in leads I, aVL, V_5, and V_6.

Left Anterior Descending Artery Occlusion

PROXIMAL TO FIRST SEPTAL BRANCH AND FIRST DIAGONAL BRANCH

- ST elevation in leads aVR and aVL.
- ST depression in leads II, III, and aVF.
- ST elevation in lead V_1 (> 2 mm) and leads V_2 to V_4.
- ST isoelectric or depressed in leads V_5 and V_6.
- Acquired intra-Hissian or RBBB may occur.

DISTAL TO FIRST SEPTAL BRANCH, PROXIMAL TO FIRST DIAGONAL BRANCH

- ST elevation in lead I and aVL.
- ST depression in lead III (lead II is isoelectric).
- ST elevation in leads V_2 to V_6 but not in lead V_1.

DISTAL TO FIRST DIAGONAL BRANCH, PROXIMAL TO FIRST SEPTAL BRANCH

- ST depression in lead aVL.
- ST elevation in inferior leads, highest in lead III.
- ST elevation in leads V_1 to V_4.

DISTAL LAD

- ST depression in aVR.
- ST elevation in inferior leads, highest in II.
- ST elevation in leads V_3 to V_6.

Left Main Coronary Artery Occlusion

- ST elevation in lead aVR.
- ST elevation in lead V_1 (lower than that of lead aVR).
- ST depression in leads II and aVF.
- ST depression in the precordial leads to the left of V_2.

[ ] EVOLUTION OF ACUTE CORONARY SYNDROMES

ECG changes indicative of *physiologic* ischemia that may progress to MI (see also Chapter 23):

1. Patients with ST-segment elevation: new or presumed new ST-segment elevation in two or more contiguous leads with the cutoff points ≥ 0.2 mV in leads V_1, V_2, or V_3 and ≥ 0.1 mV in other leads (contiguity in the frontal plane is defined by the lead sequence aVL, inverted aVR, II, aVF, III). There can be evolution into Q-wave MI or non–Q-wave MI.

2. Non–Q-wave MI may also present with ST-segment elevation as well as with T-wave abnormalities only.

[ ] LOCATION OF THE SITE OF Q-WAVE MYOCARDIAL INFARCTION

Table 2-1 shows an acceptable classification for the ECG location of MI according to leads showing abnormal Q waves, while also depicting other processes that may result in false patterns of Q-wave MI.

TABLE 2-1

Electrocardiographic Location of Infarction Sites Based on the Presence of Abnormal Q Waves

Site	Leads	False Patterns
Inferior (diaphragmatic)	II, III, aVF	WPW (PSAP), HCM
Inferolateral	II, III, aVF, VL, V_4–V_6	
"True" posterior (posterobasal)	V_1	RVH, "atypical" incomplete RBBB, WPW (LFWAP)
Inferoposterior	II, III, aVF, V_1[a]	WPW (left PSAP), HCM
Inferior–right ventricular	II, III, aVF plus V_4R–V_6R or V_1–V_3	ASMI
Anteroseptal	V_1, V_2, V_3	LVH, chronic lung disease, LBBB, chest electrode misplacement, right ventricular MI
Extensive anterior	I, aVL, V_1–V_6	
High lateral	I, aVL	Extremely vertical hearts with aVL resembling aVR
Anterior (apical)	V_3–V_4	WPW (LFWAP)
Posterolateral	V_4–V_6, V_1	
Right ventricular	V_4R with V_4R–V_6R or V_1–V_3	ASMI

ASMI, anteroseptal myocardial infarction; HCM, hypertrophic cardiomyopathy; LBBB, left bundle branch block; LFWAP, left free-wall accessory pathway; PSAP, posteroseptal accessory pathway; WPW, Wolff–Parkinson–White syndrome; RVH, right ventricular hypertrophy.

[a]Tall R wave, "reciprocal" to changes in "indicative" back leads.

PERICARDITIS

In acute pericarditis, ST segments can be elevated in all leads except aVR and, rarely, V_1. Symmetrical T-wave inversion (due to epicardial "ischemia") usually develops after the ST segments have returned to the baseline (but it can appear during the injury stage). Neither reciprocal ST-segment changes nor abnormal Q waves are seen. In most cases of acute pericarditis, the PR segment is depressed. Average ECG resolution occurs in close to 2 weeks (see also Chapter 44).

INTRAVENTRICULAR CONDUCTION DEFECTS

The following classification is the most commonly accepted and widely known. Consequently, only important pointers are presented.

【 】 LEFT ANTERIOR FASCICULAR BLOCK

1. Abnormal left superior (rarely right superior) axis with RS complexes in II, III, and aVF. Peak of R in aVL occurs before that in aVR. S wave deeper in III than in II.

2. Left precordial leads may show RS complexes when the electrical axis is markedly superior.

3. Other causes of left axis deviation—such as extensive inferior wall MI, Wolff–Parkinson–White syndrome (posteroseptal accessory pathway), hyperkalemia, ventricular pacing, and pulmonary emphysema—should be excluded.

4. QRS widening (over normal values) does not exceed 0.025 seconds.

5. Usually there are no interferences with the diagnosis of MI or RBBB.

【 】 LEFT POSTERIOR FASCICULAR BLOCK

1. Usually diagnosed only when coexisting with complete RBBB.

2. Right (and inferior) axis deviation should not be due to right ventricular hypertrophy or lateral MI.

3. The QRST pattern resembles that of inferior ischemia or infarction.

【 】 COMPLETE RIGHT BUNDLE BRANCH BLOCK

1. Does not deviate the electrical axis (determined by maximal deflections) *abnormally* to the left or to the right.

2. Although true posterior MI cannot be diagnosed in its presence, it does not interfere with the diagnosis of MI of other locations.

3. It may masquerade as LBBB when the expected wide S wave is not present in lead I, presumably because the terminal vectors are perpendicular to this lead.

4. An upright T wave in the right chest leads may be reciprocal to posterior ischemia or may reflect a primary change in repolarization in anteroseptal leads.

【 】 INCOMPLETE RIGHT BUNDLE BRANCH BLOCK

1. An r' or R' in V_1 with QRS duration of less than 0.10 seconds may be referred to as a normal incomplete RBBB (IRBBB) "pattern."

2. It need not always reflect a conduction delay in the trunk of a normal right branch, since it has been attributed to an increased conduction time due to a right ventricular enlargement or to stretch-related *delay* in an elongated right branch or in the

Purkinje–myocardial junction; an interruption of a subdivision of the right bundle branch; or a physiologic later-than-usual arrival of excitation at the crista supraventricularis.

【 】 COMPLETE LEFT BUNDLE BRANCH BLOCK

1. May simulate anteroseptal MI.
2. Interferes with the diagnosis of lateral and inferior MI but not anteroseptal MI.
3. A normal Q wave before an otherwise typical wide R wave indicates anteroseptal, not lateral, MI.
4. MI of any location may be present without any change in its basic features.
5. Acute inferior and anterolateral MIs can be diagnosed by characteristic ST-segment changes.
6. A positive T wave always reflects a primary change in repolarization.

【 】 NONSPECIFIC INTRAVENTRICULAR CONDUCTION DEFECT

This condition is associated with a wide QRS complex (with repolarization abnormalities) that does not have a characteristic left or right BBB pattern. The EA may be normal, left, or right.

WIDE QRS COMPLEXES IN PATIENTS WITH MANIFEST PREEXCITATION SYNDROMES

The classic pattern of manifest Wolff–Parkinson–White (WPW) syndrome during sinus rhythm is well known. The ventricular complex is a fusion beat resulting from ventricular activation by two wavefronts. The degree of preexcitation (amount of muscle activated through the accessory pathway) is variable and depends on many factors. Foremost among these are the distance between the sinus node and the atrial insertion of the accessory pathway and, more important, the differences in the duration of the refractory period and in conduction time through the normal pathway and accessory pathway. If there is total block at the AV node or His–Purkinje system, the impulse will be conducted using the accessory pathway exclusively. Consequently, the QRS complexes are different from fusion beats, although the direction of the delta wave remains the same. Moreover, the QRS complexes are as wide as (and really simulating) those produced by artificial or spontaneous beats arising in the vicinity of the ventricular end of the accessory pathway. Initial noninvasive determination of the anatomic position of the accessory pathway is of great clinical importance because of the introduction of surgical and catheter ablative techniques for symptomatic cases of preexcitation. Many ECG algorithms have been proposed for this task. Although useful as approximations, most are extremely complex for the average electrocardiographer, and difficult to remember. Furthermore, a new nomenclature for accessory pathway location has been recently adopted, after an expert panel discussion.

WIDE QRS COMPLEXES PRODUCED BY VENTRICULAR PACING FROM DIFFERENT SITES

In determining the location of the stimulating electrodes, what is relevant is the polarity of the *properly positioned* V_1 and V_2 electrodes and the direction of the EA. For example, endocardial or epicardial stimulation of the *anteriorly* located right ventricle at any site—apical (inferior) or mid/outflow tract (superior)—yields predominantly negative deflections in the right chest leads because of the *posterior* spread of activation. The reverse (positive deflections in V_1 and V_2) occurs when the epicardial stimulation of the superior and lateral portions of the posterior left ventricle by catheter electrodes in the distal coronary sinus or great and middle cardiac veins (or by implanted electrodes in the nearby muscle) results in *anteriorly* oriented forces. Right ventricular apical pacing may rarely produce positive deflections in V_1 specifically if this lead is (mis)placed above its usual level. On the other hand, *superior* deviation of the electrical axis indicates only that a spatially *inferior* ventricular site has been stimulated, regardless of whether this site is the apical portion of the right ventricle or the inferior part of the left ventricle, the latter being paced through the middle cardiac vein. Conversely, an *inferior* vertical axis is simply a consequence of pacing from a *superior* site, which can be the endocardium of the right ventricular outflow tract or the epicardium of the posterosuperior and lateral portions of the left ventricle. The tip of the catheter is determined by the anteroposterior and lateral x-ray views. The method discussed above to locate the site of impulse initiation during pacing is simpler than the more complicated ones used to determine the ventricular sites of exit from accessory pathways (crossing the AV junction), which require the use of right anterior oblique and especially left anterior oblique projections. Besides the utility of ECG in the location of stimulating electrodes, the ECG is useful to determine capture of the left ventricular lead in subjects with biventricular pacing, if R/S ratio ≥ 1 in V_1 and/or lead I left ventricular capture is confirmed with a high sensitivity and specificity.

LEFT VENTRICULAR HYPERTROPHY

Multiple ECG criteria have been proposed to diagnose left ventricular hypertrophy (LVH) using necropsy or echocardiographic information. Of these, the Sokolow–Lyon criterion ($SV_1 + RV_{5-6} \geq 35$ mm) is the most specific (> 95%) but is not very sensitive (around 45%). The Romhilt–Estes score has a specificity of 90% and a sensitivity of 60% in studies correlated with echocardiography. The Casale (modified Cornell) criterion ($RaVL + SV_3 > 28$ mm in men and > 20 in women) is somewhat more sensitive, but less specific than the Sokolow–Lyon criterion. The Talbot criterion ($R \geq 16$ mm in aV_L) is very specific (> 90%), even in the presence of MI and ventricular block, but not very sensitive. The Koito and Spodick criterion ($RV_6 > RV_5$) claims a specificity of 100% and a sensitivity of more than 50%. According to Hernandez Padial, a total 12-lead QRS voltage > 120 mm is a good ECG criterion for LVH in systemic hypertension and is better than those most frequently used. With echocardiography as the "gold standard," several authors have postulated ECG criteria for diagnosis of LVH in the presence of complete LBBB and left anterior fascicular block (LAFB), but these are not widely used.

PROCESSES PRODUCING OR LEADING TO RIGHT VENTRICULAR HYPERTROPHY AND ENLARGEMENT

The ECG manifestations of right ventricular hypertrophy (RVH) or enlargement can be subdivided into the following main types: (1) the posterior and rightward displacement of the QRS forces associated with low voltage, as seen in patients with pulmonary emphysema; (2) the incomplete RBBB pattern *with right axis deviation* occurring in patients with chronic lung disease and some congenital cardiac malformation resulting in volume overloading of the right ventricle; (3) the true posterior wall MI pattern with normal to low voltage of the R wave in V_1 of mitral stenosis with abnormal P wave or big F waves (which can be as large as the QRS complexes); and (4) the classic RVH and strain pattern seen in young patients with congenital heart disease (producing pressure overloading) or in adult patients with high right ventricular pressures, such as "primary" pulmonary hypertension. (See also Chapter 30.)

QT INTERVAL: NORMAL, PROLONGED, AND DISPERSED

The QT interval (considered by some to be a surrogate for action potential duration) is manually measured from the beginning of the Q wave to the point at which the T-wave downslope crosses the baseline. However, there has been considerable debate and speculation regarding the accurate measurement of the QT interval. For example, according to Coumel and associates, the human interobserver variability was 30.6 ms. Similarly, the machine interautomatic comparison of 19 systems yielded standard deviations as great as 30 ms. At present there seems to be a trend toward acceptance of the (automatic) values obtained with the QT Guard package (Marquette). With this system, the end of the T wave is determined using the intersection of the isoelectric line with the tangent to the *inflection point* of the descending part of the T. The QT interval is affected by autonomic tone and catecholamines and has day-night differences. It varies with heart rate and sex. Several formulas have been proposed to take these variables into account and provide a corrected measurement (QTc interval), of which that proposed by Bazett is the most used. In general, the unadjusted (noncorrected), usually resting QT interval decreases linearly from ± 0.42 seconds at rates of 50/min to ±0.32 seconds at 100/min to ±0.26 seconds at 150/min. However, during exercise, when the rate becomes faster, the QTc first increases until it reaches a maximum at approximately a rate of 120/min, and thereafter decreases again.

Regardless of the method of correction of QT, its measurement should be done accurately. Recommendations from an expert panel established that the QT interval should be measured manually, preferably by using one of the limb leads that best shows the end of the T wave on a 12-lead ECG. The QT interval should be measured from the beginning of the QRS complex to the end of the T wave and averaged over 3 to 5 beats. *U waves* possibly corresponding to the late repolarization of cells in the mid-myocardium should be included in the measurement *only if they are large enough to seem to merge with the T wave.*

Because the 12-lead ECG shows a normal degree of QT and QTc dispersion, indexes have been used to quantify the extent of what has been called "the heterogeneity in ventricular repolarization." The difference between the longest and shortest QT interval is referred to as *QT dispersion.* Since 1990 it has been used as a prognostic marker not only in patients with congenitally prolonged QT intervals, but also in those with acute MI and those taking drugs with proarrhythmic properties; it has also been used to predict mortality in general epidemiologic studies. However, recent reports have challenged the values of QT dispersion. The upper limits of normal vary with different investigators, but a value of 60 to 65 ms may be an acceptable compromise. Some may disagree with this range.

Coumel emphasized that QT dispersion could be an illusion or a reality. Inferred from the oncoming section on spatial vectorcardiography, the fact is that a truly spatial (Frank system) QRS-T loop cannot yield abnormal QT dispersion. In planar projections of this spatial loop (as well as in the plane of the standard and unipolar extremity leads of the ECG), the shortest interval occurs because the terminal forces are perpendicular to the plane or derived lead. On the other hand, if precordial leads are considered scalar leads that are capable of recording local potentials with different durations, then QT dispersion is a reality.

The M-cell studies of Antzelevitch allow for the differentiation of this global "dispersion" (derived from *multiple* leads, if it exists at all) from "local" transmural dispersion in *single* precordial leads (reflecting the electrical activity of the region explored by the lead) by measuring the time that elapses between the peak of the T wave and the end of the T wave (given by the end of the composite M-cell action potentials).

ELECTROLTYE IMBALANCES

〖 〗 HYPERKALEMIA

Peaked T waves are the initial effect of acute hyperkalemia. The diagnosis is almost certain when the duration of the base is less than 0.20 seconds at normal heart rates. As hyperkalemia increases, the QRS complex widens and the electrical axis deviates abnormally to the left and rarely to the right. Additionally the PR interval prolongs and the P wave flattens until it disappears. Rarely, hyperkalemia can simulate acute MI with anteroseptal ST elevation in the absence of coronary artery disease or a Brugada pattern.

〖 〗 HYPOKALEMIA

Hypokalemia manifests as QT rather than QT prolongation. With major degrees of hypokalemia, the ST segment becomes progressively more depressed, and there is gradual blending of the T wave into what appears to be a tall U wave.

〖 〗 HYPOMAGNESEMIA AND HYPERMAGNESEMIA

Isolated hypomagnesemia does not produce QU prolongation unless coexistent severe hypokalemia is present. Long-standing and severe magnesium deficiency lowers the amplitude of the T wave and depresses the ST segment. The ECG findings of hypomagnesemia are difficult to differentiate from those of hypokalemia, with which is commonly associated. Similarly, the effects of hypermagnesemia on the ECG are difficult to identify because the changes are dominated by calcium. Intravenous magnesium given to patients with torsades de pointes can control the arrhythmia without changing the prolonged QT interval significantly.

〖 〗 HYPERCALCEMIA AND OTHER CAUSES OF SHORT QT INTERVALS

Hypercalcemia produces a short QT interval during normal sinus rhythm, characterized by short Q-to-apex-of-T interval, and occasionally the ST segment disappears and the T waves become inverted. Digitalis also shortens the QT interval with the characteristic effects in leads where the R waves predominate. In addition, short QT intervals have been reported in hyperthermia, hyperkalemia, and altered autonomic tone. A congenital short QT syndrome has also been described, characterized by a QTc shorter than 300 ms and associated with malignant ventricular arrhythmia and sudden death.

SUGGESTED READING

Ammann P, Sticherling C, KaluscheD, et al. An electrocardiogram-based algorithm to detect loss of left ventricular capture during cardiac resynchronization therapy. *Ann Intern Med.* 2005;142:968–973.

Antzelevitch C, Shimizu W, Yan GX, et al. The M cell: its contribution to the ECG and to normal and abnormal electrical function of the heart. *J Cardiovasc Electrophysiol.* 1999;10:1124–1152.

Bayes de Luna A. *Clinical Electrocardiography: A Textbook.* Mt. Kisco, NY: Futura; 1993:450.

Castellanos A, Interian A Jr., Myerburg RJ. The resting electrocardiogram. In: Fuster V, O'Rourke RA, Walsh RA, et al., eds. *Hurst's The Heart.* 12th ed. New York, NY: McGraw-Hill; 2008:294–323.

Macfarlane PW, Lawrie TDV, eds. *Comprehensive Electrocardiology: Theory and Practice in Health and Disease.* New York, NY: Pergamon; 1989.

Malik M, Acar B, Gang Y, et al. QT dispersion does not represent electrocardiographic interlead heterogeneity of ventricular repolarization. *J Cardiovasc Electrophysiol.* 2000;11:835–843.

Rosenbaum MB, Elizari MV, Lazzari JO. *The Hemiblocks.* Oldsmar, FL: Tampa Tracings; 1970.

Wagner GS. *Marriott's Practical Electrocardiography.* 10th ed. New York, NY: Lippincott Williams & Wilkins; 2000.

Wellens HJJ, Conover M. *The ECG in Emergency Decision Making.* 2nd ed. St. Louis, MO: Saunders, Elsevier; 2006.

CHAPTER 3

Cardiac Roentgenography

Robert A. O'Rourke

As discussed in other chapters in this book (see Chapters 1, 2, and 5 to 7), the relatively low-cost chest roentgenogram is less commonly used than in the past as a primary diagnostic technique for determining the presence and severity of cardiac disease, even when it provides diagnostic information (e.g., pulmonary venous hypertension).

With the development of many new cardiac imaging techniques, familiarity with the altered anatomy and understanding of the underlying pathophysiology of a diseased heart are the cornerstones to appropriate interpretation of its roentgen manifestations. The conventional four-view cardiac series is tabulated in Table 3-1.

The approach to the chest roentgenogram should be thorough and objective so that no clue is overlooked and no bias is incorporated in the process of radiographic analysis. Films should initially be interpreted without any knowledge about the patient.

A secundum atrial septal defect can be incorrectly diagnosed as mitral stenosis (MS) because of similar physical signs. The split second sound can be misinterpreted as the opening snap. The diastolic rumble caused by the increased flow through a normal tricuspid valve can mimic the murmur of MS. The radiographic signs of the two entities, however, are quite different (Fig. 3-1 versus Fig. 3-2). The *final* radiologic diagnosis, however, should be made only after correlating the x-ray findings with clinical information and other laboratory data

The radiologic examination for heart disease consists of five major steps. They are (1) roentgenographic examination for anatomy, (2) comparison of serial studies, (3) statistical guidance, (4) clinical correlation, and (5) conclusion.

ROENTGENOGRAPHIC EXAMINATION FOR ANATOMY

The first step is to survey the roentgenogram and assess all the structures, searching particularly for noncardiac conditions that can reflect heart disease (Table 3-2). For instance, a right-sided stomach with an absent image of the inferior vena cava suggests the possibility of congenital interruption of the inferior vena cava with azygos continuation. A narrowed anteroposterior (AP) diameter of the thorax can be the cause of an innocent murmur.

【 】 PULMONARY VASCULATURE

The lung can often reflect the underlying pathophysiology of the heart. For example, if uniform dilatation of all pulmonary vessels is present, the diagnosis of a left-to-right shunt is more likely than a left-sided obstructive lesion. The latter typically shows a cephalic pulmonary blood flow pattern.

TABLE 3-1

Conventional Four-View Cardiac Series

Posteroanterior (PA) view	With barium
Left lateral (lateral) view	With barium
45° Right anterior oblique (RAO) view	With barium
60° Left anterior oblique (LAO) view	Without barium

【 】 LUNG PARENCHYMA

With right heart failure, the lungs become unusually radiolucent because of decreased pulmonary blood flow (PBF). Conversely, significant left heart failure is characterized by the presence of pulmonary edema and/or a cephalic blood flow pattern. Long-standing, severe pulmonary venous hypertension can lead to hemosiderosis and/or ossification of the lung. When right heart failure results from severe left heart failure, the preexisting pulmonary congestion can improve because of the decreased PBF

【 】 CARDIAC SIZE

An enlarged heart is always abnormal; however, mild cardiomegaly can reflect a higher-than-average cardiac output from a normal heart, as seen in athletes with slow heart rates. The cardiothoracic ratio remains the simplest yardstick for assessment of cardiac size; the mean ratio in the upright posteroanterior (PA) view is 44%.

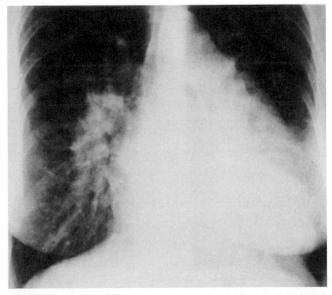

FIGURE 3-1. Roentgenographic assessment of the volume of pulmonary blood flow. Patient with a secundum atrial septal defect showing uniform increase in pulmonary vascularity bilaterally. The right descending pulmonary artery is markedly enlarged, measuring 27 mm.

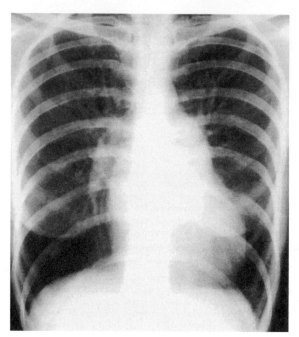

FIGURE 3-2. Abnormal pulmonary blood flow patterns. *Cephalization.* Patient with severe mitral stenosis (MS) showing dilatation of the upper vessels with constriction of the lower vessels.

TABLE 3-2

Major Steps of Roentgenologic Examination

Roentgenographic examination for anatomy
    Overview (e.g., rib notching)
    Pulmonary vascularity (e.g., shunt vascularity in ASD)
    Lung parenchyma (e.g., ossification in critical MS)
    Cardiac size (e.g., huge right heart in Ebstein's anomaly)
    Cardiac contour (e.g., boot-shaped heart in TOF)
    Abnormal densities (e.g., calcification of LV aneurysm)
    Abnormal lucency (e.g., conspicuous fat stripes in PE)
    Cardiac malpositions (e.g., dextrocardia with SS)
    Other abnormalities (e.g., Holt–Oram syndrome)
Fluoroscopic observation for dynamics
Comparison of serial studies
Statistical guidance
Clinical correlation
Conclusion

ASD, atrial septal defect; MS, mitral stenosis; TOF, tetralogy of Fallot; LV, left ventricle; PE, pericardial effusion; SS, situs solitus.

The nature of cardiomegaly can often be determined by the specific roentgen appearance. As a rule, when the PBF pattern remains normal, volume overload tends to present a greater degree of cardiomegaly than lesions with pressure overload alone. For example, patients with aortic stenosis (AS) typically show features of left ventricular hypertrophy (LVH) without dilatation. Conversely, the left ventricle both dilates and hypertrophies in the case of aortic regurgitation (AR), producing a much larger heart even before the development of heart failure.

【 】 CARDIAC CONTOUR

Any significant deviation from the normal cardiovascular contour can be a clue to the correct diagnosis. For instance, *coeur en sabot*, a "boot-shaped heart," is characteristic of tetralogy of Fallot. A bulge along the left cardiac border with a retrosternal double density is virtually diagnostic of left ventricular (LV) aneurysm. A markedly widened right cardiac contour with a straightened left cardiac border is seen frequently in patients with severe MS leading to tricuspid regurgitation (TR).

【 】 ABNORMAL DENSITIES

Besides the familiar double density cast by an enlarged left atrium (LA), other increased densities can be found within the cardiac shadow, indicating a variety of dilated vascular structures (e.g., tortuous descending aorta, aortic aneurysm, coronary artery [CA] aneurysm, pulmonary varix). Furthermore, large cardiac calcifications are readily seen, in lateral and oblique views. If smaller calcific deposits are suspected, they should be verified promptly, ruled out by cardiac fluoroscopy or CT. Any radiologically detectable calcification in the heart is clinically important. In general, the heavier the calcification, the more significant it becomes.

【 】 ABNORMAL LUCENCY

The abnormal lucent areas in and about the heart include (1) displaced subepicardial fat stripes caused by effusion or thickening of the pericardium, (2) pneumopericardium, and (3) pneumomediastinum. Pneumomediastinum is differentiated from pneumopericardium by the fact that the former shows a superior extension of the air strip beyond the confines of the pericardium.

【 】 PULMONARY VASCULARITY

Normal

The normal roentgen appearance of the pulmonary vasculature of an upright human being is typified by a caudal flow pattern because of gravity. The pressure differential between the apex and the base of the lung is approximately 22 mm Hg in adults in the upright position. Therefore, more flow under higher distending pressure is expected in the lower-lobe vessels than in the upper. Normally, one sees very little vascularity above the hilum, whereas more and larger vessels are found below the hilum. Because the pulmonary resistance is normal, all vessels taper gradually in a tree-like manner from the hilum toward the periphery of the lung. The right descending pulmonary artery measures 10 to 15 mm in diameter in males and 9 to 14 mm in females.

Abnormal

Abnormal pulmonary vascularity can be classified into two categories, either in terms of volume or in terms of distribution (Table 3-3).

> ### TABLE 3-3
>
> Pulmonary Vascularity

Normal
Caudal PBF pattern in upright position (PBF controlled by gravity)
Gradual branching, treelike
RDPA = 10–15 mm in males
RDPA = 9–14 mm in females
A/B ratio = 1

Abnormal
Volume with normal PBF pattern (distribution)
Increased, larger vessels (e.g., ASD)
Decreased, smaller vessels (e.g., TOF)
Distribution with abnormal PBF pattern
Cephalic (e.g., MS)
Centralized (e.g., Eisenmenger's syndrome)
Lateralized (e.g., Westermark's sign)
Localized (e.g., pulmonary AV fistulas)
Collateralized (e.g., severe TOF)
Combined
Decreased volume and cephalization (e.g., critical MS)
Lateralization and localization (e.g., scimitar syndrome)

A/B, artery/bronchus; ASD, atrial septal defect; AV, arteriovenous; MS, mitral stenosis; PBF, pulmonary blood flow; RDPA, right descending pulmonary artery; TOF, tetralogy of Fallot.

ABNORMALITIES IN VOLUME   In the evaluation of pulmonary vasculature, the caliber of the vessels is more important than the length or the number. As long as the PBF pattern remains normal, with a greater amount of flow to the bases than to the apices, the volume of the flow is proportional to the caliber of the pulmonary arteries. Besides measuring the right descending pulmonary artery, pulmonary blood volume can be assessed by comparing the size of the pulmonary artery with that of the accompanying bronchus where they are viewed on end. Normally, the two structures have approximately equal diameters. When the artery-bronchus ratio is greater than unity, increased blood flow is suggested. Conversely, when the ratio is smaller than unity, decreased flow is likely.

Increased Pulmonary Blood Flow   In the case of mild to moderate left-to-right shunts, for example, the vessels dilate in proportion to the increased flow with no significant change in pressure, resistance, or flow pattern. This phenomenon is also called *shunt vascularity* or *equalization*. Equalization of the PBF between the upper and lower lung zones is more apparent than real; however, the lower lobes still receive a great deal more blood than the upper lobes, although the ratio of PBF between the two zones has changed—for example, from 5:1 to 4:1 or 3:1. A mild increase in pulmonary vascularity with slight cardiomegaly is commonly found in pregnant women and trained athletes with increased cardiac output.

Decreased Pulmonary Blood Flow   Patients with tetralogy of Fallot frequently show decreased pulmonary vascularity with smaller and shorter pulmonary arteries and veins and more radiolucent lungs. Marked reduction in PBF is also encountered in patients with isolated right-sided heart failure without a right-to-left shunt. This is attributed to the significant decrease in cardiac output from both ventricles.

ABNORMALITIES IN DISTRIBUTION   An abnormal distribution of PBF (or an abnormal PBF pattern) always reflects a changed pulmonary vascular resistance, either locally or diffusely.

Cephalization   In the presence of postcapillary pulmonary hypertension (PH), physiologic disturbances begin when the total intravascular pressure exceeds the oncotic pressure of the blood. As a result, fluid leaks out of the vessels and collects in the interstitium before filling the alveoli.

Pulmonary edema interferes with gas exchange, resulting in a state of hypoxemia. Alveolar hypoxia has a profound influence on the pulmonary vessels, causing them to constrict. Because there is greater alveolar hypoxia in the lung bases than in the apices, the basilar vessels constrict significantly, forcing the blood to flow upward. This phenomenon actually represents a reversal of the normal PBF pattern: redistribution or cephalization of the pulmonary vascularity.

Cephalization occurs in any of three conditions: (1) left-sided obstructive lesions—for example, MS or AS; (2) LV failure—for example, coronary heart disease or cardiomyopathies; and (3) severe mitral regurgitation (MR) even before pump failure of the left ventricle occurs. It should be emphasized that unless there is obvious *constriction* of the lower-lobe vessels, the diagnosis of cephalization should not be made. Dilatation of the upper-lobe vessels is of secondary importance and can be found without narrowing of the basilar vessels in a number of entities, most noticeably left-to-right shunts.

Centralization   In the presence of precapillary PH, the pulmonary trunk and central pulmonary arteries dilate, whereas the distal pulmonary arteries constrict in a concentric fashion from the periphery of the lung toward the hilum. This phenomenon is called *centralization of the pulmonary vascularity*. It occurs in patients with primary PH, Eisenmenger's syndrome, recurrent pulmonary thromboembolic disease, or severe obstructive emphysema.

Lateralization   Massive unilateral pulmonary embolism can cause a lateralized PBF pattern. Because one major pulmonary artery is obstructed, the blood is forced to flow through the healthy lung only. The paucity of pulmonary vascularity in the diseased lung with the obstructed pulmonary artery is termed the *Westermark's sign*. In the case of congenital valvular pulmonary stenosis, a jet effect from the stenotic valve can cause a lateralized PBF pattern in favor of the left side.

Localization   A localized abnormal flow pattern is exemplified by a congenital pulmonary arteriovenous fistula in a cyanotic child.

Collateralization   Patients with markedly decreased PBF (e.g., severe tetralogy) tend to show numerous small, tortuous bronchial arterial collaterals in the upper medial lung zones near their origin from the descending aorta. The native pulmonary arteries are extremely small, although smooth and gracefully branching.

COMBINED ABNORMALITIES   In reality, an abnormal pulmonary vascularity is often a mixed type. There is a great variety of possible combinations—for example, cephalization plus decreased flow in severe MS or centralization with increased PBF Eisenmenger's atrial septal defect.

【 】 HEART FAILURE

In addition to specific chamber enlargement, the pulmonary vasculature uniquely portrays the underlying pathophysiology of heart failure. In the chronic setting, decreased flow with increased pulmonary lucency is the hallmark of right heart failure; striking cephalization of the pulmonary vasculature is typical for left-sided decompensation.

Left-Sided

CHRONIC   Chronic left-sided heart failure is characterized by gross cardiomegaly, striking cephalization of the pulmonary vasculature, and interstitial pulmonary edema or fibrosis with multiple distinct Kerley B lines. Pulmonary hemosiderosis, ossification, or both can result from long-standing severe postcapillary PH.

Right-Sided

ACUTE   Acute right-sided heart failure most commonly results from massive pulmonary embolism. The typical radiographic signs are rapidly developing centralization of the pulmonary vasculature and dilatation of the right-sided cardiac chambers and venae cavae. In addition, the lungs can show localized or lateralized oligemia. Eventually, opacities in either or both lungs can develop as a result of pulmonary infarction.

CHRONIC   Chronic right heart failure has many causes. The common ones include congenital pulmonary stenosis, Ebstein anomaly, severe chronic obstructive pulmonary disease, and recurrent pulmonary thromboembolic disease. Diffusely decreased pulmonary vascularity with unusually lucent lungs is seen in patients with right heart failure without PH. Centralized PBF pattern is encountered when the right-sided heart failure is secondary to precapillary PH. A cephalized flow pattern with unusually lucent lungs is found in patients with right-sided heart failure secondary to long-standing severe left heart failure. The degree of right-sided chamber enlargement is proportional to the severity of TR.

Combined

Right heart failure is caused most often by severe left heart failure. This is exemplified by patients with severe MS leading to severe TR. Other examples of bilateral heart failure are cardiac tamponade and constrictive pericarditis.

SUGGESTED READING

Chen JTT. *Essentials of Cardiac Imaging.* 2nd ed. Philadelphia, PA: Lippincott-Raven; 1997.

Chen JTT. The significance of cardiac calcifications. *Appl Radiol.* 1992;21:11–19.

Chen JTT. The plain radiograph in the diagnosis of cardiovascular disease. In: Putman C, ed. Symposium on cardiopulmonary imaging. *Radiol Clin North Am.* 1983;21: 609–621.

Chen JTT, Capp MP, Johnsrude IS, et al. Roentgen appearance of pulmonary vascularity in the diagnosis of heart disease. *AJR Am J Roentgenol.* 1971;112:559–570.

Chen JTT, Lester RG, Peter RH. Posterior wedging sign of mitral insufficiency. *Radiology.* 1974;113:451–453.

DeLeon AC, Perloff JK, Twigg HL. The straight back syndrome: clinical and cardiovascular manifestations. *Circulation.* 1965;32:193–203.

O'Rourke RA, Gilkeson RC. Cardiac roentgenography. In: Fuster V, O'Rourke RA, Walsh RA, et al., eds. *Hurst's The Heart.* 12th ed. New York, NY: McGraw-Hill; 2008:341–358.

Woodley K, Stark P. Pulmonary parenchymal manifestations of mitral valve disease. *Radiographics.* 1999;19:965–972.

CHAPTER 4

Noninvasive Testing for Myocardial Ischemia

Arie Wolak, Daniel S. Berman, Jeroen J. Bax,
Thomas H. Marwick, and Leslee J. Shaw

Myocardial ischemia is commonly detected using diverse electrocardiographic and imaging modalities. Dramatic developments in the field of cardiac imaging have paralleled improvements in microprocessor speed as well as progress in new contrast and radiopharmaceutical agents resulting in improved resolution, image quality, processing time, and quantitative interpretation programs.

PATHOGENESIS OF STRESS-INDUCED MYOCARDIAL ISCHEMIA

Myocardial ischemia is defined as a discord between oxygen supply and demand within the cardiac myocyte. Most commonly, the mechanism for demand ischemia is reduced coronary blood flow from a fixed stenosis, although impaired coronary flow reserve in nonobstructive coronary disease, as a result of endothelial dysfunction, may also elicit ischemic responses to stress. Resting blood flow is generally maintained up until 90% stenosis. When oxygen delivery fails to meet regional demand, myocardial ischemia ensues, characterized by a shift from aerobic metabolism as a dominant energy source toward anaerobic substrates and the accumulation of metabolic end-products (e.g., lactate). The shift toward anaerobic metabolism quickly results in a depletion of high-energy phosphate stores followed by impaired mechanical function.

The aim of stress testing is to provoke myocardial ischemia within a controlled environment with incremental increases in the metabolic requirements for graded physical work or as a response to a drug stressor. The manifestations of myocardial ischemia may be commonly documented through examination of regional myocardial perfusion or left ventricular wall motion, the surface electrocardiogram (ECG), and clinical observations including angina-like symptoms, exertional hypotension, or chronotropic incompetence. The sequence of occurrences and the ensuing consequences and timing of reductions in blood flow is defined as the ischemic cascade. This model for elucidating myocardial ischemia will allow us to understand the expected utility of various imaging risk markers, such as reductions in myocardial perfusion or regional wall motion abnormalities. Figure 4-1 depicts the cascade of events that occur during myocardial ischemia and the type of test that is currently applied to document each facet of the ischemic cascade. An understanding of the ischemic cascade and how it interfaces with present-day imaging allows for a more precise understanding of ischemia risk markers, their predictive accuracy, and patient populations that benefit from each type of imaging modality. The initial manifestation of myocardial ischemia is decreased perfusion followed by documented shifts toward glucose as a more prominent substrate for metabolic activity, and then by diastolic and systolic dysfunction, electrocardiographic ST-T wave changes, and

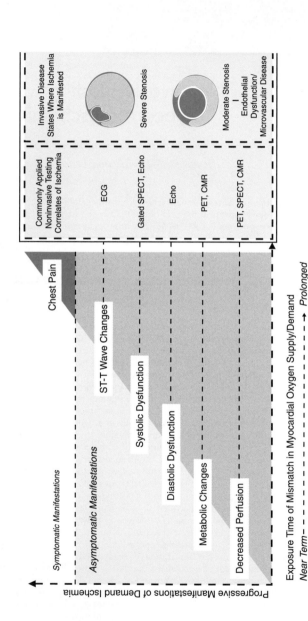

FIGURE 4-1. Progressive manifestations of myocardial ischemia as illustrated by the ischemic cascade.

ECG = Electrocardiogram, SPECT = Single Photon Emission Computed Tomography, PET = Positron Emission Tomography, Echo = Echocardiogram, CMR = Cardiovascular Magnetic Resonance Imaging finally the provocation of angina-like symptoms. Intermediate stenoses may provoke perfusion abnormalities. With more prolonged ischemia, regional wall motion abnormalities and systolic dysfunction occur. ECG and symptomatic manifestations of myocardial ischemia occur later on in this cascade.

BASICS OF PROBABILISTIC AND RISK-BASED DECISION-MAKING

【 】 OPTIMAL CANDIDATE SELECTION FOR STRESS TESTING—UNDERSTANDING PRINCIPLES OF BAYESIAN THEORY

Effective referral to noninvasive stress testing requires integrating numerous parameters from a careful patient history. Upon presentation, the type, quality, and characteristics of a patient's symptoms are an important risk stratification tool. Angina with typical exertional components generally has a higher likelihood of obstructive CAD. A thorough integration of risk markers into a global risk score comprises risk factors, symptoms, past medical history, laboratory and physical examination parameters, as well as electrocardiographic results and is a central component in decision-making for noninvasive stress testing choice. Table 4-1 provides a simple approach to risk estimation based upon the patient's symptom presentation. Determining risk or a patient's pretest likelihood of CAD provides the basis for referral for a noninvasive stress test or for invasive coronary angiography. As illustrated in Fig. 4-2, only patients with an intermediate to high likelihood of CAD are candidates for stress testing. This is based upon Bayesian theory by which CAD posttest likelihood is a function of the initial pretest risk assessment. Using this reasoning, the predictive accuracy of a test is related to disease prevalence. In low-risk populations, high rates of false positives can be expected, and the shift from pretest to posttest risk is minimal. Specifically, the overall likelihood of CAD remains relatively low in the setting of an abnormal exercise ECG (for example) for a low-risk patient. Thus, the ability to shift posttest likelihood is directly related to pretest likelihood of disease. In a low-risk population where the pretest probability of CAD is ≤ 20%, there is exceptional near-term event-free survival exceeding 99%. Thus, testing and the initiation of any intervention would yield trivial improvements in outcome. The greatest shift in posttest likelihood of disease occurs in those patients with an intermediate pretest likelihood of CAD. Using our risk-based thresholds, this population has an annual cardiac death or myocardial infarction rate ranging from 1% to 3% and expected pretest probability ranges from about 20% to 80%. Theoretically, the major benefit of stress testing in this population is that a negative test will result in a reclassification to a low-risk subset and an abnormal test will result in a reclassification to a higher risk cohort. High-risk patients, on the other hand, are often referred to stress testing for evaluation of ischemic burden as an aid to medical management decisions.

Additional key decision points in the workup of patients with stable chest pain symptoms are illustrated in Fig. 4-2; these include knowledge of the patient's functional capabilities, coronary anatomy, and resting ECG abnormalities. In addition to selecting symptomatic women and men with an intermediate to high likelihood of CAD, the second tier of decisions is an estimation of the patient's ability to perform activities of daily living. Patients who are capable of performing maximal exercise or ≥ 4 to 5 metabolic equivalents (METs) should generally be referred to treadmill or bicycle exercise testing (Table 4-2). A patient incapable of performing ≥ 4 to 5 METs of work can undergo pharmacologic stress imaging. In addition to the functionally impaired, patients with a prior CAD history or those with resting ST-T wave are often referred directly for an imaging stress test (most commonly stress echocardiography or single photon emission computed tomography).

TABLE 4-1

Comparing Pretest Likelihood of CAD in Low- to High-Risk Symptomatic Patients—Results from the ACC Guidelines for Exercise Testing

	Nonanginal Chest Pain		Atypical/Probable Angina		Typical/Definite Angina	
	Men	Women	Men	Women	Men	Women
< 40 years old	Low	Very Low	Intermediate	Very Low	Intermediate	Intermediate
40–49 years old	Low	Very Low	Intermediate	Low	High	Intermediate
50–59 years old	Intermediate	Low	Intermediate	Intermediate	High	Intermediate
60–69 years old[a]	Intermediate	Intermediate	Intermediate	Intermediate	High	High

[a]Candidates who are ≥ 70 years of age are at intermediate to high likelihood of CAD.

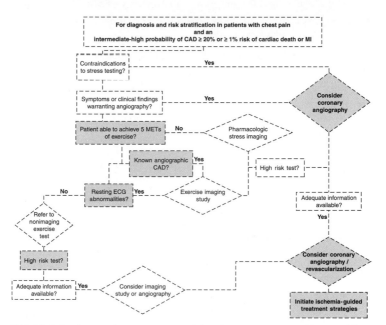

FIGURE 4-2. Choosing the appropriate candidates for stress testing—modification of the ACC/AHA Guidelines for the Evaluation of Stable Angina.

TABLE 4-2

Estimated Energy Requirements for Various Activities Derived from the AHA Exercise Testing Guidelines and Duke Activity Status Index (DASI)

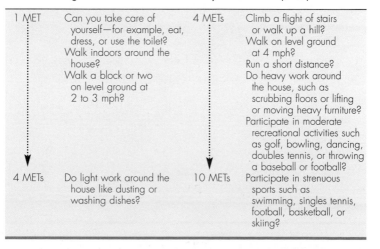

| 1 MET | Can you take care of yourself—for example, eat, dress, or use the toilet? Walk indoors around the house? Walk a block or two on level ground at 2 to 3 mph? | 4 METs | Climb a flight of stairs or walk up a hill? Walk on level ground at 4 mph? Run a short distance? Do heavy work around the house, such as scrubbing floors or lifting or moving heavy furniture? Participate in moderate recreational activities such as golf, bowling, dancing, doubles tennis, or throwing a baseball or football? |
| 4 METs | Do light work around the house like dusting or washing dishes? | 10 METs | Participate in strenuous sports such as swimming, singles tennis, football, basketball, or skiing? |

【 】 DIAGNOSTIC ACCURACY AND ISSUES OF VERIFICATION BIAS

Test accuracy has historically been defined by calculating diagnostic sensitivity and specificity. Sensitivity is the proportion of patients with an abnormal test that have obstructive CAD (or true positives / [true positives + false negatives]), while specificity is the proportion of patients who have a negative test and no obstructive CAD (or true negatives / [true negatives + false positives]). Tests where the sensitivity and specificity values exceed 80% are considered highly accurate. The diagnostic accuracy (uncorrected for workup bias) of exercise ECG, echocardiography, single photon emission computed tomography (SPECT), and cardiac magnetic resonance (CMR) is detailed in Table 4-3. During our routine workup of patients, those with abnormal studies comprise the vast majority of referrals to coronary angiography, with few patients with negative stress test results proceeding to catheterization. The differential referral to coronary angiography for patients with negative and positive stress testing results in a workup or verification bias. Thus, measures such as diagnostic sensitivity and specificity in current clinical practice more often reflect how we are applying the test as a gatekeeper to angiography (where perfect gatekeeping would result in an observed sensitivity of 100% and specificity of 0%). Methods are available for correcting verification bias.

TABLE 4-3

Compilation of Meta-analyses and Reviews on the Diagnostic Accuracy of Contemporary Noninvasive Stress Testing Including Exercise ECG, SPECT, and Echocardiography as well as Pharmacologic Stress SPECT, Echocardiography, and MRI[a]

Modality	No. Studies	No. Patients	Sensitivity (%)	Specificity (%)
Exercise ECG	58	11,691	67	72
Exercise SPECT				
Tc-99m agents only	22	2,360	87 88	73 72
Adenosine SPECT				
Tc-99m agents only	11	3,539	89 87	77 86
Dobutamine SPECT				
Tc-99m agents only	20	1,419	85 83	79 76
Exercise echocardiography	13	741	83	84
Dobutamine stress echocardiography	13	436	75	83
Stress magnetic resonance				
Dobutamine stress wall motion	10	644	84	89
Adenosine/ dipyridamole perfusion	3	108	84	85

[a]The diagnostic sensitivity and specificity values presented are uncorrected for verification bias. (Note that these are average values and wide ranges exist for most modalities.)

Despite the ability to bias correct *measures of test performance,* our current *utilization of testing results* yields a better measure of sensitivity while the exclusion of disease is problematic and can only be reliably examined through evaluation of long-term prognosis.

【 】 WHY DO STRESS TESTING RESULTS WORK SO WELL TO ESTIMATE PROGNOSIS?

The rationale for using prognosis as a measure of test performance is that an accurate assessment of patient risk is a strong determinant of the intensity of patient management. Thus, estimating prognosis has become a new standard for evaluating test performance—an evidence-based approach that requires a *larger body of evidence* on the role of testing in patient management and therapeutic decision-making. This latter notion expands beyond the idea of correlating stress testing results to a "gold standard" such as angiographic CAD extent and severity to include assessing coronary physiology, metabolism, and function that may provide added information for estimating clinical outcomes. That is, angiographic CAD extent is a major driver of prognosis, but additional measures such as regional and global ventricular function and myocardial perfusion are supplemental components to a risk assessment as well as major drivers in ischemia-guided medical management.

Simplistically stated, the estimation of prognosis is commonly defined as risk stratification, where the overall event rate is calculated for patients with normal (i.e., low risk) to severely abnormal (i.e., high risk) stress testing results. These event rates may be compared to the larger body of evidence from population studies or observational registries on CAD. Low-risk and high-risk event rate thresholds have been defined using these larger datasets; for example, an annual risk of cardiac death or nonfatal myocardial infarction of $\geq 2\%$ is equivalent to the annual risk of those with established cardiovascular disease or diabetes. These thresholds may then be applied to the review of outcome results for stress testing data (Fig. 4-3). Those with suspected CAD have an annual rate of death or myocardial infarction < 2% per year; with established CAD, of about 2% per year; and with severe or high-risk CAD, in the range of 3% to 5% or more.

SYNOPSIS OF AVAILABLE EVIDENCE ON STRESS TESTING FOR MYOCARDIAL ISCHEMIA

【 】 PREDICTIVE ACCURACY OF EXERCISE ECG—OPTIMIZING EXERCISE TREADMILL DATA

Candidates for a routine exercise treadmill exercise test include patients with suspected CAD, an interpretable 12-lead ECG, and normal physical work capacity. According to the recent stable angina guidelines, those patients with established CAD, functional disability, or resting ST-T wave changes (that preclude interpretation of peak exertional changes) are appropriate candidates for cardiac imaging testing including stress echocardiography, SPECT, and increasingly, magnetic resonance (MR) imaging. Of the current indications for a nonimaging stress test, the most challenging decision is discerning whether a patient is capable of maximal exercise. A guide to this decision-making process is whether or not a patient is capable of performing ≥ 4 to 5 METs, equivalent to routine activities of daily living (see Table 4-2). A test should be considered adequate if $\geq 85\%$ predicted maximal heart rate and ≥ 5 METs of exercise have been achieved. An accelerated heart rate response at low levels of exercise can lead to premature fatigue; consideration should then be given to repeat testing using pharmacologic stress imaging.

	Death or MI Rate (%/yr) in High Risk	Death or MI Rate (%/yr) in Low Risk	N Total	p Value
Stress Magnetic Resonance	22.9%	0.9%	466	<0.0001
Stress Echocardiography	7.0%	1.2%	32,739	<0.0001
Exercise	2.6%	0.5%	11,517	<0.0001
Dobutamine Stress	4.8%	1.7%	4,018	<0.0001
Stress SPECT	5.9%	0.9%	69,655	<0.0001
Exercise	5.6%	0.7%	58,424	<0.0001
Pharmacologic Stress	8.3%	1.2%	11,231	<0.0001
Summary Relative Risk	**6.9% (n=27,170)**	**0.7% (n=62,097)**	**89,267**	**<0.0001**

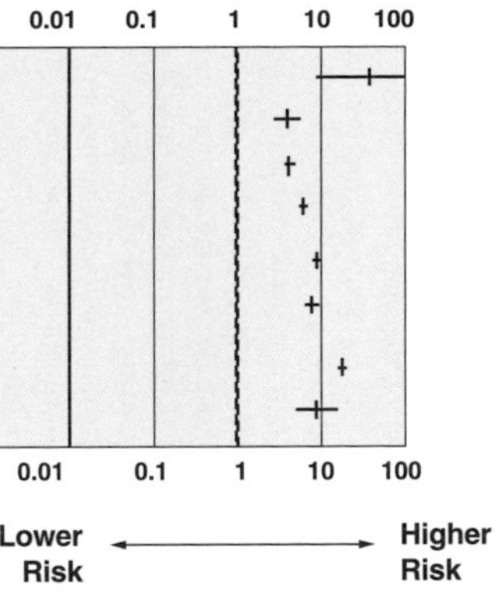

Lower Risk ← → Higher Risk

Source: CMR data is for dobutamine stress wall motion derived from SCMR and ESC Consensus Panel report (9) and related publications. Echocardiographic data is ACC/AHA guidelines for Stable angina (5) and related publications (88-97), SPECT data is ACC/AHA guidelines for SPECT imaging (5) and a recent metanalysis (30).

FIGURE 4-3. Forest plot illustrating results of a meta-analysis on the prognostic value of stress echocardiography, SPECT, and CMR. This figure examines the annual cardiac death or myocardial infarction rate in patients with low- and high-risk studies and a calculation of the relative risk (95% confidence interval) of high-risk ischemia by CMR or echocardiographic wall motion and SPECT perfusion imaging. The largest body of evidence is for stress SPECT imaging, where overall event rates are higher for patients with known CVD or diabetes and for those referred to pharmacologic stress imaging. The results for stress echocardiography have been published in several smaller series, but recently the Echo Persantine International Cooperative (EPIC) study and American Society of Echocardiography (ASE) outcome registries have been published on its prognostic value in 7,333 and 11,132 patients. Overall event rates in these larger series vary by type of stress, where annual event rates are 0.3% to 1% for low- to high-risk exercising patients and about 3% to 12% for low- to high-risk patients undergoing pharmacologic stress echocardiography. The preliminary evidence from three reports on dobutamine stress MR wall motion is promising but will require additional validation in larger series for a more definitive comparative analysis.

An impaired heart rate or blunted blood pressure response to exercise is associated with an increasing risk of events. An impaired chronotropic response to exercise should be considered when peak heart rates are < 110 to 120 beats per minute, and is often related to impaired myocardial contractility and left ventricular dysfunction. Similarly, hemodynamic impairment, defined as a blunted rise or drop in systolic blood pressure (e.g., ≤ 5 mm Hg), is also associated with a greater frequency of multivessel CAD and a depressed ejection fraction.

During stress, ECG changes with exercise should be documented, including the time to onset and offset as well as the extent and severity of ST-segment depression. A test is considered positive with ≥ 1 mm of horizontal or downsloping ST-segment depression at 60 msec post-J point; but a threshold of ≥1.5 mm is applied for upsloping ST-segment depression. As they will interfere with the provocation of ischemia, anti-ischemic drugs (e.g., beta-blockers or nitrates) should be discontinued prior to testing. High-risk patients are those who present with ST-segment changes at a low workload (i.e., < 5 METs), exhibit ≥ 2 mm ST-segment depression, and for whom the time to resolution of ≥ 1 mm ST-segment depression is ≥ 5 minutes into recovery. A Δ change of ≥ 1 mm of ST-segment deviation may be applied to patients with resting ST-T wave abnormalities. ST-segment elevation is a rare (occurring in about 1 in 10,000 patients tested) but serious occurrence during exercise testing, reflecting transmural ischemia, and consideration should be given to immediate angiography. ST-segment elevation, however, in a Q-wave lead is a marker for a preexisting wall-motion abnormality.

Care should be taken when interpreting the exercise ECG, as there are many factors that confound its interpretation including medications (i.e., anti-ischemics and other vasoactive drugs), hormonal status, resting ST-T wave changes, prior myocardial infarction, and, importantly, functional capacity. Evidence supports the fact that there are certain patient subsets where the exercise ECG is of diminished value. False-positive results can be due to lower QRS voltage, ECG abnormalities (such as left ventricular hypertrophy, left bundle branch block, or Wolff–Parkinson–White syndrome), and drug effects (e.g., digoxin); these patients should be referred to cardiac imaging. The highest relative proportion of false-positive test results is in premenopausal female patients; however, marked ST abnormalities are associated with an improved predictive accuracy. False-negative results are commonly the result of a submaximal stress test and occur commonly in patients with limited functional capacity.

Use of ST Δ / Δ Heart Rate indices (abnormality is defined as ≥ 1.6 mV/bpm), available on most commercial equipment, improves the sensitivity and specificity of imaging, in particular for women. Additionally, the Duke Treadmill Score (exercise time − [5 × ST deviation] − [4 × chest pain index (0 = none, 1 = nonlimiting, 2 = limiting)]) is readily calculable and has been shown to estimate 5-year survival and the presence and extent of significant CAD in men and women alike. Using this score, low-risk (> +5), intermediate-risk (−10 and +5), and high-risk (< −11) patients have 5-year mortality ranges from 3% to 10% for women and 9% to 30% for men.

Electrical instability, defined as a ≥ 3-beat run of ventricular tachycardia or ventricular fibrillation, is also a high-risk marker. The occurrence of premature ventricular contractions with exercise or in recovery has been studied frequently and is associated with an increased risk of coronary disease or cardiac events. Other ischemic markers, such as exertional chest pain symptoms, especially when they mimic the patient's historical symptoms, increase diagnostic certainty particularly when concurrent with ECG changes, but are of limited value in women.

Of all the risk markers available to the physician, two factors are of high priority: heart rate profile during exercise and recovery and maximal exercise capacity. One of our greatest prognosticators is a patient's physical work capability, commonly measured in METs. Patients with impaired physical work capacity are those incapable of achieving > 5 METs of exercise, who are then at increased risk of death. Additionally, a large body of evidence is available supporting the substantial prognostic value of baseline heart rate, blunted heart rate response during the exercise, and calculating a change in heart rate from peak exercise to 1 to 2 minutes postexercise (i.e., heart rate recovery). Because heart-rate responses to exercise are controlled by the autonomic nervous system, abnormalities in these parameters probably reflect defected autonomic balance and may precede dire manifestations of cardiovascular disease. The risk of sudden death from myocardial infarction is increased in subjects with a resting heart rate above 75 beats per minute; in subjects with an increase in heart rate during exercise less than 89 beats per minute; and in subjects with a decrease in heart rate of less than 25 beats per minute after the termination of exercise.

A thorough interpretation of the exercise stress test (with or without imaging) should include an evaluation of functional capacity, ECG responses to stress, ventricular ectopy, and heart rate recovery, as well as hemodynamic and chronotropic responses to stress. A synopsis of high-risk exercise test parameters is given in Table 4-4.

TABLE 4-4

Low- to High-Risk Noninvasive Stress Testing Markers from the ACC/AHA Stable Angina Guidelines

High Risk (> 3% annual mortality rate or > 5% annual cardiac death or nonfatal myocardial infarction rate)

1. Severe resting left ventricular dysfunction (LVEF < 35%).
2. High-risk Duke Treadmill Score (score ≤ –11).
3. Severe exercise left ventricular dysfunction (exercise LVEF < 35%).
4. Stress-induced large perfusion defect (particularly, if anterior).
5. Stress-induced multiple perfusion defects of moderate size.
6. Large, fixed perfusion defect with LV dilation or increased lung uptake (thallium-201 only).
7. Stress-induced moderate perfusion defect with LV dilation or increased lung uptake (thallium-201 only).
8. Echocardiographic wall-motion abnormality (involving > 2 segments) developing at low dose of dobutamine (≤ 10 mg/kg/min) or low heart rate (< 120 bpm).
9. Stress echocardiographic evidence of extensive ischemia.

Intermediate risk (1–3% annual mortality rate or 3–5% annual death or myocardial infarction rate)

1. Mild/moderate resting left ventricular dysfunction (LVEF = 35–49%).
2. Intermediate risk Duke Treadmill Score (–11 < score < 5).
3. Stress-induced moderate perfusion defect without LV dilation or increased lung uptake (thallium-201).
4. Limited stress echocardiographic ischemia with a wall-motion abnormality only at higher doses of dobutamine involving ≤ 2 segments.

Low Risk (< 1% annual mortality rate or < 1% annual death or myocardial infarction rate)

1. Low-risk Duke Treadmill Score (score ≥5).
2. Normal or small myocardial perfusion defect at rest or with stress.[a]
3. Normal stress echocardiographic wall motion or no change of limited resting wall-motion abnormalities during stress.[a]

[a]Although the published data are limited, patients with these findings should be considered at higher risk in the presence of a high-risk Duke Treadmill Score, left ventricular dysfunction, known coronary artery disease (or its risk equivalent, such as diabetes or peripheral arterial disease), or severe resting LVEF < 35%.

【 】 DECISIONS REGARDING USE OF EXERCISE VERSUS PHARMACOLOGIC STRESS IMAGING

An important decision for the referring clinician and supervising physician in the exercise testing laboratory is whether the patient is capable of performing maximal stress. A careful history and inquiry into performance of activities of daily living (e.g., using the Duke Activity Status Index) can provide insight into a patient's MET capacity. Patients capable of most common household activities generally meet this criterion and may be able to perform a graded treadmill or bicycle exercise test. However, those with activity limitations and incapable of 5 METs of exercise should be referred to a pharmacologic stress test.

A major reason for preferring exercise is to gain insight into the actual capabilities of the patient as well as the co-occurrence and timing of inducible ischemia. For a growing segment of the population, including obese or diabetic patients, choosing the correct exercise protocol is paramount to elicit a maximal myocardial stress. Although the standard Bruce protocol is commonly employed, the first stage begins at 4.7 METs (i.e., 1.7 mph / 10% grade), and is challenging for numerous subsets of the population. A modified Bruce protocol begins at about 3 METs (1.7 mph / 0% or 5% grade), and may be helpful when employed in modestly impaired patients. Not only is the Bruce protocol initially demanding, but each successive 3-minute stage increases metabolic demands by about 2 to 3 METs. Gentler protocols with less aggressive physical work demands include the Naughton and Balke protocol (see Table 4-2). Linear protocols increasing exercise demands of about 1 MET/stage with shorter exercise stages (about a minute), are commonly employed in heart failure populations but may also be of value for many patients. Many laboratories for purposes of standardization favor the use of the Bruce protocol.

For functionally impaired patients, vasodilator or inotropic pharmacologic stress testing with imaging is recommended. For SPECT imaging, vasodilator stress testing includes a short infusion of intravenous adenosine or dipyridamole and newly introduced α_{2_a} agonists. Due to the vasodilatory actions of adenosine, dipyridamole, and regadenoson, heart rate increases by around 10 to 25 beats per minute and systolic blood pressure measurements drop modestly. Side effects are common but mostly mild and transient due to the short half-life of the agents. With dipyridamole, in the event of any severe side effects, aminophylline is given to reverse the effects. Due to the short half-life of adenosine, aminophylline is seldom employed. Although side effects are more common with adenosine and regadenoson, they rapidly diminish following drug infusion (generally 30 to 45 seconds). Chest discomfort during dipyridamole or adenosine infusion is considered nondiagnostic, as it can be a side effect of the drug unrelated to ischemia. In evaluating the clinical response to vasodilator stress, the clinician is more limited than with treadmill testing, as exercise duration, heart rate, and chest pain are important factors.

Recently, in patients able to walk, low-level exercise with pharmacologic stress has become the preferred approach to vasodilator stress, reducing the side effects of the drug and improving image quality due to decreased hepatic uptake of radioactivity following stress injection.

All of the agents act by inducing arteriolar dilation and increase blood flow within the normal vasculature. For patients, in particular those who are collateral dependent, coronary steal—a shifting of blood toward areas of normal arterial dilation from arteries with impaired flow reserve—will result in inducible ischemia. Additionally, increased myocardial oxygen demand results from reflex tachycardia and vasodilator-induced regional dysfunction in chronic CAD. Because the increase in demand is slight with vasodilator stress and the coronary steal physiology occurs most often with a high-grade stenosis, for patients with angiographically insignificant CAD, the most common response to pharmacologic stress is flow heterogeneity without a wall-motion abnormality. Both adenosine and dipyridamole precipitate bronchoconstriction and should be avoided in patients with severe lung disease. Patients with severe obstructive lung disease should be referred for dobutamine SPECT or echocardiographic imaging, and there is a growing body of evidence as to the accuracy of using this pharmacologic stress agent in varying patient populations. However, the new α_{2a} agonist, regadenoson, is cardiac specific with lower rates of peripheral side effects as well as a lack of bronchoconstriction and may be helpful in lung disease patients.

Dobutamine is employed as an inotropic stress agent for echocardiographic imaging. Graded infusions of dobutamine elicit incremental increases in heart rate, similar to exercise testing. The goal of dobutamine stress is similarly to achieve maximal (i.e., $\geq 85\%$ predicted maximal heart rate [220 – patient age]). Atropine may be given in order to augment heart rate and contractility responses during the latter stages of an infusion protocol. Ventricular arrhythmias (i.e., frequent premature ventricular contractions) are common during dobutamine infusion but rarely require treatment. The frequency of serious side-effects (3/1,000) is somewhat greater than in other groups that undergo coronary vasodilator stress because of an inability to undergo exercise.

STATE-OF-THE-ART CARDIAC IMAGING

【 】 STRESS ECHOCARDIOGRAPHY

Basics of Interpretation

Stress echocardiography is based on the premise that the function of ischemic segments is less than normal segments. This has important implications that limit sensitivity (the myocardium must be sufficiently malperfused to be dysfunctional) as well as optimize specificity (few conditions other than ischemia cause stress-induced wall-motion abnormalities). Echocardiographic imaging is performed in conjunction with exercise or pharmacologic stress, most commonly in the United States, with incremental dosing of dobutamine. Multiple views are obtained at rest and immediately poststress. Traditional views include the long axis, short axis, and 2- and 4-chamber views (Fig. 4-4). For ease of comparing and evaluating changes in regional wall motion, rest and stress images are viewed in a side-by-side continuous loop format. A normal stress echocardiogram results in a decrease in left ventricular cavity size and in regional myocardial segments becoming hyperdynamic as a response to stress. Thus, a normal stress echocardiogram would include normal resting ventricular function without wall motion abnormalities associated with a hyperkinetic peak/poststress regional function.

Reduction in either the amplitude or speed of thickening denotes an abnormal echocardiogram. That is, for patients without a prior CAD diagnosis, an ischemic test is defined as a new or worsening wall-motion abnormality or delayed contraction. Regional wall motion and function is generally classified as normal, hypokinetic, akinetic, or dyskinetic. Most laboratories also employ some qualitative or semi-quantitative estimate of global left ventricular function (i.e., normal, mildly depressed, moderately depressed, or severely depressed). Although abnormal regional function is often described as "wall-motion abnormality," in fact wall thickening is the more reliable parameter, where motion is subject to translational movement. A segment is considered abnormal if a wall-motion abnormality is viewed in more than one echocardiogram view, apart from the basal inferior and septal segments, which are frequent sites of false-positive interpretations and should therefore be identified as abnormal only in the presence of an abnormality in an adjacent segment.

Resting regional-wall motion abnormalities indicate a prior myocardial infarction— these are relatively specific if the segment is thinned and akinetic, although hypokinesis is less specific; for example, cardiomyopathies may show hypokinesis with some regional variation. Moreover, in the setting of resting wall-motion abnormalities, discerning stress-induced changes becomes more difficult, unless the segment also shows viability

A

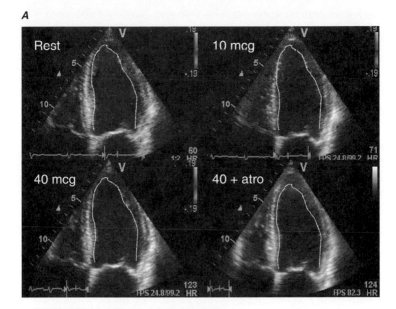

B

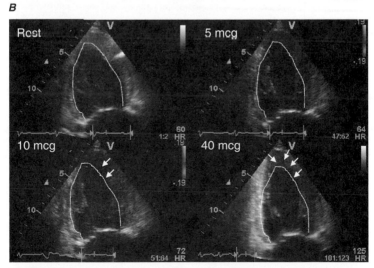

FIGURE 4-4. Appearance of a normal (**A**) and abnormal (**B**) response to dobutamine echocardiography. The display demonstrates end-systolic freeze-frames at rest (*upper left*), low-dose (*upper right*), prepeak (*lower left*), and peak stress (*lower right*). The resting end-systolic contour has been superimposed on subsequent images, showing no change in systolic cavity size in the normal study, but showing reduction of apical and anterior wall thickening (and hence shape change) in the abnormal study.

(i.e., augmentation) during low-dose dobutamine stress. In segments with resting wall-motion abnormalities, ischemia is defined as (1) deterioration from hypokinesis to akinesis or dyskinesis or (2) a biphasic response (i.e., improvement and then deterioration, even if the final level is not worse than the starting level).

Based upon the extent and severity of inducible wall-motion abnormalities or even left ventricular dilation (seen in multivessel disease), the clinician can estimate the site and extent of obstructive CAD. A 17-segment myocardial model has recently been used for interpreting the extent (number of vascular territories or segments with abnormalities) and severity (ranking of wall-motion abnormalities from normal, hypokinetic, akinetic, to dyskinetic) of ischemia, paralleling the approach taken in nuclear cardiology. Scores are then summed as the severity of hypocontractility in each of the 17 myocardial segments. An increase of such composite scores may reflect either deterioration in regional function or an increase in the number of involved segments. These scores may be integrated with clinical and stress data to produce a composite score analogous to the Duke Treadmill Score.

Intravenous Contrast Enhancement

A number of intravenous contrast agents are commercially available and approved for left ventricular opacification and endocardial border delineation in patients with initially suboptimal acoustic window, specifically those with lung disease or obese patients. These contrast agents are encapsulated gas-filled microbubbles that are generally administered as a constant infusion. For the less experienced echocardiographers and sonographers, contrast enhancement may allow for a more prompt visualization of regional function in the poststress evaluation. In patients with limited image quality, contrast enhancement has been shown to improve differentiation of low-risk and high-risk patient subsets.

Another application for contrast agents, currently under development, is the evaluation of myocardial perfusion. To evaluate myocardial perfusion, microbubbles are applied as intravascular tracers for imaging the microcirculation. Measurement of acoustic intensity of the myocardium (following background subtraction and normalized to the left ventricular cavity) provides a measure of myocardial blood volume. There are two methods of myocardial contrast echocardiogram, using either high-power ultrasound (which bursts the bubbles) and intermittent imaging at various intervals to allow them to reaccumulate; or low-power ultrasound (which permits continuous imaging as bubble destruction is minimized) together with high-power flashes to permit the same destruction-replenishment approach. The rate of replenishment of bubbles is a measure of myocardial blood flow. Although myocardial contrast echocardiography has had a long period of promising preliminary data, a number of clinical trials are being reported, with some showing incremental results with stress echocardiography alone. Moreover, myocardial contrast perfusion may provide completely new information such as the detection of subendocardial ischemia.

Although ultrasound contrast agents were proven to be efficacious by multiple studies that have established their utility in improving accuracy of stress echocardiography for the diagnosis of obstructive CAD, recently a concern was raised regarding their safety leading to contraindicating perflutren-containing ultrasound contrast agent usage in patients with acute coronary syndromes.

Current Evidence on Stress Echocardiography

DIAGNOSTIC ACCURACY   Echocardiographic visualization of left ventricular performance during stress results in dramatic improvements in diagnostic accuracy when compared with the evaluation of ST-segment changes alone. The diagnostic sensitivity and specificity for exercise echocardiography are 83% and 84%, respectively, a rate that is approximately 20% greater than for the ECG alone (see Table 4-3). In a recent head-to-head comparison, the improved diagnostic characteristics of stress echocardiography resulted in incremental cost-effectiveness when compared with exercise treadmill testing alone.

RISK STRATIFICATION   Similar to the evidence base on risk stratification with SPECT imaging, there is a developing knowledge base on the prognostic value of stress echocardiography. Using large prognostic series, a summary relative risk ratio for stress echocardiography is plotted in Fig. 4-3. This summary includes 32,739 patients undergoing stress echocardiography. For stress echocardiography, several large outcome data registries, including the Echo Persantine International Cooperative (EPIC) study and American Society of Echocardiography (ASE) outcome registries, with 7,333 and 11,132 patients, respectively, have recently been published. Annualized rates of cardiac death or myocardial infarction were, on average, 0.5% to 2.6% for low-risk (i.e., no inducible or worsening wall-motion abnormalities) to high-risk (i.e., > 1 inducible wall-motion abnormality) exercise and from 1.7% to 4.8%, respectively, for dobutamine stress echocardiography (Fig. 4-3). In addition, the prognostic value of stress echocardiography has been established in key patient subsets. For example, in women with a normal stress echocardiogram, the annual risk of death or nonfatal myocardial infarction was 0.5% ($n = 5,971$), and increased to 5.8% ($n = 1,425$) for those with a moderate to severely abnormal study.

There are several important messages that may be gleaned from Fig. 4-3. First, it appears that as we unfold evidence for commonly applied cardiac imaging modalities, the modalities appear similar with regard to prognostication. Stress echocardiography is a newer technique, and the prognostic data have only been published within the last decade. Additionally, risk stratification is a rather rudimentary method of separating subsets of the population and may be less influenced by technique differences than is thought by most clinicians. That is, low-risk studies, given an adequate stress, are generally associated with a low rate of major adverse cardiac events. An intermediate-risk stable chest pain patient has a pretest estimated annual rate of cardiac death or nonfatal myocardial infarction of 1% to 3%. Thus, if we risk-stratify from our exercise echocardiogram, we would hope to shift our patients with a negative study to a lower risk cohort with < 1% risk. As noted, the annual risk of death or myocardial infarction is approximately 0.5% for patients with a negative exercise echocardiogram.

Similar to SPECT imaging, patients undergoing pharmacologic stress echocardiography have a greater comorbidity burden and cardiovascular disease burden, which is associated with a higher rate of events, even in the setting of a normal dobutamine stress study. However, for those undergoing dobutamine stress echocardiography, all event rates are shifted higher, with effective risk stratification remaining possible in this higher-risk patient subset. That is, the event rate of a low-risk study is approximately 1.5%, which is decidedly lower than average risk in this population (~2–3%) and dramatically lower than the 5% annual risk of events in those with high-risk echocardiography results. The prevalence and associated risk of a high-risk stress echocardiogram—notably evidence of depressed left ventricular function, multiple vascular territories, or extensive areas of inducible ischemia—is increased in patients referred to pharmacologic stress testing.

Thus, the "general tenet" of risk stratification with stable chest pain populations is that low risk is < 1%, intermediate risk is approximately 3%, and high risk is approximately 5% annual risk of cardiac death or myocardial infarction, with single and multivessel CAD being more prevalent in the latter two cohorts of patients. These latter points make clear the notion that clinicians should understand the risk associated with low-risk and high-risk studies as well as the pretest population risk for a given subset of patients.

Candidates for Cardiac Catheterization

For diagnostic patient subsets, in the setting of an inducible wall-motion abnormality, anti-ischemic therapies and risk-factor modification would be initiated and consideration would also be given to coronary angiography. Of course, referral to coronary angiography is dependent on the symptom status, treatment response, comorbidities, and risk—the latter being determined in part by the extent and severity of the inducible wall-motion abnormalities. Clinicians may prefer to treat patients medically with discrete small areas of ischemia and not refer patients who are not good revascularization candidates (e.g., very elderly patients with serious comorbidity). Angiography is advised in patients with evidence of a high-risk study (Table 4-4), including those with global left ventricular dysfunction with stress or multiple vascular territories (i.e., evidence of multivessel disease) or extensive wall-motion abnormalities across the anterior myocardium (reflecting proximal LAD disease). Abnormalities in the left anterior descending coronary artery distribution had a higher event rate than patients with abnormalities elsewhere (3.2% versus 2.1% at 3 years and 10.8% versus 2.1% at 5 years; $p = 0.009$); this risk is independent of the resting ejection fraction and the extent of wall-motion abnormalities during exercise.

Several reports have noted that stress echocardiography, with only a modest increase in cost when compared to exercise ECG testing, can result in cost-effective testing as a result of improved visualization and detection of CAD. In a comprehensive evaluation of the cost effectiveness of exercise echocardiography versus ECG testing in 7,656 patients, echocardiographic imaging identified more patients as low (51% versus 24%, $p < 0.0001$) and high (22% versus 4%, $p < 0.0001$) risk. Although initial procedural cost was higher, echocardiography was associated with a greater incremental life expectancy (0.2 years) and a lower use of additional diagnostic procedures when compared with exercise ECG. Based on this analysis, echocardiography was more cost-effective than exercise ECG testing at $2,615 per life-year saved (substantially less than the efficiency threshold of <$50,000 per life-year saved).

【 】 STRESS-GATED NUCLEAR (SPECT/PET) IMAGING

Today, state-of-the-art multidetector single photon emission computed tomography (SPECT) systems allow for acquisition of rest and stress ejection fraction and regional wall motion as well as assessment of regional myocardial perfusion. Nuclear cardiology is the *most commonly performed imaging modality* for the assessment of patients with known or suspected CAD, because multiple risk markers can be measured. In contrast to two-dimensional echocardiography, SPECT and positron emission tomography (PET) provide true tomographic imaging, where all segments of the myocardium are visualized. Today, nuclear cardiology is employed in over 7 million patients annually in the United States, with annual growth rates exceeding 20%. Decades of experience and growth in the field have led to a vast array of clinical research experiences and fostered the development of large observational registries across the United States; these efforts have been successful in defining not only the diagnostic accuracy of SPECT imaging but also its prognostic value in patient cohorts exceeding 5,000 (i.e., sufficiently powered patient samples).

Basics of Interpretation

To interpret rest and stress myocardial perfusion, qualitative interpretation methods have largely been augmented by semiquantitative or quantitative methods that document the extent and severity of reversible and fixed perfusion abnormalities. Most commonly, a 17- or 20-segment myocardial model is employed that utilizes visual estimates of segmental perfusion defect severity (normal to absent perfusion on a 5-point scale within each myocardial segment; Fig. 4-5). For the rest and stress images, summing individual myocardial segment severity scores derives a global perfusion score. This semiquantitative method has been extensively evaluated and correlates well with prognosis. Extrapolation of this interpretative method to percentage of fixed or reversible myocardium is also possible, which is achieved by normalizing the score to the highest possible score, thus providing a measurement that has clinically intuitive implications and can be used for scoring systems with any number of segments. Current state-of-the-art

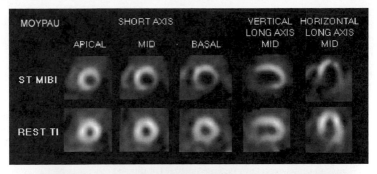

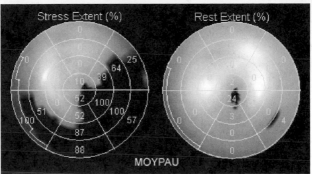

FIGURE 4-5. An example of myocardial perfusion SPECT (54-year-old male, asymptomatic, 9 minutes of exercise, ischemic ECG, reversible defect, TID 1.52, cath: LM 70%, LAD 80% prox, LCX 100% prox, RCA 100% mid).

gated SPECT imaging also includes quantitative left ventricular ejection fraction at rest and postexercise in addition to the perfusion defect analysis that serves as a backup for visual interpretation. Automated quantitative assessments of left ventricular ejection fraction and volumes at rest and postexercise are provided. Segmental wall-motion and left-ventricular volumes may also be derived and add to the prognostic information already available with SPECT imaging. The gated ventricular function parameters have also been shown to add prognostically over and above perfusion defect extent and severity. Beyond measurements of myocardial perfusion and function, indirect assessment are also made of transient ischemic dilation (TID) of the left ventricle (enlargement on the post-stress images when compared to the resting scan), a marker of severe and extensive ischemia; and increased lung uptake, a marker of increased pulmonary capillary wedge pressure. TID and increased lung uptake (considerable appearance of tracer uptake in the lung fields following stress that is absent at rest) provide valuable and added prognostic information.

Current Evidence on Gated SPECT Imaging

DIAGNOSTIC ACCURACY   A synopsis of this evidence on diagnostic accuracy is given in Table 4-3 revealing sensitivity measurements that are far superior to the exercise ECG alone. For exercise SPECT, the sensitivity and specificity from 22 reports in 2,360 patients were 87% and 73%, respectively, similar for both Tl 201 and Tc 99m agents.

For adenosine SPECT ($n = 3,539$), the diagnostic sensitivity was 89% and the specificity was 77%. It appears from numerous reviews that SPECT imaging is a highly sensitive test for the detection of a hemodynamically significant stenosis. Myocardial perfusion SPECT may also be abnormal in regions that do not appear to be hemodynamically significant if there is associated paradoxical vasoconstriction with stress that occurs with endothelial dysfunction. The principal factor affecting the specificity of myocardial perfusion SPECT, however, is soft-tissue attenuation (i.e., breast tissue artifacts in women and diaphragmatic attenuation in men) that occurs with somewhat lower frequency with the use of the higher-energy Tc-99m agents. For the clinician, however, it is critical to understand that when using stenosis thresholds of 50% to 75%, physiologically and prognostically important reduced perfusion may be noted below these cut points. Accordingly, some studies considered false positive are actually true perfusion defects. Traditionally, specificity, as a measure of diagnostic test performance, fails to consider the long-term consequences of a perfusion defect. For this and other reasons noted previously (e.g., workup bias), accuracy in estimating risk is considered by many as more critical in guiding management than diagnostic accuracy.

RISK STRATIFICATION

This latter point underscores the importance to the clinician concerning the role of gated SPECT in evaluating patient outcome and changing patient management. Much of our discussions on risk-assessment thresholds with stress echocardiography also apply to SPECT imaging. A recent meta-analysis of 19 reports in 39,173 patients notes that those with a normal or low-risk (e.g., summed stress score < 4) myocardial perfusion study had an annual cardiac event rate of 0.6% (25th to 75th percentiles = 0.5% to 0.9%). This includes evidence for all three isotopes commonly used in clinical practice today. In a multicenter registry of 10,408 patients, cardiac death rates were similar for a normal Tl-201 and Tc-99 sestamibi or tetrofosmin SPECT. Additionally, for patients with normal perfusion findings, measures of left ventricular size, function, and dilation following stress should also be integrated into the scan's interpretation and provide supplemental risk information. For example, TID with exercise or pharmacologic stress is associated with an increased risk of cardiac events, even in the setting of a normal perfusion scan.

This excellent survival in patients with normal stress SPECT findings reveals the value of evaluating the physiology of the patient's disease as supplemental information. Slightly higher event rates would be expected in patients referred to pharmacologic stress imaging, the elderly, diabetics, those with vascular disease, or other subsets of the population with greater comorbidity burdens. In these latter cohorts, the major adverse cardiac event rates would range from 1.5% to 2% per year; similar to the death or myocardial infarction rates with a negative dobutamine stress echocardiogram study. Due to this higher annual cardiac event rate, for patients with CAD or its risk equivalent (e.g., diabetics or those referred to pharmacologic stress imaging), a closer posttest evaluation may be warranted and consideration of reimaging sooner (about 1.5 years) than in lower-risk patients with normal stress scans. With any of the stress modalities, a normal stress study implies a low risk over a relatively short term (1 to 2 years) but does not imply the absence of risk for CAD progression over a longer time period.

An abnormal study is determined by the presence of perfusion defects, either fixed or reversible. When combined into summed stress scores (from the 17-segment models), higher-risk subsets may be defined as mildly abnormal (summed stress score 4 to 8), moderately abnormal (summed stress score 9 to 13), or severely abnormal (summed stress score >13). When considered as a percentage of the myocardium, from a prognostic standpoint, patients who seem to have minimal perfusion defects but > 5% of the myocardium involved are generally grouped as being normal, and those with 5% to 9% as having a mild perfusion abnormality. A cutoff of $\geq 10\%$ of the myocardium ischemic has been shown to be an important prognostic factor for providing information regarding the likelihood of benefit from revascularization. Of those in this latter subset with a moderate to severely abnormal study, there is a greater prevalence of more extensive, multivessel CAD or proximal LAD disease. In addition to the application of semiquantitative scores, a high-risk study may be defined as patients with (1) severe exercise left ventricular dysfunction (exercise LVEF < 35%), (2) stress-induced large perfusion defect (particularly if anterior), (3) stress-induced multiple perfusion defects of moderate size, (4) large, fixed perfusion defect with LV dilation or increased lung uptake, or (5) stress-induced moderate perfusion defect with LV dilation or increased lung uptake (Table 4-4). The annual rate of cardiac death or nonfatal myocardial infarction for those with high-risk perfusion findings was 5.9% (25th percentile = 4.6%, 75th percentile = 8.5%). These results are consistent with patients with angiographically severe CAD whose annualized event rates are approximately 5% per year. Those with high-risk SPECT results, diabetic patients, and those referred to pharmacologic stress have even higher event rates than other cohorts.

In addition to the estimation of risk based on an initial study, a recent report from the Clinical Outcomes Using Revascularization and Aggressive Drug Evaluation (COURAGE) trial has provided information on the prognostic value of serial changes in stress myocardial perfusion SPECT. Specifically, for CAD patients, a failure to reduce ischemia by a minimum of 5% of the myocardium or residual ischemia following 1 year of intercurrent treatment is associated with a high rate of death or nonfatal myocardial infarction.

Prognostication using perfusion defect assessment combined with measure of left ventricular function from gated SPECT has been extensively validated. As with data derived using angiographic or echocardiographic imaging, there is an inverse relationship between left ventricular ejection fraction and cardiac event rates, such that higher major adverse cardiac event rates are associated with lower ejection fraction measurements. Annualized event rates range from < 1% to > 5% for those with ejection fraction values ranging from 60% to ≤ 20%. There is a "thresholding" of risk with a clear acceleration in event rates, for any given degree of perfusion defect abnormality, for patients with ejection fraction measurements ≤ 45%.

From a recent report, end-systolic volume measurements > 70 mL were also associated with worsening event-free survival. Greater end-diastolic volume measures reflect left ventricular remodeling and are important guides for further delineation of risk.

Candidates for Cardiac Catheterization

A synthesis of available evidence notes that high-risk perfusion results (e.g., moderate to severely abnormal perfusion abnormalities, multivessel perfusion abnormalities, ≥ 10% myocardial perfusion defect, or a summed stress score > 8 for the 20-segment model) are associated with an expected rate of major adverse cardiac events ranging from 3% to 5% or more. This subset of patients has a greater prevalence of single to multivessel CAD and should be considered for referral to cardiac catheterization in addition to aggressive risk-factor modification and anti-ischemic therapy. Additionally, patients with a high-risk post-stress left ventricular ejection fraction < 45% are at an elevated risk of cardiac events. Other high-risk markers include TID, larger ventricular volumes, and increased lung uptake. Patients with mild defects have benign outcomes and may be effectively managed medically. With either stress myocardial perfusion SPECT or echocardiography, the decision to proceed with coronary angiography is complex and involves many clinical observations as well as imaging data. Factors associated with increased risk for any degree of scan abnormality include a brief duration of exercise, a high Duke Treadmill Score, an abnormal heart rate recovery, an abnormal peak/rest heart rate with adenosine stress, comorbidity (e.g., diabetes), symptoms, and exertional hypotension. Recently, Hachamovitch and associates devised a prognostic score to integrate the clinical stress test and scan information.

When strategies are employed that guide a selective use of coronary angiography based upon the extent and severity of SPECT abnormalities, substantial cost savings and a cost-effective testing pattern may ensue. In several large series, referral to angiography that was limited to patients with moderate to severely abnormal scans resulted in a reduction in evaluation costs of approximately 35%.

Moreover, for the patient with angiographic CAD, referral to coronary angiography is also indicated for those with persistent or worsening myocardial perfusion SPECT ischemia despite intensive medical management that may include prior percutaneous coronary intervention.

【 】 PET STRESS MYOCARDIAL PERFUSION

Cardiac PET imaging is a well-validated technique to assess myocardial perfusion, LV function, and viability. With more than 1,000 installed PET and PET/CT cameras in North America, clinical cardiac PET imaging is experiencing rapid expansion. In addition to the well-recognized fluorine 18 fluorodeoxyglucose (FDG) viability studies, PET stress myocardial perfusion imaging with rubidium 82 can be performed with a commercially available Rb-82 generator, obviating the need for a cyclotron. PET stress myocardial perfusion imaging utilizes radionuclide tracers (rubidium 82 and to lesser extent N-13 ammonia) which decay with the emission of a positron. The positron interacts with an electron to combined mass that is converted into the energy of two 511-keV photons traveling in opposite directions and detected by a PET camera. The new generation of high-performance dedicated PET cameras features high instrument sensitivity (about 10 to 20 times higher than SPECT), high resolution (4 to 5 mm versus 20 to 25 mm for SPECT), high speed, and larger fields of view. These technical advantages have translated to better diagnostic accuracy, thus placing PET stress myocardial perfusion as, in some cases, a superior substitute to stress SPECT. PET stress myocardial perfusion also holds the potential to assess regional myocardial blood flow, thus extending the scope of conventional scintigraphic imaging by providing insight to the subtler details of the epicardial as well myocardial coronary circulation.

With the increased clinical use of PET stress myocardial perfusion imaging, data documenting its incremental prognostic value are beginning to emerge showing that increases in the extent and severity of stress perfusion defects as well as the degree of left ventricular dysfunction are translated into proportional increases in predicted mortality.

【 】 CURRENT EVIDENCE ON CARDIOVASCULAR MAGNETIC RESONANCE IMAGING

The consistent improvement in CMR hardware and software as well as the development of innovative CMR-oriented sequences has evolved in production of CMR systems that provide high spatial resolution static images as well as high temporal and spatial resolution dynamic images. Currently, 1.5 T CMR scanners applying rapid-gradient systems enable acquisition of cine imaging of the heart at rest and under stress, allowing comparison of global as well as segmental heart function. Furthermore, assessment of a contrast agent first-pass perfusion dynamics (usually gadolinium) injected at rest and stress can provide high-quality information about the pattern of myocardial perfusion.

Because exercise is not a practical option in the scanner bore and patient movement may severely affect image quality, pharmacologic stress agents (such as adenosine) have mainly been used to elicit stress. Dobutamine is rarely used due to its unfavorable side effects profile, especially in the limited monitoring surrounding of the MR scanner.

Stress perfusion CMR studies have the capability to provide comprehensive and complementary information, that is, rest and stress cardiac function and wall motion as well as myocardial perfusion using nonionizing radiation technology that has better resolution and is attenuation freeing comparison to SPECT. Delayed enhancement images may give additional information about the presence, extent, and pattern of myocardial fibrosis.

A recent meta-analysis of 37 studies (2,191 patients) with 14 datasets (754 patients) using stress-induced wall-motion abnormality imaging and 24 datasets (1,516 patients) using perfusion imaging showed that stress-induced wall-motion abnormality imaging demonstrated a sensitivity of 83% and specificity of 86%, and perfusion imaging demonstrated a sensitivity of 91% and specificity of 81%. Moreover, in another recent a multicenter, multivendor trial that studied the diagnostic performance for stress perfusion CMR in comparison with coronary x-ray angiography and SPECT, stress perfusion CMR demonstrated equivalent and, in some cases, better diagnostic performance than SPECT.

Yet, stress perfusion CMR has several substantial downsides. It is costly, time-consuming study, highly dependent on operator and patient cooperation, and demands an experienced team and cutting-edge hardware. Also, because exercise stress is not an option, information about functional capacity and electrocardiographic and physiologic response to exercise is virtually always compromised.

CONCLUSION

We began this chapter focusing on the appropriate selection of patients based upon a global risk assessment or pretest probability of CAD. An understanding of risk assessment and a rudimentary knowledge of Bayesian theory form the basis for appropriate test selection. Of those patients presenting with symptoms suggestive of myocardial ischemia, those most appropriately referred to noninvasive stress testing include stable patients who are an intermediate pretest risk. A second tier of decision-making queries the value of an imaging or nonimaging ECG study. Current guidelines support an initial strategy using the exercise ECG alone in patients capable of performing ≥ 5 METs of work and with a normal resting ECG. Patients with an abnormal 12-lead ECG, those with established CAD, or those functionally impaired should be referred to cardiac imaging including the choice of: stress echocardiography, SPECT, or CMR techniques. Recent data from the Mayo Clinic and Cedars-Sinai Medical Center have expanded this to also include patients with a high likelihood of CAD who would benefit by direct referral to an imaging study.

As this review describes, the prognostic value of stress echocardiography and SPECT imaging is fairly comparable, and as such, test choice may be driven by local expertise. However, harkening back to our discussion of the ischemic cascade, one must also review each patient's differential diagnosis and allow test choice to be guided by those considerations. If one considers the need to document a more precise delineation of changes in myocardial blood flow that may be prompted by an underlying physiologically significant stenosis, endothelial dysfunction, or microvascular disease, then some measure of stress-induced myocardial perfusion may be in order. However, provocation of a wall-motion abnormality is also a very sensitive and specific tool for detecting an obstructive coronary lesion.

A clear paradigm shift in noninvasive testing research has been the development of risk-stratification evidence. An obvious benefit of estimating risk is that it can be coordinated with larger evidence on population-based risk as well as randomized clinical trial data to guide optimal decision-making and therapeutic interventions. Thus, our discussion of understanding risk thresholds can be essential to effectively guiding the intensity of posttest management. Furthermore, the value of any noninvasive stress test and the expected event rates is guided by the underlying hazard in the population. This fact was illustrated in the higher event rates, in the setting of normal stress test results, for patients with diabetes, established CAD, or those referred to pharmacologic stress testing. Thus, although we would expect a negative or low-risk scan to be associated with < 1% annual risk of cardiac death or nonfatal myocardial infarction, slightly higher rates would be noted in these CAD or risk equivalent populations. Similarly, one can also expect that in these higher-risk patients, with more prevalent severe CAD, a moderate to severely abnormal scan is associated with the highest rate of events at or above 5% annually. If these patients are not revascularized, it would appear appropriate to retest them following aggressive anti-ischemic and risk-modifying strategies have been initiated for assessment of the degree of residual risk.

High-risk stress results, for intermediate-risk patients, have been revealed through decades of clinical research to be associated with a high prevalence of obstructive CAD and, thus, referral to coronary angiography should be discussed and considered as part of the patient's health care plan. However, tests are not perfect, and despite all our recent improvements, problems with technical artifact and other challenges remain (e.g., soft-tissue attenuation in SPECT, poor acoustic windows in echocardiography, and false-negative or false-positive exercise ECG studies in patients taking vasoactive drugs or in premenopausal women). Thus, consideration should be given to initially excluding technical challenges as the reason for any given abnormality or lack of positivity noted. Certain patient subsets that have a higher rate of artifact or suboptimal testing include women, obese patients, those with lung disease, patients with resting ECG abnormalities or onboard medications that interfere with provocation of stress-induced ischemia, and especially, those with functional limitations who cannot provoke a central myocardial stress. Careful consideration to the challenges of testing will improve posttest decision-making and result in a more selective use of coronary angiography in appropriately diseased patients. Although this chapter covers a wide array of imaging and nonimaging tests for provoking myocardial ischemia, the reader may desire a more substantial and detailed review of the subject that is available in the larger version of *Hurst's The Heart* as well as in our suggested readings.

SUGGESTED READING

Berman DS, Hachamovitch R, Shaw LJ, et al. Nuclear cardiology. In: *Hurst's The Heart*. 11th ed. New York, NY: McGraw-Hill; 2004:563–598.

Fraker TD, Gardin JM, O'Rourke RA, et al. ACC/AHA 2002 Guideline update for the management of patients with chronic stable angina. *J Am Coll Cardiol*. 2003;41: 159–168.

Gibbons RJ, Balady, GJ, Bricker JT, et al. ACC/AHA 2002 Guideline update for exercise testing—summary article. *J Am Coll Cardiol*. 2002;106:1883–1892.

Jouven. Heart-rate profile during exercise as a predictor of sudden death. *N Engl J Med*. 2005;352:1951–1958.

Marwick TH. *Stress Echocardiography*. Boston, MA: Kluewer Academic Publishers; 1994.

Mieres JH, Shaw LJ, Arai A, et al. Diagnostic performance of stress cardiac magnetic resonance imaging in the detection of coronary artery disease: a meta-analysis. *J Am Coll Cardiol*. 2007;50:1343–1353.

O'Rourke RA, Dada M, Spertus JA, et al. Optimal medical therapy with or without percutaneous coronary intervention to reduce ischemic burden: results from the COURAGE trial nuclear substudy. *Circulation*. Feb 11 (epub).

Pennell DJ, Sechtem UP, Higgins CB, et al. Clinical indications for cardiovascular magnetic resonance: consensus panel report. *J Cardiovasc Mag Res*. 2004;6:727–765.

Redberg RF, Taubert K, Thomas G, et al. American Heart Association, Cardiac Imaging Committee consensus statement: the role of cardiac imaging in the clinical evaluation of women with known or suspected coronary artery disease. *Circulation*. 2005;111:682–696.

Shaw LJ, Berman DS, Maron DJ, et al. Prognostic value of gated myocardial perfusion SPECT. *J Nucl Cardiol*. 2004;11:171–185.

CHAPTER (5)

Noninvasive Testing for Cardiac Dysfunction

Jon C. George and Brian D. Hoit

Accurate, noninvasive assessment of global and regional left ventricular (LV) function is critical in managing most types of heart disease. The most common clinically useful parameter is the left ventricular ejection fraction (LVEF), which is the LV stroke volume normalized by LV end-diastolic volume. EF is most often *estimated* echocardiographically, but radionuclide angiography (RNA), computed tomography (CT), single photon emission computed tomography (SPECT), positron emission tomography (PET), and cardiac magnetic resonance imaging (CMR) may be employed. Whereas EF measures ventricular chamber properties, tissue velocity and strain—characterized most notably by echocardiography and CMR—measure myocardial contractility. LV diastolic function is also a clinically relevant parameter of function, which encompasses various measures of diastolic filling, myocardial relaxation, and ventricular stiffness, which are assessed by echocardiography, RNA, and CMR. In addition, various CT techniques (electron beam CT, multidetector CT) allow noninvasive coronary atherosclerosis risk stratification, complimentary to the traditional methods of echocardiographic and nuclear stress testing. This chapter discusses the various imaging modalities available for noninvasive assessment of cardiac function.

ECHOCARDIOGRAPHY

Echocardiography remains the most popular cardiac imaging modality because of its efficacy, relatively low cost, portability, versatility, and widespread availability without compromise of spatial and temporal resolution. However, limitations include the need for adequate acoustic windows, operator dependence, use of geometric assumptions in computing volumes, and inter-reader variability.

Myocardial function may be quantified using a variety of echocardiographic techniques. The M-mode (Fig. 5-1A) can be used to measure myocardial shortening and radial thickening with excellent temporal resolution, but can be used in only a limited number of myocardial segments, since the ultrasound beam has to be perpendicular to the segments being assessed. Anatomical M-mode has partly overcome this problem by allowing an operator-defined insonation angle (at the expense of a reduced temporal resolution); however, it still provides a one-dimensional view that is spatially limited and fails to provide information regarding longitudinal or circumferential function. Although M-mode echocardiography can be used to assess LV morphology, the technique is optimally suited only for ventricles with uniform geometry and wall motion. Two-dimensional echocardiography (2DE) overcomes these limitations and quantifies accurately global and regional ventricular functions (Fig. 5-1B). However, errors due to off-axis imaging, reduced interobserver variability and reproducibility, and the subjectivity inherent in mental reconstruction of tomographic 2DE images are problematic.

59

A

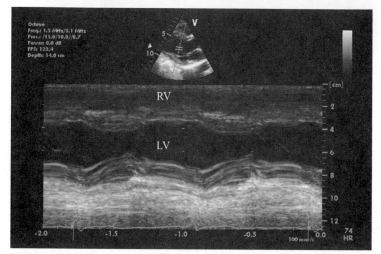

B

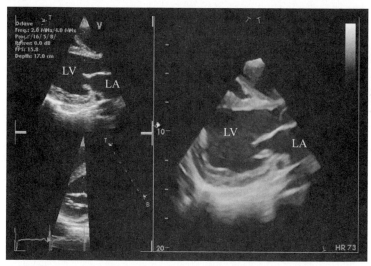

FIGURE 5-1. Left ventricular imaging by M-mode (**A**), 2D-echocardiography (**B**, *left*), and 3D-echocardiography (**B**, *right*). Annotations represent left ventricle (LV), left atrium (LA), and right ventricle (RV).

【 】 THREE-DIMENSIONAL ECHOCARDIOGRAPHY

Three-dimensional echocardiography (3DE) has added literally a new dimension to the evaluation of LV function and addresses these limitations. Although early 3DE approaches were cumbersome—involving prolonged and tedious data acquisition, time-consuming digitization, spatiotemporal registration of images, and volume rendering—advances in transducer technology, software, and computing power have made possible rapid acquisition of data from multiple, simultaneous lines of sight (matrix imaging). In this fashion, a volume of ultrasound data is reconstructed in near real time from a pyramidal ultrasound beam, providing a more accurate quantification of global and regional cardiac functions (Fig. 5-1B). To display the entire LV, a series of component volumes of the heart are acquired over 4 to 7 consecutive cardiac cycles and combined (or "stitched" together), making respiration and movement artifact a limitation in such full-volume acquisitions.

Noninvasive assessment of regional myocardial function plays a critical role in the management of ischemic heart disease. Although the echocardiographic evaluation of regional myocardial function relies largely on the visual detection of endocardial wall-motion abnormalities, this technique is subjective and demands complete visualization of the endocardium. Tissue (myocardial) velocities during systole and diastole are used to quantify ventricular function, but *measurement of strain and strain rate* (using Doppler-derived strain imaging or speckle-tracking echocardiography) *offers two important advantages*. First, within a myocardial segment, strain and strain rate (the magnitude and rate of tissue deformation, respectively), unlike tissue velocity, are less affected by translational (whole heart) movement and unaffected by "tethering" of adjacent segments; thus strain, unlike tissue Doppler, discriminates akinetic segments that are pulled (or tethered) from actively contracting segments. Second, strain and strain rate tend to be uniformly distributed across the myocardium, whereas tissue velocities tend to decrease from base to apex, making the establishment of reference values more difficult. These observations make strain and strain rate particularly well suited for the assessment of regional myocardial performance. These measures may also be useful for the determination of myocardial viability.

Diastolic function can be evaluated using M-mode and 2DE by measurement of the timing and extent of LV wall motion, wall thinning rate, and the duration of early relaxation and atrial contraction. LV filling dynamics can also be assessed by 2DE using frame-by-frame measurements of LV volume in either short-axis or apical four-chamber views; however, 2DE is limited by a low sampling rate and suboptimal lateral resolution. More commonly, Doppler echocardiographic measurements are employed. Assessment of transmitral flow (LV filling), pulmonary vein flow (LA filling), and longitudinal motion of the mitral annulus during early diastole (myocardial relaxation) are used to evaluate LV diastolic function and pressure. The normal pattern of transmitral flow is biphasic consisting of early (peak E) and late (peak A) atrial filling velocities, which is expressed as the E/A ratio and is >1 in a normal individual. The variations in this pattern along with deceleration time of E velocity (DT) and isovolumic relaxation time (IVRT) are important variables of diastolic function derived from the transmitral flow waveform (Fig. 5-2).

【 】 STRESS ECHOCARDIOGRAPHY

Recognizing abnormal regional wall-motion abnormalities (hypokinesia, akinesia, dyskinesia) is essential in the evaluation of patients with coronary artery disease. Because wall motion at rest can be normal in a patient with significant coronary artery disease, echocardiographic imaging during provoked ischemia (stress echocardiography) is needed for diagnosis. In a vessel with a flow-limiting stenosis, the increased oxygen demands of the stressed myocardium cannot be met by an increase in flow, and ischemia with impairment of diastolic function, myocardial thickening, and endocardial motion results. Stress or provoked ischemia can be induced by increasing myocardial oxygen

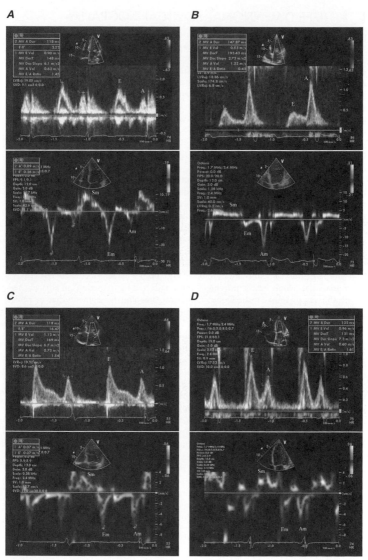

FIGURE 5-2. Diastolic function assessment by echocardiography using transmitral flow Doppler (*top*) and tissue Doppler (*bottom*). Annotations represent early diastolic flow velocity with LV relaxation (E) and late diastolic flow velocity with atrial contraction (A) for transmitral flow Doppler (*top panels*) and myocardial velocity during systole (Sm), early filling (Em), and late filling (Am) for tissue Doppler (*bottom panels*). **A** shows normal diastolic function, **B** impaired relaxation, **C** pseudonormal filling, and **D** restrictive filling, indicating a progressive impairment of LV diastolic function.

demand either with exercise or by pharmacologic interventions (Table 5-1; see also Chapter 4). In addition to the technical adequacy of the accompanying echocardiographic images and their proper interpretation, key elements in the analysis of a stress test results include duration of exercise, maximum workload (approximated by heart rate–blood pressure product), symptoms, blood pressure response, arrhythmias, and ST-segment changes on the electrocardiogram (ECG). The basic principles of image acquisition for stress echocardiography (SE) are to use standard image planes and comparable views at rest and stress, ensure that all myocardial segments are visualized, and to record images in a digital cine loop format with parallel display of rest and stress images. The cine loop format is essential, as the change in heart rate between rest and stress makes interpretation of wall motion difficult. For evaluation of regional ventricular function, optimal endocardial definition is essential, which may require careful patient positioning, use of harmonic imaging, or contrast echocardiography for opacification of the LV cavity. The sensitivity of SE for detection of coronary disease depends on acquisition of stress images at the maximal cardiac workload, which declines rapidly on cessation of exercise. 3DE acquisition systems that allow simultaneous real-time imaging in multiple image planes offer the promise of faster acquisition times at peak stress, with the potential for improved diagnostic sensitivity.

The major limitations of SE are failure to achieve an adequate workload and poor endocardial definition. In patients who cannot exercise to a maximal workload due to various conditions, pharmacologic testing can be substituted using intravenous dobutamine, which is a potent beta agonist, increasing heart rate and contractility. The infusions are started at a low dose (5 mg/kg/min) and titrated up every 3 to 5 minutes until the maximum dose (30 to 40 mg/kg/min) or a clinical end point has been reached. Atropine can be added to achieve an appropriate increase in heart rate with

TABLE 5-1

Compilation of Meta Analyses and Reviews on the Diagnostic Accuracy of Contemporary Noninvasive Stress Testing, Including Exercise ECG, SPECT, and Echocardiography as well as Pharmacologic Stress Spect, Echocardiography, and Magnetic Resonance (MR) Imaging[a]

Modality	No. Studies	No. Patients	Sensitivity (%)	Specificity (%)
Exercise ECG	58	11,691	67	72
Exercise SPECT	22	2,360	87	73
(Tc-99m agents only)			88	72
Adenosine SPECT	11	3,539	89	77
(Tc-99m agents only)			87	86
Dobutamine SPECT	20	1,419	85	79
(Tc-99m agents only)			83	76
Exercise echocardiography	13	741	83	84
Dobutamine stress echocardiography	13	436	75	83
Stress magnetic resonance:				
Dobutamine stress wall motion	10	644	84	89
Adenosine/dipyridamole perfusion	3	108	84	85

[a] The diagnostic sensitivity and specificity values presented are uncorrected for verification bias. Note that these are average values, and wide ranges exist for most modalities.

a typical goal of 85% of the maximum predicted heart rate. Reported adverse effects of dobutamine infusion include anxiety, tremulousness, palpitations, arrhythmias, paresthesias, and chest pain. Hypotension occurs rarely in patients because of peripheral β_2-receptor-mediated vasodilation or LV outflow obstruction. In patients with abnormal global or regional function at rest, SE is more difficult to interpret, decreasing its specificity for the diagnosis of coronary disease. Evaluation of areas adjacent to the resting wall-motion abnormality may be problematic due to the tethering effect by the abnormal region. Tissue velocities and strain analysis have potential in this regard. In patients with suboptimal echocardiographic windows, images can be obtained using nuclear perfusion imaging. Vasodilator stress using persantine or adenosine is used less often with echocardiography than with nuclear medicine techniques (see Chapter 4).

RADIONUCLIDE ANGIOGRAPHY

Radionuclide angiography (RNA) may be performed using equilibrium or first-pass methods; both can assess ventricular volumes, EF, and regional wall motion. With the first-pass approach, imaging is performed during the initial transit of radionuclide. Equilibrium radionuclide angiocardiography, also referred to as multiple gated acquisition (MUGA) or gated blood pool imaging, is usually regarded as the most accurate technique for measurement of LVEF. MUGA is performed by labeling the patient's red blood cell pool with a radioactive tracer and measuring radioactivity over the anterior chest with a suitably positioned gamma camera. The number of counts recorded per unit of time is proportional to the blood volume, giving a direct volumetric assessment of the cardiac chambers throughout the cardiac cycle. Blood pool labeling is routinely performed with technetium Tc 99m, which achieves high red cell labeling, has a relatively short half-life (6 hours), and has an emission photo peak (140 keV) close to the maximal sensitivity of the gamma camera crystal. Labeling can be performed in vitro by incubating a small autologous blood sample with Tc 99m or, more commonly, in vivo with the direct intravenous injection of Tc 99m pertechnetate. The in vivo labeling technique is more convenient for most patients because it involves only one venipuncture, is less time consuming, and is less costly. Although red blood cell labeling is generally more efficient with the in vitro techniques, more than 80% of the injected radionuclide usually binds to red blood cells with the in vivo approach. Shortly after injection, the labeled red blood cells equally distribute throughout the entire blood pool. Image acquisition is performed for 800 to 1,000 heartbeats for each projection, corresponding to a time period of 5 to 10 minutes. The RR interval is divided into 16 to 32 equal phases (gating windows), and counts are recorded separately for each phase. At the end of the acquisition, the counts are summed for all cardiac cycles, and images obtained for each phase are then displayed in sequence, creating a cine-loop of the entire cardiac cycle. Images are obtained in the anterior, left posterior oblique, and modified left anterior oblique projections to best visualize all cardiac chambers and provide indirect information for all left ventricular walls. The left anterior oblique projections are used for measurements of ejection fraction because the LV is free of any overlap with other cardiac chambers. Left ventricular time–volume curves are used to derive a number of indices of systolic and diastolic function.

MUGA scans are *contraindicated* in lactating and pregnant women because of the concern of ionizing radiation exposure, although quite small (620 mrem). ECG gating also becomes unreliable in patients with arrhythmias and significant variability of the RR interval, which can be corrected to an extent with modified acquisition and post-processing protocols. Obtaining the optimum projection for separation of the ventricles and defining the ventricular contours is operator dependent, and poor technique can introduce measurement errors.

COMPUTED TOMOGRAPHY

Both *multidetector* computed tomography (MDCT) and *electron beam* computed tomography (EBCT) can provide anatomic and functional data on both ventricles using various protocols specific to the information of interest, and allow precise measurement of ventricular volumes, function, regional wall motion, and mass. MDCT is *not* a first-line method of EF measurement, but may be useful if echocardiographic images are poor and CMR is contraindicated. Evaluation by CT for ischemic heart disease includes CT angiography with intravenous contrast injection for assessment of coronary atherosclerotic burden and calcium scoring without contrast enhancement for identification and quantification of calcification within the coronary arteries, which has a high predictive value for cardiac events. The data obtained during coronary CT angiography can be further used to create multiplanar reconstruction (Fig. 5-3) cine images in the LV short axis from the cardiac base to the apex to evaluate LV function and calculate EF in addition to other parameters, which is likely to provide useful additional information; when compared to CMR, MDCT is an adequate alternative for functional assessment. Moreover, with dynamic contrast administration and fast scanning capability, myocardial perfusion defects can be identified at rest in regions of myocardial infarction. CT has also been used to assess myocardial infarction location and size by using delayed contrast-enhanced methods, which are performed 5 to 10 minutes after intravenous iodinated contrast injection.

The major limitations of CT include contrast-related nephropathy and radiation dose exposure. Although the radiation dose for calcium scoring is relatively low, coronary CT angiography and functional imaging methods provide a radiation dose of 8 to 10 mSv on 16-detector and 14 to 18 mSv on 64-detector systems.

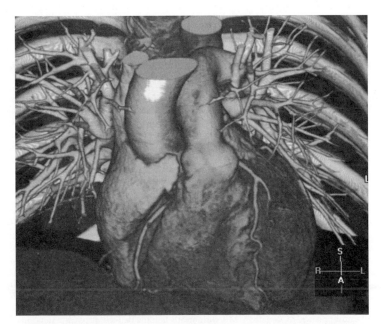

FIGURE 5-3. CT angiography with three-dimensional reconstruction of a normal heart.

SINGLE PHOTON EMISSION COMPUTED TOMOGRAPHY

Single photon emission computed tomography (SPECT) is a tomographic nuclear medicine technique in which a radionuclide is injected and its distribution through the body imaged using a gamma camera (see also Chapter 4). Two-dimensional projections from multiple angles are acquired and reconstructed using specific algorithms to yield three-dimensional images. The use of ECG-gated SPECT allows simultaneous assessment of LV wall motion and myocardial perfusion with good correlation with other imaging techniques and high reproducibility. Automated methods are used to quantify global systolic and diastolic function; regional wall motion and thickening are usually assessed by semiquantitative visual analysis. LV volumes and EF by thallium Tl 201 SPECT correlate highly with Tc 99 sestamibi SPECT, which in turn have been validated against a number of nonnuclear methods. Gated SPECT further allows the detection of coronary artery disease and myocardial viability by combining the evaluation of regional wall motion and thickening with the assessment of perfusion (Fig. 5-4). Disadvantages of SPECT include the relatively low spatial resolution compared to other techniques, moderate cost, and complexity of quantification due to the presence of considerable image noise.

Myocardial perfusion imaging in conjunction with exercise or pharmacologic stress testing has been validated as an alternative modality for noninvasive assessment of coronary artery disease (see also Chapter 4). Exercise stress testing is performed using protocols similar to those for SE, followed by SPECT scan to assess regional myocardial perfusion. As an alternative, pharmacologic stress testing can be performed in those patients who cannot exercise, using vasodilating agents such as adenosine and dipyridamole, or less often, catecholamines such as dobutamine. Pharmacologic vasodilator stress imaging does not provoke ischemia, but rather induces a differential pattern of coronary blood flow (see also Chapter 4). This flow disparity translates into relative hypoperfusion of the ischemic myocardium, which can be detected on the radionuclide myocardial perfusion images.

POSITRON EMISSION TOMOGRAPHY

Positron emission tomography (PET) images the decay of an injected radioactive tracer as it distributes in the body. Although it lacks high spatial resolution, important quantitative physiologic parameters, such as perfusion and metabolism, can be imaged, making PET the gold standard for these measurements. Major disadvantages include the limited availability of PET imaging centers, a high complexity of obtaining measurements, increased cost, and limited spatial resolution compared to other imaging techniques.

【 】 CARDIAC MAGNETIC RESONANCE IMAGING

Cardiac magnetic resonance imaging (CMR) is recognized as the most accurate noninvasive imaging modality for the assessment of LV function and is now the *gold standard* for determination of cardiac EF. ECG-gated cine images from state-of-the-art magnetic resonance imaging scanners depict LV function with high contrast and excellent spatial and temporal resolution (Fig. 5-5), and are readily acquired in breath-holds of 5 to 10 heartbeats. For patients in whom breath-holding and ECG gating are difficult, real-time cine imaging without ECG gating and breath-holding can be performed. Both ECG-gated and cine CMR acquire one segment of image raw data per heartbeat for each cardiac phase, which over multiple heartbeats comprises a complete set of raw data for all cardiac phases. ECG-gated CMR with breath-holding delivers a spatial resolution of approximately 1.5×2 mm^2, slice thickness of 5 to 10 mm, and temporal resolution of

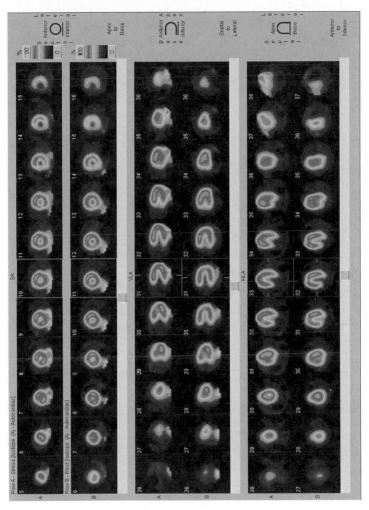

FIGURE 5-4. Rest and stress images of regional myocardial perfusion by SPECT.

30 to 50 ms per frame compared to cine CMR, which has lower spatial and temporal resolution with shorter data acquisition times and typically more artifacts. Cine CMR is also suitable for quantitative analysis from multi-slice images covering the LV, including myocardial mass, volumes, EF, and wall thickness and thickening. These parameters are commonly computed after manual planimetry of the LV epicardial and endocardial borders at end-diastole and end-systole. Cardiac volumes are calculated by multiplying the blood pool area by the slice thickness and summing over slices; myocardial mass is computed as the difference between the volumes determined by the epicardial and endocardial borders multiplied by the specific gravity of myocardium.

Beyond conventional CMR, a variety of tissue-tracking methods exist for quantifying tissue displacement, velocity, strain, strain rate, twist, and torsion by measuring

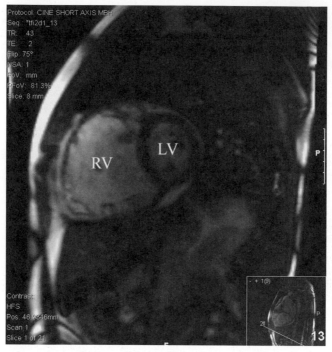

FIGURE 5-5. CMR with a short-axis view of the left ventricle (LV) in a patient with a grossly dilated right ventricle (RV).

motion of small regions of tissue within the myocardium. Tissue-tracking techniques include myocardial tagging, velocity-encoded phase contrast CMR, harmonic phase analysis, and displacement encoding with stimulated echoes. Phase contrast CMR can also be applied to measure early and late diastolic ventricular inflow for assessment of diastolic dysfunction (see also Chapter 4).

However, CMR has a number of disadvantages, the greatest one being the exclusion of patients with pacemakers or implantable cardiac defibrillators due to the high magnetic fields, which can tamper with the function of these devices. Other limitations include the need for breath-holding, the gantry's claustrophobic environment, high cost, increased complexity of data analysis, and limited availability of the technology.

SUGGESTED READING

Bogaert J, Dymarkowski S, Taylor AM. *Clinical Cardiac MRI*. Berlin: Springer-Verlag; 2005.

Budoff MMJ, Shinbane JS. *Cardiac CT Imaging: Diagnosis of Cardiovascular Disease*. London: Springer-Verlag; 2006.

Epstein FH. MRI of left ventricular function. *J Nucl Cardiol*. 2007;14:729–744.

Heller GV, Hendel RC. *Nuclear Cardiology: Practical Applications*. New York, NY: McGraw-Hill; 2004.

Otto CM. *Textbook of Clinical Echocardiography*. 3rd ed. Philadelphia, PA: Elsevier Saunders; 2004.

Teske AJ, De Boeck BWL, Melman PG, et al. Echocardiographic quantification of myocardial function using tissue deformation imaging, a guide to image acquisition and analysis using tissue Doppler and speckle tracking. *Cardiovasc Ultrasound*. 2007;5:27.

Woodard PK, Bhalla S, Javidan-Nejad C, et al. Non-coronary cardiac CT imaging. *Semin Ultrasound CT MRI*. 2006;27:56–75.

CHAPTER 6

Cardiac CT and MRI

Steve L. Liao and Valentin Fuster

COMPUTED TOMOGRAPHY OF THE HEART

Although best known for its ability to noninvasively provide information about the epicardial coronary arteries, computed tomography (CT) is a technique that, in actuality, can fully evaluate both cardiac structure and function. Advances in spatial and temporal resolution and image reconstruction software have helped in the evaluation of cardiac structures including coronary veins, pulmonary veins, atria, ventricles, aorta, and thoracic arterial and venous structures.

【 】 TECHNICAL CONSIDERATIONS

Multirow Detector Computed Tomography

Multidetector computed tomography (MDCT) scanners produce images by rotating an x-ray tube around a circular gantry through which the patient advances on a table. By increasing the numbers of detectors, a reduction in the time to image the entire cardiac anatomy has been achieved. Additionally, the introduction of multirow spiral CT detector systems currently allows acquisition of 4 to 64 simultaneous images, with slice thickness reduced to 0.5 to 0.625 mm. Retrospective electrocardiography (EECG) gating with MDCT employs acquisition of multiple images throughout each cardiac cycle. Prospective gating during either spiral or nonspiral acquisitions employs image triggering only at a specific temporal location of the cardiac cycle, thereby significantly reducing radiation exposure.

Electron-Beam Computed Tomography

Electron-beam computed tomography (EBCT) uses an electron beam deflected via a magnetic coil and focused to strike a series of four tungsten targets located beneath the patient. As they pass through the patient, the x-rays are attenuated and recorded by two detector arrays. As there are no moving parts, the image is aquired within 50 msec.

【 】 EVALUATION OF CORONARY ARTERY DISEASE

Detection of Coronary Artery Calcification

A calcified lesion is generally defined as either two or three adjacent pixels (0.68 to 1.02 mm^2 for a 512^2 reconstruction matrix and camera field size of 30 cm) of >130 Hounsfield units (HU). Using the traditional Agatston method, each calcified lesion is multiplied by a density factor as follows: 1 for lesions with a maximal density between 130 and 199 HU; 2 for lesions between 200 and 299 HU; 3 for lesions between 300 and 399 HU; and 4 for lesions > 400 HU. The total coronary artery calcium score

(CACS) is calculated as the sum of each calcified lesion in the four main coronary arteries over all the consecutive tomographic slices.

MDCT imaging protocols vary among different camera systems and manufacturers. Generally 40 consecutive 2.5- to 3-mm-thick images are acquired per cardiac study. Calcified lesions are defined as two or three adjacent pixels with a tomographic density of either > 90 or > 130 HU. Calcium scoring is usually based on the traditional Agatston method (i.e., initial density of > 130 HU). As with EBCT scoring, the total CACS is calculated as the sum of each calcified plaque over all the tomographic slices.

Coronary Artery Calcification and Atherosclerotic Plaque Burden

The presence of CAC is an indicator of coronary atherosclerosis. Furthermore, its severity is directly related to the total atherosclerotic plaque burden present in the epicardial coronary arteries. Thought to begin early in life, CAC progresses more rapidly in older individuals who have advanced atherosclerotic lesions. Calcification is an active, organized, and regulated process occurring during atherosclerotic plaque development where calcium phosphate precipitates in atherosclerotic coronary arteries in a similar fashion as observed in bone mineralization. Although lack of calcification does not exclude the presence of atherosclerotic plaque, calcification occurs exclusively in atherosclerotic arteries and is not found in normal coronary arteries. The total calcium area underestimates total plaque area, with approximately *five times as many noncalcified as calcified plaques.*

Coronary Artery Calcification and Stenosis Severity

Significant (> 50%) coronary artery stenosis by angiography is almost universally associated with the presence of coronary artery calcium. However, the severity of angiographic coronary artery stenosis is not directly related to the total CACS. The poor *specificity of coronary calcium scanning* can be reconciled by the fact that the coronary calcification confirms the presence of atherosclerotic plaque but it may not necessarily be obstructive. There appears to be a threshold CACS above which most patients will have significant coronary artery stenosis. The accuracy for identifying significant CAD based on CACS may be further improved by incorporating age, gender, and traditional risk-factor information. The current American College of Cardiology/American Heart Association (ACC/AHA) guidelines on coronary angiography *do not recommend coronary angiography on the basis of a positive EBCT but do suggest angiography may be avoided with the finding of a negative (zero score) study.*

Coronary Artery Calcification: Prognostic Implications

The likelihood of plaque rupture and the development of acute cardiovascular events is related to the total atherosclerotic plaque burden. Although controversy exists as to whether calcified or noncalcified plaques are more prone to rupture, extensive calcification indicates the presence of both plaque morphologies. There is a direct relationship between the CACS severity, the extent of atherosclerotic plaque, and the presence of silent myocardial ischemia. Therefore, the CACS could be useful for risk assessment of asymptomatic individuals and potentially guide therapeutics.

Traditional risk-factor analysis is commonly used to identify individuals who are at increased risk for developing cardiovascular disease based on standard clinical criteria. Because the development of symptomatic cardiovascular disease occurs almost exclusively in patients with atherosclerosis, CAC score appears to provide complementary prognostic information to that obtained by the Framingham risk model.

Several recent trials in both symptomatic and asymptomatic patients have studied whether the extent of CAC can predict subsequent patient outcome. The calcium score seems to predict cardiovascular events independently of standard risk factors. In addition to the risk conferred by a high calcium score, an increase in CAC over time also increases risk of a major coronary event.

[ ] COMPUTED TOMOGRAPHY ANGIOGRAPHY

Assessment of Native Coronary Arterial Disease

Noninvasive detection of CAD is one of the most interesting but most challenging applications of coronary CT angiography. Invasive coronary angiography carries procedural risk as well as high procedural cost. It was estimated that approximately 20% to 27% of patients who undergo coronary angiography have normal angiograms, and many patients with significant CAD do not require revascularization procedures.

Because of its high negative predictive value, the consensus among many imaging experts is that MDCT may be used as a reliable filter before invasive coronary angiography in the assessment of symptomatic patients with intermediate risk of CAD and in patients with uninterpretable or equivocal stress tests. A recent scientific statement from the American Heart Association on cardiac CT concluded, "CT coronary angiography is reasonable for the assessment of obstructive disease in symptomatic patients (Class IIa, Level of Evidence B)." Use of CT angiography in asymptomatic persons as a screening test for atherosclerosis (non-calcific plaque) is not recommended (Class III, Level of Evidence C). (See Chapter 57).

Careful selection of patients is crucial to increase the diagnostic yield of coronary CTA using MDCT. Three major limitations of spiral coronary CT angiography are relatively fast heart rate (i.e., more than 70 beats/min), irregular heart rhythm, and extensive CAC. Heavy calcification does not affect the negative predictive value of MDCT on a segment-based analysis, and the newer generation of MDCT technology with even faster gantry rotation may further reduce the blooming artifact associated with coronary calcification. The recent appropriateness criteria for coronary CT angiography do not endorse the use of coronary CTA in the evaluation of patients with a body mass index (BMI) > 40 kg/m^2.

Assessment of Coronary Bypass Grafts

Coronary CT angiography demonstrated good diagnostic accuracy for evaluating graft stenosis; however, the assessment of bypass graft stenosis has several important limitations, namely the image artifacts caused by surgical clips and the presence of extensive coronary calcification in the native coronary arteries.

Presently, coronary CTA may be used for the evaluation of coronary bypass grafts and coronary anatomy in symptomatic patients. In the case of reoperation, coronary CTA may provide critically important information on the status and anatomy of the bypass grafts. The AHA Scientific Statement on Cardiac CT states, "It might be reasonable in most cases to not only assess the patency of bypass graft but also the presence of coronary stenoses in the course of the bypass graft or at the anastomotic site as well as in the native coronary artery system (Class IIb, Level of Evidence C)." In summary, coronary CTA using MDCT may be appropriate in properly selected patients by providing useful information on the overall status and the patency of the bypass grafts without exposing them to an invasive diagnostic approach

Assessment of In-Stent Restenosis

Despite promising results, assessment of symptomatic patients with implanted coronary stents using current CT technology is one of the uncertain areas in terms of its overall clinical utility. The problems faced by the current imaging technology relates to the partial volume effect caused by the metallic stents with or without the coexistence of coronary calcification. Such artifact limits the overall visibility of the inner lumen of a deployed stent. The expert consensus thus far does not advocate the routine use of MDCT in ruling out in-stent restenosis except for highly selected cases.

【 】 EVALUATION OF CARDIAC STRUCTURE

Although echocardiography is generally used to assess native and prosthetic valvular heart disease, CT can be an alternative for patients with poor acoustic windows who cannot undergo CMR or transesophageal echocardiography. Cardiac CT has been used to evaluate mitral and aortic valve calcification, bicuspid aortic valves, as well as other structures such as the atrial and ventricular septum. Use of MDCT to evaluate valvular flow abnormalities, however, continues to remains more challenging.

In addition to cardiac MRI, cardiac CT has been used increasingly for the assessment of congenital heart disease. Both modalities can be rendered into three-dimensional (3D) images that are useful in clarifying the often complex anatomic relationships in patients with congenital heart disease. Additionally, the development of four-dimensional (4D) capability has accelerated over the last few years. The heart is a dynamic organ best understood when studied throughout the cardiac cycle. Hence, the development of 4D CT cineangiography (time being the fourth dimension) is a milestone in the clinical application of this technology.

【 】 EVALUATION OF CORONARY ANOMALIES

Anomalies of the coronary arteries are reported in 0.3% to 1% of healthy individuals, and despite usually being benign, they can be hemodynamically significant and some lead to abnormalities of myocardial perfusion and/or sudden death. The coronary anomalies that may be associated with significant clinical symptoms or adverse outcomes including sudden death are those that course between the pulmonary artery and the aorta.

Until recently, invasive coronary artery angiography has been the gold standard for the detection of such anomalies. However, MDCT angiography has proven its worth in diagnosing these anomalies. Coronary CTA is considered the preferred imaging modality in patients with suspected coronary artery anomalies and in patients in whom an invasive diagnostic procedure was inconclusive.

【 】 EVALUATION OF PERICARDIAL DISEASE

CT scanning provides excellent visualization of the pericardium and associated mediastinal structures. CT is aided by the fact that epicardial and extrapericardial fat often outline the normal pericardium. Fat, being of very low density, serves as a natural contrast agent. Therefore, even minimal pericardial thickening (4 to 5 mm) is well recognized by cardiac CT. The high density of pericardial calcium makes its detection relatively easy. The 3D representation of anatomy by CT provides the surgeon with precise detail of the extent of calcification and the degree of myocardial invasion. CT scanning can be useful particularly when visualization of the pericardium is suboptimal with echocardiography. CT scanning can readily detect pericardial effusion and can help determine the characteristics of the fluid based on CT density. Additionally, CT scanning is useful in accurately diagnosing constrictive pericarditis and distinguishing it from similar conditions, such as restrictive myopathy. Cine mode images of the right atrium and RV can also detect diastolic collapse when pericardial tamponade is present. Enlargement of the superior and inferior venae cavae can also be identified when either constriction or tamponade is present.

【 】 DISEASES OF THE GREAT VESSELS

Conventional CT scanning is widely used for diagnosing thoracic aortic aneurysms and dissections. With the introduction of MDCT scanners, hundreds of images of approximately 0.625 to 2.5 mm thickness can be acquired within a single breath-hold. A complete study of the thoracic aorta can be completed in only 10 to 15 seconds. Following scan acquisition, 3D reconstructions are readily produced, which can be rotated in multiple views.

Aortic dissection, aneurysms, and coarctation can be readily diagnosed with CT angiography. In patients undergoing *redo* coronary artery bypass surgery, CT scanning has several advantages. CT angiography may guide the surgical approach by defining the position of the sternum to the right ventricle, existing grafts, and aorta, and thereby avoid unnecessary bleeding. CT is an excellent modality to evaluate the aorta for plaque and atherosclerotic disease, allowing the surgeon to plan an arterial revascularization rather than depending on saphenous vein grafting.

Finally, CT angiography of the pulmonary arteries may be particularly useful in the diagnosis of acute pulmonary embolism, replacing the nuclear ventilation perfusion scan in many centers.

【 】 SUMMARY

CAC is helpful in risk stratifying intermediate-risk patients as well as ruling out obstructive disease in the symptomatic patient with low probability of disease. CTA with detection of both luminal stenosis and calcified and noncalcific plaque, should significantly aid in improving risk stratification and diagnoses. CTA is likely to become an initial test in the symptomatic patient with a low to intermediate probability of obstructive CAD. Given a consistent negative predictive power > 97% in multiple studies, CTA is unlikely to misclassify a patient at risk for CAD. It affords significant clinical information but must be used in context of other tests and in specific clinical situations, because the current radiation dose and contrast requirements preclude its use as a screening test. MDCT angiography can be a powerful tool in assessing structural abnormalities of the heart, including coronary anomalies and pulmonary veins.

MAGNETIC RESONANCE IMAGING OF THE HEART

Advances in technical abilities and clinical utilization of cardiovascular magnetic resonance (CMR) imaging has allowed CMR to provide dynamic, rapid, and high-resolution imaging of ventricular function, valvular motion, and myocardial perfusion. Moreover, CMR is now considered the gold standard for the assessment of regional and global systolic function, myocardial infarction and viability, and the assessment of congenital heart disease.

【 】 BASIC PRINCIPLES

Magnetic resonance imaging (MRI) acquires images through the transmission and reception of energy. However, unlike other modalities, MRI offers the ability to modulate both the emitted and received signals so that a multitude of tissue characteristics can be examined and differentiated without the need to change scanner hardware. As a result, from a single imaging session, a wide variety of information about cardiac function and morphology, perfusion and viability, hemodynamics, and large vessel anatomy can be obtained. This information is gathered from multiple short acquisitions, each requiring different pulse sequences (software programs that drive the scanner) with specific operational parameters and optimal settings.

【 】 MAGNETIC RESONANCE PHYSICS

An MRI scanner is not a single device, but rather consists of multiple separate components that perform three basic operations: (1) the generation of a static magnetic field, (2) the transmission of energy within the radiofrequency (RF) range to the patient, and (3) the reception of the MR signal following the transmission of RF energy. When a patient is placed within the bore of the scanner, hydrogen protons within the patient's body align parallel or antiparallel to the static magnetic field. More protons align parallel to the field than against the field, leading to a small net magnetization vector. While aligned in the magnetic field, these protons rotate or precess about the field (in the same way a spinning top precesses in a gravitational field) at a rate known as the *Larmor frequency*. This frequency (ω_o) depends on magnetic field strength (B_0) and a nuclei specific physical constant, known as the gyromagnetic ratio (γ), by the formula, $\omega_o = \gamma B_0$.

With the absorption of the energy from the RF pulse, the net magnetization vector is tilted from its equilibrium orientation parallel to the static magnetic field (longitudinal direction) into the transverse plane. Following the RF excitation, two independent relaxation processes return the net magnetization vector to its thermal equilibrium (realigned with the static magnetic field). Longitudinal relaxation time (T1) results from the transfer of energy from the excited protons to surrounding molecules in the local environment. The time constant, T1, describes the exponential regrowth of longitudinal magnetization. The second process, known as *transverse* or *spin-spin relaxation*, describes the decay of the magnetization vector in the transverse (x-y) plane. The T1 and T2 are intrinsic properties of any given tissue. Pulse sequences use differences in T1 and T2 to generate image contrast between tissues.

【 】 IMAGE ACQUISITION AND SIGNAL PROCESSING

The MR signals following RF excitation are localized in 3D space by the use of magnetic fields generated by three sets of gradient coils. These gradient coils alter the strength of the static magnetic field as a linear function of distance from the isocenter of the magnet in each of three orthogonal directions (x-, y-, and z-axes). The variation in field strengths across space produces differences in proton precessional frequencies along each axis. The raw data from the scanner consists of a two-dimensional grid of data (also known as *k-space*), which is converted to an MR image by an inverse two-dimensional Fourier transform by the image reconstruction computer.

【 】 CREATING CONTRAST IN MAGNETIC RESONANCE IMAGES

One of the important advantages of MRI is the ability to generate substantial soft-tissue contrast by the use of pulse sequences and the administration of contrast media. In general, pulse sequences are adjusted to emphasize differences in tissue T1 and T2, which can be inherent or altered by the presence of contrast media. The administration of intravenous contrast agents can also be used to affect image contrast by altering tissue T1 and/or T2. The magnitude of T1 and/or T2 change depends on the specific relaxivities of the contrast media, the distribution characteristics (i.e., intravascular, extracellular, or targeted to a specific tissue), and tissue perfusion. Gadolinium-based contrast media is commonly used in CMR imaging. When administered, it primarily shortens the T1 in the tissues where it is distributed.

【 】 CMR IMAGING SAFETY

The CMR imaging environment has the potential to pose serious risks to patients and facility staff in several ways. Injuries can result from the static magnetic field (projectile impact injuries), very rapid gradient-field switching (induction of electric currents leading to peripheral nerve stimulation), RF-energy deposition (heating of the imaged portion of the body), and acoustic noise. Patients with medical devices or implants can face additional potential hazards, including device heating, movement, or malfunction. Recently, in several small case series, it has been reported that a small subset of patients with end-stage renal disease, receiving gadolinium contrast, may be at risk for developing nephrogenic systemic fibrosis (NSF). NSF is characterized by an increased tissue deposition of collagen, often resulting in thickening and tightening of the skin and predominantly involving the distal extremities. A policy statement regarding the use of gadolinium contrast agents in the setting of renal disease has been published by the American College of Radiology.

【 】 THE CARDIOVASCULAR EXAMINATION

Function and Volumes

The assessment of cardiac function and volumes is a fundamental component of the core examination. Cine MRI has been shown to be highly accurate and reproducible in the measurement of ejection fraction, ventricular volumes, and cardiac mass. In recent years, cine MRI has become widely accepted as the gold standard for the measurement of these parameters. Moreover, it is also increasingly used as an end point in studies of left ventricular (LV) remodeling and as a reference standard for other imaging techniques.

Cine MRI can be acquired in real-time, single-shot, free-breathing mode or by means of a segmented k-space data acquisition approach, which is performed using a breath-hold and offers substantial improvement in image quality with superior spatial and temporal resolution. Thus, in clinical practice, segmented imaging is usually preferred. In segmented acquisition, data is collected over multiple, consecutive heartbeats (typically 5–10). During each heartbeat, blocks of data (segments) are acquired with reference to ECG timing, which represent the separate phases or frames of the cardiac cycle. Following the full acquisition, data from a given phase, collected from the multiple heartbeats, are combined to form the complete image of the particular cine frame. For the core examination, a short-axis stack from the mitral-valve plane through the apex and two-, three-, and four-chamber long-axis views are obtained.

Perfusion at Stress and Rest

The goal of perfusion imaging is to create a movie of the transit of contrast media (typically gadolinium based) with the blood during its initial pass through the LV myocardium (*first-pass contrast enhancement*). After scout and cine imaging, adenosine is infused under continuous electrocardiography and blood pressure monitoring for at least 2 minutes prior to the initiation of perfusion imaging. Gadolinium contrast is then administered, followed by a saline flush. The perfusion images are observed as they are acquired, with breath-holding starting from the appearance of contrast in the RV cavity. Once the contrast bolus has transited the LV myocardium, adenosine is stopped, and imaging is completed 5 to 10 seconds later. Prior to the rest perfusion scan, a waiting period of approximately 15 minutes is required for gadolinium to sufficiently clear from the blood pool. Approximately 5 minutes after rest perfusion, delayed enhancement imaging (see the following section) can be performed.

Viability and Infarction

Myocardial viability and infarction are simultaneously examined using the technique known as delayed enhancement magnetic resonance imaging (DEMRI). In the literature, DEMRI is used interchangeably with late gadolinium-enhancement CMR imaging or delayed hyperenhancement imaging. Although at first glance, the utility of DEMRI appears to be limited to those with coronary artery disease, new applications are steadily arising over a wide range of cardiovascular disorders. Thus, DEMRI is an essential component of the core examination.

Following an intravenous bolus, gadolinium distributes throughout the intravascular and interstitial space, while simultaneously being cleared by the kidneys. In normal myocardium, where the myocytes are densely packed, tissue volume is predominately intracellular. Because gadolinium is unable to penetrate intact sarcolemmal membranes, the volume of distribution is small, and one can consider viable myocytes as actively excluding gadolinium media. In acute myocardial infarction, myocyte membranes are ruptured, allowing gadolinium to passively diffuse into the intracellular space. This results in an increased gadolinium volume of distribution, and thus increased tissue concentration compared with normal myocardium. Similarly in chronic infarction, as necrotic tissue is replaced by collagenous scar, the interstitial space is expanded, and gadolinium tissue concentration is increased. T1-weighted can depict infarcted regions as bright or *hyperenhanced* whereas viable regions appear black or *nulled.* Compared with other imaging techniques that are currently used to assess myocardial viability, an important advantage of DEMRI is the high spatial resolution.

Flow and Velocity

Depending on the clinical question, the core examination can include velocity-encoded cine MRI (VENC MRI) to measure blood velocities and flows in arteries and veins, and across valves and shunts. Also known as phase-contrast velocity mapping, the underlying principle is that signal from moving blood or tissue will undergo a phase shift relative to stationary tissue, if a magnetic-field gradient is applied in the direction of motion. Encoding velocity in the slice gradient direction allows measurement of *through-plane* velocities, and encoding in either the frequency or phase-encode gradient directions allows *in-plane* measurement of velocity components directed either vertically or horizontally within the image plane.

VENC MRI allows blood flow through an orifice to be directly measured on an en-face image of the orifice with *through-plane* velocity encoding. With echocardiography there are two limitations. First, the blood flow profile is not directly measured but assumed to be flat (i.e., velocity in the center of the orifice is the same as near the edges) so that, hopefully, one sampling velocity would indicate average velocity. Additionally, the cross-sectional area of the orifice is estimated from a diameter measurement of the orifice at a different time from when Doppler velocity was recorded using a different examination (M-mode or two-dimensional imaging). Conversely, VENC MRI has some disadvantages. Perhaps most importantly, VENC MRI is not performed in real time and requires breath-holding to minimize artifacts from respiratory motion. One consequence is that it is difficult to measure changes in flow that occur with respiration.

【　】 CLINICAL APPLICATIONS

Coronary Artery Disease and Ischemia

DOBUTAMINE-STRESS CINE MRI　Analogous to echocardiography, cine MRI during dobutamine stimulation can be used to detect ischemia-induced wall-motion abnormalities. Dobutamine cine MRI can yield higher diagnostic accuracy than dobutamine echocardiography and can be effective in patients not suited for echocardiography because of poor acoustic windows. Limitations include the need to administer dobutamine while the patient is inside the magnet, the risk of inducing ischemia with dobutamine, and the diminished diagnostic utility of the ECG as it is altered by the magnetic field.

ADENOSINE STRESS-PERFUSION MRI　The diagnostic performance of stress-perfusion MRI has shown good correlations with radionuclide imaging and x-ray coronary angiography, although there have been some variable results. On average, the sensitivity and specificity of perfusion MRI for detecting obstructive CAD were 83% (range, 44% to 93%) and 82% (range, 60% to 100%), respectively. Likely on the basis of these studies, the most recent consensus report on clinical indications for CMR imaging classified perfusion imaging as a Class II indication for the assessment of CAD (provides clinically relevant information and is frequently useful).

CORONARY MR ANGIOGRAPHY　Coronary magnetic resonance angiography (MRA) is technically demanding for several reasons. The coronary arteries are small (3 to 5 mm) and tortuous compared with other vascular beds that are imaged by MRA, and there is nearly constant motion during both the respiratory and cardiac cycles. Currently, the only clinical indication that is considered appropriate for coronary MRA is the evaluation of patients with suspected coronary anomalies.

VIABILITY AND INFARCTION   Abundant animal model data demonstrate a nearly exact relationship between the size and shape of infarcted myocardium by DEMRI to that by histopathology. Human studies demonstrate that DEMRI is effective in identifying the presence, location, and extent of myocardial infarction in both the acute and chronic settings. DEMRI can also distinguish between acute infarcts with only necrotic myocytes and acute infarcts with necrotic myocytes and damaged microvasculature. The latter, termed the *no-reflow phenomenon*, indicates the presence of compromised tissue perfusion despite epicardial artery patency. Importantly, if imaging is repeated over time, no-reflow regions can gradually become hyperenhanced, as contrast slowly accumulates in these regions.

Clinically, DEMRI is used to differentiate patients with potentially reversible ventricular dysfunction from those with irreversible dysfunction. In the setting of ischemic heart disease, it is primarily the former group that will benefit from coronary revascularization. Kim and coworkers published the initial study demonstrating that DEMRI done before coronary revascularization could be used to predict functional improvement after revascularization, as measured by improved wall motion and global function.

Prior reports have concluded that in patients with CAD and ventricular dysfunction regions with thinned myocardium represent scar tissue and cannot improve in contractile function after revascularization. However, data from case reports and a pilot study indicate that thinning should not be equated with the absence of viability, and that in some patients, these regions can improve after revascularization. Additional studies will be needed to elucidate these provocative initial findings.

Because DEMRI is a relatively new technique, there is a paucity of data regarding the prognostic importance of myocardial infarction or scarring detected by this technique. However, this is an area of intense investigation, and the literature is growing rapidly. Recent work demonstrated that the presence of unrecognized myocardial scarring detected by DEMRI was associated with poor outcomes, even after accounting for common clinical, angiographic, and functional predictors. Additional investigation is needed to determine the full prognostic significance of DEMRI findings.

Heart Failure and Cardiomyopathies

In patients with heart failure, it is important to determine the etiology of heart failure to appropriately plan therapy and provide prognostic information. The utility of DEMRI in the setting of cardiomyopathy is based on the understanding that rather than simply measuring viability, the presence and pattern of hyperenhancement (nonviable myocardium) hold additional information. A stepwise algorithm has been proposed:

1. The presence or absence of hyperenhancement is determined. In patients with severe cardiomyopathy but without hyperenhancement, the diagnosis of idiopathic dilated cardiomyopathy should be strongly considered.

2. If hyperenhancement is present, the location and distribution of hyperenhancement should be classified as a CAD or non-CAD pattern.

3. If hyperenhancement is present in a non-CAD pattern, further classification should be considered.

DILATED CARDIOMYOPATHY   The clinical presentation of ischemic and nonischemic dilated cardiomyopathy (DCM) can be indistinguishable. However, chronic ischemic cardiomyopathy demonstrates myocardial scarring consistent with prior infarcts. Conversely, prior infarction in DCM is uncommon. DEMRI hyperenhancement was the best clinical parameter in noninvasively discriminating ischemic from nonischemic cardiomyopathy.

HYPERTROPHIC CARDIOMYOPATHY   CMR imaging is proving to be increasingly valuable in the clinical evaluation of hypertrophic cardiomyopathy (HCM). Echocardiography often underestimates the magnitude of hypertrophy in comparison with cine MRI. This finding may be of clinical relevance since extreme hypertrophy (wall thickness $\geq$ 30 mm) is recognized as an important risk factor for sudden death. Because scarring is observed in the majority of patients with HCM, the clinical importance of detecting scar by DEMRI in HCM patients is currently being investigated by several groups. The presence of scarring can be helpful in distinguishing LV hypertrophy because of HCM from hypertension or physiologic hypertrophy. In the latter, unless there is coexisting CAD, scarring is usually absent (see Chapter 40).

ANDERSON–FABRY DISEASE   Unlike patients with classical systemic Fabry disease, who present with multiple organ involvement, patients with the cardiac variant can manifest few or no symptoms and present only with idiopathic LV hypertrophy. In these patients, the cardiac phenotype is similar to that seen in HCM, and the diagnosis can be difficult. In these patients, hyperenhancement was most frequently observed in the basal inferolateral wall, and often the subendocardium was spared. Histologically, hyperenhanced regions appear to correspond to areas of replacement of viable myocardium with collagenous scar.

SARCOIDOSIS   Autopsy studies have shown that cardiac involvement is found in 20% to 30% of patients with sarcoidosis. However, in vivo, cardiac involvement is recognized in < 10% of patients, as current diagnostic tools are insensitive. Under-recognition of cardiac involvement can be important clinically because sudden cardiac death is one of the most common causes of mortality in sarcoid patients. Hyperenhancement was found isolated to the mid-myocardial wall or epicardium, indicative of a non-CAD pattern. However, subendocardial or transmural hyperenhancement was also observed, mimicking the pattern of myocardial infarction.

AMYLOIDOSIS   Cardiac amyloidosis is a common cause of restrictive cardiomyopathy and is associated with poor prognosis. DEMRI can demonstrate diffuse LV hyperenhancement in these patients. Although the subendocardium is preferentially involved, hyperenhancement is clearly in a non-CAD pattern because the distribution often is global and does not match any specific coronary artery perfusion territory. Practically speaking, it can be difficult to determine the optimal inversion time that will null normal myocardium, as there can be few areas that are completely normal. Therefore, it may be helpful to acquire multiple images using different inversion times. If a large portion of myocardium goes through the null point earlier than the blood pool, infiltrative involvement of the myocardium is highly likely.

MYOCARDITIS   The pattern of hyperenhancement observed in myocarditis is an evolution from a focal to a disseminated process during the first 2 weeks of symptoms. Although some investigators have interpreted this finding as evidence that hyperenhancement in the setting of acute myocarditis can represent viable myocardium, a more likely explanation is that hyperenhanced regions decrease in size because the volume of nonviable myocardium shrinks. As part of the normal healing process, necrotic regions undergo involution as they remodel and are replaced by dense collagenous scar.

CHAGAS' DISEASE   An inflammatory disease caused by the protozoan, *Trypanosoma cruzi*, Chagas' disease starts with an acute phase. Patients then remain asymptomatic for many years, and 20% eventually develop chronic heart failure. DEMRI demonstrated that the prevalence of myocardial scarring progressively increased from 20% in asymptomatic patients without structural heart disease by echocardiography to 100% in patients with left ventricular dysfunction and ventricular tachycardia. Scarring occurred most commonly in the LV apex and inferolateral wall. Both non-CAD (isolated epicardial or midwall involvement) and CAD type (indistinguishable from prior myocardial infarction) scar patterns were observed.

ARRHYTHMOGENIC RIGHT VENTRICULAR CARDIOMYOPATHY   Traditionally, a major focus in the evaluation of arrhythmogenic right ventricular cardiomyopathy (ARVC) by CMR has been to identify fatty infiltration of RV myocardium using spin-echo sequences. However, there is growing realization that this focus can be misplaced because of technical as well as physiologic reasons. The primary goal of the CMR-imaging examination should be to determine global and regional RV morphology and function. Cine imaging should be performed, with high spatial and temporal resolution and complete anatomic coverage including the RV outflow tract.

Hemodynamics

ATRIAL SEPTAL DEFECT   CMR-imaging evaluation of atrial septal defect (ASD) has focused on hemodynamic severity as measured indirectly by VENC MRI of the pulmonary artery and aorta (i.e., Qp/Qs). From the *en face* view, the rim of tissue separating the ASD from the base of the aorta (retroaortic rim), tricuspid valve, venae cavae, and coronary sinus can be viewed from a single image plane. Flow across the ASD can also be measured directly from the *en face* view by VENC MRI. Failure to capture the optimal *en face* view, however, leads less accurate measurements than measuring flow in the pulmonary artery and aorta.

VALVULAR LESIONS   Measurements of aortic valve area in aortic stenosis assessed by planimetry on cine MRI agree with those values obtained by echocardiography and cardiac catheterization. Planimetry for valve area is performed on cine MRI with higher spatial and temporal resolution than usual for standard imaging. On cine MRI, regurgitant jets appear as signal voids associated with nonlaminar flow (turbulence, acceleration, etc.). Similar to echocardiography, the size and extent of the regurgitant jet can be used to semiquantitatively grade the severity of regurgitation. For quantitative assessment of regurgitation, the regurgitation fraction can be calculated from data derived from VENC MRI sometimes in combination with cine MRI. For example, with MR the regurgitant volume can be obtained by subtracting the effective forward flow across the proximal ascending aorta from the diastolic inflow across the mitral valve from two separate through-plane VENC MRI acquisitions.

Pericardial Disease and Cardiac Masses

CONSTRICTIVE PERICARDITIS   Older CMR sequences could accurately determine the thickness of the pericardium, thereby was helpful in confirming the diagnosis of constrictive pericarditis, if the pericardial thickening was found to be extreme (> 5 mm). Newer real-time cine MRI can be used to demonstrate increased ventricular interdependence, a hemodynamic hallmark of pericardial constriction. Specifically, abnormal ventricular septal motion toward the left ventricle in early diastole is seen during the onset of inspiration. Although the number of patients that have been studied is quite small, this finding appears helpful in distinguishing between constrictive pericarditis and restrictive cardiomyopathy.

PERICARDIAL EFFUSION   Both loculated and circumferential pericardial effusions are readily identified by CMR imaging. Simple (transudate) effusions typically appear bright and homogenous on T2-weighted images and dark on T1-weighted images. Complex effusions can appear heterogeneous and darker on T2 imaging.

MASSES   In the past, characterization of cardiac masses by CMR imaging focused primarily on comparing image intensities on T1-, T2-, and proton-density weighted images. Presently, a typical protocol for the evaluation of a cardiac mass should consist of multiple pulse sequences where the aim is to assess morphology, motion, perfusion, and delayed enhancement, in addition to inherent differences in T1 and T2. For example, perfusion MRI can demonstrate increased vascularity, which can be prominent in malignancies such as angiosarcoma; DEMRI can identify areas of tissue necrosis within the core of a malignant tumor, which appear as areas of hyperenhancement.

LEFT VENTRICULAR THROMBUS   Although most common in the LV apex, thrombus can occur elsewhere, with predilection for locations with stagnant blood flow such as adjacent to akinetic, infarcted myocardium. The presence of LV thrombus can be apparent on cine MRI, if the thrombus is clearly intracavitary. However, layered mural thrombus can be difficult to detect because image intensity differences between thrombus and myocardium are minimal. Recent studies suggest that DEMRI following contrast administration can be an improved method for detecting LV thrombus. The basic principle utilized is that thrombus is avascular and has essentially no contrast uptake. Thus, it should be easily distinguished as a nonenhancing defect surrounded by bright ventricular blood pool and contrast-enhanced myocardium.

【 】 CONCLUSION

Cardiovascular magnetic resonance provides a multifaceted approach to cardiac diagnosis by enabling the assessment of morphology, function, perfusion, viability, tissue characterization, and blood flow during a single comprehensive examination.

SUGGESTED READING

Budoff MJ, Achenbach S, Blumenthal RS, et al. Assessment of coronary artery disease by cardiac computed tomography: a scientific statement from the American Heart Association Committee on Cardiovascular Imaging and Intervention, Council on Cardiovascular Radiology and Intervention, and Committee on Cardiac Imaging, Council on Clinical Cardiology. *Circulation.* 2006;114:1761–1791.

Califf RM, Armstrong PW, Carver JR, et al. 27th Bethesda conference: matching the intensity of risk factor management with the hazard for coronary disease events. Task Force 5. Stratification of patients into high, medium and low risk subgroups for purposes of risk factor management. *J Am Coll Cardiol.* 1996;27:1007–1019.

Detrano R, Guerci AD, Carr JJ, et al. Coronary calcium as a predictor of coronary events in four racial or ethnic groups. *N Engl J Med.* 2008;358:1336–1345.

Fuster V, Kim RJ. Frontiers in cardiovascular magnetic resonance. *Circulation.* 2005;112:135–144.

Hendel RC, Patel MR, Kramer CM, et al. ACCF/ACR/SCCT/SCMR/ASNC/NASCI/SCAI/SIR 2006 appropriateness criteria for cardiac computed tomography and cardiac magnetic resonance imaging: a report of the American College of Cardiology Foundation Quality Strategic Directions Committee Appropriateness Criteria Working Group, American College of Radiology, Society of Cardiovascular Computed Tomography, Society for Cardiovascular Magnetic Resonance, American Society of Nuclear Cardiology, North American Society for Cardiac Imaging, Society for Cardiovascular Angiography and Interventions, and Society of Interventional Radiology. *J Am Coll Cardiol.* 2006;48:1475–1497.

Kim RJ, Wu E, Rafael A, et al. The use of contrast-enhanced magnetic resonance imaging to identify reversible myocardial dysfunction. *N Engl J Med.* 2000;343:1445–1453.

CHAPTER 7

Cardiac Catheterization and Coronary Angiography

Marco A. Costa and Joseph Jozic

INDICATIONS AND CONTRAINDICATIONS FOR CATHETERIZATION

The benefits need to outweigh the inherent risks of any invasive procedure, and such risk-benefit relationship must be carefully evaluated in each patient. Cardiac catheterization is an invasive testing modality used to evaluate and diagnose conditions such as coronary artery disease (CAD), cardiomyopathies, pulmonary hypertension, and valvular and congenital heart abnormalities by catheter-based hemodynamic monitoring and contrast angiography. Table 7-1 lists the indications for coronary angiography. Given the invasive nature of cardiac catheterization, it is equally important to consider contraindications to the procedure. Patient refusal is the only absolute contraindication; however, there are a number of relative contraindications. Table 7-2 lists the contraindications to cardiac catheterization.

【 】 PATIENT PREPARATION

Prior to the procedure, a complete explanation of the risks and benefits of the procedure should be given to the patient. The risk of complications should be addressed. Overall risk of a major complication is less than 2%, the risk of death is 0.11%, myocardial infarction 0.05%, and cerebrovascular accident 0.07%. The risk of a vascular complication was found to be 0.43%, contrast reaction 0.37%, and a hemodynamic complication 0.26%. Prior to the procedure or administration of any sedation, a written consent must be signed by a competent patient or legal patient representative (if the patient is not able to sign). Some patients, such as the elderly, those requiring an urgent or emergent procedure, patients with cardiogenic shock or acute myocardial infarction, and patients with renal insufficiency or congestive heart failure, are at a higher risk for developing complications. In patients with renal insufficiency or a known allergy to iodine contrast, treatment prior to catheterization minimizes the risk associated with the procedure and medical condition. Table 7-3 lists specific pretreatment regimens used.

【 】 VASCULAR ACCESS

Arterial Access

Percutaneous arterial access may be obtained from either the upper or lower extremities. In the upper extremity, radial, brachial, or even axillary arteries are utilized, while the common femoral artery is the preferred site in the lower extremity. The pulsation of the femoral artery is palpated 1 to 2 cm below the inguinal ligament. This site is proximal to the bifurcation of the superficial femoral and profunda arteries.

TABLE 7-1

Class I Recommendations for Coronary Angiography

	Level of Evidence
Stable Angina or Asymptomatic Individuals	
1. CCS Class III and IV angina on medical treatment.	B
2. High-risk criteria on noninvasive testing regardless of anginal severity.	A
3. Patients who have been successfully resuscitated from sudden cardiac death or have sustained (> 30 s) monomorphic ventricular tachycardia or nonsustained (< 30 s) polymorphic ventricular tachycardia.	B
Unstable Coronary Syndromes	
1. High or intermediate risk for adverse outcome in patients with unstable angina refractory to initial adequate medical therapy or with recurrent symptoms after initial stabilization. Emergent catheterization is recommended.	B
2. High risk for adverse outcome in patients with unstable angina. Urgent catheterization is recommended.	B
3. High- or intermediate-risk unstable angina that stabilizes after initial treatment.	A
4. Initially low short-term risk unstable angina that is subsequently high risk on noninvasive testing.	B
5. Suspected Prinzmetal's angina.	C
During Initial Management of Acute MI (MI Suspected and ST Elevation or BBB Present): Coronary Angiography Coupled with Intent to Perform Primary PTCA	
1. As an alternative to thrombolytic therapy in patients who can undergo angioplasty of the infarct artery within 12 h of the onset of symptoms or beyond 12 h if ischemic symptoms persist, if performed in a timely fashion[a] by individuals skilled in the procedure and supported by experienced personnel in an appropriate laboratory environment.	A
2. In patients who are within 36 h of an acute ST elevation/Q-wave or new LBBB MI who develop cardiogenic shock, are < 75 years of age, and in whom revascularization can be performed within 18 h of the onset of shock.	A
During Risk-Stratification Phase of MI (Patients with All Types of MI)	
Isclschhemia at low levels of exercise with ECG changes (1-mm ST-segment depression or other predictors of adverse outcome) and/or imaging abnormalities.	B
Perioperative Evaluation Before (or After) Noncardiac Surgery: Patients with Suspected or Known CAD	
1. Evidence for high risk of adverse outcome based on noninvasive test results.	C
2. Angina unresponsive to adequate medical therapy.	C
3. Unstable angina, particularly when facing intermediate- or high-risk noncardiac surgery.	C
4. Equivocal noninvasive test result in a high-clinical-risk patient undergoing high-risk surgery.	C

TABLE 7-1

Class I Recommendations for Coronary Angiography (*Continued*)

	Level of Evidence
Patients with Valvular Heart Disease	
1. Before valve surgery or balloon valvotomy in an adult with chest discomfort, ischemia by noninvasive imaging, or both.	B
2. Before valve surgery in an adult free of chest pain but of substantial age and/or with multiple risk factors for coronary disease.	C
3. Infective endocarditis with evidence of coronary embolization C.	C
Patients with CHF	
1. CHF due to systolic dysfunction with angina or with regional wall motion abnormalities and/or scintigraphic evidence of reversible myocardial ischemia when revascularization is being considered.	B
2. Before cardiac transplantation.	C
3. CHF secondary to postinfarction ventricular aneurysm or other mechanical complications of MI.	C

BBB, bundle branch block; CCS, Canadian Cardiovascular Society; CHF, congestive heart failure; LBBB, left bundle branch block; MI, myocardial infarction; PTCA, percutaneous transluminal coronary angioplasty.

*a*Performance standard: within 90 min. Individuals who perform > 75 PTCA procedures per year. Centers that perform > 200 PTCA procedures per year and have cardiac surgical capability.

Modified and reproduced with permission from the American College of Cardiology: Scanlon PJ, Faxon DP, Audet AM, et al. ACC/AHA Guidelines for Coronary Angiography: A report of the American College of Cardiology/American Heart Association Task Force on Practice Guidelines (Committee on Coronary Angiography). *J Am Coll Cardiol.* 1999;33:1756–1824 (See also Chapter 59).

The inguinal ligament courses from the anterior superior iliac spine to the superior pubic ramus (Fig. 7-1). The inguinal ligament should be used as a landmark, not the inguinal crease, as the skin crease may be misleading especially in obese patients. The site of anticipated arterial puncture may be confirmed with fluoroscopy of the right groin with a metal clamp overlying the proposed site of puncture. The site of arterial puncture should overlie the middle of the head of the femur, as this location will allow for ideal compression of the arteriotomy site during manual compression. After administration of 10 to 20 mL of 1% lidocaine, an 18-gauge introducer needle is passed into the skin and directed at a 30-degree angle toward the palpated femoral artery pulsation. Before inserting the needle, a small skin incision may be made with a scalpel to facilitate passage of the needle through the skin. A single-wall arterial puncture should be made, with blood return through the needle being pulsatile and brisk. Then a 0.035-in J-tip guidewire is carefully advanced through the needle. If resistance is felt during this maneuver, the wire should be withdrawn, intraluminal position of the needle tip should be reconfirmed by pulsatile blood flow, and readvancement of the wire should be performed under fluoroscopic guidance. Once the wire is advanced up to the level of the iliac artery or aorta, the needle is removed and replaced, over the guidewire, with an appropriately sized vascular sheath. The size of the sheath used is determined by the size

TABLE 7-2

Relative Contraindications for Cardiac Catheterization

Acute renal failure
Chronic renal failure secondary to diabetes
Active gastrointestinal bleeding
Unexplained fever, which may be due to infection
Untreated active infection
Acute stroke
Severe anemia
Severe uncontrolled hypertension
Severe symptomatic electrolyte imbalance
Severe lack of cooperation by patient due to psychologic or
    severe systemic illness
Severe concomitant illness that drastically shortens life
    expectancy or increases risk of therapeutic interventions
Refusal of patient to consider definitive therapy such as PTCA,
    CABG, or valve replacement
Digitalis intoxication
Documented anaphylactoid reaction to angiographic contrast
    media
Severe peripheral vascular disease limiting vascular access
Decompensated congestive heart failure or acute pulmonary
    edema
Severe coagulopathy
Aortic valve endocarditis
PTCA, percutaneous transluminal coronary angioplasty; CABG, coronary
artery bypass graft.

Modified and reproduced with permission from the American College of Cardiology:
Scanlon PJ, Faxon DP, Audet AM, et al. ACC/AHA Guidelines for Coronary Angiography:
A Report of the American College of Cardiology/American Heart Association Task Force on
Practice Guidelines (Committee on Coronary Angiography). *J Am Coll Cardiol.*
1999;33:1756–1824.

of the catheters being used. For diagnostic coronary angiography, catheters with diameters varying from 4 to 6 Fr are commonly used, although complex anatomic scenarios may require 7 or 8 Fr catheters for extra support.

Radial artery access allows for more rapid patient ambulation and is associated with fewer bleeding complications. Adoption of this technique is somewhat limited, because coronary catheterization is technically more challenging from the upper extremity. Prior to obtaining vascular access in the radial artery, patency of the palmar arch needs to be assessed, as occlusion of the radial artery during or following the procedure can lead to digit injury if the palmar arch in not intact. Patency should be assessed with a modified Allen's test using a pulse oximeter. This approach places a pulse oximeter on the thumb while compressing the radial artery. The presence of an arterial waveform, even one with reduced amplitude or delayed reappearance, and a hemoglobin saturation of greater than 90% (Barbeau type A, B, C), confirm the adequacy of palmar arch blood flow. Following confirmation of the palmar arch flow, the radial artery is accessed 1 to 2 cm proximal to the radial styloid with a 4 Fr radial artery micropuncture kit. The radial artery, particularly in large males, can accommodate up to a 7 or 8 Fr vascular sheath. We recommend use of a sheath with a hydrophilic coating, and infusion of heparin and intra-arterial vasodilators immediately after access is confirmed to avoid spasm and thrombosis and facilitate removal of the sheath.

TABLE 7-3

Pretreatment Regimens for Patients Undergoing Cardiac Catheterization/ Coronary Angiography

Patients with Renal Insufficiency

Withholding nephrotoxic medications prior to the procedure and until renal function
normalizes following the procedure (e.g., metformin, NSAIDs).
Hydration
    Isotonic solution (normal saline or sodium bicarbonate) given optimally for
       12 h before the procedure and continued for 6–12 h after, with a goal of
       1 L to be given before the procedure and rates of 100–150 mL/h.
N-Acetylcysteine
    600-mg orally dosed BID for 2 doses prior to and after catheterization.
Other considerations
    Use of isoosmolar contrast.
    Adjusting the dose of contrast received to the renal function.
    MRCD (maximum radiographic contrast dose) = 5 mL × weight (kg)/serum
      creatinine.

Patients with Radiographic Contrast Allergy

Corticosteroids
    Oral corticosteroids (methylprednisone 32 mg or prednisone 50 mg) given
      6–24 h and 2 h prior to contrast. Two or three doses may be given. Two-dose
      regimen is given 12 and 2 h prior to contrast. Three-dose regimen is given
      13, 7, and 1 h prior to contrast administration.
H1 antagonists
    Diphenhydramine 50 mg IV/IM/PO given 1 h prior to contrast.

Data compiled from Schweiger MJ, Chambers CE, Davidson CJ, et al. Prevention of contrast induced nephropathy: recommendations for the high risk patient undergoing cardiovascular procedures. *Catheter Cardiovasc Interv.* 2007;69:135–140; and Tramer MR, von Elm E, Loubeyre P, et al. Pharmacological prevention of serious anaphylactic reactions due to iodinated contrast media: systemic review. *BMJ.* 2006;333:675–681.

Venous Access

Femoral vein access is obtained approximately 1 cm medial and 1 cm inferior to the site of arterial access. An 18-gauge needle is used with a syringe attached to its hub. Following a small skin incision, the needle is advanced at a 30- to 45-degree angle with slight suction applied to the syringe. Dark venous blood should be easily aspirated upon entering the vein. A 0.035-in J-tipped guidewire is the advanced, and following removal of the needle, a vascular access sheath is placed into the vein over the guidewire.

【　】 HEMOSTASIS

Hemostasis following the procedure is extremely important. The most common complications of diagnostic coronary angiography are associated with the vascular entry site.

Manual Pressure

Manual pressure is applied to an area 3 finger-breadths above the site of skin puncture. For venous access, light manual pressure applied for 5 to 10 minutes following sheath removal is usually sufficient to effect hemostasis. For arterial access, firm manual pressure

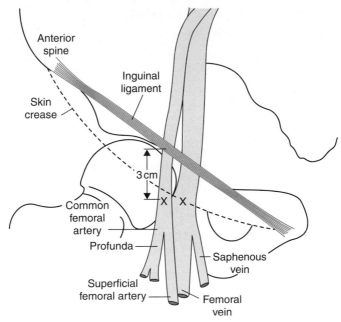

FIGURE 7-1. The right femoral artery and vein course underneath the inguinal ligament, which connects the anterior-superior iliac spine and pubic tubercle. The arterial skin incision (indicated by 10) should be placed approximately 3 cm below the inguinal ligament and directly over the femoral artery pulsation. The venous skin incision should be made at the same level but approximately 1 finger-breadth medial. (Reproduced with permission from Baim DS, Simon DI. Percutaneous approach, including trans-septal and apical puncture. In: Baim DS, ed. *Grossman's Cardiac Catheterization, Angiography, and Intervention.* 7th ed. Philadelphia, PA: Lippincott Williams & Wilkins; 2006.)

is applied following sheath removal over the area of femoral artery pulsation and arterial puncture, usually 2 finger-breadths above the site of skin puncture. Pressure should be initially firm enough to obliterate the pedal pulse and is slowly eased after 10 minutes. Duration of manual pressure is dependent on the size of the sheath and use of anticoagulant or antithrombotic medications. A useful rule of thumb is manual pressure should be applied for 3 minutes for every French size; for example, a 6 Fr hemostasis sheath would require 18 minutes of manual compression, with longer hold times being required for patients who are anticoagulated. The application of manual pressure should not be interrupted. If bleeding is noted after releasing the pressure, the manual compression process must be restarted from time zero. Pressure maybe fully released only after the predetermined amount of time has elapsed.

Vascular Closure Devices

There are a number of devices available on the market today to facilitate arterial hemostasis following completion of a cardiac catheterization. Closure devices allow for more rapid ambulation of the patient, but have not been shown to lower bleeding or vascular complications. These devices should be use with extreme caution in patients with a low arterial puncture, below the bifurcation of the femoral artery, and in patients with peripheral arterial disease.

【 】 HEMODYNAMIC MEASUREMENTS

During a right heart catheterization, hemodynamic measurements, such as direct measurements of blood pressure, are taken from the right atrium, ventricle, and pulmonary artery and in the wedge position in a pulmonary artery. Hemodynamic measurements are important in the assessment of fluid status, evaluation of valvular lesions or shunt fractions, and calculation of cardiac output. A right heart catheterization is performed, by accessing a central vein, usually the femoral or internal jugular vein, advancing a balloon-tipped catheter, like a Swan-Ganz catheter, to the right atrium. Care is taken to steer the catheter from the right atrium into the right ventricle and with a clockwise turn advance the catheter across the pulmonic valve and into the pulmonary artery. A 0.021-in wire may be necessary to support advancement of the catheter into the pulmonary artery. Further advancement of the catheter will allow the inflated balloon of the catheter tip to wedge into a smaller branch of the pulmonary artery there by transducing an approximation of the left atrial pressure via the end-hole of the catheter.

Table 7-4 lists normal values associated with a right heart catheterization.

In addition to obtaining pressure measurements, which can aid in assessing fluid status of a patient, blood samples are obtained from the superior and inferior venae cavae, right atrium and ventricle, and the pulmonary artery and in the wedge position. Hemoglobin saturation measurements obtained from the blood sample can identify and assess an intracardiac shunt, and can be used in the calculation of cardiac output and systemic and pulmonary vascular resistance.

Cardiac Output and Vascular Resistance

Cardiac output, which is the volume of blood expelled from the heart over a period of time, may be calculated by two methods in the cardiac catheterization laboratory: the thermal dilution method and using the Fick calculation. The thermal dilution method uses a known volume of saline, 10 mL, at room temperature, which is rapidly injected into the proximal port of a pulmonary artery catheter. A thermistor at the distal tip of the catheter records the temperature decrease as the fluid is moved past the catheter by the pumping action of the heart. The computer in the catheterization lab, using the thermodilution equation, will calculate a cardiac output. In general, thermodilution cardiac output measurements may have an error of 5% to 10% even when performed carefully. The other common method to calculate cardiac output is the Fick equation. For the Fick equation and shunt calculations, the patient should not be receiving supplemental oxygen. The Fick equation is as follows:

$$\text{Cardiac Output} = \frac{O_2 \text{ Consumption (mL/min)}}{(\text{Arterial Saturation} - \text{Mixed Venous Saturation}) \times \text{Hgb} \times 1.35 \times 10}$$

TABLE 7-4

Normal Values Associated with Right Heart Catheterization

Right atrium	8–10 mm Hg
Right ventricle	25/4 mm Hg
Pulmonary artery	25/9 mm Hg
Pulmonary capillary wedge pressure	9 mm Hg
Cardiac output	3–7 L/min
Cardiac index	2.5–4 L/min/m^2
Systemic vascular resistance	900–1300 dyne·sec/cm^5
Pulmonary vascular resistance	155–250 dyne·sec/cm^5

O_2 consumption may be measured; however, many catheterization laboratories will assume an O_2 consumption of 125 mL/m^2 in adults and 110 mL/m^2 in older patients. Mixed venous saturation is calculated using the hemoglobin saturations from the superior vena cava (SVC) and inferior vena cava (IVC). IVC blood has a higher hemoglobin oxygen saturation than blood from the SVC because the kidneys use less oxygen relative to their blood flow:

$$\text{Mixed Venous Saturation} = \frac{2\,\text{SVC} + \text{IVC}}{3}$$

A normal mixed venous saturation is 60% to 80%. The cardiac output may be corrected for body size and expressed as the cardiac index:

$$\text{Cardiac Index} = \frac{\text{Cardiac Output}}{\text{Body Surface Area (m}^2)}$$

With the cardiac output calculated, systemic vascular resistance and pulmonary vascular resistance can be calculated:

$$\text{Systemic Vascular Resistance} = \frac{\text{Mean Arterial Pressure} - \text{Central Venous Pressure}}{\text{Cardiac Output}}$$

$$\text{Pulmonary Vascular Resistance} = \frac{\text{Mean Pulmonary Artery Pressure} - \text{Left Atrial Pressure}}{\text{Cardiac Output}}$$

Shunt and Valve Area Calculations

Hemoglobin oxygen saturations are used to assess for the presence of an intracardiac shunt. A left-to-right shunt is suspected when > 6% difference is noted between the mixed venous and pulmonary artery saturations. A simplified formula for the calculation of the flow ratio, between systemic and pulmonary systems, can be used to estimate the magnitude of a left-to-right shunt:

$$\frac{Qp}{Qs} = \frac{(\text{SA O}_2 - \text{MV O}_2)}{(\text{PV O}_2 - \text{PA O}_2)}$$

A shunt ratio less than 1.5 denotes a small left-to-right shunt. A shunt ratio greater than 2.0 denotes a large left-to-right shunt and is considered sufficient evidence to recommend repair of the defect.

Direct pressure measurements can also be used to calculate stenotic valve orifice area. By using pressure measurements proximal and distal to the stenotic valve and one of either two formulas, one can estimate the valve area of a stenotic aortic or mitral valve.

The Gorlin formula is as follows:

$$A = \frac{\text{CO/(DFP or SEP)(HR)}}{44.3\text{C}\sqrt{\Delta P}}$$

Where A is the valve area (cm^2), CO is cardiac output (cm^3/min), DFP is the diastolic filling period (s/beat) for mitral valve areas, SEP is the systolic ejection period (s/beat) for aortic valve areas, HR is heart rate (beats/min), C is an empirical constant (0.85 for mitral valve calculations), and (P is the pressure gradient. A simplified formula developed by Hakki and associates is also available:

$$A = \frac{\text{CO}}{\sqrt{\Delta P}}$$

【 】 CORONARY ANGIOGRAPHY

Coronary angiography remains the gold standard diagnostic modality to detect coronary artery disease. Angiography provides a visual representation of vascular structures. During a cardiac catheterization, the patient is placed in a supine position on the catheterization, table. At the cranial end is the x-ray source below the table and the image intensifier, or digital flat panel detector in newer machines, above the table. These components move in tandem but in opposite directions allowing for the imaging of coronary arteries and other vascular structures in multiple views. The orientation of the view obtained is described by the detector's position relative to the patient. Cranial angulation means the detector is tilted toward the patient's head and caudal means the detector is angled toward the feet. In right anterior oblique (RAO) position, the detector is tilted to the patient's right side; and in left anterior oblique (LAO) position, the detector is tilted to the patient's left side. Radiopaque contrast is used to opacify the coronary arteries. The contrast is selectively injected into the coronary arteries through specially preformed catheters. Initially, cardiac catheterization was performed via brachial cutdown using a single catheter (Sones) that was maneuvered to engage both right and left coronary artery systems as well as perform ventriculography. Subsequently, numerous preformed catheters have been developed to cannulate the left and right coronary arteries (Fig. 7-2). The most commonly used are the Judkins left and right catheters. Other commonly used catheters are Amplatz right or left, and multipurpose catheters. The catheters are advanced from the site of vascular access over a 0.035-in J-tipped guidewire to the ascending aorta. Basic principles of optimal coronary angiography include having a coaxial alignment of the catheter and coronary ostium, full opacification of the coronary lumen, no vessel or other structures (catheters, ECG patch, wires, etc.) overlapping the coronary image, and a minimum of two orthogonal projections for each vessel with minimal foreshortening of the target segments.

Left Coronary Artery

The left coronary artery originates from the left sinus of Valsalva near the sinotubular ridge. The left main coronary artery (LM) bifurcates into the left anterior descending (LAD) artery, which courses in the intraventricular groove giving off septal perforators and diagonal branches that supply the lateral wall; and the left circumflex (LCx) artery, which courses in the atrioventricular (AV) groove and gives off obtuse marginal branches supplying the lateral and posterolateral walls. The LM can be cannulated in most patients with a Judkins left catheter with a 4-cm curve (JL 4) by advancing the catheter down from just distal of the sinotubular junction, while viewing the catheter in a RAO or LAO angulation. The JL 4 catheter should advance easily and the tip will "jump" after passing the sinotubular ridge, placing the catheter tip at the ostium of the LM. In imaging the left coronary artery system, cranial images are able to visualize the mid and distal LAD segments, and caudal images are for the LM, LCx, and proximal LAD segments, with RAO and LAO angulation used to minimize overlap and better visualize specific segments of the artery. The initial image taken is in the RAO/caudal projection. This view allows for visualization of the entire LM and proximal segments of the LAD/LCx vessels, which represent > 70% of the myocardium. RAO/cranial and LAO/cranial projections demonstrate the mid to distal LAD well, with a straight lateral (90-degree LAO) angulation being used to visualize an LAD that is overlapped in other traditional views. Either RAO or LAO caudal projections allow for visualization of the LCx as well as the left main and proximal LAD.

Right Coronary Artery

The right coronary artery arises from the right sinus of Valsalva, near the sinotubular junction; however, its position of origin can be variable within the sinus. The artery courses along the right AV groove to the posterior LV wall, where in 85% of patients it

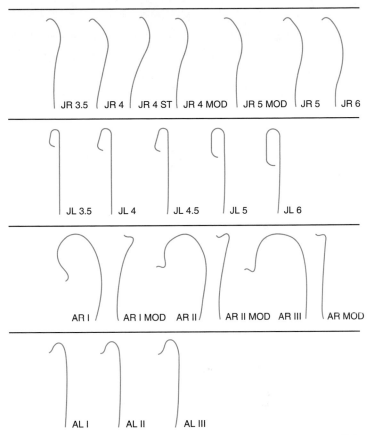

JR 3.5 JR 4 JR 4 ST JR 4 MOD JR 5 MOD JR 5 JR 6

JL 3.5 JL 4 JL 4.5 JL 5 JL 6

AR I AR I MOD AR II AR II MOD AR III AR MOD

AL I AL II AL III

FIGURE 7-2. A schematic diagram demonstrating the Judkins and Amplatz variety of left and right coronary catheters, and their differing sizes.

will supply the posterior descending artery (PDA), which gives off perforating branches supplying the basal and posterior third of the septum, AV nodal artery, and posterolateral left ventricular (PLLV) branches. Dominance of the coronary arteries is ascribed to the vessel from which the PDA, PLLV, and AV nodal artery arise. In a right-dominant system, the PDA, PLLV, and AV nodal artery arise from the RCA; and in a left-dominant system they arise from the LCX. The LAO/cranial view can be used to easily determine if the LCX is dominant.

The RCA is cannulated by advancing a Judkins right catheter with a 4-cm curve (JR 4) to the cusps of the aortic valve. Gently withdrawing the catheter, while making a clockwise rotation, turns the tip of the catheter anteriorly and causes it to cannulate the right coronary artery. RAO or LAO projections demonstrate the proximal portions of the RCA. But the distal vessel and bifurcation of the PDA and PLLV branches are best visualized with a cranial angulation.

Figure 7-3 demonstrates views useful in assessing specific segments of each coronary artery.

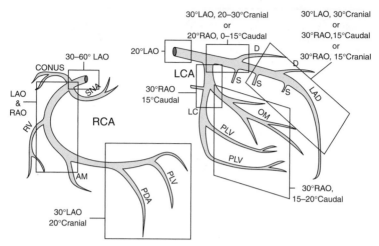

FIGURE 7-3. A schematic representation of the right and left coronary arteries. Approximate frontal and sagittal plane projections and angulations for visualization of various portions of the coronary arteries are indicated. (Reproduced with permission from Pepine CJ, Hill JA, Lambert CR. Coronary angiography. In: Pepine CJ, ed. *Diagnostic and Therapeutic Coronary Catheterization.* 3rd ed. Baltimore, MD: Lippincott Williams & Wilkins; 1998.

Bypass Grafts

Saphenous vein grafts and radial artery grafts mostly originate off of the ascending aorta. Occasionally radiopaque markers are sutured near the site of implantation marking their location. The grafts can be engaged using a JR 4 catheter. Grafts are arranged, proximal to distal, on the ascending aorta in the following order: grafts to RCA, grafts to LAD, then diagonals, and then grafts to obtuse marginal branches. Grafts to the RCA or LCX branches should be imaged in a RAO caudal and LAO cranial projection. This will allow for simple identification of the native vessels supplied by the particular bypass graft. The internal mammary arteries, typically the left internal mammary artery (LIMA), are also used as bypass grafts, often to the LAD. The LIMA arises anteriorly from the caudal portion of the subclavian artery distal to the origin of the vertebral artery. It can be cannulated for selective angiography with a JR 4 catheter or with a specially formed IMA catheter. After the catheter is advanced to the distal subclavian artery over a 0.035-in J-tipped guidewire using a LAO view, the catheter is slowly withdrawn until it engages the IM artery. This maneuver is performed in the AP view. The preformed IMA catheter is frequently able to easily engage the left internal mammary artery.

Left Ventriculography

Ventriculography is used when assessment of left ventricular wall motion or function is needed. An angled pigtail catheter is advanced to the aortic valve, and the catheter prolapsed across the valve leaflets. Occasionally a straight guidewire is needed to facilitate passage across a stenotic valve, but such a procedure should be performed by experienced operators because of the risk of coronary injury and cerebral embolic events. Once in the left ventricle, the catheter is positioned in a stable location to avoid induction of arrhythmias, including ventricular fibrillation. Contrast (at least 20 mL, optimal 30 to 40 mL) is injected into the ventricle by a power injector using a rate of 10 to 15 mL/s and 450 to 600 psi. A 30-degree RAO angulation will allow for visualization of the anterior and inferior walls as well as the left atrium. Mitral regurgitation is assessed by the amount of contrast visualized in the left atrium. A 60-degree LAO angulation is utilized to visualize septal and lateral walls, which are difficult to distinguish in RAO.

Aortography

Aortography is used to visualize the aortic root, ascending aorta, and origin of the great vessels. A LAO of 30 to 45 degrees with 10-degrees cranial orientation of the detector, with an injection of 40 to 60 mL of contrast injected at 20 mL/s at 600 psi, allows for opacification of the aorta to assess for aortic regurgitation, the width of the aortic root and ascending aorta, and origin of the great vessels. The use of digital subtraction might be useful. The patient should be instructed to hold his or her breath during this procedure so as to minimize motion artifact.

FINAL REMARKS

The catheterization laboratory is a place for thoughtful, timely, and meticulous execution of procedures Careful patient preparation and appropriate selection of devices are essential for successful outcomes. One must make sure that the catheterization laboratory is equipped with all necessary tools to treat potential complications prior to starting the procedure. Judicious manipulation of all intravascular devices and monitoring of the arterial pressure waveform and electrocardiography tracings are extremely important to avoid procedural complications. Gentle, slow, and purposeful movements of the catheter will usually engage the desired vessel. If a vessel is not engaged in the first attempt, return the catheter to a neutral position and repeat the maneuver once again. If you do not succeed in three or four attempts, exchange for a catheter with a different shape or curvature. Contrast should be restricted to the minimum necessary to obtain the diagnosis. Never inject contrast into an artery from which you see a damped waveform, as doing so could cause a dissection, or in the case of the RCA, ventricular fibrillation. The arterial sheath should be aspirated and subsequently flushed with heparinized saline following each catheter exchange, to avoid the formation of clots.

SUGGESTED READING

Baim DS. Coronary angiography. In: Baim DS, ed. *Grossman's Cardiac Catheterization, Angiography, and Intervention*. 7th ed. Philadelphia, PA: Lippincott Williams & Wilkins; 2006.

Baim DS, Simon DI. Percutaneous approach, including trans-septal and apical puncture. In: Baim DS, ed. *Grossman's Cardiac Catheterization, Angiography, and Intervention*. 7th ed. Philadelphia, PA: Lippincott Williams & Wilkins; 2006.

Barbeau GR, Arsenault F, Dugas L, et al. Evaluation of the ulnopalmar arterial arches with pulse oximetry and plethysmography: comparison with the Allen's test in 101 patients. *Am Heart J*. 2004;147:489–493.

Gorlin R, Gorlin G. Hydraulic formula for calculation of area of stenotic mitral valve, other cardiac valves and central circulatory shunts. *Am Heart J*. 1951;41:1.

Hakki AH, Iskandrian AS, Bemis CE, et al. A simplified valve formula for the calculation of stenotic cardiac valve areas. *Circulation*. 1981;63:1050–1055.

Kern MJ, King III SB. Cardiac catheterization, cardiac angiography, and coronary blood flow and pressure measurements. In: Fuster V, O'Rourke RA, Walsh R, et al. *Hurst's The Heart*. 12th ed. New York, NY: McGraw-Hill; 2008.

Pepine CJ, Hill JA, Lambert CR. Coronary angiography. In: Pepine CJ. *Diagnostic and Therapeutic Cardiac Catheterization*. 3rd ed. Baltimore, MD: Lippincott Williams & Wilkins; 1998.

Scanlon PJ, Faxon DP, Auden AM, et al. A report of the American College of Cardiology/American Heart Association Task Force on the Practice Guideline (Committee on Coronary Angiography). Developed in collaboration with the Society for Cardiac Angiography and Interventions Committee members. ACC/AHA Guidelines for Coronary Angiography: executive summary and recommendations. *Circulation*. 1999;99:2345–2357.

Schweiger MJ, Chambers CE, Davidson CJ, et al. Prevention of contrast-induced nephropathy: recommendations for the high risk patient undergoing cardiovascular procedures. *Catheter Cardiovasc Interv*. 2007;69:135–140.

Tramer MR, von Elm E, Loubeyre P, et al. Pharmacological prevention of serious anaphylactic reactions due to iodinated contrast media: systemic review. *BMJ*. 2006;333:675–681.

CHAPTER (8)

Mechanisms of Cardiac Arrhythmias and Conduction Disturbances

Alexander Burashnikov and Charles Antzelevitch

A cardiac arrhythmia can be defined as a variation from the normal heart rate and/or rhythm that is not physiologically justified. Recent years have witnessed important advances in our understanding of the electrophysiologic mechanisms underlying the development of a variety of cardiac arrhythmias (Table 8-1) and conduction disturbances. The mechanisms responsible for cardiac arrhythmias are generally divided into two major categories: (1) enhanced or abnormal impulse formation (i.e., focal activity) and (2) conduction disturbances (i.e., reentry).

ABNORMAL IMPULSE FORMATION

【 】 NORMAL AUTOMATICITY

Automaticity is the property of cardiac cells to generate spontaneous action potentials. Spontaneous activity is the result of diastolic depolarization caused by a net inward current flowing during phase 4 of the action potential, which progressively brings the membrane potential to threshold (Fig. 8-1A). The sinoatrial (SA) node normally displays the highest intrinsic rate. All other pacemakers are referred to as subsidiary or latent pacemakers, because they take over the function of initiating excitation of the heart only when the SA node is unable to generate impulses or when these impulses fail to propagate. These include latent pacemakers at the atrioventricular (AV) junction and His–Purkinje system, as well those within the crista terminalis and Bachmann's bundle. The automaticity of all subsidiary pacemakers within the heart is inhibited when they are overdrive-paced. This inhibition is called overdrive suppression. In general, sympathetic influences (largely through beta-adrenergic receptor stimulation) and hyperkalemia increase, whereas parasympathetic influences (through muscarinic receptor stimulation) reduce the rate of phase 4 depolarization and, therefore, spontaneous activity.

The ionic mechanism underlying normal SA and AV nodes and Purkinje system automaticity includes: (1) a hyperpolarization-activated inward current (I_f) and/or (2) decay of outward potassium current (I_K). The contribution of I_f and I_K differs in SA/AV nodes and Purkinje fiber because of the different potential ranges of these two pacemaker types (i.e., −70 to −35 mV and −90 to −65 mV, respectively). L-type calcium current (ICa) participates in the late phase of diastolic depolarization in SA and AV nodes, but not in Purkinje fibers. In atrial pacemaker cells, low voltage-activated T-type ICa has been shown to contribute by sarcoplasmic reticulum calcium release, which in turn stimulates the inward Na-Ca exchange current (INa-Ca).

TABLE 8-1

Characteristics and Presumed Mechanisms of Cardiac Arrhythmias

	Mechanism	Origin	Rate Range, bpm	AV or VA Conduction
Sinus tachycardia	Automatic (normal)	Sinus node	≥100	1:1
Sinus node reentry	Reentry	Sinus node and right atrium	110–180	1:1 or variable
Atrial fibrillation	Reentry, fibrillatory conduction, automatic	Atria, pulmonary veins, SVC	260–450	Variable
Atrial flutter	Reentry	Right atrium, left atrium (infrequent)	240–350, usually 300 ± 20	2:1 or variable
Atrial tachycardia	Reentry, automatic, triggered activity	Atria	150–240	1:1, 2:1, or variable
AV nodal reentry tachycardia	Reentry	AV node with an atrial component	120–250, usually 150–220	1:1
AV reentry (WPW or concealed accessory AV connection)	Reentry	Circuit includes accessory AV connection, atria, AV node, His–Purkinje system, ventricles	140–250, usually 150–220	1:1
Accelerated AV junctional tachycardia	Automatic	AV junction (AV node and His bundle)	61–200, usually 80–130	1:1 or variable
Accelerated idioventricular rhythm	Abnormal automaticity	Purkinje fibers	> 60	Variable, 1:1, or AV dissociation

Ventricular tachycardia	Reentry, automatic, triggered activity	Ventricles	120–300, usually 140–240	AV dissociation, variable
Ventricular fibrillation	Reentry, automatic, triggered activity	Ventricles	> 240, irregular	AV dissociation, variable
Bundle branch reentrant tachycardia	Reentry	Bundle branches and ventricular septum	160–250, usually 195–240	AV dissociation, variable, or 1:1
Right ventricular outflow tract	Automatic, triggered activity	Right ventricular outflow tract	120–200	AV dissociation, variable, or 1:1
Torsades de pointes tachycardia	Reentry	Ventricles	> 200	AV dissociation

AV, atrioventricular; DAD, delayed afterdepolarization; WPW, Wolff–Parkinson–White syndrome; EAD, early afterdepolarization; bpm, beats per minute; SVC, superior vena cava.

Data from Waldo AL, Wit AL. Mechanisms of cardiac arrhythmia and conduction disturbances. In: Fuster V, Alexander RW, O'Rourke RA, eds. Hurst's The Heart. 11th ed. New York, NY: McGraw-Hill; 2004: 787–816.

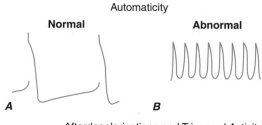

Automaticity

Normal   **Abnormal**

A   *B*

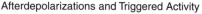

Afterdepolarizations and Triggered Activity

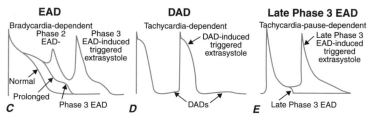

EAD   **DAD**   **Late Phase 3 EAD**

Bradycardia-dependent   Tachycardia-dependent   Tachycardia-pause-dependent

Phase 2 EAD-   Phase 3 EAD-induced triggered extrasystole   DAD-induced triggered extrasystole   Late Phase 3 EAD-induced triggered extrasystole

Normal

Prolonged

C   Phase 3 EAD   *D*   DADs   *E*   Late Phase 3 EAD

FIGURE 8-1. Automaticity and afterdepolarizations. **A, B.** Normal and abnormal automaticity. **C.** Phase 2 and 3 early afterdepolarizations (EADs). **D.** Delayed afterdepolarization (DAD). **E.** Late phase 3 EAD. Reproduced with permission from Burashnikov A, Antzelevitch C. Late-phase 3 EAD. A unique mechanism contributing to initiation of atrial fibrillation. *PACE.* 2006;29:290–295, Blackwell Publishers, Ltd (**C, D**); and Reproduced with permission from Burashnikov A, Antzelevitch C. *Circulation.* 2003;107:2355–2360 (**E**).

【 】 ABNORMAL AUTOMATICITY

Abnormal automaticity or depolarization-induced automaticity is observed under conditions of reduced resting membrane potential, such as ischemia and infarction (Fig. 8-1B). The membrane potential at which abnormal automaticity develops ranges between −70 and −30 mV. Abnormal automaticity may occur in tissues that normally develop diastolic depolarization (i.e., Purkinje fiber), as well as those that normally do not display this feature (e.g., ventricular or atrial myocardium). Compared to normal automaticity, abnormal automaticity in Purkinje fibers or ventricular and atrial myocardium shows little to no overdrive suppression. The rate of abnormal automaticity is substantially higher than that of normal automaticity. Similar to normal automaticity, abnormal automaticity is enhanced by beta-adrenergic agonists and by hyperkalemia. The ionic basis for diastolic depolarization in abnormal automaticity may be in part similar to that of normal automaticity in intrinsically depolarized tissues (SA and AV nodes).

【 】 AUTOMATICITY AS A MECHANISM OF CARDIAC ARRHYTHMIAS

Sinus bradycardia and tachycardia can be caused by simple alteration of the rate of impulse initiation by the normal SA node pacemaker (Table 8-1). Alterations in sinus rate may be accompanied by shifts of the origin of the dominant pacemaker within the sinus node or to subsidiary pacemaker sites elsewhere in the atria. Impulse conduction out of the SA mode may be impaired or blocked as a result of disease or increased vagal activity leading to development of bradycardia. AV junctional rhythms occur when atrioventricular junctional pacemakers located either in the AV node or in the His bundle take control of the heart, usually in the presence of AV block. Normal or subsidiary pacemaker activity also may be enhanced (due to sympathetic nerve activity, hypokalemia, or acute stretch), leading to sinus tachycardia or a shift to ectopic sites within the atria, giving rise to atrial tachycardia. Accelerated idioventricular rhythms have been attributed to enhanced normal automaticity in the His–Purkinje system. Various forms of parasystolic activity are thought to be caused by latent pacemakers protected by entrance block. Common clinical conditions like hypertrophy and heart failure promote automaticity. Automaticity can precipitate or trigger rapid reentrant arrhythmias. Atrial fibrillation can be triggered by rapid automaticity arising in the pulmonary vein muscular sleeves.

【　】 AFTERDEPOLARIZATIONS AND TRIGGERED ACTIVITY

Oscillatory depolarizations that attend or follow the cardiac action potential and depend on preceding transmembrane activity for their manifestation are referred to as afterdepolarizations (Fig. 8-1C through E). Two subclasses are traditionally recognized: (1) early and (2) delayed. Early afterdepolarizations (EADs) interrupt or retard repolarization during phase 2 and/or phase 3 of the cardiac action potential, whereas delayed afterdepolarizations (DADs) arise after full repolarization. When EAD or DAD amplitude suffices to bring the membrane to its threshold potential, a spontaneous action potential referred to as a triggered response results, and may be responsible for extrasystoles and tachyarrhythmias.

【　】 EARLY AFTERDEPOLARIZATIONS AND TRIGGERED ACTIVITY

Although conditions and mechanisms of EAD induction may differ, a critical prolongation of repolarization and bradycardia/pauses accompany most, but not all, EADs. Fig. 8-1C illustrates the two types of EAD generally encountered in Purkinje fiber. Oscillatory events appearing at potentials positive to −30 mV are generally referred to as phase 2 EADs. Those occurring at more negative potentials are termed phase 3 EADs. In contrast to Purkinje fibers, EAD activity recorded in ventricular preparations are always phase 2 EADs. In the case of prolonged repolarization, beta-adrenergic stimulation and/or acceleration from an initially slow rate may transiently facilitate the induction of EADs (due to intracellular calcium loading). EADs develop more readily in Purkinje fibers and in cells in the midmyocardial region than in epicardial or endocardial regions of the ventricles.

Most pharmacologic interventions or pathophysiologic conditions associated with EADs can be categorized as acting predominantly through one of four different mechanisms: (1) a reduction of repolarizing potassium currents (I_{Kr}, class IA and III antiarrhythmic agents; IKs, chromanol 293B); (2) an increase in the availability of calcium current (Bay K 8644, catecholamines); (3) an increase in the sodium–calcium exchange current due to augmentation of intracellular calcium activity or upregulation of the exchanger; and (4) an increase in late sodium current (late I_{Na}) (aconitine, anthopleurin-A, and ATX-II). Combinations of these interventions (i.e., calcium loading and I_{Kr} reduction) or pathophysiologic states may act synergistically to facilitate the development of EADs.

【　】 DELAYED AFTERDEPOLARIZATIONS AND TRIGGERED ACTIVITY

The conditions and mechanisms responsible for DADs are invariably related to cellular calcium loading, which generally occurs at rapid activation rates and is commonly facilitated by digitalis, beta-adrenoreceptor stimulation, and low extracellular potassium (Fig. 8-1D). DADs are initiated by spontaneous sarcoplasmic reticulum calcium release following the end of the action potential. DADs are believed to be induced by a transient inward current (I_{ti}) generated by (1) a nonselective cationic current (I_{ns}), (2) activation of an electrogenic Na/Ca exchanger, or (3) calcium-activated Cl⁻ current. All are secondary to the release of calcium from the overloaded sarcoplasmic reticulum.

【 】 LATE PHASE 3 EADs

Recent studies have uncovered a novel mechanism giving rise to triggered activity, termed *late phase 3 EADs*, which combine properties of both EADs and DADs but have their own unique character (Fig. 8-1E). Late phase 3 EAD-induced triggered extrasystoles represent a new concept of arrhythmogenesis in which abbreviated repolarization permits "normal sarcoplasmic reticulum calcium release" to induce an EAD-mediated triggered response, under conditions of intracellular calcium loading. In contrast to previously described DADs or intracellular calcium-dependent EADs, it is *normal,* not spontaneous sarcoplasmic reticulum calcium release that is responsible for the generation of late phase 3 EADs.

【 】 ROLES OF TRIGGERED ACTIVITY IN THE DEVELOPMENT OF CARDIAC ARRHYTHMIAS

EAD-induced triggered activity is thought to be involved in precipitating torsades de pointes under condition of congenital and acquired long QT syndromes (Table 8-1). Clinical arrhythmias postulated to be caused by DAD-induced triggered activity include (1) idiopathic right and left ventricular outflow tract ventricular tachyarrhythmias and (2) idioventricular rhythms—accelerated AV junctional escape rhythms that occur as a result of digitalis toxicity or in a setting of myocardial infarction. Other possible DAD-mediated arrhythmias include exercise-induced adenosine-sensitive ventricular tachycardia (VT); repetitive monomorphic VT caused presumably by cAMP-mediated triggered activity; some adrenergic-dependent supraventricular tachycardias and fibrillation; some tachyarrhythmias associated with nonischemic and ischemic cardiomyopathy, as well as heart failure; and catecholaminergic or familial polymorphic ventricular tachycardia. EAD and DAD activity may also be involved in the genesis of cardiac arrhythmias associated with hypertrophy and heart failure. It is noteworthy that EADs developing in select transmural subtypes (such as M cells) can exaggerate transmural dispersion of repolarization, thus setting the stage for reentry. Late phase 3 EAD-induced triggered beats may be responsible for the immediate reinitiation of AF following termination of AF. The conditions that give rise to late phase 3 EADs may also occur immediately following termination of other tachyarrhythmias. Late phase 3 EAD may be involved in the initiation of some forms of AF associated with an interaction of sympathetic and parasympathetic systems, particularly in pulmonary vein muscular sleeves.

REENTRANT ARRHYTHMIAS

The circuitous propagation of an impulse around an anatomic or functional obstacle leading to reexcitation of the heart describes a circus movement reentry. Several *conceptually* different forms of reentry have been described: (1) the ring model (Fig. 8-2A); (2) the leading circle model (Fig. 8-2B); and (3) the spiral wave model. The ring model of reentry differs from the other three in that an anatomic obstacle is required.

Electrical heterogeneity and the wavelength are pivotal concepts for understanding the development of circus movement reentry. The wavelength, the distance along the reentrant path occupied by the active response, is calculated as the product of conduction velocity and refractory period. The wavelength must be shorter than the pathlength for reentry to be initiated and maintained. In healthy hearts, conduction velocity in most areas of the heart is too rapid and the refractory period is too long to accommodate a reentrant circuit within the atria or ventricles. A structurally and electrically normal heart seldom develops reentrant arrhythmias. Slowing conduction velocity and/or abbreviating repolarization generally promote the appearance of reentrant arrhythmias by reducing wavelength. Augmentation of electrical heterogeneity greatly predisposes

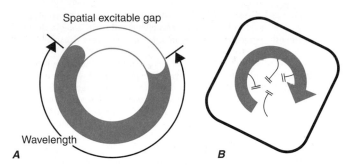

FIGURE 8-2. Reentrant mechanisms. **A.** Schematic of a ring model of reentry. **B.** The activation pattern of leading circle of reentry and the converging centripetal wavelets.

the heart for the appearance of reentry as well, by increasing the probability of conduction block (i.e., wavebreak). Cardiac disease is commonly associated with an increase in electrical heterogeneity, slowing of conduction velocity, and changes in refractory period, explaining the predisposition of the abnormal heart to reentrant arrhythmias. The development of reentry typically requires a trigger as well as a substrate. The precipitating extrasystole or trigger may be automatic, triggered, or reentrant. The substrate is generally due to electrical and/or structural heterogeneities.

【 】 RING MODEL

The ring model is the simplest form of reentry (Fig. 8-2A). The criteria developed more than a century ago for identification of circus movement reentry remain in use today: (1) an area of unidirectional block must exist; (2) the excitatory wave progresses along a distinct pathway, returning to its point of origin and then following the same path again; and (3) interruption of the reentrant circuit at any point along its path should terminate the circus movement. A reentrant circuit formed about an anatomic obstacle normally has a fully excitable gap allowing entrainment.

【 】 LEADING CIRCLE MODEL

Allessie and coworkers in 1973 were the first to experimentally demonstrate a reentrant arrhythmia without anatomic obstacle (Fig. 8-2B). Using multiple intracellular electrodes, they showed that although the basic beats elicited by stimuli applied near the center of the tissue spread normally throughout the preparation, premature impulses propagate only in the direction of shorter refractory periods. An arc of block thus develops around which the impulse is able to circulate and reexcite the tissue. The functionally refractory region that develops at the vortex of the circulating wavefront prevents the centripetal waves from short circuiting the circus movement and thus serves to maintain the reentry. Because the head of the circulating wavefront usually travels on relatively refractory tissue, a fully excitable gap of tissue may not be present; unlike other forms of reentry, the leading circle model may not be readily influenced by extraneous impulses initiated in areas outside the reentrant circuit and thus may not be easily entrained.

【 】 SPIRAL WAVES AND ROTORS

The concept of spiral waves has attracted a great deal of interest over the past decade. Although leading circle and spiral wave reentry are considered by some to be similar, a number of conceptual distinctions have been suggested. Curvature of the activation front determines the core of the reentrant circuit in the spiral wave model (due to sink-source mismatch), but not in the leading circuit model. A major difference between the leading circle and spiral wave also is the state of the core; in the former it is kept permanently refractory, whereas in the latter the core is excitable but not excited.

A role for spiral waves in atrial (AF) and ventricular (VF) fibrillation is likely to be most common. There are two major theories to explain AF/VF generation. The first, originally suggested by Gordon Moe and colleagues, proposes that fibrillation is maintained by the continuing development of *multiple unstable reentrant wavelets*. The other theory, "single source hypothesis," proposes that AF/VF can be maintained by a single high-frequency source, giving rise to fibrillatory conduction in the remainder of the ventricle or atria. A reentrant mechanism is believed to underlie a single source maintaining AV/VF in most cases (the so-called mother rotor). However, a rapidly activating focal source (automatic or triggered activity) can cause some forms of AF/VF as well.

Whether fibrillation is caused by a single or multiple reentrant sources, wavebreak (i.e., conduction block) is an indispensable requirement for reentry to develop. Wavebreak occurs when a propagated activating waveform encounters an anatomic or functional (refractory state) obstacle. Anatomic heterogeneity is well recognized as promoting wavebreak, reentry, and AF/VF in healthy and particularly in structurally abnormal ventricles. There are two fundamental hypotheses to explain wavebreak occurring in the absence of anatomic obstacles. The first involves spatial refractory period heterogeneity. Gordon Moe's multiple-wavelet concept is fundamentally based on spatial inhomogeneity of refractory periods, providing the substrate for conduction block and wavefront fragmentation (wavebreaks), leading to continuous appearance and disappearance of multiple wandering reentrant wavelets. The second concept, referred to as the restitution hypothesis, invokes temporal dynamic electrical heterogeneity (which is essentially determined by electrical restitution properties of the myocardium) to explain spiral wave instability and breakup during AF/VF. In addition to action potential duration and conduction velocity restitution, a number of other "functional" factors have been shown to contribute to wavebreak during VF/AF, including cardiac memory and anisotropy.

【　】 SPECIFIC REENTRANT MECHANISMS

Reflection involves the to and fro electrotonic propagation of an impulse across an electrically depressed or inactive segment of cardiac tissue. *Phase 2 reentry* may occur when the dome of the action potential, most commonly epicardial, propagates from sites at which it is maintained to sites at which it is abolished, causing local reexcitation of the myocardium.

【　】 CARDIAC ARRHYTHMIAS CAUSED BY REENTRY

Reentrant mechanisms are thought to underlie the maintenance of most of rapid cardiac arrhythmias (Table 8-1). Among the most representative clinical reentrant ring model equivalents are various forms of atrial flutter, involving superior or inferior venae cavae, tricuspid annulus, and so forth, as anatomic barriers to circulate around. Bundle-branch reentry and reentrant tachyarrhythmias in Wolff–Parkinson–White (WPW) preexcitation syndrome are also caused by the anatomically determined pathway. Many forms of ventricular tachycardia occurring under conditions of structural heart diseases (such as ischemia, infarct, and heart failure) are often maintained by anatomically predetermined reentrant pathways. Ventricular Purkinje fiber networks are thought to provide anatomic reentrant circuits as well. Reflection has been suggested as the mechanism underlying reentrant extrasystolic activity in infarcted ventricles and in some cases of ventricular bigeminy. Phase 2 reentry is believed to initiate ventricular fibrillation in Brugada syndrome as well as ventricular arrhythmias during the acute phase of myocardial infarction. Atrial and ventricular fibrillation (occurring under practically all encountered conditions, such as ischemia, infarct, remodeling, hypertrophy, and stress) is mostly maintained by reentrant mechanisms. Polymorphic ventricular tachycardias (torsades de pointes) associated with various forms of QT syndrome are thought to be maintained by reentrant mechanisms as well.

SUGGESTED READING

Antzelevitch C. Mechanisms of cardiac arrhythmia and conduction disturbances. In: Fuster V, O'Rourke RA, Walsh RA, Poole-Wilson P, eds. *Hurst's The Heart.* 12th ed. New York, NY: McGraw Hill; 2007:913–945.

Antzelevitch C, Burashnikov A, Di Diego JM. Mechanisms of cardiac arrhythmias. In: Gussak I, Antzelevitch A, eds. *Electrical Diseases of the Heart.* London: Springer-Verlag; 2008:65–132.

Burashnikov A, Antzelevitch C. Late-phase 3 EAD. A unique mechanism contributing to initiation of atrial fibrillation. *PACE.* 2006;29:290–295.

Nattel S. New ideas about atrial fibrillation 50 years on. *Nature.* 2002;415:219–226.

Rho RW, Page RL. Ventricular arrhythmias. In: Fuster V, O'Rourke RA, Walsh RA, et al., eds. *Hurst's The Heart.* 12th ed. New York, NY: McGraw Hill; 2007:1003–1019.

Waldo AL, Wit AL. Mechanisms of cardiac arrhythmia and conduction disturbances. In: Fuster V, Alexander RW, O'Rourke RA, eds. *Hurst's The Heart.* 11th ed. New York, NY: McGraw Hill; 2004: 787–816.

Wit AL, Rosen MR. Afterdepolarizations and triggered activity: Distinction from automaticity as an arrhythmogenic mechanism. In: Fozzard HA, Haber E, et al., eds. *The Heart and Cardiovascular System.* 2nd ed. New York, NY: Raven; 1992:2113–2163.

CHAPTER (9)

Approach to the Patient with Cardiac Arrhythmias*

Robert A. O'Rourke

HISTORY

It is imperative that a complete history of the patient's symptoms be obtained. Important elements include: (1) documentation of initial onset of symptoms; (2) complete characterization of symptoms; (3) identifying conditions that appear to initiate symptoms; (4) duration of episodes; (5) frequency of episodes; (6) pattern of symptoms over time, for example, better or worse; (7) effect of any treatment; and (8) family history of a similar problem. It is also important to ascertain any pertinent past medical history. This might include history of myocardial infarction (MI), especially in a patient who presents with palpitations and syncope, or the recent initiation of an antihypertensive agent in a patient who now presents with dizzy spells.

PHYSICAL EXAMINATION

Observations from the physical examination are helpful primarily to define whether cardiovascular disease is present. For example, in a patient who presents with dizzy spells or syncope, the presence of orthostatic hypotension, a carotid bruit, or decreased carotid pulses may be important findings that lead to a diagnosis of coronary artery disease. Most importantly, the presence of specific cardiac murmurs or an S_3 or S_4 gallop may direct the clinician toward a cardiac cause for the patient's symptoms. Also pay attention to the patient's gender, age, and physiognomy. Paroxysmal supraventricular tachycardia (PSVT) that occurs in a 12-year-old boy is more likely caused by atrioventricular reentry tachycardia, whereas PSVT presenting in a 45-year-old woman more commonly is caused by atrioventricular (AV) node reentry.

【 】 SYNCOPE, PRESYNCOPE, DIZZINESS

Patients with syncope, presyncope, or dizziness are often referred to the electrophysiologist for evaluation for fear that the symptoms are caused by an arrhythmia. Unless an ECG rhythm strip is recorded at the time of the patient's event, it is impossible to positively eliminate an arrhythmic cause. Regardless, a detailed history typically points in the correct direction. The ECG may disclose many clues to the cause of syncope, including MI, cardiac hypertrophy, sinus node dysfunction, conduction abnormality, Wolff–Parkinson–White syndrome, long or short QT interval, or Brugada syndrome. Evaluation of the echocardiogram may lead to a variety of cardiac diagnoses (see Chapter 4).

*Adapted from Chapter 36 by Eric N. Prystowsky and Richard I. Fogel in Fuster V, O'Rourke RA, Walsh RA, et al., eds. *Hurst's The Heart*. 12th ed. New York, NY: McGraw-Hill; 2008, with permission of authors and publisher.

Neurally mediated syncope is very common. Typically the patient is in an upright position, either sitting or standing, and may recount a feeling of being hot or warm with or without concomitant nausea prior to loss of consciousness. Sweating is a common feature, but the patient may state that it occurred on regaining consciousness rather than prior to syncope. Normally the patient is alert on regaining consciousness but may feel fatigued. Although patients often state that their heart was *pounding* or faster than usual on awakening, they do not give a history of a rapid regular pulse that persists for minutes after the event. This latter feature should direct one to a possible arrhythmic cause for syncope.

Cardiac syncope is often sudden in onset and frequently unaccompanied by any prodrome. In some circumstances patients relate a feeling of rapid palpitations prior to loss of consciousness, and these individuals should be evaluated for a cardiac arrhythmia regardless of whether heart disease is present. One should remember that rapid PSVT as well as ventricular tachycardia can cause syncope. Unfortunately, a sudden loss of consciousness without prodrome is not specific for an arrhythmia, and patients with an arrhythmia can present with some features of a vasovagal syncope.

For patients who present with dizziness or presyncope, it is important to distinguish between vertigo and true light-headedness. Ask patients whether they feel like the room is spinning or they are spinning, compared with a sensation that *the lights are going out* or they are about to lose consciousness, especially if they are taking medication.

【 】 PALPITATIONS

Palpitations are described by patients in many ways including skipped beats, a sudden thump, hard beating, fluttering in the chest, a jittery sensation, a rapid pulse, or as merely a vague feeling that their heart is irregular. The authors have noted that many patients equate a *strong heartbeat* with palpitations, and it is important to distinguish this from irregular heartbeats. A premature atrial or ventricular complex often cannot be felt by the patient, and what they experience is the strong heartbeat that follows the pause. It may be useful to tap out various cadences for the patient. For example, to distinguish between atrial fibrillation (AF) and PSVT, tap out a rapid, irregular cadence compared with a rapid regular cadence—patients often recognize one over the other. Similarly, tap out a cadence of extra beats with a pause. Palpitations are often more prominent at night, especially when patients lie on their left side. Although these may be premature beats, often it is simply sinus rhythm.

Other historic features often tailor the initial workup. A rapid regular rhythm that occurs a few times per year and has been ongoing for many years is likely a form of PSVT. In the absence of a previous correlation with an ECG rhythm strip or 12-lead ECG, an electrophysiologic study typically is required for diagnostic and/or therapeutic reasons. Noninvasive monitoring for such infrequent arrhythmias is usually futile, and an electrophysiologic study is preferred over prescription of an implantable loop recorder. In contrast, for patients with more frequent symptoms, noninvasive event recorder monitoring is often our choice, and a unique new form of technology using wireless outpatient continuous monitoring can even identify asymptomatic arrhythmic episodes. Even if sinus rhythm is identified as the cause of palpitations, the results are valuable to the patient.

Women might present with palpitations during the week prior to menstruation. It is commonly believed that alcohol and caffeine are arrhythmogenic; and although this may be so in certain patients, it has been our experience that these agents typically play a minor role in patients who have arrhythmias. Obviously, patients with AF might have episodes during heavy alcohol intake, but such is usually not the case for PSVT and sustained ventricular tachycardia.

【 】 FATIGUE, CHEST PAIN, AND DYSPNEA

Patients may present with symptoms such as fatigue, chest pain, or dyspnea that seem unrelated to an arrhythmia. This is particularly true for those who have AF. It is surprising how many patients with AF do not experience palpitations and present with either fatigue or shortness of breath. Thus, although these symptoms typically direct the clinician down another diagnostic road, remember that they might be caused by an arrhythmia. Of particular importance are patients who present with AF and symptoms of heart failure without palpitations. Often these individuals have tachycardia-mediated cardiomyopathy, and with appropriate control of the ventricular rate the ventricular function might even normalize.

ADJUNCTIVE TESTS

【 】 ELECTROCARDIOGRAM

The ECG is covered elsewhere (Chapter 2), but two specific findings on the 12-lead ECG during PSVT should be emphasized. A pseudo r′ in ECG lead V_1 is very typical for patients who present with AV node reentry. The r′ results from superimposition of the P wave on the end of the QRS complex and is noted best in ECG lead V_1. In contrast, the typical finding in patients with AV reentry caused by retrograde conduction over an accessory pathway (Wolff–Parkinson–White syndrome). The P wave is positioned in the early ST segment

【 】 HEAD-UP TILT TABLE TESTING

Head-up tilt (HUT) table testing is a diagnostic technique to assess the susceptibility of an individual to neurally mediated syncope. The protocol for HUT generally involves footrest-supported head-up tilting at 70 to 80 degrees for 30 to 45 minutes (Fig. 9-1).

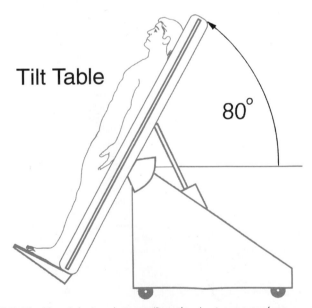

FIGURE 9-1. Tilt table with footboard support. (Reproduced with permission from Prystowsky EN, Klein GT. *Cardiac Arrhythmias: An Integrated Approach for the Clinician.* New York, NY: McGraw-Hill; 1994:353.)

If HUT is negative, the test may be repeated following pharmacologic provocation. Most laboratories use isoproterenol at a dose of 1 to 3 μg/min. Repeat tilting is generally performed for 10 minutes after a steady state has been reached. Higher doses of isoproterenol, especially when coupled with longer durations of tilt, significantly decrease the specificity of the test. In control patients with no history of syncope, 70-degree head-up tilting has a specificity of approximately 90%.

【 】 RISK STRATIFICATION AFTER MYOCARDIAL INFARCTION

Risk stratification after MI may be divided into two categories. The first category includes signal-averaged electrocardiography (SAECG) to identify high-frequency potentials at the end of the QRS complex (late potentials) and microvolt changes in T-wave amplitude. The second category assesses autonomic tone by analyzing spontaneous and induced changes in heart rate and blood pressure.

【 】 SIGNAL-AVERAGED ELECTROCARDIOGRAPHY

SAECG allows the identification of small potentials in the surface ECG that are not seen because their amplitude is less than the noise intrinsic to the ECG signal. A more detailed description of the technique may be found elsewhere. In brief, orthogonal surface XYZ ECG leads are acquired for approximately 200 beats and digitally stored. High-pass filtering minimizes the contribution of low-frequency content. The X, Y, and Z leads are then combined into a vector magnitude referred to as the *filtered QRS complex* (Fig. 9-2). Most commonly the SAECG has been used to identify late potentials appearing at the end of the QRS complex. These potentials correspond to fragmented electrical activity that is generated in areas of slow conduction either within or at the border zone of infarcts, which may be arrhythmogenic and prone to reentry.

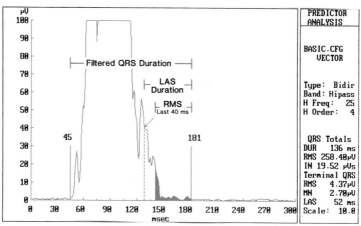

FIGURE 9-2. Positive signal-averaged electrocardiogram in a patient with sustained ventricular tachycardia. All three measured parameters are abnormal. Filtered QRS duration (DUR) is 136 msec; and the root-mean-square (RMS) voltage of the last 40 msec of the QS complex is 4.37μV. (LAS, low-amplitude signal.) (Reproduced with permission from Prystowsky EN, Klein GT. *Cardiac Arrhythmias: An Integrated Approach for the Clinician.* New York, NY: McGraw-Hill; 1994:345.)

Three parameters have been identified to describe late potentials:

1. Filtered QRS duration (QRSd).
2. Root-mean-square voltage of the terminal 40 msec of the QRS complex (RMS40).
3. The duration of the low-amplitude signal (LAS) > 40 mV.

The latter two parameters represent the amplitude and duration of the late potential, respectively. With 40-Hz filtering, a QRSd >114 msec, RMS40 < 20 mV, and LAS >38 msec are considered abnormal. The interpretation of the SAECG is problematic in the presence of a significant baseline intraventricular conduction defect.

Late potentials are hypothesized to be associated with an increased incidence of ventricular arrhythmias and sudden death. In some studies of patients after MI, the incidence of an arrhythmic event was 17% to 29% when late potentials were present. When late potentials were absent, the incidence of sudden death was 3.5% to 5%. Late potentials were an independent risk factor when assessed along with left ventricular ejection fraction (EF). The combination of an abnormal SAECG, reduced EF, and high-grade ectopy identified a population with a 50% risk in the same study.

【 】 MICROVOLT T-WAVE ALTERNANS

Microvolt T-wave alternans (MTWA) is a technique that measures small changes in T-wave amplitude that occur on an alternating beat-to-beat basis. These changes have been associated with an increased risk of malignant ventricular arrhythmias and are thought to be caused by exaggerated repolarization heterogeneity. Several techniques have now been developed to detect and quantify these subtle variations in T-wave amplitude. The most common method involves the spectral analysis of a large number of beats. Using this technique, an *alternans power* and *alternans voltage* can be determined. The alternans voltage represents the magnitude of the variation of the alternans T-wave amplitude from the mean T-wave amplitude.

The most significant limitation of this technique is the requirement of atrial pacing to elevate heart rate. Because MTWA is heart rate dependent, other techniques that used exercise were developed. Patients who developed MTWA at lower heart rates had a higher risk. Patients who developed MTWA only at high heart rates or did not develop MTWA were felt to be a lower risk.

Subsequent clinical studies identified exercise-induced microvolt T-wave alternans as a predictor of arrhythmic risk. The test is considered positive if the onset of sustained MTWA occurs at < 110 beats/min, and negative if sustained MTWA does not occur at heart rates 105 beats/min. The most common causes of an indeterminate test are failure to attain an adequate heart rate, frequent ectopy, nonsustained alternans, and excessive background electrocardiographic noise. The predictive power of MTWA appears to be independent of other risk-stratifying techniques including heart rate variability, SAECG, baroreceptor sensitivity testing, ejection fraction, and electrophysiologic testing.

Gehi and coworkers performed a metaanalysis of 19 prospective studies involving 2,608 patients with an average follow up of 21 months for a variety of cardiac problems and found the positive predictive value for arrhythmic events was 19.3%. The negative predictive value was 97.2%. The RR of a positive test for an arrhythmic event was 3.77. In patients with congestive heart failure and a nonischemic cardiomyopathy (7 studies), the predictive value of a positive test was 21.3% and of a negative test was 95.2%. In this population the RR was 3.67. In patients with congestive heart failure and an ischemic cardiomyopathy, the positive predictive value was 29.7% and the negative predictive value was 91.6%. However, this analysis included data from only 2 studies.

More recently, Chow and colleagues reported the use of MTWA for risk stratification in 768 consecutive patients with an ischemic cardiomyopathy (EF < 35%) and no history of ventricular arrhythmias. Of the 768 patients studied, 514 (67%) had a nonnegative (positive or indeterminate) MTWA test. After multivariate analysis a nonnegative MTWA test was associated with a higher risk of all cause mortality (hazard ratio 2.24) and arrhythmic mortality (hazard ratio 2.24).

【 】 HEART RATE VARIABILITY

Heart rate variability (HRV) analysis is based on subtle variations in sinus cycle length and has been used to assess cardiac autonomic status by two methods. The time-domain methods identify the RR-interval sequences and then apply statistical techniques to express the variance. The most commonly employed measure is the standard deviation of normal-to-normal beats (SDNN), or of all RR intervals; however, multiple other measures have been used.

Frequency domain methods apply the fast Fourier transform to the RR-interval sequence to develop a power spectral density that describes how the variance of the signal (i.e., power) is distributed as a function of frequency. Three main spectral components have been identified: (1) very-low-frequency < 0.04 Hz, (2) low-frequency 0.04 to 0.15 Hz, and (3) high-frequency 0.15 to 0.40 Hz.

HRV has been used for post-myocardial risk stratification. Several studies have shown that decreased heart rate variability is associated with an increased risk of sudden death. Additionally, heart rate variability increases with beta-blocker treatment and is consistent with the protective effects of beta-adrenergic-blocking agents post-MI.

【 】 BAROREFLEX SENSITIVITY

Baroreflex sensitivity (BRS) testing is another technique to assess the cardiac autonomic nervous system. Typically, as carotid pressure rises, the RR interval is prolonged. The increase in carotid pressure is detected by the carotid sinus baroreceptors and results in vagal activation offsetting the rise in systemic blood pressure. Under normal circumstances there is resting vagal predominance and sympathetic inhibition. The theory underlying BRS sensitivity testing is that decreased BRS may be present post-MI and that a substantial reduction in BRS is a marker of increased risk for ventricular fibrillation.

Most commonly, BRS is assessed by measuring the heart rate response following infusion of a vasoactive agent. Usually phenylephrine is given in doses to increase systolic blood pressure 20 to 40 mm Hg. The changes in RR intervals are plotted against systolic blood pressure changes, and the slope is considered the BRS. In a group of normal controls, the average BRS was 14.8 ± 9 msec/mm Hg. Overall baroreceptor sensitivity decreases when the sympathetic nervous system is activated. An alternative technique employs neck collar suction to activate carotid baroreceptors.

CONCLUSION AND IMPLICATIONS

In the evaluation of patients with reduced left ventricular function to identify those at highest risk for arrhythmic death, the various noninvasive tests either alone or in combination have shown some value. They typically have relatively high negative predictive value, but a weakness is their rather low positive predictive value. The *optimum* risk stratification is yet to be found.

SUGGESTED READING

Bloomfield DM, Bigger JT, Steinman RC, et al. Microvolt T-wave alternans and the risk of death or sustained ventricular arrhythmias in patients with left ventricular dysfunction. *J Am Coll Cardiol.* 2006;47:456–463.

Cain ME, Anderson JL, Arnsdorff MF, et al. American College of Cardiology expert consensus document: signal averaged electrocardiography. *J Am Coll Cardiol.* 1996;27:238–249.

Chow T, Kereiakes DJ, Bartone C, et al. Prognostic utility of microvolt T wave alternans in risk stratification of patients with ischemic cardiomyopathy. *J Am Coll Cardiol.* 2006;47:1820–1827.

Farrell TG, Bashir Y, Gipps T, et al. Risk stratification for arrhythmic events in postinfarction patients based on heart rate variability, ambulatory electrocardiographic variables and signal averaged electrocardiogram. *J Am Coll Cardiol.* 1991;18:687.

Gehi AK, Stein RH, Metz LD, et al. Microvolt T-wave alternans for the risk stratification of ventricular tachyarrhythmic events. *J Am Coll Cardiol.* 2005;46:75–82.

Gomes JA, Cain ME, Buxton AE, et al. Prediction of long-term outcomes by signal-averaged electrocardiography in patients with unsustained ventricular tachycardia, coronary artery disease, and left ventricular dysfunction. *Circulation.* 2001;104: 436–441.

Hohnloser SH, Klingenheben T, Yi-Gang L, et al. T wave alternans as a predictor of recurrent ventricular tachyarrhythmias in ICD recipients: prospective comparison with conventional risk markers. *J Cardiovasc Electrophysiol.* 1989;9:1258–1268.

Hohnloser SH, Klinenheben T, Zabel M, et al. T wave alternans during exercise and atrial pacing in humans. *J Cardiovasc Electrophysiol.* 1997;8:987–993.

Narayan SM. T-wave alternans and the susceptibility to ventricular arrhythmia. *J Am Coll Cardiol.* 2006;47:269–281.

Rosenbaum DS, Jackson LE, Smith JM, et al. Electrical alternans and vulnerability to ventricular arrhythmias. *N Engl J Med.*1994;330:235–241.

CHAPTER (10)

Atrial Fibrillation, Atrial Flutter, and Supraventricular Tachycardia*

Robert A. O'Rourke

Atrial fibrillation, atrial flutter, and supraventricular tachycardia are common arrhythmias associated with a variety of cardiac conditions. Indeed, atrial fibrillation is the most commonly sustained cardiac arrhythmia encountered in clinical practice and is increasing in prevalence. These arrhythmias may be associated with deterioration of hemodynamics, a wide spectrum of symptoms, and significant morbidity, mortality, and medical costs. Perhaps because no single therapy has been shown to be ideal for all patients, there are a variety of treatment strategies that may be applied to these arrhythmias. These include no therapy at all, rhythm control, and rate control, and these treatment strategies have both pharmacologic and nonpharmacologic options available. This chapter describes the epidemiology, electrophysiologic mechanisms, and approach to management of patients with atrial fibrillation, atrial flutter, and atrial tachycardia.

ATRIAL FIBRILLATION

Atrial fibrillation (AF) is characterized by disorganized atrial electrical activation and uncoordinated atrial contraction. The surface electrocardiogram characteristically demonstrates rapid fibrillatory waves with changing morphology and rate and a ventricular rhythm that is irregularly irregular (Fig. 10-1). Most AF originates in one or more of the pulmonary veins (PVs), and because of disparate atrial refractory periods the rapid firing focus in the left atrium (LA) cannot be conducted in a 1:1 manner to the right atrium, which leads to fibrillatory conduction. Additionally, it is thought that a driver, perhaps a reentrant focus in the LA, acts in a similar manner. Although the ECG has the characteristic appearance of disorganized atrial activation, further analysis may reveal what appears to be a regular rapid atrial rhythm, often seen best in lead V_1 (Fig. 10-1). Careful measurement will disclose variability in the P-P intervals, and this should not be misinterpreted as atrial flutter, or so-called *atrial fibrillation-flutter*. Atrial flutter, as discussed later, is a very regular rhythm with monotonous repetition of similar P waves with each cycle.

The ventricular rate during AF can be quite variable, and depends on autonomic tone, the electrophysiologic properties of the atrioventricular (AV) node, and the effects of medications that act on the AV conduction system.

The ventricular rate may be very rapid (> 300 beats per min [bpm]) in patients with Wolff–Parkinson–White (WPW) syndrome, with conduction over accessory pathways (wide preexcited QRS complexes) having short antegrade refractory periods. A regular, slow ventricular rhythm during AF suggests a junctional rhythm, either as an escape mechanism with complete AV block or as an accelerated junctional pacemaker.

---

*Adapted in part from Chapter 37 by Prystowsky EN, Waldo AI. Atrial fibrillation, atrial flutter, and atrial tachycardia. In: Fuster V, O'Rourke RA, Walsh RA, et al., eds. Hurst's The Heart. 12th ed. New York: McGraw-Hill; 2008, with permission of authors and publisher.

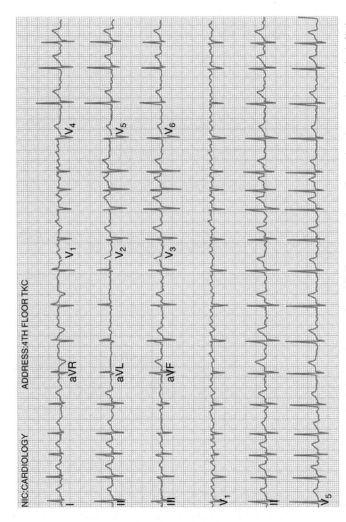

FIGURE 10-1. Twelve-lead electrocardiogram of atrial fibrillation. Note the rapid, irregular, changing, low-amplitude fibrillatory waves and an irregularly irregular ventricular response.

[ ] CLASSIFICATION

At the initial detection of AF, it may be difficult to be certain of the subsequent pattern of duration and frequency of recurrences. Thus, a designation of *first detected* episode of AF is made on the initial diagnosis. When the patient has experienced two or more episodes, atrial AF is classified as *recurrent*. After the termination of an episode of AF, the rhythm can be classified as *paroxysmal* or *persistent*. Paroxysmal AF is characterized by self-terminating episodes that generally last < 7 days (most < 24 hours), whereas persistent AF generally lasts > 7 days and often requires electrical or pharmacologic cardioversion.

AF is classified as *permanent* when it has failed cardioversion or when further attempts to terminate the arrhythmia are deemed futile. It might be more appropriate to use the term *established* rather than permanent, because these patients can undergo successful ablation to restore and maintain sinus rhythm precluding the concept of *permanent*. Although this classification scheme is generally useful, the pattern of AF may change in response to treatment. Thus, AF that has been persistent may become paroxysmal during pharmacologic therapy with antiarrhythmic medications.

[ ] EPIDEMIOLOGY

AF is the most common arrhythmia requiring treatment, with estimates of 2.2 to 5.0 million Americans and 4.5 million in the European Union experiencing paroxysmal or persistent AF. The incidence and prevalence of AF steadily increase with age, such that this arrhythmia occurs in < 0.5% of the population < 50 years of age, and increases to approximately 2% for ages 60 to 69 years, 4.6% for ages 70 to 79 years, and 8.8% for ages 80 to 89 years.

Familial AF can also occur. In most circumstances the molecular abnormality is unknown. However, specific genetic defects have been identified in a few families.

AF confers an increased relative risk of overall mortality ranging from 1.4 times controls in the Manitoba study to 2.3 times controls in the Whitehall study, and is predominantly caused by stroke. In the absence of anticoagulation, the relative risk of stroke in patients with rheumatic AF is increased approximately 17-fold. The Framingham study demonstrated that the risk of stroke in AF is clearly related to age.

[ ] PATHOPHYSIOLOGY

AF is associated with a wide variety of predisposing factors (Table 10-1). In the developed world, the most common clinical diagnoses associated with AF are hypertension and coronary artery disease.

Two concepts of the underlying mechanism of AF have received considerable attention: factors that *trigger* the onset and factors that *perpetuate* this arrhythmia. Triggering foci of rapidly firing cells within the sleeve of atrial myocytes extending into the pulmonary veins have been clearly shown to be the underlying mechanism of most paroxysmal AF. In animal models, these pulmonary vein foci manifest delayed after-potentials and triggered activity in response to catecholamine stimulation, rapid atrial pacing, or acute stretch. The pulmonary veins of patients with paroxysmal AF demonstrate abnormal properties of conduction such that there is a markedly reduced effective refractory period within the pulmonary veins, progressive conduction delay within the pulmonary veins in response to rapid pacing or programmed stimulation, and often conduction block between the pulmonary veins and the LA (Fig. 10-2).

For patients with pulmonary vein foci, a primary increase in adrenergic tone followed by a marked vagal predominance has been reported just prior to the onset of paroxysmal AF. A similar pattern of autonomic tone has been reported in an unselected group of patients with paroxysmal AF and a variety of cardiac conditions. Vagal stimulation

TABLE 10-1

Anatomic and Electrophysiologic Substrates Promoting the Initiation and/or Maintenance of Atrial Fibrillation

Diseases	Anatomic	Cellular	Electrophysiologic
Part A. Substrate develops during sinus rhythm (remodeling related to stretch and dilatation). The main pathways involve the RAAS, TGF-α, and CTGF.			
Hypertension	Atrial dilatation	Myolysis	Conduction abnormalities
Heart failure	PV dilatation	Apoptosis, necrosis	ERP dispersion
Coronary disease	Fibrosis	Channel expression change	Ectopic activity
Valvular disease			
Part B. Substrate develops because of tachycardia (tachycardia-related remodeling, downregulation of calcium channel, and calcium handling).			
Focal AF	None or[b]	None or[b]	Ectopic activity
Atrial flutter	Atrial dilatation[a]	Calcium-channel down-regulation	Microentry
	PV dilatation		Short ERP[c]
	Large PV sleeves	Myolysis	ERP dispersion[d]
	Reduced contractility[e]	Connexin down-regulation	Slowed conduction
	Fibrosis	Adrenergic supersensitivity	
		Changed sympathetic innervation	

CTGF, connective tissue growth factor; ERP, effective refractory period; PV, pulmonary vein; RAAS, renin–angiotensin–aldosterone system; TGF-α, transforming growth factor α.

[a]Substrate develops either while in sinus rhythm, usually caused by ventricular remodeling, atrial pressure overload, and subsequent atrial dilatation (Part A), or because of the rapid atrial rate during atrial fibrillation (AF), according to the principle that "AF begets AF."
[b]The listed changes may only occur with prolonged episodes of AF at high atrial rate.
[c]Short ERP and slow conduction may produce short wavelength, thereby promoting further AF.
[d]ERP dispersion together with spontaneous or stretch-induced ectopic activity may initiate AF. Long ERPs occur in Bachmann bundle among other tissues.
[e]The reduction of atrial contractility during AF may enhance atrial dilatation, leading to persistent AF.

Fuster V, Rydén LE, Cannon DS, et al. ACC/AHA/ESC 2006 guidelines for the management of patients with atrial fibrillation: a report of the American College of Cardiology/American Heart Association Task Force on Practice Guidelines and the European Society of Cardiology Committee for Practice Guidelines (Writing Committee to Revise the 2001 Guidelines for the Management of Patients With Atrial Fibrillation). *Eur Heart J.* 2006;27:1979–2030. (See also Chapter 59.)

Adapted in part from Chapter 37 by Prystowsky EN, Waldo AI. Atrial fibrillation, atrial flutter, and atrial tachycardia. In: Fuster V, O'Rourke RA, Walsh RA, et al., eds. *Hurst's The Heart.* 12th ed. New York, NY: McGraw-Hill; 2008, with permission of authors and publisher.

shortens the refractory period of atrial myocardium but with a nonuniform distribution of effect. These factors support the importance of vagal stimulation in the induction of paroxysmal AF.

Long-standing AF results in loss of myofibrils, accumulation of glycogen granules, disruption in cell-to-cell coupling at gap junctions, and organelle aggregates.

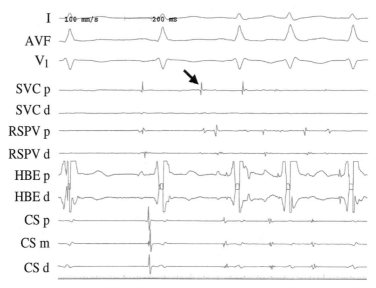

FIGURE 10-2. A rapidly firing focus in the superior vena cava (SVC) that induces atrial fibrillation. Surface leads I, aVF, and V₁ are recorded simultaneously with intracardiac bipolar electrograms from the SVC proximal (SVC p) and distal (SVC d) pairs, right superior pulmonary vein (RSPV p and RSPV d), His bundle (HBE p and HBE d), and coronary sinus (CS p, CS m, CS d). The *arrow* indicates early activation in the superior vena cava.

In a population-based study of elderly patients without AF at baseline, Tsang and coworkers demonstrated that AF developed in direct relations to the echocardiographic left atrial volume index. An even stronger predictor of the development of nonvalvular AF was a restrictive transmitral Doppler flow pattern. Thus, clinical evidence for diastolic dysfunction strongly supports the concept that myocardial stretch is an important mechanism of AF in the elderly. Altered stretch on atrial myocytes results in opening of stretch-activated channels.

【 】 HEMODYNAMIC EFFECTS

AF produces several adverse hemodynamic effects, including loss of atrial contraction, a rapid ventricular rate, and an irregular ventricular rhythm. The loss of mechanical AV synchrony may have a dramatic impact on ventricular filling and cardiac output when there is reduced ventricular compliance, as with left ventricular (LV) hypertrophy from hypertension, restrictive cardiomyopathy, hypertrophic cardiomyopathy, or the increased ventricular stiffness associated with aging. In addition, patients with mitral stenosis, constrictive pericarditis, or right ventricular infarction typically experience marked hemodynamic deterioration at the onset of AF. The loss of AV synchrony results in a decrease in LV end-diastolic pressure (LVEDP) as the loading effect of atrial contraction is lost, thereby reducing stroke volume and LV contractility by the Frank–Starling mechanism. Although there is a reduction in the LVEDP, there is an increase in the left atrial mean diastolic pressure. Patients with significant restrictive physiology may experience pulmonary edema and/or hypotension with the onset of AF.

The irregular ventricular rhythm has adverse hemodynamic effects that are independent of the ventricular rate. Irregularity significantly reduces cardiac output and coronary blood flow compared with a regular ventricular rhythm at the same average heart rate. The effect of ventricular irregularity on coronary blood flow may explain in part why some patients with AF experience precordial pain in the presence of normal coronary arteriography.

【 】 THROMBOEMBOLISM

Stroke is the most feared consequence of AF, and its prevention is a major focus of the management of patients with this condition. Most thrombi associated with AF arise within the left atrial appendage. Flow velocity within the left atrial appendage is reduced during AF because of the loss of organized mechanical contraction. Compared with transthoracic echocardiogram, the transesophageal echocardiogram offers a much more sensitive and specific means of assessing left atrial thrombi and spontaneous echo contrast, an indicator of reduced flow. Several factors contribute to the enhanced thrombogenicity of AF. Nitric oxide (NO) production in the left atrial endocardium is reduced in experimental AF, with an increase in levels of the prothrombotic protein plasminogen activator inhibitor 1 (PAI-1).

In the Stroke Prevention in Atrial Fibrillation (SPAF) III study, increased plasma levels of Von Willebrand factor (vWF) were strongly correlated with the clinical predictors of stroke in AF (age, prior cerebral ischemia, CHF, diabetes, and body mass index). There was a stepwise increase in vWF with increasing clinical risk of stroke in this population.

【 】 CLINICAL MANIFESTATIONS

Episodes of AF may be relatively short and self-terminating, or persistent for weeks or months. Even in the same patient there is substantial variability, making it difficult at times to label the patient as one with *paroxysmal* or *persistent* AF. However, most patients have a dominant pattern over time and are classified in that manner.

The clinical manifestations of AF range from no symptoms at all to profound hemodynamic deterioration (Table 10-2).

【 】 TREATMENT

Anticoagulation

STROKE RISK AND STRATIFICATION SCHEMES FOR PATIENTS WITH ATRIAL FIBRILLATION
The recognized risk factors for stroke are prior stroke or transient ischemic attack (TIA), hypertension, diabetes, heart failure, and age older than 75 years (Table 10-3). Other stroke-risk factors are mechanical prosthetic valve, mitral stenosis, coronary artery disease, thyrotoxicosis and female gender, LV dysfunction, and age older than 65 years. Not all stroke-risk factors have the same degree of association with stroke in patients with AF, which is factored in when considering indications for oral anticoagulation therapy.

The CHADS$_2$ stroke-risk stratification scheme, which is based on analysis of 1,773 patients in the National Registry for Atrial Fibrillation, has gained considerable favor and is used in the ACC/AHA/ESC 2006 management guidelines to tailor therapy for stroke prevention. The *C* in CHADS stands for recent CHF, *H* for hypertension, *A* for age older than 75 years, *D* for diabetes, and *S* for prior stroke or transient ischemic attack. Each category gets 1 point except stroke, which gets 2 because it is the most serious risk factor. The adjusted stroke rate per 100 patient-years increases from 1.9 with a score of 1 to 18.2 with a score of 6 (Table 10-3). Table 10-4 gives the new recommendations on antithrombotic therapy to prevent thromboembolism in patients with AF. There is widespread consensus that all patients with rheumatic valvular heart disease and AF require anticoagulation with warfarin unless there is an absolute contraindication.

TABLE 10-2

Clinical Evaluation of Atrial Fibrillation

Minimum Evaluation	Additional Testing (one or several tests may be necessary)

1. To define history and physical examination
    Presence and nature of symptoms associated with AF
    Clinical type of AF (first episode, paroxysmal, persistent, or permanent)
    Onset of the first symptomatic attack or date of discover of AF
    Frequency, duration, precipitating factors, and modes of termination of AF
    Response to any pharmacologic agents that have been administered
    Presence of any underlying heart disease or other reversible conditions (e.g., hyperthyroidism or alcohol consumption)
2. To identify electrocardiogram rhythm (verify AF)
    LV hypertrophy
    P-wave duration and morphology or fibrillatory waves
    Preexcitation
    Bundle-branch block
    Prior MI
    Other atrial arrhythmias
    To measure and follow the R-R, QRS, and QT intervals in conjunction with antiarrhythmic drug therapy
3. To identify transthoracic echocardiogram
    Valvular heart disease
    LA and RA size
    LV size and function
    Peak RV pressure (pulmonary hypertension)
    LV hypertrophy
    LA thrombus (low sensitivity)
    Pericardial disease
4. Blood tests of thyroid, renal, and hepatic function
    For a first episode of AF, when the ventricular rate is difficult to control
	1. Six-minute walk test
	    If the adequacy of rate control is in question
	2. Exercise testing
	    If the adequacy of rate control is in question (permanent AF)
	    To reproduce exercise-induced AF
	    To exclude ischemia before treatment of selected patients with a type 1C antiarrhythmic drug
	3. Holter monitoring or event recording
	    If diagnosis of the type of arrhythmia is in question
	    As a means of evaluating rate control
	4. Transesophageal echocardiography
	    To identify LA thrombus (in the LA appendage)
	    To guide cardioversion
	5. Electrophysiological study
	    To clarify the mechanism of wide-WRS-complex tachycardia
	    To identify a predisposing arrhythmia such as atrial flutter or paroxysmal supraventricular tachycardia
	    To seek sites for curative ablation or AV conduction block/modification
	6. To evaluate chest radiograph
	    Lung parenchyma, when clinical findings suggest an abnormality
	    Pulmonary vasculature, when clinical findings suggest an abnormality

AF, atrial fibrillation; AV, atrioventricular; LA, left atrial; LV, left ventricular; MI, myocardial infarction; RA, right atrial; RV, right ventricular. Type 1C refers to the Vaughn Williams classification of antiarrhythmic drugs.

TABLE 10-3

Stroke Risk in Patients with Nonvascular Atrial Fibrillation Not Treated with Anticoagulation According to the CHADS$_2$ Index

CHADS$_2$ Risk Criteria	Score
Prior stroke or TIA	2
Age > 75 y	1
Hypertension	1
Diabetes mellitus	1
Heart failure	1
Patients (N = 1,733)	

Warfarin is remarkably effective at reducing stroke risk in patients with AF. This was clearly demonstrated by a meta-analysis by the investigators of five randomized, controlled clinical trials comparing warfarin versus placebo in patients with AF:

1. Copenhagen Atrial Fibrilaltion Aspirin and Anticoagulation (AFASAK) trial
2. SPAF trial
3. Boston Area Anticoagulation Trial for Atrial Fibrillation (BAATAF)
4. Canadian Atrial Fibrillation trial
5. Stroke Prevention in Nonrheumatic Atrial Fibrillation (SPINAF) trial (Fig. 10-3)

Using an intention-to-treat analysis that compared warfarin therapy with placebo, there was a 68% risk reduction in stroke for patients taking warfarin compared with patients taking placebo ($p < 0.001$). Moreover, a subsequent on-treatment analysis demonstrated an 83% risk reduction in stroke when patients were taking warfarin compared with placebo. Warfarin should be administered to achieve an international normalized ratio (INR) between 2 and 3, with a target INR of 2.5 to provide both efficacy and safety (Fig. 10-3).

TABLE 10-4

Antithrombotic Therapy for Patients with Atrial Fibrillation

Risk Category	Recommended Therapy
No risk factors	Aspirin, 81–325 mg daily
One moderate-risk factor	Aspirin, 81–325 mg daily, or warfarin
Any high-risk factor or > 1	(INR 2.0–3.0, target 2.5)
moderate-risk factor	Warfarin (INR 2.0–3.0, target 2.5)

Less Validated or Weaker Risk Factors	Moderate-Risk Factors	High-Risk Factors
Female gender	Age 75 y	Previous stroke, TIA, or embolism
Age 65–74 y	Hypertension	Mitral stenosis
Coronary artery disease	Heart failure	Prosthetic heart valvae
Thyrotoxicosis	LV ejection fraction 35% or less	
	Diabetes mellitus	

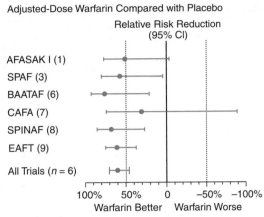

FIGURE 10-3. Effects of warfarin versus placebo on risk of stroke in six randomized, placebo-controlled clinical trials in nonvalvular atrial fibrillation. AFASAK I (*1*), the Copenhagen Atrial Fibrillation, Aspirin, and Anticoagulant Therapy Study; BAATAF (*6*), Boston Area Anticoagulation Trial for Atrial Fibrillation; CAFA (*7*), Canadian Atrial Fibrillation Anticoagulation; EAFT (*9*), European Atrial Fibrillation Trial; SPAF (*3*), Stroke Prevention in Atrial Fibrillation; and SPINAF (*8*), Stroke Prevention in Atrial Fibrillation. (CI, confidence interval.) (Adapted with permission from Hart RG, Benavente O, McBride R, Pearce LA. Antithrombotic therapy to prevent stroke in patients with atrial fibrillation: a meta-analysis. *Ann Intern Med.* Oct 5, 1999;131(7):492–501.)

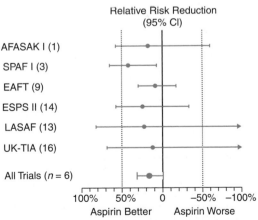

FIGURE 10-4. Effects of aspirin versus placebo on risk of stroke in six randomized, placebo-controlled trials in nonvalvular atrial fibrillation. AFASAK I (*1*), the Copenhagen Atrial Fibrillation, Aspirin, and Anticoagulant Therapy Study; EAFT (*9*), European Atrial Fibrillation Trial; ESPS II (*14*), European Stroke Prevention Study; LASAF (*13*), Alternate-Day Dosing of Aspirin in Atrial Fibrillation Pilot Study Group; SPAF I (*3*), Stroke Prevention in Atrial Fibrillation; and UK-TIA (*16*), United Kingdom Transient Ischaemic Attack Trial. (CI, confidence interval.) (Adapted with permission from Hart RG, Benavente O, McBride R, Pearce LA. Antithrombotic therapy to prevent stroke in patients with atrial fibrillation: a meta-analysis. *Ann Intern Med.* Oct 5, 1999;131(7):492–501.)

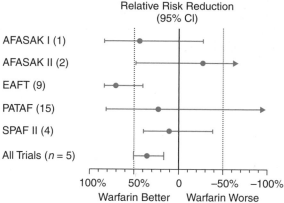

Warfarin Compared with Aspirin

FIGURE 10-5. Effects of aspirin versus warfarin on risk of stroke in five randomized, controlled clinical trials in nonvalvular atrial fibrillation. AFASAK I (*1*) and AFASAK II (*2*), the Copenhagen Atrial Fibrillation, Aspirin, and Anticoagulant Therapy Study; EAFT (*9*), European Atrial Fibrillation Trial; PATAF (*15*), Primary Prevention of Arterial Thromboembolism in Nonrheumatic Atrial Fibrillation; and SPAF II (*3*), Stroke Prevention in Atrial Fibrillation. (Adapted with permission from Hart RG, Benavente O, McBride R, Pearce LA. Antithrombotic therapy to prevent stroke in patients with atrial fibrillation: a meta-analysis. *Ann Intern Med.* Oct 5, 1999;131(7):492–501.)

In summary, it is important that the risks of bleeding versus the benefits on stroke prevention always be weighed for each patient. However, the risk of stroke typically is greater than the risk of bleeding for most patients with AF at substantial risk for stroke. Thus, even though the ACC/AHA/ESC guidelines allow aspirin or warfarin therapy for patients who have one moderate-risk factor (see Table 10-4), we generally prefer warfarin for such patients. It is also important to remember that there is no difference in the indications for antithrombotic therapy between paroxysmal, persistent, and permanent AF.

Cardioversion

Cardioversion can be accomplished using either antiarrhythmic drugs or the direct-current approach. In situations where urgent cardioversion is needed, such as marked hypotension, the direct-current approach is preferred. The need for anticoagulation prior to cardioversion must be considered. There is general consensus that AF that has been present for < 48 hours can be cardioverted without prior anticoagulation, but there are no randomized trial data to support this, and probable systemic emboli can occur in this situation. Because often it is impossible to time accurately the onset of AF, anticoagulation therapy is recommended for AF of uncertain duration.

There are two basic strategies to deal with cardioversion: (1) oral warfarin with a therapeutic INR (2–3) for 3 to 4 weeks before cardioversion followed by continued warfarin thereafter, or (2) transesophageal echocardiography (TEE) and heparin immediately before cardioversion followed by oral warfarin thereafter.

Successful electrical cardioversion requires attention to details. Always be sure the patient is adequately anticoagulated. Rather than use handheld paddles, adhesive gel electrodes should be placed anteriorly over the sternum (with the upper edge at the sternal angle) and posteriorly (just to the left of the spine).

The duration of AF is a major factor for cardioversion success using antiarrhythmic drugs, and AF lasting approximately 1 week has a substantial chance of cardioversion using oral flecainide, propafenone, dofetilide, and intravenous ibutilide. For longer duration AF, only dofetilide seems to have a reasonable chance of success, but amiodarone and ibutilide may be useful. A single oral dose of propafenone (e.g., 600 mg) or flecainide (e.g., 300 mg) can be useful to convert recent-onset AF to sinus rhythm. A recent study demonstrated the safety of the pill-in-the-pocket approach to outpatient conversion of AF in some patients. Select patients were observed in hospital while being given a single oral loading dose of either propafenone or flecainide to convert AF. Those with success were allowed to self-administer the drug if they had a recurrence of AF, and few complications occurred during follow-up. Because a type 1C drug may convert AF to atrial flutter, an AV nodal blocking agent should usually be administered concomitantly.

Rate-Control Versus Rhythm-Control Strategies

Several prospective, randomized trials have been published comparing the strategies of rate control and rhythm control in patients with AF. The AFFIRM trial enrolled 4,060 patients aged older than 65 years or with risk factors for stroke, randomizing them to rate versus rhythm control. Over a mean follow-up period of 3.5 years, there was no significant difference in overall mortality between the two groups.

CONTROL OF VENTRICULAR RATE   Control of the ventricular rate involves both acute and chronic phases. In the acute phase, intravenous diltiazem, metoprolol, esmolol, and verapamil have all been demonstrated to provide slowing of AV nodal conduction within 5 minutes; these drugs are indicated for patients with severe symptoms related to a rapid ventricular rate. Intravenous digoxin requires a longer duration to achieve rate control and is less useful. For patients with only mild or moderate symptoms, oral medications that slow AV nodal conduction should be prescribed. After control of the resting ventricular rate has been achieved, attention is paid to the ambulatory heart rate. There is no overall agreement on what constitutes optimum rate control.

Digoxin may provide effective control of the resting heart rate but is often ineffective during exertion. Beta-adrenergic blockers or calcium-channel antagonists provide much better control of the ventricular rate during exercise and should be considered for most patients.

ABLATION OF THE ATRIOVENTRICULAR NODE   Some patients may continue to experience significant symptoms from a rapid or irregular ventricular rhythm despite drug therapy. Chronically elevated ventricular rates (usually > 120 bpm) despite adequate trials of AV nodal blocking agents can cause a tachycardia-induced cardiomyopathy. Catheter ablation of the AV conduction system and permanent pacemaker implantation is a highly effective means of establishing permanent control of the ventricular rate during AF in selected patients. Despite the many favorable effects of this procedure, there are several limitations. First, AV nodal ablation does not change the long-term need for anticoagulation. Second, although an adequate junctional escape rhythm is typically present after ablation, patients should be considered permanently pacemaker dependent. Third, because this procedure does not restore AV synchrony, patients who are highly dependent on mechanical atrial contraction often do not experience as much improvement as other patients. Fourth, right ventricular pacing produces an abnormal LV contraction sequence, and acute worsening of hemodynamics has been observed in some patients. In the Post AV Node Ablation Evaluation (PAVE) trial, patients who received biventricular versus RV apical pacing, especially those with abnormal LV ejection fractions before ablation, had longer 6-minute walking distances and higher LV ejection fractions after ablation.

MAINTENANCE OF SINUS RHYTHM   When a rhythm-control strategy is chosen for patients with paroxysmal or persistent AF, prophylactic treatment with antiarrhythmic drugs is usually needed to maintain sinus rhythm. Although the ideal of pharmacologic therapy would be to prevent all recurrences of AF, this is unrealistic for many patients. Rather, marked reduction of the frequency, duration, and symptoms of AF may be a very acceptable clinical goal. In addition, the use of pharmacologic agents to prevent AF does not change the indication for anticoagulation.

As compared with drug therapy for life-threatening arrhythmias, the choice of pharmacologic agent is largely determined by the potential side effects of a given drug in an individual patient.

ANTIARRHYTHMIC DRUG SELECTION   Antiarrhythmic drugs are selected on a safety-first basis (Fig. 10-6). The ACC/AHA/ESC guidelines suggest for patients with no or minimal heart disease to start with flecainide, propafenone, or sotalol, agents with minimal noncardiac toxicity. The second-line therapy is either amiodarone/dofetilide or catheter ablation. Patients with hypertension who do not have substantial LV hypertrophy have a similar treatment algorithm; but those with substantial LV hypertrophy are considered at increased proarrhythmia risk with most drugs other than amiodarone, which becomes first-line therapy here. Catheter ablation is second-line treatment. Safety of drugs in coronary artery disease has been demonstrated for dofetilide/sotalol (first-line) and amiodarone (second-line), and catheter ablation is also second-line treatment.

Surgical Treatment

Several surgical treatments for the prevention of AF have been developed. Success rates have ranged from 70% to 95%. For patients with AF who are undergoing cardiac surgery, consideration should be given to concomitant AF surgery. Otherwise, its role is typically for patients who require sinus rhythm for symptom relief and have failed to respond to antiarrhythmic drugs and catheter ablation.

CATHETER ABLATION   Recent approaches to catheter ablation of AF, especially paroxysmal AF, have been to eliminate triggering foci, primarily within the pulmonary veins but also in the LA posterior wall, superior vena cava, crista terminalis, vein of Marshall, and coronary sinus. Various techniques have been employed to isolate the pulmonary veins, including the use of intracardiac echocardiography or an electroanatomical mapping system to guide delivery of radiofrequency energy circumferentially outside of the pulmonary veins.

ATRIAL FLUTTER

【 】 CLASSIFICATION AND MECHANISMS

There are several types of atrial flutter, all having rapid, regular atrial rates, generally 240 to 340 bpm, because of a reentrant mechanism in the atria. Typical atria flutter, also called *counterclockwise atrial flutter,* is characterized by negative sawtooth flutter waves (Fig. 10-7); and reverse typical atria flutter, also called *atypical* or *clockwise atrial flutter,* is characterized by positive flutter waves in ECG leads II, III, and aVF These two atrial flutter types share the same right atrial reentrant circuit.

【 】 EPIDEMIOLOGY

Atrial flutter often is a persistent rhythm, but more typically it is paroxysmal, lasting for variable periods. In most patients it is spontaneously induced by a premature atrial beat or beats that produce a transitional rhythm, resembling AF. Atrial flutter commonly occurs in patients in the first week after open-heart surgery. Atrial flutter is also associated with chronic obstructive pulmonary disease, mitral or tricuspid

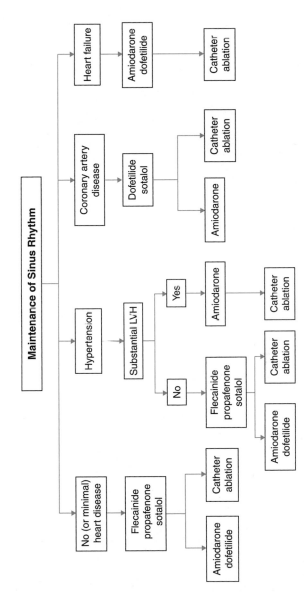

FIGURE 10-6. Proposed strategy for use of antiarrhythmic drugs to maintain sinus rhythm in patients with atrial fibrillation. (LVH, left ventricular hypertrophy.) (Modified with permission from Fuster V, Rydén LE, Cannom DS, et al. ACC/AHA/ESC 2006 guidelines for the management of patients with atrial fibrillation: a report of the American College of Cardiology/American Heart Association Task Force on Practice Guidelines and the European Society of Cardiology Committee for Practice Guidelines (Writing Committee to Revise the 2001 Guidelines for the Management of Patients With Atrial Fibrillation). *Eur Heart J.* 2006;27(16):1979–2030.)

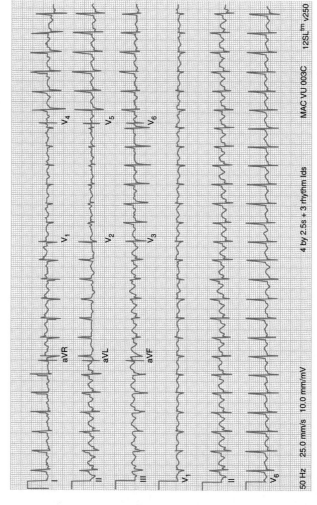

FIGURE 10-7. Twelve-lead electrocardiogram of typical atrial flutter. Note the negative flutter waves in leads II, III, and aVF, and the upright flutter waves in lead V₁. This is characteristic of counterclockwise, isthmus-dependent atrial flutter.

valve disease, thyrotoxicosis, and postsurgical repair of certain congenital cardiac lesions (e.g., atrial septal defect, the Mustard procedure, the Senning procedure, or the Fontan procedure), as well as enlargement of the atria for any reason, especially the right atrium.

【 】 DIAGNOSIS

Atrial flutter usually can be diagnosed from the ECG (see Fig. 10-7). The standard for the diagnosis of atrial flutter is the presence of atrial complexes of constant morphology, polarity, and cycle length. On occasion, the identification of atrial flutter complexes in the ECG may be difficult because of their temporal superimposition on other ECG deflections, such as the QRS complex or the T wave, or because of their very low amplitude. Use of vagal maneuvers or the intravenous administration of adenosine to prolong transiently AV conduction may result in AV nodal block and reveal atrial flutter complexes in the ECG if they are present.

【 】 MANAGEMENT

Acute Treatment

Usually, atrial flutter should be treated acutely to restore sinus rhythm, or at the very least to control the ventricular response rate as needed. Transthoracic direct current (DC) cardioversion of atrial flutter to sinus rhythm has a very high likelihood of success. Antiarrhythmic drug therapy to restore sinus rhythm is primarily intravenous ibutilide, which is associated with a 60% likelihood of converting recent atrial flutter to sinus rhythm. Intravenous procainamide may also be useful in converting atrial flutter to normal sinus rhythm.

Drug therapy may also be used to slow the ventricular response rate as needed. Useful agents include beta-blockers, verapamil, diltiazem, and digitalis, alone or in combination. It is often difficult to achieve sufficient AV nodal block to slow adequately the ventricular response during atrial flutter, and 2:1 AV conduction frequently recurs. For this reason cardioversion to sinus rhythm is the best option, if possible. When using a class I antiarrhythmic drug, especially a IC agent, to treat atrial flutter, care must be taken to provide adequate AV block.

Long-Term Treatment

CATHETER ABLATION THERAPY   Catheter ablation is highly successful, typically 9% or greater, to cure atrial flutter. This coupled with the recognized difficulty in achieving adequate long-term suppression with antiarrhythmic drug therapy make catheter ablation a first-line treatment option for many patients. Because classical atrial flutter is usually preceded by a variable period of AF, successful ablation of the atrial flutter reentrant circuit per se may not prevent either the new appearance or the recurrence of AF.

ANTIARRHYTHMIC DRUG THERAPY   Selection of an antiarrhythmic drug to treat atrial flutter mirrors that to treat AF. However, this form of therapy is no longer the treatment of choice for long-term therapy in most patients with atrial flutter, because catheter ablation to cure atrial flutter has superceded it.

ANTICOAGULANT THERAPY   In patients with atrial flutter, daily warfarin therapy to achieve an INR between 2 and 3 (target 2.5) is recommended using the same criteria as for AF. In addition, several studies indicate that the incidence of stroke associated with atrial flutter approaches that of AF.

FOCAL ATRIAL TACHYCARDIA

【 】 CLASSIFICATION

The term atrial tachycardia refers to rapid (usually 130 to 250 bpm), relatively regular rhythms that originate in the atria, do not require participation of either the sinus node or the AV node for maintenance, and are neither AF nor atrial flutter (Fig. 10-8). Focal atrial tachycardia is characterized by atrial activation starting rhythmically at a small area (focus). Potential mechanisms include reentry, automaticity, and triggered activity. Foci are most frequently found in the pulmonary veins in the LA and the crista terminalis in the right atrium, but can occur at various sites in both atria. When incessant, they may be associated with a dilated cardiomyopathy and CHF.

【 】 MECHANISM

An automatic focus may demonstrate progressive rate increase at tachycardia onset (warm-up) and/or progressive rate decrease before termination (cool down), does not respond to vagal maneuvers, and often displays an incessant nature.

【 】 EPIDEMIOLOGY

The incidence of focal atrial tachycardia increases with age, reportedly occurring in up to 13% of elderly subjects. An increased incidence has been reported in patients with myocardial infarction, nonischemic heart disease, obstructive lung disease, serum electrolyte disorders, and drug toxicity, especially caused by digitalis. However, focal atrial tachycardia may occur in normal individuals, and nonsustained episodes have been noted in 2% of healthy young adults. Most episodes of focal atrial tachycardia are paroxysmal (deemed largely caused by reentry or triggered activity), but some episodes may be incessant (considered largely caused by automaticity).

【 】 DIAGNOSIS

A standard way to determine the presence or absence of an AV nodal independent atrial tachycardia is to demonstrate that despite the presence of conduction block at the AV node, the rhythm continues. Termination of a supraventricular tachycardia by a drug such as adenosine that causes transient AV node block generally supports the diagnosis of an underlying AV nodal-dependent reentrant tachycardia—for example, AV node reentry. However, adenosine is known to terminate some atrial tachycardias, so that termination of an atrial tachyarrhythmia after the administration of intravenous adenosine cannot be used per se to characterize the rhythm as AV nodal dependent. The same seems true for beta-blockers. A useful sign of AV nodal dependence is consistent termination of tachycardia with a P wave without conduction to the ventricles. Unfortunately, termination with a conducted P wave and no further arrhythmia can occur with AV nodal dependent and independent arrhythmias, and provides little diagnostic utility.

【 】 TREATMENT

For focal atrial tachycardia, especially in patients with clinically important (usually symptomatic, incessant, or both) atrial tachycardia, catheter ablation is usually the primary therapy regardless of the underlying mechanism. Reports of catheter ablation therapy for reentrant atrial tachycardia demonstrate a success rate > 75%.

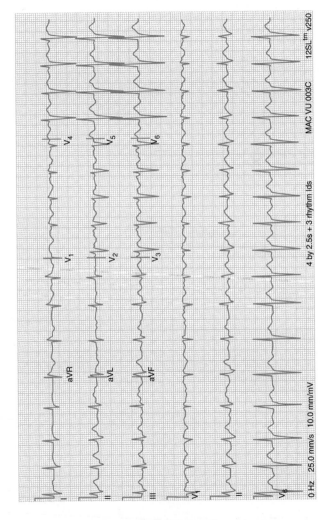

FIGURE 10-8. Surface electrocardiogram of an atrial tachycardia involving the right atrium. Note the discrete P waves with 2:1 AV conduction.

MULTIFOCAL ATRIAL TACHYCARDIA

Multifocal atrial tachycardia (MAT) remains largely a descriptive entity with a need for better characterization. MAT is usually diagnosed by ECG criteria that include an atrial rate greater that 100 bpm with P waves of at least three distinct morphologies. The diagnosis of MAT can be difficult. The chaotic nature of the P-wave morphology with varying AV intervals makes confusion with AF common.

【 】 MECHANISM

The mechanism underlying MAT is unknown. Several reports have noted that MAT cannot be induced or initiated by programmed stimulation. Thus, reentry seems an unlikely mechanism. Anecdotal reports of successful treatment of MAT with calcium-channel blockers or beta-blockers are consistent with both automatic and triggered mechanisms.

【 】 EPIDEMIOLOGY

MAT is often observed in patients with acute pulmonary disorders and associated hypoxia. Patients with MAT are usually acutely ill and often are receiving agonists or theophylline preparations. As such, both agonists and theophylline have been causally implicated.

【 】 TREATMENT

The therapeutic issues revolve around the extent to which the rapid ventricular response rate during MAT affects the clinical condition of the patient. If the ventricular response is controlled (usually difficult), MAT per se probably shouldn't affect the patient's clinical course.

The basis for therapy should principally be correction of the underlying pulmonary problem. DC cardioversion has not provided successful therapy in patients with MAT. There is limited experience reported with the use of standard antiarrhythmic drugs. Blockers have been used with success in selected patients. Precipitation of bronchospasm may be a potentially fatal complication when blockers are used in acutely ill patients. Thus, short-acting 1-specific agents like esmolol seem most appropriate for initial use. Beta-blockers have been used with limited success. In selected patients, blockers may have a role in the treatment of patients with MAT. It remains questionable whether or not antiarrhythmic drug therapy will affect outcome in this dramatically ill group of patients.

APPENDIX 10-1

Class I (Positive) and Class III (Negative) Recommendations for Management of Atrial Fibrillation[a]

Pharmacologic Rate Control During Atrial Fibrillation
Class I
1. Measurement of the heart rate at rest and control of the rate using pharmacologic agents (either a beta-blocker or nondihydropyridine calcium-channel antagonist, in most cases) are recommended for patients with persistent or permanent AF. (Level of Evidence: B)
2. In the absence of preexcitation, IV administration of beta-blockers (esmolol, metoprolol, or propranolol) or nondihydropyridine calcium-channel antagonists (verapamil, diltiazem) is recommended to slow the ventricular response to AF in

the acute setting, exercising caution in patients with hypotension or heart failure (HF). *(Level of Evidence: B)*

3. IV administration of digoxin or amiodarone is recommended to control the heart rate in patients with AF and HF who do not have an accessory pathway. *(Level of Evidence: B)*

4. In patients who experience symptoms related to AF during activity, the adequacy of heart rate control should be assessed during exercise, adjusting pharmacologic treatment as necessary to keep the rate in the physiologic range. *(Level of Evidence: C)*

5. Digoxin is effective following oral administration to control the heart rate at rest in patients with AF, and is indicated for patients with HF, left ventricular (LV) dysfunction, or for sedentary individuals. *(Level of Evidence: C)*

Class III

1. Digitalis should not be used as the sole agent to control the rate of ventricular response in patients with paroxysmal AF. *(Level of Evidence: B)*

2. Catheter ablation of the AV node should not be attempted without a prior trial of medication to control the ventricular rate in patients with AF. *(Level of Evidence: C)*

3. In patients with decompensated HF and AF, intravenous administration of a nondihydropyridine calcium-channel antagonist may exacerbate hemodynamic compromise and is not recommended. *(Level of Evidence: C)*

4. IV administration of digitalis glycosides or nondihydropyridine calcium-channel antagonists to patients with AF and a preexcitation syndrome may paradoxically accelerate the ventricular response and is not recommended. *(Level of Evidence: C)*

Preventing Thromboembolism

Class I

1. Antithrombotic therapy to prevent thromboembolism is recommended for all patients with AF, except those with lone AF or contraindications. *(Level of Evidence: A)*

2. The selection of the antithrombotic agent should be based upon the absolute risks of stroke and bleeding and the relative risk and benefit for a given patient. *(Level of Evidence: A)*

3. For patients without mechanical heart valves at high risk of stroke, chronic oral anticoagulant therapy with a vitamin K antagonist is recommended in a dose adjusted to achieve the target intensity international normalized ratio (INR) of 2.0 to 3.0, unless contraindicated. Factors associated with highest risk for stroke in patients with AF are prior thromboembolism (stroke, transient ischemic attack [TIA], or systemic embolism) and rheumatic mitral stenosis. *(Level of Evidence: A)*

4. Anticoagulation with a vitamin K antagonist is recommended for patients with more than one moderate risk factor. Such factors include age 75 y or greater, hypertension, HF, impaired LV systolic function (ejection fraction 35% or less or fractional shortening less than 25%), and diabetes mellitus. *(Level of Evidence: A)*

5. INR should be determined at least weekly during initiation of therapy and monthly when anticoagulation is stable. *(Level of Evidence: A)*

6. Aspirin, 81–325 mg daily, is recommended as an alternative to vitamin K antagonists in low-risk patients or in those with contraindications to oral anticoagulation. *(Level of Evidence: A)*

7. For patients with AF who have mechanical heart valves, the target intensity of anticoagulation should be based on the type of prosthesis, maintaining an INR of at least 2.5. *(Level of Evidence: B)*

8. Antithrombotic therapy is recommended for patients with atrial flutter as for those with AF. *(Level of Evidence: C)*

Class III

Long-term anticoagulation with a vitamin K antagonist is not recommended for primary prevention of stroke in patients below the age of 60 y without heart disease (lone AF) or any risk factors for thromboembolism. *(Level of Evidence: C)*

Cardioversion of Atrial Fibrillation

Pharmacologic Cardioversion
Class I

Administration of flecainide, dofetilide, propafenone, or ibutilide is recommended for pharmacologic cardioversion of AF. *(Level of Evidence: A)*

Class III

1. Digoxin and sotalol may be harmful when used for pharmacologic cardioversion of AF and are not recommended. *(Level of Evidence: A)*
2. Quinidine, procainamide, disopyramide, and dofetilide should not be started out of hospital for conversion of AF to sinus rhythm. *(Level of Evidence: B)*

Direct-Current Cardioversion
Class I

1. When a rapid ventricular response does not respond promptly to pharmacologic measures for patients with AF with ongoing myocardial ischemia, symptomatic hypotension, angina, or HF, immediate R-wave synchronized direct-current cardioversion is recommended. *(Level of Evidence: C)*
2. Immediate direct-current cardioversion is recommended for patients with AF involving preexcitation when very rapid tachycardia or hemodynamic instability occurs. *(Level of Evidence: B)*
3. Cardioversion is recommended in patients without hemodynamic instability when symptoms of AF are unacceptable to the patient. In case of early relapse of AF after cardioversion, repeated direct-current cardioversion attempts may be made following administration of antiarrhythmic medication. *(Level of Evidence: C)*

Class III

1. Frequent repetition of direct-current cardioversion is not recommended for patients who have relatively short periods of sinus rhythm between relapses of AF after multiple cardioversion procedures despite prophylactic antiarrhythmic drug therapy. *(Level of Evidence: C)*
2. Electrical cardioversion is contraindicated in patients with digitalis toxicity or hypokalemia. *(Level of Evidence: C)*

Pharmacologic Enhancement of Direct-Current Cardioversion
Class I

1. For patients with AF of 48-h duration of longer, or when the duration of AF is unknown, anticoagulation (INR 2.0–3.0) is recommended for at least 3 wk prior to and 4 wk after cardioversion , regardless of the method (electrical or pharmacologic) used to restore sinus rhythm. *(Level of Evidence: B)*
2. For patients with AF or more than 48-h duration requiring immediate cardioversion because of hemodynamic instability, heparin should be administered concurrently (unless contraindicated) by an initial intravenous bolus injection followed by a continuous infusion in a dose adjusted to prolong the activated partial thromboplastin time to 1.5–2 times the reference control value. Thereafter, oral anticoagulation (INR 2.0–3.0) should be provided for at least 4 wk, as for patients undergoing elective cardioversion. Limited data support subcutaneous administration of low-molecular-weight heparin in this indication. *(Level of Evidence: C)*

3. For patients with AF of less than 48-h duration associated with hemodynamic instability (angina pectoris, myocardial infarction [MI], shock, or pulmonary edema), cardioversion should be performed immediately without delay for prior initiation of anticoagulation. (Level of Evidence: C)

Maintenance of Sinus Rhythm

Class I
Before initiating antiarrhythmic drug therapy, treatment of precipitating or reversible causes of AF is recommended. (Level of Evidence: C)

Class III
1. Antiarrhythmic therapy with a particular drug is not recommended for maintenance of sinus rhythm in patients with AF who have well-defined risk factors for proarrhythmia with that agent. (Level of Evidence: A)
2. Pharmacologic therapy is not recommended for maintenance of sinus rhythm in patients with advanced sinus node disease or atrioventricular (AV) node dysfunction unless they have a functioning electronic cardiac pacemaker. (Level of Evidence: C)

Special Considerations

Postoperative Atrial Fibrillation
Class I
1. Unless contraindicated, treatment with an oral beta-blocker to prevent postoperative AF is recommended for patients undergoing cardiac surgery. (Level of Evidence: A)
2. Administration of AV nodal blocking agents is recommended to achieve rate control in patients who develop postoperative AF. (Level of Evidence: B)

Acute Myocardial Infarction

Class I
1. Direct-current cardioversion is recommended for patients with severe hemodynamic compromise or intractable ischemia, or when adequate rate control cannot be achieved with pharmacologic agents in patients with acute MI and AF. (Level of Evidence: C)
2. Intravenous administration of amiodarone is recommended to slow a rapid ventricular response to AF and improve LV function in patients with acute MI. (Level of Evidence: C)
3. Intravenous beta-blockers and nondihydropyridine calcium antagonists are recommended to slow a rapid ventricular response to AF in patients with acute MI who do not display clinical LV dysfunction, bronchospasm, or AV block. (Level of Evidence: C)
4. For patients with AF and acute MI, administration of unfractionated heparin by either continuous intravenous infusion of intermittent subcutaneous injection is recommended in a dose sufficient to prolong the activated partial thromboplastin time to 1.5 to 2 times the control value, unless contraindications to anticoagulation exist. (Level of Evidence: C)

Class III
The administration of class IC antiarrhythmic drugs is not recommended in patients with AF in the setting of acute MI. (Level of Evidence: C)

Management of Atrial Fibrillation Associated with Wolff-Parkinson-White (WPW) Preexcitation Syndrome

Class I

1. Catheter ablation of the accessory pathway is recommended in symptomatic patients with AF who have WPW syndrome, particularly those with syncope due to rapid heart rate or those with a short bypass tract refractory period. *(Level of Evidence: B)*
2. Immediate direct-current cardioversion is recommended to prevent ventricular fibrillation in patients with a short anterograde bypass tract refractory period in whom AF occurs with a rapid ventricular response associated with hemodynamic instability. *(Level of Evidence: B)*
3. IV procainamide or ibutilide is recommended to restore sinus rhythm in patients with WPW in whom AF occurs without hemodynamic instability in association with a wide QRS complex on the ECG (greater than or equal to 120-ms duration) or with a rapid preexcited ventricular response. *(Level of Evidence: C)*

Class III

IV administration of digitalis glycosides or nondihydropyridine calcium-channel antagonists is not recommended in patients with WPW syndrome who have preexcited ventricular activation during AF. *(Level of Evidence: B)*

Hyperthyroidism

Class I

1. Administration of a beta-blocker is recommended to control the rate of a ventricular response in patients with AF complicating thyrotoxicosis, unless contraindicated. *(Level of Evidence: B)*
2. In circumstances when a beta-blocker cannot be used, administration of a nondihydropyridine calcium-channel antagonist (diltiazem or verapamil) is recommended to control the ventricular rate in patients with AF and thyrotoxicosis. *(Level of Evidence: B)*
3. In patients with AF associated with thyrotoxicosis, oral anticoagulation (INR 2.0 –3.0) is recommended to prevent thromboembolism, as recommended for AF patients with other risk factors for stroke. *(Level of Evidence: C)*
4. Once a euthyroid state is restored, recommendations for antithrombotic prophylaxis are the same as for patients without hyperthyroidism. *(Level of Evidence: C)*

Management of Atrial Fibrillation During Pregnancy

Class I

1. Digoxin, a beta-blocker, or a nondihydropyridine calcium-channel antagonist, is recommended to control the rate of ventricular response in pregnant patients with AF. *(Level of Evidence: C)*
2. Direct-current cardioversion is recommended in pregnant patients who become hemodynamically unstable due to AF *(Level of Evidence: C)*
3. Protection against thromboembolism is recommended throughout pregnancy for all patients with AF (except for those with lone AF and/or low thromboembolic risk). Therapy (anticoagulant or aspirin) should be chose according to stage of pregnancy. *(Level of Evidence: C)*

Management of Atrial Fibrillation in Patients with Hypertrophic Cardiomyopathy (HCM)

Class I

Oral anticoagulation (INR 2.0–3.0) is recommended in patients with HCM who develop AF, as for other patients at high risk of thromboembolism. *(Level of Evidence: B)*

Management of Atrial Fibrillation in Patients with Pulmonary Disease

Class I

1. Correction of hypoxemia and acidosis is the recommended primary therapeutic measure for patients who develop AF during an acute pulmonary illness or exacerbation of chronic pulmonary disease. *(Level of Evidence: C)*
2. A nondihydropyridine calcium-channel antagonist (diltiazem or verapamil) is recommended to control the ventricular rate in patients with obstructive pulmonary disease who develop AF. *(Level of Evidence: C)*
3. Direct-current cardioversion should be attempted in patients with pulmonary disease who become hemodynamically unstable as a consequence of AF. *(Level of Evidence: C)*

Class III

1. Theophylline and beta-adrenergic agonist agents are not recommended in patients with bronchospastic lung disease who develop AF. *(Level of Evidence: C)*
2. Beta-blockers, sotalol, propafenone, and adenosine are not recommended in patients with obstructive lung disease who develop AF. *(Level of Evidence: C)*

°See also Chapter 59

Data compiled from Fuster V, Rydén LE, Cannom DS, et al. ACC/AHA/ESC 2006 guidelines for the management of patients with atrial fibrillation: a report of the American College of Cardiology/American Heart Association Task Force on Practice Guidelines and the European Society of Cardiology Committee for Practice Guidelines (Writing Committee to Revise the 2001 Guidelines for the Management of Patients with Atrial Fibrillation). *Circulation.* 2006;114:e257–e354.

SUPRAVENTRICULAR ARRHYTHMIAS

【 】 SINUS RHYTHM AND SINUS TACHYCARDIA

Normal sinus rhythm is defined as a rate of 60 to 100 bpm, originating in the sinus node; the rhythm is regular. Sinus arrhythmia is present when the variation between the longest and the shortest cycle on a resting tracing is above 0.12 seconds. This is a normal variant occuring most commonly in the young.

Sinus tachycardia is characterized by normal sinus P waves at a rate greater than 100 per minute. It usually does not exceed 130 to 140 bpm under resting conditions, but can be as high as 180 to 200 bpm, particularly during exercise. Sinus tachycardia is a normal physiologic response to exercise or emotional stress or may be pharmacologically induced by such drugs as epinephrine, ephedrine, or atropine. Exposure to alcohol, caffeine, or nicotine can also cause sinus tachycardia. Vagotonic maneuvers, such as carotid sinus massage or Valsalva maneuver, may help differentiate sinus tachycardia from other supraventricular tachycardias (SVTs). Gradual slowing of the rapid rate followed by gradual return to that rate is typical for sinus tachycardia. In contrast, vagal maneuvers may abruptly terminate other SVTs by blocking conduction in the AV node. Sinus tachycardia usually requires no specific treatment; management should be directed toward the underlying disorder.

【 】 PREMATURE ATRIAL CONTRACTIONS

Atrial extrasystoles or premature atrial contractions (PACs) are impulses that arise in an ectopic atrial focus and are premature in relation to the prevailing sinus rate. The early P wave has a different vector from the sinus P wave, and the PR interval of the conducted PAC may be normal or prolonged. If the coupling interval of the PAC to the previous sinus P wave is short, aberrant intraventricular conduction may occur, making the diagnosis dependent on recognition of the P wave distorting the previous T wave. The hallmark of the timing of PACs is the less than fully compensatory pause; however, this may not always occur. The significance of atrial extrasystoles depends on the clinical setting in which they occur. Often they are found in completely normal individuals.

【 】 SUPRAVENTRICULAR TACHYARRHYTHMIAS

All tachyarrhythmias that originate above the bifurcation of the bundle of His are classified as supraventricular arrhythmias. The atrial rate must be 100 or more bpm for a diagnosis, but the ventricular rate may be less when AV conduction is incomplete. SVTs usually have narrow QRS configurations, but they may be wide because of aberrant conduction through the intraventricular conduction tissue, preexisting bundle branch block, or conduction via an accessory pathway. Atrial activity may be identified by using a long rhythm strip with multiple leads. Recording the rhythm strip at a rapid paper speed (e.g., 50 mm/s) may be helpful. Other diagnostic aids include vagal maneuvers or drug therapy to slow the AV conduction rate or an esophageal lead to identify atrial activity (Table 10-1). Intraatrial electrograms are occasionally required.

SVTs may be classified as *paroxysmal* (lasting seconds to hours), *persistent* (lasting days to weeks), or *chronic* (lasting weeks to years). Consideration not only of the duration of the tachyarrhythmia but also of its electrophysiologic mechanism is essential to appropriate management. Paroxysmal SVT (PSVT) may occur in the presence or absence of heart disease and in patients of all ages. It is most often due to reentry involving the AV node or an accessory pathway; infrequently, sinus node reentry or intra-atrial reentry is the mechanism.

【 】 SUPRAVENTRICULAR TACHYCARDIA DUE TO ATRIOVENTRICULAR NODAL REENTRY

AV nodal reentry is the most common mechanism of SVT and is characterized electrophysiologically by two functionally distinct pathways within or near the AV node. In the common form of AV nodal reentrant tachycardia, antegrade conduction occurs over the slow pathway and retrograde conduction over the fast pathway, resulting in almost simultaneous activation of the atria and ventricles. Electrocardiographically, retrograde P waves are hidden within the QRS complex or appear immediately after it. In the uncommon form, in which antegrade conduction occurs over the fast pathway, the retrograde P wave occurs well after the end of the QRS complex and is characterized by a long R-P interval and a short PR interval with an inverted P wave in II, III, and aVF. In the absence of structural heart disease, PSVT due to AV nodal reentry is a benign rhythm and may be treated acutely with rest, sedation, and vagotonic maneuvers. If these physiologic interventions are unsuccessful, intravenous adenosine, intravenous calcium antagonists, digoxin, or beta-adrenergic blockers may be used. Adenosine, 6 mg intravenously, followed by one or two 12-mg boluses if necessary, has an extremely short half-life (10 sec), causes no hemodynamic complications, and is the *first choice* for treatment of PSVT (Table 10-5).

Long-term therapy for control of recurrent SVT due to AV nodal reentry is most frequently achieved today with either pharmacologic methods or catheter-ablation techniques. No chronic therapy may be necessary in patients who have infrequent, short-lived, well-tolerated attacks and/or who respond to physiologic maneuvers. Patients who have more frequent attacks, who are intolerant to medications, and/or whose SVTs cause hemodynamic compromise are offered *radiofrequency catheter ablation* for curative therapy. Ablation of AV nodal reentry is achieved by selective ablation of the slow pathway to abolish the reentrant loop. Less commonly, ablation of the fast pathway will be performed, but the risk of iatrogenic heart block is higher. In either case, experience has demonstrated that this is a safe and effective technique for the management of AV nodal reentry (Table 10-6).

Pharmacologic therapy is an alternative for patients who do not desire radiofrequency ablation or who have few, well-tolerated occurrences. Beta-adrenergic blocking agents, verapamil, or digoxin in standard doses may be used. In patients with no structural heart disease, class IC agents may be used (Table 10-7).

TABLE 10-5

Differentiation of Various Narrow-Qrs-Complex Tachycardias Using ECG[a] and Response to Carotid Sinus Pressure (CSP) or IV Adenosine (A)

1. Irregular tachycardia
   a. Atrial fibrillation: ventricular rate transiently slows with CSP or A
   b. Atrial flutter with varying AV conduction: ventricular rate slows with CSP or A, and flutter waves seen at ≥ 240/min
   c. Multifocal atrial tachycardia: different P-wave morphologies
2. Regular tachycardia with no visible P waves
   AVNRT: rate 140–250/min. No change or terminates with CSP or A
3. Regular tachycardia, atrial rate greater than ventricular (baseline, CSP or A)
   a. Atrial flutter: regular flutter waves at ≥ 240/min
   b. Atrial tachycardia with block: abnormal P waves at 100–240/min
4. Regular tachycardia with RP shorter than PR
   a. AVNRT: P at the end of QRS, with RP < 70 msec. No change or terminates with CSP or A
   b. Orthodromic AVRT: RP > 70 msec; no change or terminates with CSP or A
   c. Atrial tachycardia with first-degree AV block: RP > 70 msec, AV block worsens with CSP or A
5. Regular tachycardia with RP longer than PR
   a. Ectopic atrial tachycardia: abnormal P waves, AV block with CSP or A
   b. Atypical AVNRT: abnormal P wave, no change or terminates with CSP or A
   c. Sinus node reentry: paroxysmal P wave similar to sinus, terminates with premature atrial beats, CSP or A
   d. Sinus tachycardia: normal P waves, transient slowing with CSP or A
6. AV dissociation present
   Paroxysmal junctional tachycardia

AVNRT, AV nodal reciprocating tachycardia; AVRT, AV reciprocating tachycardia; CSP, carotid sinus pressure.

[a]Twelve-lead ECG is necessary to identify P waves.

TABLE 10-6

Drugs for Acute Management of Supraventricular Tachycardia

Drug	Dosage
Adenosine	IV: 6 mg rapidly; if unsuccessful within 1–2 min, 12 mg rapidly
Diltiazem	IV: 0.25 mg/kg body wt over 2 min; if response inadequate, wait 15 min, then 0.35 mg/kg over 2 min; maintenance of 10–15 mg/h
Digoxin[a]	IV: 0.5 mg over 10 min; if response inadequate, 0.25 mg q 4 h to a maximum of 1.5 mg in 24 h
Esmolol	IV: 500 µg/kg per min × 1 min followed by 50 µg/kg per min × 4 min, repeat with 50-µg increments to maintenance dose of 200 µg/kg/min
Procainamide	IV: 10–15 mg/kg at 25 mg/min as loading dose, then 1–4 mg/min
Propranolol	IV: 0.1 mg/kg in divided 1-mg doses
Vorapamil	IV: 5 mg over 1 min; if unsuccessful, one to two 5-mg boluses 10 min apart

[a]Contraindicated in patients with Wolff–Parkinson–White syndrome.

TABLE 10-7

Antiarrhyhmic Drugs: Dosage and Kinetics

Drug		Usual Dosing Range[a]	Half-Life	Therapeutic Range (μg/mL)	Plasma Protein Binding (%)	Major Route of Excretion
Class IA	Quinidine	Oral sulfate: 200–600 mg q6h Oral longacting: 330–660 mg, q8h or q6h	5–7 h	2.3–5	80	H
	Procainamide	Oral: 250–750 mg, q4h or q6h Oral longacting: 500–1500 mg, q8h or q6h IV: 10–15 mg/kg at 25 mg/min, then 1–6 mg/min	3–5 h	4–10	15	R[b]
	Disopyramide	Oral: 100–200 mg q8h or q6h	8–9 h	2–5	35–95	H/R
	Moricizine[c]	Oral: 150–300 mg q12h to q8h	6–13 h	—	95	H
Class IB	Lidocaine	IV: 1–3 mg/kg at 20–50 mg/min, then 1–4 mg/min	1–2 h	1–5	60	H
	Tocainide	Oral: 400–600 mg 8–12 h	15 h	4–10	10	H
	Mexiletine	Oral: 200–400 mg q8h	10–12 h	0.5–2.0	55	H
Class IC	Flecainide	Oral: 100–200 mg q12h	20 h	0.4–1.0	40	H
	Encainide	Oral: 25–50 mg q8h	3–4+ h	0.5–1.0[d]	80	H
	Propafenone[a]	Oral: 150–300 mg q8h	2–10 h	0.5–1.5[d]	95	H
Class II	Propranolol	Oral: 10–100 mg q6h	4–6 h	0.04–0.10	95	H
	Esmolol	IV: 0.1 mg/kg in divided 1 mg doses IV: 500 μg/kg per min × 1 min followed by 50 μg/kg per min × 4 min, repeat with 50μg increments to maintenance dose to 200 μg/kg per min	9 min	—	55	H
Class III	Acebutolol	Oral: 200–600 mg bid	3–4 h	—	26	H/R
	Amiodarone	Oral: 600–1600 mg/day × 1–3 weeks, then 200–400 mg/day IV: 5 mg/min × min, then 1 mg/min × 6 h, then maintenance at 0.5 mg/min	50 days ?	1–2.5 ?	96	H

136

	Dosing	Half-life		Bioavailability	Elimination
Bretylium	IV: 5–10 mg/kg at 1–2 mg/kg, then 0.5–2.0 mg/min	8–14 h	0.5–1.5	—	R
Sotalol[d]	Oral: 80–320 mg q12h	10–15 h	—	0	R
Ibutilide	IV: (for > 60 kg): 1 mg over 10 min, may repeat × 1. 10 min after completion of initial dose[c]	2–12 h	—	40	H
Class IV Verapamil	Oral: 80–32 mg q6–8h; IV: 5–10 mg in 1–2 min	3–8 h	0.1–0.15	90	H
Diltiazem	IV: 0.25 mg/kg body wt over 2 min; if response inadequate, wait 15 min, then 0.35 mg/kg over 2 min; maintenance 10–15 mg/h	3.5–5.0 h	0.1–3.0	70–80	H
Other Digoxin	Oral: 1.25–1.5 mg in divided doses over 24 h followed by 0.125–0.375 mg/day IV: Approximately 70% of oral dose	36 h	0.8–1.4 mg/ml	30	R
Adenosine	IV: 6 mg rapidly; if unsuccessful within 1–2 min, 12 mg rapidly	10 s	—	—	—

H, hepatic; R, renal.

[a] All dosing should follow FDA-approved guidelines as outlined in package insert or *Physicians' Desk Reference*. See also Chap. 43. Does not include pediatric use in infants and young children.
[b] Parent compound metabolized to active metabolite (NAPA) in liver; both active metabolite and unmetabolized parent compound excreted by kidneys.
[c] Shares classes IB, IC activities.
[d] Active metabolite limits significance of these measurements.

【 】 SUPRAVENTRICULAR TACHYCARDIA DUE TO WOLFF–PARKINSON–WHITE SYNDROME

This is the second most common form of reentrant SVT. When conduction during an SVT occurs antegrade through the AV node and retrograde through the accessory pathway, it is referred to as an *orthodromic* reciprocating tachycardia. This is the common form of SVT in Wolff–Parkinson–White (WPW) syndrome; the ECG pattern is a narrow-QRS tachycardia at rates ranging from 160 to 240 bpm. *Antidromic* SVT, referring to antegrade conduction using an accessory pathway and retrograde conduction through the normal pathway, is uncommon; the QRS complexes are wide and are similar to fully preexcited impulses during sinus rhythm or premature atrial contractions.

Intracardiac EP studies permit characterization of the accessory pathway and its associated tachyarrhythmias. Electrophysiologic testing is recommended for patients who have frequent or poorly tolerated tachyarrhythmias or a history of atrial fibrillation or atrial flutter (particularly with antegrade bypass tract conduction). *Radiofrequency catheter ablation* of the accessory pathway has revolutionized the treatment of SVT due to WPW syndrome, and today it is the preferred method. Intracardiac mapping utilizing multielectrode catheters allows for localization of the accessory pathway and the subsequent application of radiofrequency energy to abolish the reentrant loop, preventing the recurrence of arrhythmias. Medical therapy with class IC agents may be used temporarily in patients without structural heart disease while the patient awaits ablative therapy or in patients who do not desire ablation.

ECTOPIC ATRIAL TACHYCARDIAS

Ectopic atrial tachycardias are characterized by an abnormal P-wave vector, a tendency to low P-wave amplitude, and rapid atrial rates (range, 160–240 bpm). Ectopic atrial rates in excess of 200 bpm are usually accompanied by 2:1 AV conduction. An ectopic atrial rhythm associated with a high-grade block and a relatively slow ventricular rate (so-called paroxysmal atrial tachycardia [PAT] with block) suggests digitalis intoxication.

Antiarrhythmic agents may provide effective treatment if no reversible cause can be found. Cardioversion is rarely helpful. Ectopic atrial tachycardias commonly have precipitating factors; therefore, correction of the inciting factors (e.g., digitalis intoxication, decompensated chronic obstructive pulmonary disease, electrolyte imbalance, metabolic abnormalities, hypoxia, and thyrotoxicosis) is the primary therapy. In patients in whom no reversible cause can be identified, intracardiac localization of the arrhythmia's focus and subsequent radiofrequency ablation may be attempted.

MULTIFOCAL ATRIAL TACHYCARDIA

This tachycardia is identified electrocardiographically by three or more P-wave morphologies and a chaotic, irregular rhythm. The rate is usually < 150 bpm. When the average rate is < 100 bpm, it is not a tachycardia and is referred to as a chaotic or multifocal atrial *rhythm,* but the implications are similar. It occurs most commonly in chronic lung disease but is also seen in patients with severe metabolic abnormalities or sepsis. Although calcium-channel antagonists have been tried with some success, the most effective approach to therapy has been to correct the underlying hypoxia or other metabolic disturbance. There is no role for cardioversion, surgery, or catheter ablation.

ATRIOVENTRICULAR JUNCTIONAL AND ACCELERATED VENTRICULAR RHYTHMS

AV junctional rhythms originate within or just distal to the immediate vicinity of the AV node. This category includes premature AV junctional impulses, accelerated junctional rhythms, and AV junctional tachycardias that may be automatic or reentrant. In AV junctional rhythm, the impulse travels antegrade and retrograde at the same time from the AV junction and is characterized by a normal QRS complex (unless coexistent BBB or aberrancy is present) and a retrograde P wave. Depending on the site of origin and the rate of conduction in each direction, the P wave may occur shortly before the QRS complex, follow the QRS complex, or be lost within it. The rates of AV junctional escape rhythms are usually in the range of 40 to 60 bpm; therefore, these rhythms become manifest only when the sinus impulse fails to reach the AV node within physiologic ranges of rate. These rhythms are secondary, occurring as a result of sinus depression or sinoatrial block, and are a normal physiologic phenomenon. Failure of these escape rhythms can result in significant bradycardia. This is discussed in the section on bradyarrhythmias later in this chapter.

Another type of secondary rhythm is an *accelerated ventricular rhythm*. This occurs because the sinus rate is slow enough to permit an ectopic ventricular rhythm to escape. The ectopic pacemaker is accelerated above its normal physiologic rate of 20 to 40 bpm and overrides the sinus rate, which may be relatively depressed. The rate of an accelerated ventricular rhythm is usually between 50 and 100 bpm, and the QRS complexes are wide. The rhythm commonly begins with one or two fusion beats and then is regular; however, it may show progressive acceleration or deceleration until it terminates spontaneously.

【 】 ACCELERATED JUNCTIONAL AND VENTRICULAR RHYTHMS

If the AV junctional rate exceeds 60 bpm but is less than 100 bpm, it is referred to as an *accelerated junctional rhythm*. These rhythms are seen commonly in patients with acute myocardial infarction (MI), particularly when the inferior wall is involved. They have also been associated with digitalis intoxication, electrolyte abnormalities, hypertensive heart disease, cardiomyopathy, and congenital and rheumatic heart disease. This rhythm usually requires no specific treatment; in fact, the use of antiarrhythmic agents may suppress the subordinate pacemaker required for maintenance of an adequate rate. If a faster ventricular rate is required to maintain adequate hemodynamics, atropine, 0.6 to 1.2 mg intravenously, may be given to increase the sinus rate, or temporary pacing may be used.

【 】 ATRIOVENTRICULAR JUNCTIONAL TACHYCARDIA

Occasionally, the rate of accelerated AV junctional rhythm increases abruptly to the tachycardia range (i.e., ≥ 100 bpm). This phenomenon probably represents an autonomic focus firing at the faster rate, often with AV dissociation. Usually no treatment is needed except in ischemia, when faster heart rates are unacceptable. Persistent AV junctional tachycardia (sometimes referred to as *nonparoxysmal* junctional tachycardia) occasionally occurs in patients with chronic heart disease. The response to treatment is unpredictable, and the rhythm may be resistant to conventional antiarrhythmics. Catheter ablation has been utilized in some patients.

SUGGESTED READING

AFFIRM investigators. A comparison of rate control and rhythm control in patients with atrial fibrillation. *N Engl J Med.* 2002;347:1825–1833.

Blomstrom-Lundqvist C, Scheinman MM, Aliot EM. ACC/AHA/ESC guidelines for the management of patients with supraventricular arrhythmias. *Circulation.* 2003;108:1871–1909.

Cox JL. Cardiac surgery for arrhythmias. *J Cardiovasc Electrophysiol.* 2004;15:250–262.

DiMarco JP. Implantable cardioverter-defibrillators. *N Engl J Med.* 2003;349:1836–1847.

Fuster V, Rydén LE, Cannom DS, et al. ACC/AHA/ESC 2006 guidelines for the management of patients with atrial fibrillation: a report of the American College of Cardiology/American Heart Association Task Force on Practice Guidelines and the European Society of Cardiology Committee for Practice Guidelines (Writing Committee to Revise the 2001 Guidelines for the Management of Patients With Atrial Fibrillation). *Eur Heart J.* 2006;27:1979–2030.

Gregoratos G, Cheitlin MD, Conill A, et al. ACC/AHA guidelines for implantation of cardiac pacemakers and antiarrhythmia devices. *J Am Coll Cardiol.* 1998;31:1175–1209.

Hsu LF, Jais P, Sanders P, et al. Catheter ablation for atrial fibrillation in congestive heart failure. *N Engl J Med.* 2004;351:2373–2383.

Myerburg RJ, Kloosterman EM, Castellanos A. Recognition, clinical assessment, and management of arrhythmias and conduction disturbances. In: Fuster V, Alexander RW, O'Rourke RA, et al., eds. *Hurst's The Heart.* 11th ed. New York, NY: McGraw-Hill; 2004:797–873.

Oral H, Scharf C, Chugh A, et al. Catheter ablation for paroxysmal atrial fibrillation: segmental pulmonary vein ostial ablation versus left atrial ablation. *Circulation.* 2003;108:2355–2360.

CHAPTER (11)

Ventricular Arrhythmias

Mohan N. Viswanathan, Robert W. Rho,
and Richard L. Page

Ventricular arrhythmias occur commonly in clinical practice and range from benign asymptomatic premature ventricular complexes (PVCs) to ventricular fibrillation (VF) resulting in sudden death (Table 11-1). The presence or absence of structural heart disease and left ventricular function (ejection fraction) play a major role in risk stratification; however, it is important to recognize that potentially lethal arrhythmias may occur in structurally normal-appearing hearts. Management depends on the associated symptoms, hemodynamic consequences, and long-term prognosis. The electrocardiographic (ECG) pattern of the ventricular arrhythmia provides important guidance in selecting appropriate management strategies.

PREMATURE VENTRICULAR COMPLEXES

Premature ventricular complexes are frequent in clinical practice. The significance of PVCs depends on their frequency, the presence and severity of structural heart disease, and the presence of associated symptoms.

【 】 PREMATURE VENTRICULAR COMPLEXES IN THE ABSENCE OF STRUCTURAL HEART DISEASE

In general, PVCs that occur in patients without structural heart disease are not associated with excess risk of sudden death, and as such warrant no therapy, unless significant symptoms are present. Therapy is directed toward removal of precipitating factors; occasionally, low-dose beta-adrenergic receptor blockers can offer symptomatic benefit.

【 】 PREMATURE VENTRICULAR COMPLEXES AFTER ACUTE MYOCARDIAL INFARCTION

The relationship between PVCs following myocardial infarction (MI) and sudden death has been studied extensively. In general, the presence of PVCs after an MI is associated with an increased risk of sudden death when the frequency of PVCs exceeds 10 per hour. Patients with larger MIs and lower left ventricular ejection fractions (LVEFs) are at the greatest risk of sudden death.

Despite the risk associated with postinfarct ectopy, the routine use of antiarrhythmic agents in the acute or more remote postinfarct period does not convey benefit, and in some cases increases risk. Thus, the routine prophylactic use of antiarrhythmics following an MI *is not recommended*. Likewise, *treatment of PVCs and nonsustained ventricular tachycardia (VT) with antiarrhythmics is also not recommended* unless they are associated with hemodynamic compromise. If frequent and persistent ventricular ectopy results in hemodynamic instability, a beta-blocker or amiodarone is the preferred agent.

TABLE 11-1

Ventricular Arrhythmias: Mechanisms and Clinical Features

Ventricular Arrhythmia	ECG Features	Mechanism	Clinical Features
Premature ventricular complexes (PVCs)	Variable: CAD: RBBB morphology RVOT PVCs: LBBB morphology	Reentry focal triggered	Significance depends on structural heart disease
Ischemic ventricular tachycardia	Variable: usually RBBB morphology	Reentry most common	Significance depends on etiology/ hemodynamic consequences/EF
VT in ARVD	LBBB VT morphology	Reentry most common	Multiple morphologies progressive disease
VT in cardiac sarcoid	Usually RBBB VT morphology	Reentry most common	Associated with conduction abnormalities
VT in Chagas' disease	Variable: usually RBBB VT morphology	Reentry most common often epicardial	LV dysfunction/aneurysm South American protozoa: *T. cruzi*
BBR VT	Usually LBBB pattern but may be RBBB pattern (in ischemic cardiomyopathy)	Reentry	A sustained monomophic VT in dilated cardiomyopathy Amenable to RF ablation
RVOT VT	LBBB VT with left Inferior axis	Triggered activity Increased automaticity	Benign. Treat symptoms or tachycardia
Idiopathic left VT	RBBB VT with left superior axis	Probably reentry involving left ant/post fascicles Functional reentry	Benign. Treat symptoms or tachycardia Sensitive to Verapamil
Ventricular fibrillation	Rapid and irregular No discernable QRS complex		Fatal unless immediate defibrillation associated with ischemia
Torsades de Pointes	Polymorphic VT twisting around central axis	Triggered activity initiates and functional reentry maintains VT	Associated with Long QT syndrome drugs prolonging QT must be identified and disconinued

Lidocaine may be considered temporarily when hemodynamically significant ventricular arrhythmias occur in the setting of acute MI. In all cases, electrolyte and acid–base imbalance should be vigilantly corrected.

The use of amiodarone in patients during and following an acute MI has increased but is still controversial. In this acute setting, prospective randomized trials have shown that amiodarone use for the treatment of hemodynamically significant ventricular arrhythmias or other arrhythmias, such as atrial fibrillation, appears to be safe but does not confer survival benefit.

【 】 PREMATURE VENTRICULAR COMPLEXES AND NONSUSTAINED VENTRICULAR TACHYCARDIA IN NONISCHEMIC CARDIOMYOPATHY

The association between PVCs in nonischemic cardiomyopathy and sudden death is less clear. Prospective clinical trials have found that nonsustained VT (NSVT) is a risk factor for sudden death in this population. In general, sudden and total cardiac death rates are increased in patients with high-grade PVCs (> 10/hr) and nonischemic cardiomyopathy, as in patients with ischemic cardiomyopathy, hypertensive heart disease, and hypertrophic cardiomyopathy.

VENTRICULAR TACHYCARDIA IN PATIENTS WITH CORONARY ARTERY DISEASE

Ventricular tachycardia in patients with coronary disease ranges from NSVT to sustained VT that leads to hemodynamic compromise and sudden death. The anatomic substrate supporting sustained monomorphic VT usually involves healthy and damaged myocardium interlaced with fibrous scar primarily at the border zone of a myocardial scar. The risk of VT is thought to be highest during the first year after an MI, but new onset of VT may occur many years later. In general, patients with larger infarctions and lower EFs are at highest risk of fatal ventricular arrhythmias.

【 】 MANAGEMENT OF SUSTAINED VENTRICULAR TACHYCARDIA ASSOCIATED WITH CORONARY ARTERY DISEASE

Sustained VT is a series of continuous ventricular impulses ≥100 beats per minute, for longer than 30 seconds or resulting in hemodynamic instability in < 30 seconds. On ECG, differentiating VT from a supraventricular tachycardia (SVT) with aberrant intraventricular conduction can be difficult. The presence of atrioventricular dissociation with clearly discernible P waves unrelated to ventricular activity, single QRS complexes (usually narrowed in relation to the VT) likely representing a fusion complex between the VT and a conducted supraventricular impulse (fusion beats), QRS duration > 140 msec, and a concordantly positive or negative QRS complex across the precordium, all favor VT over an SVT with aberrant conduction (Table 11-2).

Patients with VT and hemodynamic compromise, congestive heart failure, and/or ischemia, should be treated promptly with DC cardioversion. In patients with stable sustained VT, intravenous procainamide is a reasonable first choice; however, it may cause hemodynamic instability because of its negative inotropic effects. In the setting of VT associated with hemodynamic instability, amiodarone is the treatment of choice over lidocaine or procainamide. All patients with VT should be treated with a beta-blocker unless precluded by hypotension, bradycardia, or other clinical factors. Reversible factors contributing to VT should be corrected.

Long-term management in patients with sustained VT is directed to preventing recurrent VT and sudden death, and usually involves a combination of antiarrhythmic

TABLE 11-2

Electrocardiographic Features that Favor Ventricular Tachycardia in Comparison to Supraventricular Tachycardia with Aberrant Conduction

Atrioventricular (AV) dissociation
Fusion and capture beats
Positive or negative concordance of QRS morphology across the precordial leads (V_1-V_6)
Superiorly directed QRS axis, especially if directed toward right upper quadrant between -90 degrees and $+180$ degrees
RBBB pattern with QRS duration longer than 140 msec, or LBBB pattern with QRS duration longer than 160 msec
RBBB pattern QRS with monophasic R wave in V_1
LBBB pattern QRS with one of the following:
1. Notching in S-wave downstroke in V_1 or V_2
2. Any Q wave in V_6
3. QRS onset to nadir of S wave in V_1 greater than 60 msec
Polymorphic tachycardias

Adapted from Simmons JD, Chakko SC, Myerburg RJ. Arrhythmias and conduction disturbances. In: O'Rourke RA, Fuster V, Alexander W, eds. *Hurst's The Heart Manual of Cardiology.* 11th ed. New York, NY: McGraw-Hill; 2005:93.

therapy and implantation of an internal cardioverter-defibrillator (ICD). Patients who present with sustained VT and an LVEF < 35% generally should receive an ICD. In patients with preserved LV function, amiodarone is a reasonable alternative in selected individuals. It is important that VT be clinically well-controlled in order to prevent multiple shocks from the ICD; this is often achieved with a combination of beta-blockers and antiarrhythmic medications. Ventricular tachycardia that is refractory to medications may be successfully treated with *radiofrequency catheter ablation* techniques, but such ablation is palliative.

【　】 MANAGEMENT OF NONSUSTAINED VENTRICULAR TACHYCARDIA

Patients with preserved LV function and NSVT (three consecutive ventricular impulses up to 30 seconds of nonsustained VT) are generally at low risk and require no further treatment, but patients with low EF are at high risk of sudden death. Based on recent randomized studies, those who are post-MI and have an LVEF < 35% should *be considered* for ICD implantation for primary prevention of sudden death regardless of whether they have clinically documented NSVT.

VENTRICULAR TACHYCARDIA IN PATIENTS WITH NONISCHEMIC CARDIOMYOPATHY

Sustained VT or VF is thought to be the most common cause of death in dilated cardiomyopathy. Nonsustained VT is relatively common and can be seen in up to 50% to 60% of these patients. The mechanisms underlying VT in this setting include myocardial or bundle branch reentry (BBR, a type of VT using the conduction system, namely the left and right bundle branches as part of the VT circuit); increased automaticity; or triggered activity. Clinical recognition of BBR is important as this arrhythmia may be treated successfully with radiofrequency catheter ablation. Sustained VT can also be seen in cardiac sarcoidosis and in Chagas' disease, two less frequent causes of nonischemic cardiomyopathy. As in patients with ischemic cardiomyopathy, patients with nonischemic cardiomyopathy, an LVEF < 35%, and NYHA class II to III heart failure symptoms, should receive an ICD for primary prevention of sudden cardiac death. The role of amiodarone therapy in these individuals is unclear.

VENTRICULAR TACHYCARDIA IN ARRHYTHMOGENIC RIGHT VENTRICULAR DYSPLASIA

Arrhythmogenic right ventricular dysplasia (ARVD) is characterized by fatty infiltration, fibrosis, and thinning of the right ventricle and is associated with ventricular arrhythmias and sudden death. Magnetic resonance imaging, echocardiography, electrocardiography, and signal-averaged electrocardiography may be helpful in the diagnosis. On ECG, T-wave inversion may be present in leads V_1 to V_3, and an increased QRS duration > 140 msec can be seen, as well as epsilon waves, small deflections found in the terminal portion of the QRS complex. There is a paucity of clinical data on the efficacy of antiarrhythmic therapy for sustained VT in ARVD; however, amiodarone, beta-blockers, and/or sotalol are first-line agents for treatment. Patients who have had sustained VT or have suffered a cardiac arrest should receive an ICD.

IDIOPATHIC VENTRICULAR TACHYCARDIA

Idiopathic VT occurs in patients with structurally normal hearts, and may represent approximately 10% of patients referred for evaluation of VT. The two main clinical entities of idiopathic VT include repetitive monomorphic VT arising from the right ventricular outflow tract (named RMVT or RVOT VT) and idiopathic left VT (fascicular VT or verapamil-sensitive VT). RMVT has a characteristic ECG pattern with a left bundle branch block morphology and inferior axis and usually a single VT morphology. The fascicular VTs usually have a right bundle branch block-morphology and have a QRS width < 140 msec. The differentiation of these VTs from VTs associated with structural heart disease is important because they often respond well to drug therapies, are associated with an excellent prognosis, and can be cured with catheter ablation.

POLYMORPHIC VENTRICULAR TACHYCARDIA

Polymorphic VT is characterized by a tachycardia with continuously varying QRS morphology that is often seen in acute ischemic states, or in the setting of catecholamine excess. A specific variant of polymorphic VT is torsades de pointes (TdP), a rapid polymorphic VT that constantly changes (cycle length, axis, and morphology) in a pattern that appears to "twist" around a central axis. TdP is defined as occurring in the setting of a prolonged QT interval and can be precipitated by bradycardia, heart block, hypokalemia, and drugs known to prolong the QT interval. Treatment includes correcting the precipitating factors and rapid defibrillation for hemodynamically unstable TdP. In select patients with bradycardia, cautious use of temporary cardiac pacing may be indicated.

TdP may also be caused by the congenital long-QT syndrome, a heterogeneous group of genetic disorders resulting from defects in ion channels that are involved in membrane repolarization. The acquired (drug-induced) causes are much more common than the congenital long-QT syndrome. Beta-blockade may be indicated for symptomatic ventricular arrhythmias, and ICD placement should be considered in high-risk individuals with long-QT syndrome.

VENTRICULAR FIBRILLATION

VF is associated with rapid hemodynamic collapse, and is the most common arrhythmia resulting in out-of-hospital cardiac arrest. Ventricular fibrillation requires immediate defibrillation, as minimizing the delay to defibrillation is critical to survival. After successful defibrillation, underlying causes should be addressed and management is aimed at preventing recurrences of VF. In most individuals, initial workup should include an assessment of LV function and coronary angiography with revascularization in selected cases. Based on clinical trial data, most all cardiac arrest survivors should be considered for ICD implantation after the initial workup is completed and underlying causes have been identified.

SUGGESTED READING

ACC/AHA/ESC 2006 Guidelines for Management of Patients with Ventricular Arrhythmias and the Prevention of Sudden Cardiac Death. *J Am Coll Cardiol.* 2006;48:e247–e346. Available at www.content.onlinejacc.org/cgi/content.

Antiarrhythmics versus Implantable Defibrillators (AVID) investigators. A comparison of antiarrhythmic-drug therapy with implantable defibrillators in patients resuscitated from near-fatal ventricular arrhythmias. *N Engl J Med.* 1997;337:1576–1584.

Bardy GH, Lee KL, Mark DB, et al. Amiodarone or an implantable cardioverterdefibrillator for congestive heart failure. *N Engl J Med.* 2005;352:225–237.

Buxton AE, Lee KL, Fisher JD, et al. A randomized study of the prevention of sudden death in patients with coronary artery disease. *N Engl J Med.* 1999;341:1882–1890.

Echt DS, Liebson PR, Mitchell LB, et al. Mortality and morbidity in patients receiving encainide, flecainide, or placebo. The Cardiac Arrhythmia Suppression Trial. *N Engl J Med.*1991;324:781–788.

Moss AJ, Zareba W, Hall WJ, et al. Prophylactic implantation of defibrillators in patients with myocardial infarction and reduced ejection fraction. *N Engl J Med.* 2002;346:877–883.

CHAPTER (12)

Bradyarrhythmias and Pacing

Raul D. Mitrani, Robert J. Myerburg, and
Agustin Castellanos

Bradyarrhythmias are generally caused by abnormalities of impulse formation in the sinus node or by atrioventricular (AV) conduction abnormalities. The bradyarrhythmias may be persistent or intermittent. These abnormalities may be secondary to extrinsic factors, such as drugs with negative chronotropic or dromotropic properties; or may be secondary to intrinsic factors such as fibrosis and disease in the sinus node, AV node, or bundle branch/His–Purkinje conduction system. The indications for permanent pacers depend on the underlying cause, as well as the presence of associated symptoms, in most cases (Table 12-1).

ACUTE TREATMENT OF BRADYARRHYTHMIAS

Acute treatment of bradyarrhythmias depends on the patient's blood pressure and symptoms such as syncope, near-syncope, dizziness, and light-headedness. The hemodynamic response to bradyarrhythmias is complex and dependent on underlying systolic and diastolic function, systemic vascular resistance, and the time course over which the bradyarrhythmia developed. Some patients with heart block and rates in the high 20s may be asymptomatic, whereas other patients with rates in the 40s could have symptoms of hypoperfusion. The decision to acutely intervene should not be solely based on the actual heart rate.

Atropine 1 mg intravenously, with repeat doses up to 3 mg, may be administered acutely. This is more often useful in patients with sinus node (SN) dysfunction rather than patients with high-degree AV block. In fact, for patients with second-degree or high-degree AV block, atropine may have the potential of increasing the sinus rate and increasing the level of block, which may paradoxically *lower* the heart rate. For persistent bradyarrhythmias, particularly arrhythmias associated with SN dysfunction, a sympathomimetic amine such as isoproterenol 0.5 to 2 µg/min, or dobutamine 1 to 5 µg/kg/min, may be used carefully to increase the heart rate on a temporary basis. Patients need careful blood-pressure monitoring during infusion, and these drugs should be avoided in patients with acute coronary syndromes, ischemic symptoms, hypertrophic cardiomyopathy, or other conditions where excess sympathetic tone is contraindicated.

Temporary pacing is used when patients experience intermittent or persistent hemodynamically relevant bradyarrhythmias or to provide standby pacing for patients at increased risk for sudden asystole or heart block. The end point for temporary pacing is either resolution of a temporary indication for pacing or implantation of a permanent pacemaker for a persisting bradyarrhythmia.

TABLE 12-1

Indications for Pacing

	Class I	Class II	Class III
Acquired AV block	Advanced second- or third-degree AV block with: • Bradycardia and symptoms, or exercise induced • Requirement of drugs that result in symptomatic bradycardia • Catheter ablation of the AV junction or postoperative AV block not expected to resolve • Neuromuscular diseases • Escape rhythm < 40 bpm or asystole > 3 s or pauses > 5 s during atrial fibrillation in awake symptom-free patients, or escape > 40 bpm with left ventricular dysfunction • Second-degree AV block, permanent or intermittent, with symptomatic bradycardia	**Class IIa** Asymptomatic complete AV block with average awake ventricular rate > 40 bpm Asymptomatic type II second-degree AV block (permanent or intermittent) Asymptomatic second-degree AV block at or below the bundle or His (documented by electrophysiology study) First or second-degree AV block with associated symptoms **Class IIb** AV block in the setting of drug use or toxicity when the block is expected to recur after drug withdrawal Neuromuscular disease with any degree of AV block where there is concern for progression of AV block	Asymptomatic first-degree AV block Asymptomatic type I second-degree AV block above the level of the bundle of His AV block expected to resolve

148

After myocardial infarction	Persistent second- or third-degree AV block in the His–Purkinje system Transient advanced infranodal AV block and associated bundle branch block Symptomatic second- or third-degree AV block at any level	Class IIb Persistent advanced AV block at the AV node level	Transient AV conduction disturbances without intraventricular conduction defects or with isolated left anterior fascicular block New bundle branch block in absence of AV block Persistent first-degree AV block in the presence of bundle branch or fascicular block
Bifascicular or trifascicular block	Intermittent complete heart block associated with symptoms Type II second-degree AV block Alternating bundle branch block	Class IIa Bifascicular or trifascicular block with syncope not proven to be due to AV block but other causes of syncope not identifiable HV interval > 100 ms or pacing-induced infra-His block Class IIb Neuromuscular diseases with or without symptoms	Fascicular block without AV block or symptoms Fascicular block with first-degree AV block without symptoms

TABLE 12-1

Indications for Pacing (Continued)

	Class I	Class II	Class III
Sinus node dysfunction	Sinus node dysfunction with documented symptomatic bradycardia (in some patients, this will occur as a result of long-term essential drug therapy of a type and dose for which there is no acceptable alternative) Symptomatic chronotropic incompetence	Class IIa Sinus node dysfunction, occurring spontaneously or as a result of necessary drug therapy, with heart rates < 40 bpm without clear association between symptoms and bradycardia Syncope of undetermined etiology with sinus node dysfunction during electrophysiology study Class IIb In minimally symptomatic patients, awake heart rate < 40 bpm	Sinus node dysfunction in asymptomatic patients, Sinus node dysfunction in patients in whom symptoms suggestive of bradycardia are clearly documented not to be associated with a slow heart rate Sinus node dysfunction with symptomatic bradycardia due to nonessential drug therapy
Hypersensitive carotid sinus and neurocardiac syndromes	Recurrent syncope associated with clear, spontaneous events provoked by carotid sinus stimulation; minimal carotid sinus pressure induces asystole > 3 s duration in the absence of any medication that depresses the sinus node or AV conduction	Class IIa Recurrent syncope without clear, provocative events and with a hypersensitive cardioinhibitory response Class IIb Recurrent syncope with spontaneous or tilt-test induced bradycardia	A hyperactive cardioinhibitory response to carotid sinus stimulation in the absence of symptoms or with vague symptoms Vasovagal syncope where avoidance therapy is effective

Class I refers to conditions where there is agreement that pacer therapy is beneficial, useful, and effective. Class II refers to conditions where there is conflicting evidence and/or divergence of opinion about usefulness of pacer therapy. Class IIa refers to conditions where opinion is in favor of usefulness, and class IIb indicates conditions where evidence and opinion are less well established. Class III refers to conditions for which there is evidence and agreement that a pacer is not indicated and could possibly be harmful.

Transcutaneous pacing is a common rapid method for noninvasively pacing patients who require a prophylactic temporary pacer or require emergent pacing. The unit incorporates two large pads placed in an anterior and posterior position. However, its main drawback is the high energy requirement (50–100 mA at 20–40 ms), which may cause skeletal muscle stimulation and pain.

TYPES OF BRADYARRHYTHMIAS AND INDICATIONS FOR PACEMAKERS

【 】 SINUS BRADYCARDIA

Sinus bradycardia (SB) is a rhythm in which atrial depolarization initiates from the SN at a rate less than 60/min. The P-wave morphology is similar to that observed in normal sinus rhythm. Resting sinus bradycardia due to high vagal tone is normal in otherwise healthy well-conditioned adults. Other etiologies of SB include medication with negative chronotropic properties, hypothyroidism, inferior ischemia or infarction, hypothermia, hyperkalemia, or autonomic disorders producing increased vagal tone relative to sympathetic tone. Patients are often asymptomatic and require no therapy. However, those who are unable to increase the sinus rate during exercise are generally considered abnormal, and may require permanent pacing.

【 】 SICK SINUS SYNDROME AND SINUS NODE DYSFUNCTION

Sick sinus syndrome and SN dysfunction encompass a group of disorders that have in common the presence of abnormally slow sinus rate, and may have associated intermittent atrial tachyarrhythmias such as atrial fibrillation. *This is the most common indication for pacing in the United States.* Some patients exhibit fixed or intermittent SB, others have SB alternating with normal sinus rhythm and/or supraventricular tachyarrhythmias such as atrial fibrillation (the "tachy/brady syndrome"). Many patients are at risk of periods of asystole or marked bradyarrhythmias following cessation of the tachyarrhythmia.

The guidelines for pacing therapy generally require correlation of symptoms to bradyarrhythmias. However, some symptoms are nonspecific, such as fatigue and dyspnea. *After appropriate evaluation*, pacing is indicated for symptomatic SN dysfunction or when bradycardia or pauses are documented that may be secondary to essential long-term drug therapy.

【 】 FIRST-DEGREE ATRIOVENTRICULAR BLOCK

Isolated first-degree AV block is characterized electrocardiographically (ECG) by a PR interval exceeding 200 ms. It may occur as the result of increased vagal tone, vagotonic drugs, digitalis, beta-adrenergic receptor blockade, hypokalemia, acute carditis, tricuspid stenosis, Chagas' disease, and some forms of congenital heart disease. Isolated first-degree AV block is rarely symptomatic and therefore rarely requires therapy.

【 】 SECOND-DEGREE ATRIOVENTRICULAR BLOCK

Mobitz type I AV block, or the Wenckebach phenomenon, is characterized electrocardiographically by consecutively conducted impulses with progressively increasing PR intervals until an impulse is blocked and the P wave is not followed by a QRS complex. This is the most common form of second-degree AV block and is usually not symptomatic. *It usually does not progress to high-grade AV block;* therefore, pacing is not necessary.

In contrast, the less common Mobitz type II block is generally associated with significant distal or infrahisian conduction system disease. It is characterized by consecutively conducted impulses with fixed PR intervals and a sudden block of impulse conduction. Paroxysmal AV block, characterized by a series of nonconducted P waves, is considered a variant of the Mobitz type II pattern. The QRS complex is typically wide in Mobitz type II block, and is almost always associated with organic heart disease, including disease in the AV conduction system distal to the AV node. It may progress to complete AV block. For this reason, permanent pacing is often indicated. In some cases an electrophysiology study may be necessary to define the level of block and guide the decision for pacing therapy.

Pacing is indicated for either type of second-degree AV block in symptomatic patients.

【 】 COMPLETE ATRIOVENTRICULAR BLOCK

Complete heart block, or third-degree AV block, is characterized by a complete interruption of antegrade AV conduction; supraventricular impulses are unable to propagate to and activate the ventricles. The ventricles are subsequently activated by a subsidiary junctional or idioventricular pacemaker at a rate of 20 to 50 bpm. Two independent pacemakers then control the rhythm of the heart: one for the atria and one for the ventricles. The two rhythms are independent. *In general, complete heart block*, permanent or intermittent, at any anatomic level associated with symptoms such as dizziness, lightheadedness, congestive heart failure, and confusion is *an indication for a permanent pacemaker*. Pacing should also be considered for complete or advanced AV block in asymptomatic patients in the absence of reversible causes. In the presence of bifascicular or trifascicular block, intermittent third-degree or type II second-degree AV block usually indicates the need for a permanent pacemaker. Patients who present with syncope and bifascicular or trifascicular block may require a pacemaker; however, further evaluation of the syncope, including electrophysiology study, may be required.

In the setting of inferior infarction, AV block typically occurs at the level of the AV node and may be due to reversible injury and/or poor autonomic tone; thus, AV block usually subsides if one waits a sufficient time. In contrast, complete or intermittent AV block in association with acute anterior wall myocardial infraction (MI) may be permanent and require permanent pacing. Transient advanced infranodal AV block with associated bundle-branch block is also an indication for pacing; however, electrophysiology studies may be required to determine the level of block.

【 】 CONGENITAL AV BLOCK

The site of AV block in congenital heart block is usually at the level of the AV node. However, congenital AV block often is associated with serious complications, including syncope and sudden death. Some develop a cardiomyopathy over time in the absence of permanent pacing. Cardiac pacing is indicated in all symptomatic patients as well as in patients with associated wide QRS escape rhythm, complex ventricular ectopy, ventricular dysfunction, or other cardiac structural abnormalities. Pacing is indicated in most asymptomatic adult patients because of an increased mortality risk from persistent bradycardia and/or cardiomyopathy.

【 】 ATRIOVENTRICULAR DISSOCIATION

AV dissociation is characterized by the absence of a fixed temporal relationship between atrial and ventricular activation. The causes of AV dissociation include marked slowing of normal pacemaker activity such that the normal escape rhythm of a subsidiary focus predominates, acceleration of a subordinate focus, or third-degree AV block. The diagnosis of *AV dissociation*, however, is *not synonymous with complete AV block*. The ECG diagnosis is made when the P waves of sinus rhythm are dissociated from the QRS complexes of an ectopic junctional or idioventricular rhythm. Fortuitously timed P waves may "capture" the ventricles when AV block is not the mechanism for dissociation. If a patient with AV dissociation is symptomatic, the underlying rhythm disturbance that is responsible for the symptoms must be identified and treatment directed toward that rhythm disturbance.

OTHER INDICATIONS FOR PACING

【 】 PACING FOR CAROTID SINUS SYNDROME AND NEUROCARDIOGENIC SYNCOPE

The diagnosis of carotid sinus syndrome is typically made by demonstrating asystolic pauses > 3 sec with carotid sinus massage or a vasodepressor response > 50 mm Hg associated with clear symptoms provoked by carotid sinus stimulation, such as wearing a tight shirt or turning one's head. Improvement of symptoms and prevention of syncope has been demonstrated by treating patients with dual-chamber pacing. *Pacing* is indicated in patients with syncope associated with hypersensitive carotid sinus responses in the absence of an alternative cause, *but is not indicated in asymptomatic patients with hypersensitive carotid sinus responses.*

For patients with neurocardiogenic syncope, cardiac pacing is limited to recurrent syncope with clear associated bradycardias/asystole. However, pacing is rarely used in these patients because even with pacing, many patients still experience vasodepressor responses with hypotension and persistent symptoms.

【 】 CARDIAC RESYNCHRONIZATION THERAPY

Biventricular pacing is being used to resynchronize ventricular contraction in patients with class III or IV heart failure, ejection fraction < 35%, and wide QRS complex ≥ 130 ms, typically but not necessarily in a left bundle-branch block pattern. Left ventricular (LV) stimulation can be achieved by placing a transvenous pacing lead into a branch of the coronary sinus or through direct placement on the LV epicardial surface. Resynchronization of the LV activation in these patients with wide QRS complexes often leads to more efficient ventricular systolic function, decreasing symptoms of congestive heart failure (CHF), and in one study, reduction of total mortality. However, in practice, many of these patients also have standard indications for implantable defibrillators; therefore, these patients would likely benefit from, and usually receive, a combined biventricular pacer-defibrillator unit.

PACEMAKERS

Pacemakers are coded by a specific abbreviation according to the *type of pacemaker* and *mode of pacing.* The first letter refers to the chamber(s) being paced and the second to the chamber(s) being sensed. The letters A and V indicate atrial or ventricular pacing and/or sensing. If both atrial and ventricular chambers are paced and/or sensed, the designation D is used. The third letter refers to the response to a sensed event. The pacemaker inhibits (I) pacing output from one or both of its leads, or triggers (T) pacing at a programmable interval after the sensed event. If a pacer can inhibit atrial output and trigger a ventricular paced complex after a sensed atrial complex, then the designation D is used for the third letter. A fourth letter R denotes rate responsiveness, that is, changes in paced rate in response to changing levels of activity.

To stimulate myocardial tissue, a minimal threshold of current is necessary. The current delivered is a function of the pacemaker voltage and pulse width, which is generally programmed to deliver two to four times the threshold current in order to have an adequate safety margin. Some pacers can automatically check thresholds, and therefore can adjust outputs to deliver less current, thereby prolonging battery longevity while preserving safety.

A pacemaker senses intrinsic cardiac activity by the intracardiac electrograms. The range for atrial and ventricular electrograms is 0.5 to 5 mV and 5 to 20 mV, respectively; therefore pacemaker sensitivities are programmed at 0.25 to 2 mV in the atrial channel and 2 to 4 mV in the ventricular channel in order to provide an adequate safety margin for sensing.

【 】 HARDWARE

Pacemaker leads can be unipolar or bipolar. Unipolar leads use a distal electrode in the catheter as the cathode and the shell of the pacemaker generator as the anode. Therefore, the myocardium and adjacent tissue complete the circuit. Because the unipolar lead uses body tissue to complete the circuit, there is the possibility of causing muscle stimulation. Unipolar sensing is also far more likely to detect extracardiac signals, including myopotentials, remote cardiac potentials (far-field sensing), and electromagnetic interference. A bipolar lead consists of two separate conductors and electrodes within the lead. Since the electrodes for sensing in a bipolar lead are much closer together, bipolar signals are sharper and subject to less extraneous interference. Most new pacer systems use bipolar leads; *however, unipolar leads are occasionally used for LV pacing through the coronary sinus due to their smaller diameter.*

【 】 FUNCTION AND MODES

Magnet Mode

Magnets cause asynchronous pacing in virtually all pacemakers. The specific magnet rate and response varies according to manufacturer, pacemaker model, and battery voltage. In patients who are pacemaker-dependent and experiencing oversensing, thereby inhibiting pacemaker output, a magnet is a convenient short-term method of ensuring pacing.

VVI Mode

VVI mode ensures that a minimum ventricular rate is maintained by ventricular pacing at the pacemaker rate unless there is an intrinsic ventricular rate greater than the pacemaker's lower rate. This is useful in patients with atrial fibrillation or for those who need backup pacing.

Hysteresis is a programmable function in which the ventricular escape interval is longer after a sensed ventricular event than after a paced ventricular event. This feature is intended to conserve battery life and maintain an intrinsic rhythm, *because the effective rate at which a pacer begins to pace is lower than the actual lower rate of the pacemaker.*

DDD Pacing

DDD pacing is the most common pacing mode for dual-chamber pacemakers. This mode is used for patients with AV node and/or sinus node dysfunction.

1. *Patients with AV block and normal sinus node function.* In the DDD mode, if the lower rate of the pacer is programmed at a sufficiently low value to permit atrial tracking, the pacemaker stimulates the ventricle synchronously in response to intrinsic P waves with a programmed AV interval. If the pacer's programmed lower rate exceeds the patient's intrinsic atrial rate, than AV sequential pacing occurs.

2. *DDD pacing in patients with sinus node dysfunction.* These patients may have intermittent or chronic sinus bradycardia requiring intermittent or continuous atrial pacing. If patients have intact AV conduction, the pacemaker functions as an AAI pacer, since intrinsic conduction would inhibit pacer ventricular output. However, because

patients with sinus node dysfunction may also have AV conduction system disease, DDD pacemakers frequently can pace the ventricles. Depending on intrinsic conduction and the programmed AV interval, there may be a paced ventricular complex, a fused ventricular complex combining ventricular stimulation with intrinsic AV conduction system, or a pacing spike in the middle of the QRS complex, termed "pseudofusion" (consistent with normal pacemaker function).

AAI Pacing

AAI pacing is similar to VVI pacing except that the pacemaker is stimulating the atrium. AAIR is a useful pacing mode in a patient with sinus node dysfunction and normal AV conduction. Some pacers may automatically switch from AAI mode to DDD mode if second- or third-degree AV block develops.

DDI Pacing

DDI pacing is a useful mode for patients with a tachycardia–bradycardia pattern of sick sinus syndrome who have intact AV conduction. During atrial tachyarrhythmias, a pacer in the DDI mode will pace the ventricles at the lower rate. During episodes of bradyarrhythmia, the pacer functions in an atrial or AV pacing mode. DDI pacing is inappropriate for patients with permanent or intermittent AV block.

【　】 USE OF PACEMAKERS IN DIFFERENT CLINICAL SITUATIONS

Paroxysmal Atria Fibrillation, Flutter, or Other Tachycarrhythmias

In order to prevent inappropriate upper tracking behavior during atrial tachyarrhythmias, a pacer can be reprogrammed to AAI[R] or DDI[R] if the patient has intact AV conduction. Alternatively, pacers have a programmable feature, an *automatic mode switch*, that changes the pacer mode from DDD[R] to VVI[R] or DDI[R] during episodes of atrial tachyarrhythmias.

Some studies have demonstrated that atrial-based pacing (DDD, DDI, AAI) may reduce the frequency of atrial fibrillation compared with ventricular-based pacing (VVI).

Patients with Complete or Intermittent Third-Degree AV Block

Patients with complete or intermittent third-degree AV block generally receive a dual-chamber pacemaker programmed in the DDD mode. *Occasionally, some patients have a single-lead VDD pacer that paces the ventricle but senses and tracks the atrial activity.*

Patients with Carotid Sinus Syndrome and Vasovagal Syncope

Patients with the neurally mediated syncope syndromes require only intermittent AV pacing unless they have concomitant sinus node dysfunction. In the absence of sinus node dysfunction, the pacing strategy involves an algorithm that tracks a drop in instrinsic heart rate to a programmable lower rate (e.g., 40–50 bpm), at which time an interventional pacing rate of 75 to 100 bpm is activated for 1 to 5 minutes. This interventional rate is intended to overcome the vagal effects and prevent syncope.

Avoiding Right Ventricular Pacing

Right ventricular pacing may cause dyssynchrony that may lead to systolic dysfunction and heart failure. Table 12-2 shows programmable strategies to avoid or minimize ventricular pacing.

TABLE 12-2

Strategies to Minimize Ventricular Pacing

Strategy	Advantage	Disadvantage
Program long AV intervals	Available in all pacers	Pacing may occur at long AV intervals
DDI mode	No tracking of atrial rhythm when rate above lower rate	No tracking mode if patient goes into second- or third-degree AV block
AV search hysteresis	Pacing occurs with physiologic AV interval	May not minimize RV pacing
AAI pacing (with backup DDD)	No ventricular pacing unless second- or third-degree AV block	Excessively long PR intervals may result

【 】 COMPLICATIONS

Early infections related to pacemaker implantation occur in approximately 1% of implants. Early infections may be caused by *Staphylococcus aureus* and can be aggressive. Late infections are commonly related to *Staphylococcus epidermidis* and may have a more indolent course. Signs of infection include local inflammation and abscess formation, erosion of the pacer, and fever with positive blood culture but without an identifiable focus of infection. Transesophageal echocardiography may help to determine whether vegetations are present on the pacemaker lead. If the pacemaker is infected, removal of the pacemaker leads and generator is usually required.

The insulation of pacer leads may break or leads may fracture, leading to problems with oversensing (due to electrical noise), undersensing, and failure to capture (due to current leak). This problem often manifests itself intermittently and may be difficult to detect during a routine pacer check. The patient may complain of pectoral muscle stimulation due to current leak around an insulation break.

Pacemaker Syndrome

The pacemaker syndrome is a constellation of signs and symptoms representing adverse reaction to VVI pacing or dual-chamber pacing with very long AV intervals. The basis for pacemaker syndrome involves loss of AV synchrony and inappropriate timing of the atrial complex, which follows rather than precedes the ventricular complex. Symptoms include orthostatic hypotension, near syncope, fatigue, exercise intolerance, malaise, awareness of heartbeat, chest fullness, headache, chest pain, and other nonspecific symptoms. Strategies to minimize ventricular pacing (Table 12-2) can infrequently lead to these symptoms. Restoration and optimization of AV synchrony often clears the symptoms.

Electromagnetic Interference with Pacemaker Function

Unipolar pacemakers are usually more susceptible to electromagnetic interference (EMI) than bipolar pacemakers because the sensing circuit encompasses a larger area. Most magnetic resonance imaging (MRI) is contraindicated in patients with pacers. However, there are recent data demonstrating safe MRI scanning using 1.5-T MR systems in non-pacer-dependent patients with cardiac monitoring during their procedure. Cellular phones can rarely adversely affect pacemaker function. It is therefore recommended that patients keep cellular phones at least 20 cm away from their pacemakers.

【 】 PACEMAKER MALFUNCTION

Pacemaker malfunction can be categorized as loss of capture, abnormal pacing rate, undersensing, oversensing, or other erratic behavior. The approach to diagnosing pacemaker malfunction is to carefully inspect the ECG; interrogate the pacemaker; check pacing and sensing thresholds, lead impedances, and battery voltage/magnet rate; and perform a chest x-ray.

Abnormal pacing rates can be due to normal or abnormal pacing function. Failure of the pacemaker output is usually due to oversensing (Fig. 12-1). Occasionally, the pacemaker output is not visible because bipolar pacing produces pacing artifacts of very low amplitude. Conversely, absence of pacing stimuli may be due to interruption of current flow from a lead fracture, an insulation break, or a loose set screw.

Abnormally fast pacing rates usually occur in the context of normal pacing function. They may occur in response to rate-adaptive sensors. In DDD pacing, upper-rate pacing may be due to sinus tachycardia, atrial tachyarrhythmias, or pacemaker-mediated tachycardia. Application of a magnet can terminate pacemaker-mediated tachycardia.

Loss of pacemaker capture occurs when there is a visible pacing stimulus and no atrial or ventricular depolarization (Fig. 12-1). This may be intermittent or persistent. Etiologies include elevation of pacing threshold, lead dislodgment, lead fracture or insulation break, and loose set screws. Battery depletion also leads to pacing failure.

Oversensing leads to inappropriate pauses. The cause can be intracardiac or extracardiac or due to EMI. Analysis of the ECG, especially with pacemaker interrogation and pacemaker marker channels, may help to determine the cause. Oversensing due to lead fracture, insulation break, or other electrode problems will be random and erratic. Oversensing can occasionally be solved by reprogramming pacer sensitivity. Application of a magnet to a pacer may ensure continuous pacing in pacer-dependent patients who demonstrate inappropriate pauses. Occasionally, newer algorithms can cause the appearance of abnormal pacer function (Fig. 12-2).

Undersensing an intracardiac signal can lead to inappropriate pacing. Etiologies include inflammation or scar formation at the tissue–lead interface, drugs, electrolyte abnormalities, infarction, ischemia, lead fracture or insulation breaks, and cardiac defibrillation. Usually, undersensing is a greater problem in the atrium than in the ventricle. The optimal solution is to program an enhanced sensitivity (decrease the sensing level).

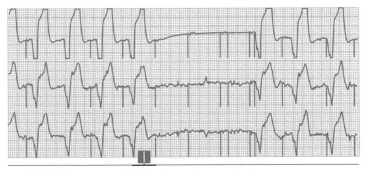

FIGURE 12-1. Three consecutive complexes with absent QRS complexes. In the first two of these complexes, there is no ventricular pacing artifact, suggesting that oversensing inhibited ventricular pacing output. However, in the third complex with absent QRS complex, there is a ventricular pacing artifact without QRS complex. This suggests lead failure (insulation break or conductor fracture that could account for either oversensing and/or failure to capture).

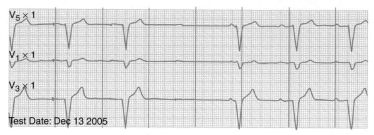

FIGURE 12-2. AV pacing with a single complex showing lack of ventricular output. This is a normal function of a pacer that has an algorithm that periodically checks for AV conduction to determine whether it should pace DDD versus AAI, and therefore allows one atrial paced complex to have an absent QRS complex.

Other etiologies for undersensing arise when intrinsic atrial or ventricular complexes fall within one of the programmed refractory periods. Undersensing can also result when a pacer functions in an asynchronous mode (as occasionally happens with battery depletion or resetting of the pacemaker generator).

SUGGESTED READING

Cleland JDF, Daubert JC, Erdmann E, et al. The effect of cardiac resynchronization on morbidity and mortality in heart failure. *N Engl J Med*. 2005;352:1539–1549.

Epstein AE, DiMarco JP, Ellenbogen KA, et al. ACC/AHA/HRS guidelines for device-based therapy of cardiac rhythm abnormalities. A report of the ACC/AHA Task Force on Practice Guidelines (Writing Committee to Revise the ACC/AHA/NASPE 2002 Guidelines Update for Implantation of Cardiac Pacemakers and Antiarrhythmia Devices). *Circulation* . Oublished online May 15, 2008.

Vijayaraman P, Ellenbogen KA. Bradyarrhythmias and pacemakers. In: Fuster V, O'Rourke RA, Walsh RA, et al., eds. *Hurst's The Heart*. 12th ed. New York, NY: McGraw-Hill; 2008:1020–1054.

CHAPTER (13)

Long-Term Continuous Electrocardiographic Recording*

Robert A. O'Rourke

Long-term electrocardiographic (ECG) recording is a method of recording the ECG over an extended time period. Technological advances in the past few years have provided a diversity of recording, transmitting, and analysis systems.

INDICATIONS

Ambulatory ECG recording may be helpful in diagnosing and, less frequently, quantitating cardiac arrhythmias. The recording of an arrhythmia during a patient's symptoms may be the only means of diagnosis, particularly when the two are relatively infrequent (Fig. 13-1). The recording of a normal rhythm during symptoms may prove equally valuable in excluding an arrhythmia as the cause for the symptoms.

Detection of asymptomatic arrhythmias using ambulatory ECG recordings (e.g., nonsustained ventricular tachycardia) may be indicated in certain patients for assessing risk for future cardiac events. These may include patients with hypertrophic cardiomyopathy and those post–myocardial infarction with left ventricular (LV) dysfunction. Patients who are treated for arrhythmias, such as atrial fibrillation or ventricular tachycardia, may benefit from ambulatory ECG recordings for assessing the efficacy of therapy. Other potential uses of ambulatory ECG are detection of myocardial ischemia from ST-segment or T-wave changes, and measurement of heart rate variability and QT dispersion. However, technical limitations, including nonstandard lead positioning and low-fidelity recordings, lead to uncertainty of the significance of ST-segment and T-wave changes. Even more important than these technical considerations are certain physiologic limitations. For instance, standing, hyperventilation, eating, anxiety, use of drugs, and changes in autonomic tone are all daily events that may result in depression of the ST segment or inversion of the T wave to simulate ischemic changes. The American College of Cardiologists/American Heart Association (ACC/AHA) clinical practice *Guidelines for Ambulatory Electrocardiography* provide a more complete consideration of clinical indications for ambulatory ECG recordings (see App. 13-1).

---

*Adapted from Chapter 41 by Prystowsky EN, Padanilam BJ. In: Fuster V, O'Rourke RA, Walsh RA, et al., eds. *Hurst's The Heart*. 12th ed. New York, NY: McGraw-Hill; 2008, with permission of authors and publisher.

Rapid Heartbeat Symptom

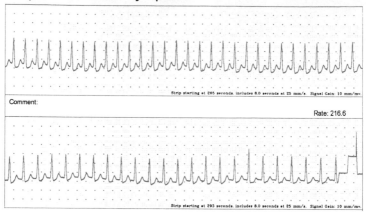

Comment:

Rate: 216.6

FIGURE 13-1. An episode of rapid paroxysmal supraventricular tachycardia captured with a handheld even recorder during a typical period of symptoms.

APPENDIX 13-1

ACC/AHA Guidelines for Ambulatory Electrocardiography*

A. Indications for Ambulatory ECG (AECG) to Assess Symptoms Possibly Related to Rhythm Disturbances

---

Class I

1. Patients with unexplained syncope, near syncope, or episodic dizziness in whom the cause is not obvious.
2. Patients with unexplained recurrent palpitation.

Class IIb

3. Patients with episodic shortness of breath, chest pain, or fatigue that is not otherwise explained.
4. Patients with neurologic events when transient atrial fibrillation or flutter is suspected.
5. Patients with symptoms such as syncope, near syncope, episodic dizziness, or palpitation in whom a probable cause other than an arrhythmia has been identified but in whom symptoms persist despite treatment of this other cause.

Class III

6. Patients with symptoms such as syncope, near syncope, episodic dizziness, or palpitation in whom other causes have been identified by history, physical examination, or laboratory tests.
7. Patients with cerebrovascular accidents, without other evidence of arrhythmia.

B. Indications for AECG Arrhythmia Detection to Assess Risk for Future Cardiac Events in Patients Without Symptoms from Arrhythmia

Class IIb

1. Post–myocardial infarction (MI) patients with LV dysfunction (ejection fraction < 40%).
2. Patients with congestive heart failure (CHF).
3. Patients with idiopathic hypertrophic cardiomyopathy.

Class III

4. Patients who have sustained myocardial contusion.
5. Diabetic subjects to evaluate for diabetic neuropathy.
6. Patients with rhythm disturbances that preclude HRV analysis (e.g., atria fibrillation).

D. Indications for AECG to Assess Antiarrhythmic Therapy

Class I

1. To assess antiarrhythmic drug response in individuals in whom baseline frequency of arrhythmia has been characterized as reproducible and of sufficient frequency to permit analysis.

Class IIa

2. To detect proarrhythmic responses to antiarrhythmic therapy in patients at high risk.

Class IIb

3. To assess rate control during atrial fibrillation.
4. To document recurrent or asymptomatic nonsustained arrhythmias during therapy in the outpatient setting.

E. Indications for AECG to Assess Pacemaker and Intracardiac Cardioverter-Defibrillator (ICD) Function

Class I

1. Evaluation of frequent symptoms of palpitation, syncope, or near syncope to assess device function to exclude myopotential inhibition and pacemaker-mediated tachycardia and to assist in the programming of enhanced features such as rate responsivity and automatic mode switching.
2. Evaluation of suspected component failure or malfunction when device interrogation is not definitive in establishing a diagnosis.
3. To assess the response to adjunctive pharmacologic therapy in patients receiving frequent ICD therapy.

Class IIb

4. Evaluation of immediate postoperative pacemaker function after pacemaker or ICD implantation as an alternative or adjunct to continuous telemetric monitoring.
5. Evaluation of the rate of supraventricular arrhythmias in patients with implanted defibrillators.

Class III

6. Assessment of ICD/pacemaker malfunction when device interrogation, ECG, or other available data (chest radiograph and so forth) are sufficient to establish an underlying cause/diagnosis.
7. Routine follow-up in asymptomatic patients.

F. Indications for AECG for Ischemia Monitoring

Class IIa

1. Patients with suspected variant angina.

Class IIb

2. Evaluation of patients with chest pain who cannot exercise.
3. Preoperative evaluation for vascular surgery of patient who cannot exercise.
4. Patients with known coronary artery disease (CAD) and atypical chest pain syndrome.

Class III

5. Initial evaluation of patients with chest pain who are able to exercise.
6. Routine screening of asymptomatic subjects.

G. Indications for AECG Monitoring in Pediatric Patients

Class I (Chapter 59)

1. Syncope, near syncope, or dizziness in patients with recognized cardiac disease, previously documented arrhythmia, or pacemaker dependency.
2. Syncope or near syncope associated with exertion when the cause is not established by other methods.
3. Evaluation of patients with hypertrophic or dilated cardiomyopathies.
4. Evaluation of possible or documented long QT syndromes.
5. Palpitations in the patient with prior surgery for congenital heart disease and significant residual hemodynamic abnormalities.
6. Evaluation of antiarrhythmic drug efficacy during rapid somatic growth.
7. Asymptomatic congenital complete AV block, nonpaced.

Class IIa

8. Syncope, near syncope, or sustained palpitation in the absence of a reasonable explanation and where there is not overt clinical evidence of heart disease.
9. Evaluation of cardiac rhythm after initiation of an antiarrhythmic therapy, particularly when associated with a significant proarrhythmic potential.
10. Evaluation of cardiac rhythm after transient AV block associated with heart surgery or catheter ablation.
11. Evaluation of rate-responsive or physiologic pacing function in symptomatic patients.

Class IIb

12. Evaluation of asymptomatic patients with prior surgery for congenital heart disease, particularly when there are either significant or residual hemodynamic abnormalities, or a significant incidence of late postoperative arrhythmias.
13. Evaluation of the young patient (< 3 year old) with a prior tachyarrhythmia to determine if unrecognized episodes of the arrhythmia recur.
14. Evaluation of the patient with a suspected incessant atrial tachycardia.
15. Complex ventricular ectopy on ECG or exercise test.

Class III

16. Syncope, near syncope, or dizziness when a noncardiac cause is present.
17. Chest pain without clinical evidence of heart disease.
18. Routine evaluation of asymptomatic individuals for athletic clearance.
19. Brief palpitation in the absence of heart disease.
20. Asymptomatic Wolff–Parkinson–White syndrome.

---

* See also Chapter 59

Reproduced with permission from Crawford MH, Berstein SJ. ACC/AHA Guidelines for Ambulatory Electrocardiography. A report of the American College of Cardiology/American Heart Association Task Force on Practice Guidelines (Committee to revise the guidelines for ambulatory electrocardiography). Developed in collaboration with the North American Society for Pacing and Electrophysiology. *J Am Coll Cardiol.* Sept 1999;34(3):912–948.

RECORDING TECHNIQUES

Four general types of devices are currently available: continuous recorders, intermittent or event recorders, instruments for real-time recording and transmission of ECGs, and implantable recorders (Table 13-1).

【 】 CONTINUOUS RECORDERS

The ECG can be recorded continuously on cassette tape or digitally in solid-state memory. The tape recorder is a battery-powered, miniature device with a very slow tape speed that is small enough to be suspended by a strap over the shoulder or around the waist. The leads are usually attached to the patient's precordial skin using adhesive patches.

All digital recording systems amplify, digitize, and store the ECG in solid-state memory. Two types of digital recorders are available. In the first, each QRS complex is recorded, similar in this sense to the continuous tape recording. "Full disclosure" of the ECG is provided by enhanced storage capacity on a memory card the size of a credit card. With the second, microcomputers and microelectronic circuits sample the cardiac rhythm in real time as it is being recorded, convert the analog signal into a digital signal, and analyze the data in terms of maximal and minimal rates, RR intervals, and changes in RR intervals. This instrument differs in that the actual ECG has not been recorded on tape; only the histogram has been stored. Selected brief segments of the patient's ECG can also be stored, however. Microcomputers are available that can analyze electronic data over periods of up to several days.

【 】 EVENT RECORDERS

This alternative method records not continuously, but only when the patient activates the device. There are two basic types of event recorders, which differ on the basis of their memory—post-event recorders and pre-event recorders. In the post-event recorder, without memory, the patient usually wears the recorder continuously, activating it when symptoms appear. The device does not record the ECG until it is activated. Alternatively, the patient may carry a miniature solid-state recorder with which the symptomatic rhythm can be recorded simply by placing the unit on the precordium or, in some cases, on the wrist. The recorded data are stored in memory until the patient submits the information either directly or transtelephonically to an ECG recorder. With a pre-event recorder, employing a memory loop, the rhythm is monitored continuously. Patients activate the unit when they experience symptoms and the loop recorder is capable of recording an ECG several seconds or minutes before and after a recognized event; the number of events that can be recorded and the allotment of recording time prior to and after activation of the unit are programmable.

The limitations of traditional event recorders include their inability to record asymptomatic arrhythmias, inability for the patient to transmit specific symptoms with each event,

TABLE 13-1

Types of Electrocardiographic Recording Instruments

Type	Recording	Scanning	Transmitting
Continuous			
Analog	All ECG complexes, "full disclosure"	Technician with computer assistance, templating, area determination, and superimposition	None
Digital—continuous recording	All ECG complexes, "full disclosure"	Technician with computer assistance, templating, area determination, and superimposition	Transtelephonic
Digital—real-time analysis	Computer analysis of ECG and selected ECG printouts	Real time by microprocessor with retrospective technician editing	None
Event Recorder			
"Postevent," nonlooping, without memory, handheld or worn	ECG, selected by patient activation	Direct visualization	Transtelephonic
"Pre-event," looping, with memory, monitor worn with attached electrodes	ECG, selected by patient activation, with memory of pre-event	Direct visualization	Transtelephonic
Continuous mobile outpatient telemetry system	ECG, selected by patient or automatic	Direct visualization; technician with computer assistance	Transtelephonic

Implantable Devices			
Subcutaneous, implanted digital recorder	ECG, selected by patient activation with memory of preevent or automatic	Direct visualization	Direct telemetry
Automatic electronic sensor in ICD or pacemaker	ECG, when activated by ICD discharge or recognized by sensor in pacemaker, with memory	Direct visualization of analysis or ECG	Direct telemetry
Real Time			
Real-time transtelephonic monitoring	ECG at central monitoring station — no recording at device	Direct visualization	Transtelephonic

and missed events because of patient error in activating the device. A newer mobile cardiac outpatient telemetry system consists of a three-electrode, two-channel sensor transmitting wirelessly to a portable monitor, which analyzes and stores ECG data. Significant arrhythmias, whether symptomatic or asymptomatic, are transmitted automatically by the wireless network to a central monitoring station and analyzed by trained personnel.

【　】 IMPLANTABLE RECORDERS

A miniaturized event recorder can be implanted subcutaneously on the precordium. It can be manually activated by the patient to record an ECG when symptoms occur, and high and low heart rate limit parameters can be programmed for the device to record events automatically. These devices are particularly useful to capture events that occur relatively infrequently—for example, a few times per year. Event recording is also provided by some newer-generation pacemakers and implantable cardioverter/defibrillators that automatically recognize and record abnormal rhythms.

【　】 REAL-TIME MONITORING

Real-time monitoring devices acquire data and transmit the ECG information directly and transtelephonically, in real time, without recording the data in the unit. The patient's ECG can be transmitted daily, or even multiple times each day, to a recording station. Routine transtelephonic pacemaker evaluations use such systems.

SCANNING AND ANALYSIS TECHNIQUES

The recording can be analyzed by scanning the tape or digital record at high speed, by printing it out directly, or—as in the case of microcomputers—by processing during the recording and printing out the analysis at the end of sampling. Scanning techniques include technician-dependent analysis, in which a technician interprets the cardiac rhythm as it is played back at high speed on an oscilloscope at 30 to 240 times the speed of the actual event. One technique superimposes each QRS complex on the immediately preceding complex so that identical QRS contours present as a stationary image. Variations in QRS contour then become readily apparent. A computer can be interfaced with the scanner to quantitate the data even more accurately. The playback analysis can occur at up to 240 times the normal rate. Electronic analyzers and scanners can be programmed to recognize the patient's own QRS complex template and then to recognize any deviation from normal. The computer program can provide summaries of heart rates, heart rate variability, frequency of premature atrial or ventricular extrasystoles, coupling intervals, arrhythmias, and variations in QRS, ST, QT, or T-wave pattern during any time period. When arrhythmias or pattern changes are detected, an automatic ECG printout can be triggered.

SELECTION OF DEVICE AND DURATION OF RECORDING

The selection of a long-term ECG recording system depends on the individual patient's needs. If a precise count of ectopy is required, a continuous recorder with computer-based analysis is essential. If the purpose of the recording is to detect episodic arrhythmic events such as ventricular tachycardia or atrial fibrillation, an event recorder would be an excellent choice. An event recorder provides an opportunity to monitor over prolonged periods of time and is of benefit to the patient whose symptoms do not occur on a daily basis. When the goal is to correlate the patient's ECG pattern with symptoms that are very infrequent (e.g., every few months) an implantable loop recorder may be the best choice. A pre-event loop recorder is needed for evaluation of symptoms of brief duration (such as syncope without warning), and allows the patient to activate the recorder after the event. The monitoring period must be extended sufficiently to incorporate a symptomatic period, which may be hours to months. For assessment of ventricular rate control for a patient with atrial fibrillation, a 24-hour ECG monitoring period is usually sufficient. However, continuous outpatient telemetry monitoring, performed for 1 to 2 weeks, may be advantageous in the titration of oral medications (e.g., betablockers, calcium-channel blockers, digoxin) in patients with atrial fibrillation and uncontrolled ventricular rates.

ARTIFACTS AND ERRORS

Artifacts registered during prolonged ECG recording have mimicked virtually every variety of cardiac arrhythmias and have led to misdiagnosis and inappropriate treatment. Artifacts can occur at different levels of the recording process. *Patient-related* artifacts may result from involuntary muscle contractions (e.g., tremors, rigors, hiccoughs) and body movements (e.g., changing body position, brushing teeth, combing hair). The Parkinson disease tremor often has a frequency of 4 to 5 per second and when captured on an ECG, can be mistaken for atrial flutter or ventricular tachycardia.

A second type of artifact may occur during *data recording and processing*. Recording system artifacts can occur for a variety of reasons, including loose skin–electrode contact, lead fractures, processing errors, altered tape speed in the recorder, and incomplete erasure of a previous recording. The most common artifact probably is that resulting from a loose electrode or mechanical "stimulation" of the electrode. High-frequency signal dropout or generation of a high-frequency signal mimicking pacing artifacts can occur from processing errors, especially in digital systems. Failure of either the battery or the motor of the recorder generally results in a slowing of the tape speed as the ECG is recorded. When played back, the heart rate appears fast, mimicking a tachycardia (Fig. 13-2). The interpreter may be alerted to the artifact by the concomitant shortening of all ECG intervals (PR, QRS, QT, and RR). Conversely, transient slowing or sticking of the tape during playback may mimic bradycardia, atrioventricular (AV) block, and intraventricular conduction delays. Recording an ECG on a previously used tape that is incompletely erased can result in the simultaneous registration of two ECGs and possible misinterpretation of a "parasystolic" ectopic rhythm. The artifact can be identified by "looking through" longer rhythm strips where nonphysiologic QRS coupling intervals may become apparent. *Rare clinical scenarios where this can occur without being an artifact are Siamese twins and "piggyback heart transplantations," where two independent cardiac rhythms are simultaneously recorded.*

External interferences also offer a very common cause for ECG artifacts. "Noise" can occur in the recordings because of external sources, such as 60 Hz from alternating current or electromagnetic interference from mechanical devices. Simultaneous use of a variety of medical equipment (e.g., infusion pumps, transcutaneous or implanted nerve stimulators) may result in ECG artifacts mimicking atrial or ventricular arrhythmias. Implanted or external nerve stimulators in some patients can result in an atrial flutter-like appearance, but can be distinguished by its rate, "spike-like" nature of the artifacts, and appearance of sinus P waves in some recording leads.

Most of these artifacts are readily identifiable from their characteristic appearance. One should "look through" the artifacts for normal background ECG appearance. Quite often QRS complexes can be identified and "marched out" at cycle lengths similar to the sinus rhythm cycle lengths before the beginning of the artifacts. Look for high-frequency (spike-like activity) or low-frequency signals inconsistent with the normal PQRST waves. Nonphysiologic (e.g., < 140 ms) coupling intervals between QRS complexes and unstable ECG baselines are sometimes more apparent at the beginning or the ending of the recorded artifacts. Lack of clinical correlation to an identified "arrhythmia" may be a useful feature, but beware that some serious cardiac arrhythmias can be asymptomatic. Ultimately, the keys to identifying artifacts are the clinician's familiarity with the various types of artifacts and the careful analysis of the ECG.

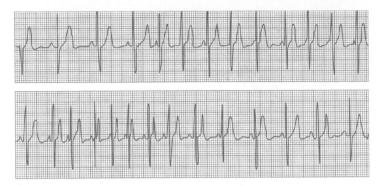

FIGURE 13-2. Deceleration of tape during recording. Supraventricular tachycardia is simulated toward the end of the top and beginning of the second trace as the tape, which transiently slowed as a result of battery failure during recording, was played back on recording paper at proper speed. Note the foreshortening of the duration of the P wave, PR interval, QRS complex, and QT interval.

SUGGESTED READING

Fogel R, Evans J, Prystowsky E. Utility and cost of even recorders in the diagnosis of palpitations, presyncope and syncope. *Am J Cardiol.* 1997;79:207–208.

Holter NJ. New method for heart studies: continuous electrocardiography of active subjects over long periods is now practical. *Science.*1961;134:1214–1220.

Joshi AK, Kowey PR, Prystowsky EN, et al. First experience with a mobile cardiac outpatient telemetry (MCOT) system for the diagnosis and management of cardiac arrhythmias. *Am J Cardiol.* 2005;95:878–881.

Knight BP, Pelosi F, Michaud GF, et al. Clinical consequences of electrocardiographic artifact mimicking ventricular tachycardia. *N Engl J Med.* 1999;341:1270–1274.

Krahn A, Klein G, Yee R, et al. Use of an extended monitoring strategy in patients with problematic syncope. *Circulation.* 1999;99:406–410.

Krasnow AZ, Bloomfield DK. Artifacts in portable electrocardiographic monitoring. *Am Heart J.* 1976;91:349–357.

Myerburg JR, Chaitman BR, Ewy GA, et al.Training in electrocardiography, ambulatory electrocardiography, and exercise testing *J Am Coll Cardiol.* 2008;51:384.

Prystowsky EN. Assessment of rhythm and rate control in patients with atrial fibrillation. *J Cardiovasc Electrophysiol.* 2006;17:S7–S10.

CHAPTER 14

Techniques of Electrophysiologic Evaluation

M. Eyman Mortada and Masood Akhtar

The regular, surface 12-lead electrocardiogram (ECG) provides extensive information about the heart's rhythm and its abnormalities. However, it cannot determine the exact diagnosis, mechanism, or location of a dysrhythmia to direct appropriate management. For the past few decades, the recording of intracavitary electrocardiographic signals and various forms of pacing programs have experienced enormous growth.

TECHNIQUES OF INTRACARDIAC ELECTROPHYSIOLOGIC STUDIES

The exact type of electrical signal recordings, specific equipment used, and pacing protocol depend on the nature of the clinical problem, type of electrophysiologic assessment, and anticipated course of action. Routine cardiac electrophysiology studies (EPS) are performed while patients are in a nonsedated postabsorptive state.

The typical electrode catheters used for both recording and cardiac stimulation are multipolar, inserted via peripheral veins. They are placed under fluoroscopic guidance in the high right atrium, at the His bundle, in the right ventricular, and sometimes in the region of the coronary sinus (Fig. 14-1). Transseptal catheterization is invaluable when accessing the pulmonary veins via the right atrium during ablation of atrial fibrillation (AF). Left-sided heart catheterization is seldom necessary, but used therapeutically in ablating ventricular tachycardia (VT) or left-sided accessory pathway. Heparin may be given as needed, unless left-heart catheterization is desirable; then continuous heparinization is required to avoid thromboembolic complications.

【 】 ELECTROPHYSIOLOGIC RECORDINGS

Once the electrode catheters are placed appropriately, the connections are made via a junction box. Electrograms are displayed simultaneously on a multichannel oscilloscopic recorder. Filter settings between 30 to 40 and 500 Hz are best suited for sharp intracardiac signals. In addition to the intracardiac signals, several surface electrocardiographic leads are recorded. All equipment is reliably grounded.

Catheters have evolved into different shapes. Some of them have multiple electrodes that help localize special areas, mainly during AF ablation (e.g., Basket and Lasso catheters used in isolating the pulmonary veins, Pentarrays used to locate fractionated recordings in the left atrium, and balloon catheters used in noncontact mapping).

【 】 ELECTROPHYSIOLOGIC MAPPING

More recently, several mapping/recording systems have emerged that facilitate more accurate location of the arrhythmia. They create three-dimensional (3D) color-coded

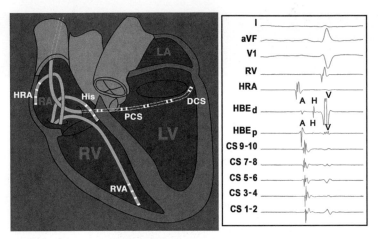

FIGURE 14-1. Standard catheter position for a "four-wire" diagnostic EP study (*left panel*). Electrograms display during standard four-wire study in sinus rhythm (*right panel*). Although all 12 surface ECG leads are recorded, only 3 approximately orthogonal leads are shown, for clarity. The right ventricular apex (RV) and high right atrium (HRA) leads show sharp single-chamber electrograms. The His bundle catheter records activity adjacent to the AV node; the distal bipole (HBE$_d$) favoring the His bundle electrogram (H) and the adjacent ventricular myocardium (V), while the proximal bipole (HBE$_p$) shows a large atrial electrogram (A.) The electrograms recorded by the bipoles of the decapolar coronary sinus catheter are labeled *CS 9-10* (proximal) to *CS 1-2* (distal); each shows a sharp atrial electrogram followed by a smaller ventricular electrogram. (Murgatroyd FD, Krahn AD, Yee R, et al. *Handbook of Cardiac Electrophysiology.* London: ReMEDICA; 2002:8–9. Reproduced with permission from the publisher and authors.)

activation and/or voltage maps, making it possible to manipulate the ablation catheter without the use of fluoroscopy.

Biosense CARTO System

The CARTO system consists of a magnetic field generator locator pad placed under the patient table, a sensor-mounted catheter and a reference catheter placed intracardially, a mapping system, and a graphic computer. The catheter tip allows orientation in relation to the reference signal. By moving the sensor sequentially, one can generate a 3D activation map (Fig. 14-2).

EnSite System

NavX System (St. Jude Medical, Minneapolis, MN)   Based on the LocaLisa (Medtronic Inc., St. Paul, MN) technology, the NavX system combines catheter location and tracking features of the LocaLisa with the ability to create a 3D anatomic model of the cardiac chamber using only a single, conventional electrophysiology catheter and skin patches (Fig. 14-3).

EnSite Array System (Noncontact Mapping)   Noncontact mapping can be done using the Endocardial Solutions system. The EnSite catheter uses a balloon design with a 64-electrode array arranged over the outside of the balloon. This balloon

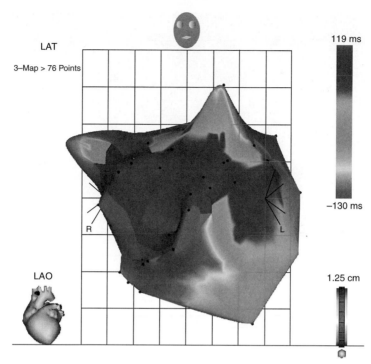

FIGURE 14-2. Left anterior oblique view of the left atrium during left atrial flutter using the Biosense CARTO system. The red shows the earliest activation with respect to the timing reference (typically the proximal coronary sinus recording), and the blue and the violet represent areas of late activation. There are two areas where early activation meets late activation, a characteristic of dual-loop reentrant tachycardias. Both share one arm that runs through the lateral wall of the left atrium (mitral isthmus).

is positioned in the center of the chamber and does not come in contact with the walls of the chamber being mapped. Employing data from the 64-electrode-array catheter, the computer uses sophisticated algorithms to compute an *inverse solution* to determine the activation sequence on the endocardial surface.

Intracardiac Ultrasound

Intracardiac ultrasound is useful in locating the fosa ovalis to perform transseptal puncture; in visualizing the mitral valve annulus, left atrial appendage, and pulmonary veins; in guiding the catheter position and its tip-to-tissue contact; and finally, in monitoring lesion formation to prevent microbubbles. Recently, it has been used with other mapping systems (e.g. CARTOSOUND) to create more accurate anatomical images.

Computed Tomography and Magnetic Resonance Imaging

Both computed tomography (CT) and magnetic resonance imaging (MRI) can reproduce and segment a 3D model of a specific heart chamber. This model can then be used as a reference, or can even be imported directly into the mapping application and synchronized

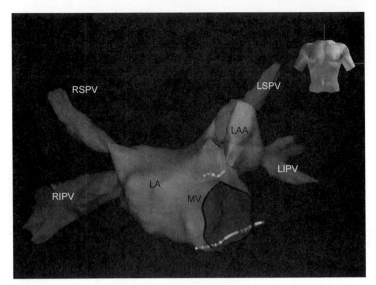

FIGURE 14-3. Anatomic reconstruction of the left atrium in a patient using NavX, anterior–posterior projection. A cutout is shown at the location of the mitral valve. The coronary sinus and radiofrequency ablation catheters are shown in the image. (LA, left atrium; LAA, left atrial appendage; LSPV, left superior pulmonary vein; LIPV, left inferior pulmonary vein; MV, mitral valve; RIPV, right inferior pulmonary vein; RSPV, right superior pulmonary vein.)

or registered for real-time catheter location and tracking in a patient-specific anatomic model of the cardiac chamber (e.g., CARTO-Merge, EnSite Fusion, and CT-fluoroscopy registration) (Fig. 14-4).

【 】 ELECTROPHYSIOLOGIC STEERING TECHNIQUES

The conventional technique to advance recording catheters and manipulate ablation catheters in the cardiac chambers is manual. Almost all ablation catheters and a few sheaths and recording catheters are deflectable, aiding movement to the desired location. New technology has evolved using robotic catheter navigation, where the operator can steer the catheter remotely: the Hansen robotic system and a remote magnetic navigation system.

【 】 PROGRAMMED ELECTRICAL STIMULATION

Two formats of pacing protocol are common. The first is incremental atrial or ventricular pacing, which is pacing at a constant cycle length with gradual shortening until the occurrence of a desirable event, such as induction of a tachycardia or production of atrioventricular (AV) or ventriculoatrial (VA) block. Bursts of pacing at a constant cycle length are also used.

The second pacing format is premature (or extra) stimulation from atrial or ventricular sites. For induction of supraventricular tachycardias (SVTs), single, double, or more extra stimuli may be delivered (Fig. 14-5). For the induction of VT, up to three ventricular extra stimuli are employed. The sensitivity of pacing protocols seems to be directly related to the number of extrastimuli used. This occurs, however, at the expense of specificity, when polymorphic VT/VF can be induced at very short coupling intervals by using multiple extra stimuli.

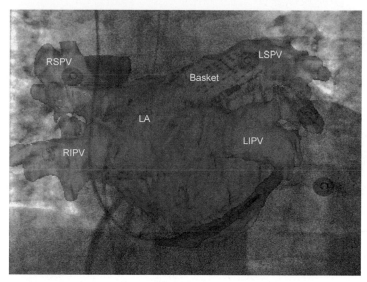

FIGURE 14-4. Real-time CT-fluoroscopy registration image. Anterior-posterior fluoroscopy view of the cardiac silhouette with ablation catheter and basket recording catheter in the left superior pulmonary vein. The coronary sinus, high atrial, and His bundle catheters are in their designated locations. The CT image is posterior-anterior overlapping the fluoroscopy image with sophisticated ECG-gated registration technique. (LA, left atrium; LSPV, left superior pulmonary vein; LIPV, left inferior pulmonary vein; RIPV, right inferior pulmonary vein; RSPV, right superior pulmonary vein.)

During routine EPSs, a variety of electrophysiologic parameters are measured, including sinus node function and intra-atrial, AV nodal, and His–Purkinje system conduction. Initiation of SVT and VT is attempted to determine the mechanisms, site of origin, prognostication, and potential of overdrive termination as a therapy option. After baseline studies, intravenous drugs may be administered to facilitate induction of tachycardias, aggravation of sinus node function, or production of AV block.

INVASIVE ELECTROPHYSIOLOGIC STUDIES FOR DIAGNOSIS

【 】 SINUS NODE DYSFUNCTION

Electrophysiologic studies are performed to detect suspected sinus node dysfunction in patients with dizziness, presyncope, and/or syncope, in which the diagnosis cannot be made noninvasively. The most frequently performed test is that of sinus node suppression, using overdrive atrial pacing for approximately 30 seconds or longer. The resultant escape interval, which is called *sinus node recovery time,* is measured. By deducting the predominant sinus cycle length from this interval, one can obtain the so-called *corrected sinus node recovery time.* A value of corrected sinus node recovery time of more than 525 ms is found in patients with overt sinus node dysfunction.

In the vast majority of patients with true sinus node disease, sinoatrial conduction abnormalities are the predominant reason for sinus node dysfunction. It is measured by

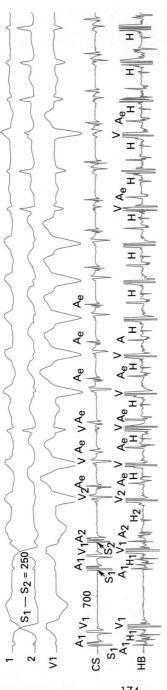

FIGURE 14-5. Induction of supraventricular tachycardia (SVT) in Wolff-Parkinson–White syndrome. The tracings are labeled. Atrial pacing from coronary sinus (CS) is done at a 700-ms basic cycle. During the basic drive pacing, left free-wall accessory pathway conduction to the ventricle produces ventricular preexcitation. A single premature beat (S_2) blocks in the accessory pathway (AP) and conducts over the normal pathway with a left bundle-branch block morphology, and the SVT is initiated. Note the intermittent normalization of the QRS complex during this SVT. (Jazayeri M, Caceres J, Tchou P, et al. Electrophysiologic characteristics of sudden QRS axis deviation during orthodromic tachycardia. *J Clin Invest.* 1989;83:952–959. Reproduced with permission from the publisher and authors.)

atrial extra-stimuli maneuvers, with normal conduction time of less than 100 ms. It is important to test AV conduction in patients with sinus node dysfunction, as the former is also frequently abnormal.

【 】 ATRIOVENTRICULAR BLOCK

In asymptomatic individuals with second-degree AV block (Mobitz I and/or Mobitz II), electrophysiologic assessment is used to find the site of the block by discernible His bundle recording (Fig. 14-6). Patients with intra- or infra-Hisian block tend to have a more unpredictable course, and permanent pacing is desirable. In symptomatic patients with second-degree AV block, the role of EPS is limited because permanent pacing is the appropriate intervention. On the other hand, if the patient's symptoms cannot be

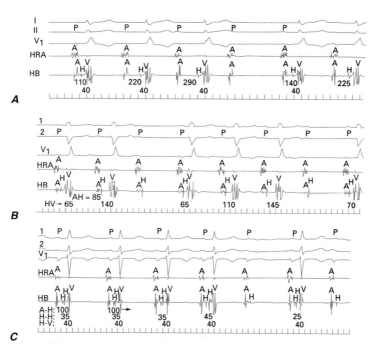

FIGURE 14-6. His bundle (HB) electrograms in atrioventricular (AV) block. The tracings are from three different patients with second-degree AV block. In **A** and **B**, the conducted QRS complexes are wide and associated with bundle branch block. In **A**, the block is within the AV node (i.e., the A wave on the HB is not followed by an HB deflection). In **B**, it can be appreciated that the block is distal to the HB even though the surface ECG demonstrates a Wenckebach phenomenon. The latter can obviously occur in the His–Purkinje system as well, as depicted in this figure. In **C**, the site of the block is within the HB. This is suggested by split HB potentials (labeled H and H+), and the block is distal to the H but proximal to the H+. Intra-His block is difficult to diagnose from the surface ECG but can be suspected when a Mobitz type II occurs in association with a normal PR interval and a narrow QRS complex. (Aklilar M. Invasive cardiac electrophysiologic studies: an introduction. In: Parmley WW, Chatterjee K, eds. *Cardiology.* Vol. 1. *Physiology, Pharmacology, Diagnosis.* Philadelphia, PA: Lippincott Williams & Wilkins; 1991:6.54–56.67. Reproduced with permission from the publisher and authors.)

explained on the basis of AV block and may be related to another arrhythmia, such as VT, EPS should be considered. EPS are rarely required for the other types of AV block.

If 1:1 AV conduction is noted during EPS in patients suspected of intermittent AV block, incremental atrial pacing should be done to see whether AV block can be reproduced.

【 】 NARROW QRS TACHYCARDIA

Narrow QRS tachycardia is supraventricular in origin. It includes sinus and atrial tachycardia, atrial flutter, AF, AV nodal reentrant tachycardia, junctional tachycardia, and orthodromic AV reentrant tachycardia via an accessory pathway. Baseline characteristics (e.g., intracardiac activation sequence, and the initiation and termination of the tachycardia) may help in identifying the etiology of the tachycardia. To confirm the diagnosis, pacing maneuvers (e.g., entrainment and/or extrastimuli during His refractory period) are required most of the time.

【 】 WIDE QRS TACHYCARDIA

Wide QRS tachycardia occurs as a consequence of a variety of electrophysiologic mechanisms, both from supraventricular and ventricular origins in the presence or absence of accessory pathways (Fig. 14-7). Defining the underlying nature of the wide QRS tachycardia is

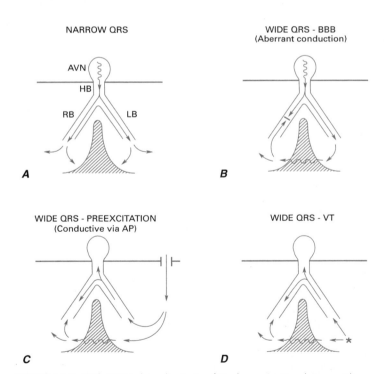

FIGURE 14-7. Wide QRS tachycardia. Routes of impulse propagation during a wide QRS tachycardia in various settings are depicted. It should be noted that only in **A** and **B** is His bundle activation expected to precede ventricular activation. This helps the delineation from other causes of wide QRS tachycardia shown in **C** and **D**.

critical for both prognosis and therapy. With few exceptions, when the nature of the arrhythmic problem is not known and the direction of therapy is not clear, patients with wide QRS tachycardia should undergo EPS.

【 】 UNEXPLAINED SYNCOPE

Syncope may be caused by cardiovascular mechanisms. Electrophysiologic evaluation constitutes an integral part of the evaluation of patients with unexplained syncope, especially those with heart disease. Neurocardiogenic mechanisms constitute the most common cause of syncope in patients without structural heart disease, especially in younger patients (< 50 years of age) with syncope and documented bradycardia (sinus arrest or AV block) and can be unmasked on a tilt table. The triage of patients toward one or the other—that is, electrophysiologic testing versus head-up tilt—is a fairly simple choice, determined by the clinical history and the presence or absence of structural heart disease.

【 】 RISK STRATIFICATION FOR SUDDEN CARDIAC ARREST

Within the last decade, implantable cardioverter defibrillators (ICDs) have been approved for primary and secondary prevention of sudden cardiac arrest (SCA). Therefore, use of EPS for justification of ICD implantation has been abandoned, except in a few scenarios where risk stratification for SCA is required. EPS is indicated in patients with left ventricular (LV) dysfunction (LV ejection fraction ≤ 40%) and recorded nonsustained VT occurring during the waiting period for ICD implantation; in patients with symptoms suggestive of VT/VF (e.g., palpitation, presyncope, or syncope); or in patients with high risk of sudden cardiac death (SCD), such as those with hypertrophic obstructive cardiomyopathy or Brugada syndrome, where an ICD implant may be beneficial. In a few cases, EPS is required to reduce the frequency of ICD shocks, and to help define a strategy for mapping and ablating the cause (SVT, bundle branch reentry VT, or ischemic VT).

INVASIVE CARDIAC ELECTROPHYSIOLOGIC STUDIES FOR THERAPEUTIC INTERVENTION

【 】 SUPRAVENTRICULAR TACHYCARDIA

Therapeutic intervention for most SVT is very successful. In this instance, EPS and transvenous catheter-based ablation are first-line therapy. On the other hand, this is considered a second-line therapy after pharmacologic therapy fails in some SVT (e.g., atrial tachycardia, atypical atrial flutter, and AF). It has been shown that ablation success is optimized with the use of 3D mapping systems. Three-dimensional mapping aids in locating the foci in atrial tachycardia, the macroreentrant circuit in atrial flutter, and the anatomic model or electrical fractionation of the left atrium in AF.

The introduction of catheter ablation techniques has made it rare for patients to undergo surgery for SVT. Some individuals with resistant atrial fibrillation and flutter, and those who fail catheter ablative therapy, may still be considered candidates for a surgical approach.

【 】 VENTRICULAR TACHYCARDIA

In patients with an ICD, electrophysiologic evaluation and therapy can be accomplished through the permanent leads of the ICD. Pacing, antitachycardia function, low-energy cardioversion, and cardiac defibrillation can all be programmed through the device. When problems are encountered following discharge of a patient with an ICD, electrophysiologic reassessment via ICD is frequently necessary, and sometimes transvenous catheterization may be required.

EPS is essential in all patients undergoing therapeutic intervention (ablation) for VT, regardless of the etiology (normal heart structure VT, scar-related VT, or even idiopathic VF). Conventional electrical mapping (e.g., pace mapping or entrainment mapping) and 3D mapping are tools to facilitate successful outcome. Catheter-based ablation is performed mainly via a percutaneous transvascular approach; if that fails, a nonsurgical transthoracic epicardial catheter ablation approach may be necessary to eliminate ventricular dysarrhythmia.

Patients with coronary artery disease and VT that can be mapped are also candidates for VT surgery if the VT cannot be managed with an ICD, antiarrhythmic drugs, and/or catheter ablation. Preoperative EPS for this eventuality is important.

CATHETER ABLATION TECHNIQUES

The realization that the origin of VT and SVT can be effectively mapped (pace map, entrainment, or 3D map) has made the catheter ablation technique a rational approach. The radiofrequency or cryoablation forms of energy delivered through a catheter permit controlled trauma to cardiac tissue to abolish or modify reentrant circuits in both SVT and VT. Unifocal atrial tachycardia, isthmus-dependant atrial flutter, AV nodal reentry of all varieties, and accessory pathways, including atriofascicular fibers, can be cured in over 95% of patients with radiofrequency catheter ablation. The success rate of AF and atypical atrial flutter ablation ranges between 60% and 80%. Patients with monomorphic VT, associated with normal heart structure, can also be considered candidates, particularly when they fail drug therapy. Bundle-branch reentrant VT is an ideal substrate for catheter ablation in patients with abnormal heart structure. Additionally, in patients with incessant VT or frequent VT with inadequate control despite antiarrhythmic and ICD therapy, VT ablation should be considered.

IATROGENIC PROBLEMS ENCOUNTERED DURING ELECTROPHYSIOLOGIC STUDIES

Mechanical irritation from catheters during placement, even when they are not being manipulated, can cause a variety of arrhythmias and conduction disturbances. These include induction of atrial, junctional, and ventricular ectopic beats and multiple types of AV block. Ventricular stimulation can also occur from physical movement of the ventricular catheter coincident with atrial contraction, producing electrocardiographic patterns of ventricular preexcitation.

Certain types of arrhythmias must be avoided, such as atrial fibrillation and VF. Catheter trauma resulting in abolition of accessory pathway conduction or the reentrant pathway may make the curative ablation difficult or impossible.

RISK AND COMPLICATIONS

The complication rate of EPS is relatively low, with almost negligible mortality. Complications include deep venous thrombosis, intracavitary thrombosis, pulmonary or systemic embolism, infection at catheter sites, systemic infection, pneumothorax, hemothorax perforation of a cardiac chamber or coronary sinus, pericardial effusion, and tamponade.

SUGGESTED READING

Akhtar M, Damato AN, Gilbert-Leeds CJ, et al. Induction of iatrogenic electrocardiographic patterns during electrophysiologic studies. *Circulation.* 1977;56:60–65.

Akhtar M, Mahmud R, Tchou P, et al. Normal electrophysiologic responses of the human heart. *Cardiol Clin.* 1986;4:365–386.

Dhingra RC, Wyndham C, Bauernfeind R, et al. Significance of block distal to the His bundle induced by atrial pacing in patients with chronic bifascicular block. *Circulation.* 1979;60:1455–1464.

Gomes JA. The sick sinus syndrome and evaluation of the patient with sinus node disorders. In: Parmley WW, Chatterjee K, eds. *Cardiology.* Vol. 1. *Physiology, Pharmacology, Diagnosis.* Philadelphia, PA: Lippincott Williams & Wilkins; 1991:100–106.

Knight B, Ebinger M, Oral H, et al. Diagnostic value of tachycardia features and pacing maneuvers during paroxysmal supraventricular tachycardia. *J Am Coll Cardiol.* 2000;36:574–582.

Lee KW, Badhwar N, Scheinman MM. Supraventricular Tachycardia. *Curr Probl Cardiol.* 2008;33:553–662.

Mortada ME, Akhtar M. Sudden cardiac death. In: Jeremias A, Brown DL, eds. *Cardiac Intensive Care.* 2nd ed. St. Louis, MO: Elsevier; in press.

Sra J, Akhtar M. Mapping techniques for atrial fibrillation ablation. *Curr Probl Cardiol.* 2007;32:669–767.

Sra JS, Anderson AJ, Sheikh SH, et al. Unexplained syncope evaluated by electrophysiologic studies and head-up tilt testing. *Ann Intern Med.* 1991;114:1013–1019.

Stevenson WG, Friedman PL, Kocovic D, et al. Radiofrequency catheter ablation of ventricular tachycardia after myocardial infarction. *Circulation.* 1998;98:308–314.

Zipes DP, DiMarco JP, Gillette PC, et al. Guidelines for clinical intracardiac electrophysiological and catheter ablation procedures. A report of the American College of Cardiology/American Heart Association Task Force on Practice Guidelines (Committee on Clinical Intracardiac Electrophysiologic and Catheter Ablation Procedures), developed in collaboration with the North American Society of Pacing and Electrophysiology. *J Am Coll Cardiol.* 1995;26:555–573.

CHAPTER 15

Treatment of Cardiac Arrhythmias with Ablation Therapy

Usha B. Tedrow and William G. Stevenson

Successful catheter ablation requires precise localization of the source of the arrhythmia, accurate placement of the ablation catheter, and achievement of an adequate ablation lesion. Catheter positioning is assisted primarily by fluoroscopy. Sophisticated mapping systems can also display catheter position and a three-dimensional (3D) depiction of the anatomy. Magnetic resonance imaging (MRI), computed tomography (CT), and echocardiographic data can also be integrated with these systems. Radiofrequency (RF) energy is most commonly used, but freezing with cryoablation catheters is a potential alternative. Serious complications of catheter ablation are infrequent and most often related to the catheterization procedure, usually including vascular injury and cardiac perforation with tamponade.

REENTRANT SUPRAVENTRICULAR TACHYCARDIA

【 】 ATRIOVENTRICULAR NODAL REENTRANT TACHYCARDIA

Ablation for atrioventricular nodal reentrant tachycardia (AVNRT) is recommended when episodes are poorly tolerated or resistant to medical therapy, or if the patient cannot tolerate medications. The atrioventricular (AV) node consists of a compact portion and adjoining lobes. In patients with AVNRT, the lobe extending toward the coronary sinus likely forms a functional pathway for slow conduction between the os of the coronary sinus and the septal leaflet of the tricuspid valve that can be ablated safely. Success is achieved in more than 95% of patients. Heart block is the major risk, occurring in approximately 0.8% of patients and requiring permanent pacemaker implantation. Cryoablation may be associated with a lower risk of heart block, but has lower long-term success rates.

【 】 ATRIOVENTRICULAR RECIPROCATING TACHYCARDIA

Patients with atrioventricular reciprocating tachycardia (AVRT) have an accessory pathway connecting atrium and ventricle and bypassing the His–Purkinje system. If the pathway has manifest antegrade conduction, the electrocardiogram (ECG) shows preexcitation, a hallmark of the Wolff–Parkinson–White syndrome. Accessory pathways conducting only from ventricle to atrium are termed *concealed* because during sinus rhythm preexcitation is absent, but AVRT still can occur. Catheter ablation is the standard of care for symptomatic Wolff–Parkinson–White syndrome, or for concealed accessory pathways causing symptomatic tachycardias when pharmacologic therapy is ineffective or not desirable.

Pathway location along the mitral or tricuspid annulus determines whether an arterial, venous, or transseptal approach is required (Fig. 15-1). Success rates are 95%, and serious complications are uncommon. Heart block can occur with ablation of septal pathways located close to the AV node.

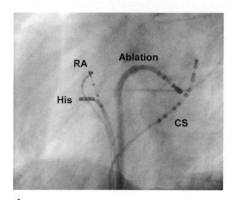

A

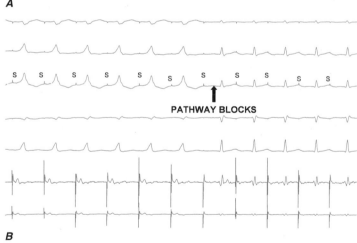

B

FIGURE 15-1. A. Ablation of a left-sided accessory pathway in a patient with Wolff–Parkinson–White syndrome. Shown is a left anterior oblique fluoroscopic image depicting catheter position for catheter ablation of a left-sided accessory pathway by a transeptal approach. A decapolar catheter is seen in the coronary sinus (CS). The ablation catheter (Ablation) is passed through a sheath that crosses the fossa ovalis into the left atrium for mapping along the tricuspid valve annulus. **B.** Five surface ECG leads and two intracardiac leads depict ablation of a left lateral accessory pathway during atrial pacing. The right atrium is being paced (pacing stimuli indicated by S). Pacing stimuli initially conduct from the atrium to the ventricles over the AV node and an accessory pathway producing a pattern of ventricular preexcitation with a wide QRS and a slurred initial delta wave. The pathway blocks within seconds of the application of radiofrequency energy with sudden narrowing of the QRS complex indicating that conduction to the ventricles is occurring only over the normal conduction system of AV node and His bundle.

REGULAR ATRIAL ARRHYTHMIAS

【 】 FOCAL ATRIAL TACHYCARDIA

Focal atrial tachycardia (AT) tends to occur in specific anatomic locations: along the crista terminalis, tricuspid or mitral annulus, coronary sinus musculature, atrial appendages, and in the pulmonary veins. The tachycardia must be present or provocable to be successfully localized for ablation. Ablation is successful in more than 80% of patients. Significant complications occur in 1% to 2% of patients.

【 】 SINUS NODE MODIFICATION FOR INAPPROPRIATE SINUS TACHYCARDIA

Patients with inappropriate sinus tachycardia have sinus tachycardia without a discernible cause. Catheter ablation can be a last resort when severe symptoms do not respond to pharmacologic therapy. Ablation of the rapidly firing regions along the crista terminalis can slow the sinus rate. Ablation of the entire sinus node, with permanent pacemaker implantation, can require epicardial ablation, but long-term success is limited, as many patients have recurrent symptoms, some despite improvement in heart rate. Potential complications include narrowing of the superior vena cava, right phrenic nerve paralysis, and the need for chronic pacing.

【 】 ATRIAL FLUTTER AND OTHER MACROREENTRANT ATRIAL TACHYCARDIAS

Common atrial flutter is caused by a large macroreentrant circuit with a wavefront revolving around the tricuspid annulus. In typical counterclockwise atrial flutter, the wavefront proceeds up the atrial septum and down the right atrial free wall. Reentry is dependent on conduction through the cavotricuspid isthmus bounded by the tricuspid valve, inferior vena cava, eustachian ridge, and coronary sinus os. Once the diagnosis is confirmed by entrainment and activation mapping, a series of ablation lesions is placed across the cavotricuspid isthmus, creating a line of conduction block (Fig. 15-2). Success is achieved in more than 95% of patients. Approximately 20% to 30% of patients also have atrial disease that leads to atrial fibrillation in the next 20 months.

Other macroreentrant circuits can occur in the left or right atrium not involving the cavotricuspid isthmus. Arrhythmias from reentry occurring around atrial scars from prior heart surgery, such as atrial septal defect repair, are referred to as "scar-related" macroreentrant ATs. Catheter ablation is more difficult, with success rates of 80% to 85%, and more frequent late recurrences than are observed for common flutter.

ATRIAL FIBRILLATION

【 】 ATRIOVENTRICULAR JUNCTION ABLATION FOR RATE CONTROL

In patients with atrial fibrillation (AF), catheter ablation of the AV junction to produce complete heart block with implantation of a permanent pacemaker can be used to control the ventricular rate. The strategy is generally reserved for older patients who may already have an implanted pacemaker or defibrillator, who cannot tolerate rate-control medications, and who are not candidates for other rhythm-control strategies. Anticoagulation for thromboembolic risk is still required. For patients with previously uncontrolled ventricular rates, quality of life, exercise tolerance, and ejection fraction can improve. However, following the abrupt decrease in heart rate, cases of sudden death

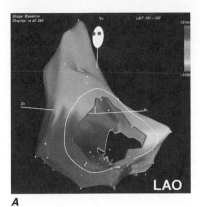

A

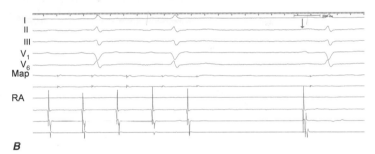

B

FIGURE 15-2. Mapping and ablation of typical counterclockwise atrial flutter. **A.** It is an activation map of the right atrium during counterclockwise atrial flutter as viewed in a left anterior oblique projection. Activation circulates up the interatrial septum, across the roof, down the free wall, and through the cavotricuspid isthmus. A line of RF lesions was placed across this isthmus, which blocked conduction in the isthmus terminating atrial flutter. **B.** The tracing shows surface ECG leads and intracardiac recordings from the mapping catheter (Map) and lateral right atrium (RA) during RF ablation. Atrial flutter terminates and is followed by sinus rhythm (*arrow*).

have occurred, likely as a result of polymorphic ventricular tachycardia. Pacing the ventricle at 90 beats per minute for the first several weeks and then gradually reducing the rate over time reduces the risk. Right ventricular (RV) pacing can have adverse hemodynamic consequences in some patients with poor left ventricular (LV) function. Biventricular pacing likely reduces this risk.

【 】 ATRIAL FIBRILLATION ABLATION FOR MAINTAINING SINUS RHYTHM

The majority of focal triggers that initiate paroxysmal AF originate in the pulmonary veins. Although ablation strategies vary, most target areas within the atrium that encircle the pulmonary veins, often with the goal of electrically isolating these regions without ablating in the veins themselves. Extensive series of lesions are usually placed in the left atrium. Intracardiac echocardiography and 3D mapping systems that incorporate anatomy from MRI or CT images are helpful adjuncts to facilitate ablation strategies.

Success varies with the type of AF and severity of underlying heart disease. Successful maintenance of sinus rhythm after the initial healing phase is achieved in more than 70% to 80% of young patients with paroxysmal AF without structural heart disease, but reported follow-ups are still relatively short, with few studies reporting data beyond 1 year. Success rates are lower for patients with persistent or permanent AF.

For several weeks following ablation, atrial arrhythmias can occur as ablation lesions heal and the atrium remodels, but these often subsequently resolve. A second procedure is required in 20% to 50% of patients. Antiarrhythmic medications are often continued for 1 to 3 months after ablation. Anticoagulation with warfarin is required.

Major procedural complications include myocardial perforation with tamponade (1–2%) and stroke (0.5–1%). Severe pulmonary vein stenosis has been reported in 2% to 6% of patients. Death from atrioesophageal fistulae, presenting days to a few weeks after the procedure with endocarditis, septic emboli, or gastrointestinal bleeding, has been reported (< 0.1% estimated). Appropriate patient selection requires adequate assessment of risks and benefits for each individual patient. The risks and benefits can be expected to improve as this relatively new procedure continues to evolve.

VENTRICULAR TACHYCARDIA

【 】 IDIOPATHIC VENTRICULAR TACHYCARDIA

Idiopathic ventricular tachycardia (VT) occurs in the absence of structural heart disease and is often amenable to catheter ablation. The most common form originates from a focus in the RV outflow tract, beneath the pulmonary valve and may cause exercise-induced VT, repetitive bursts of monomorphic VT, or symptomatic premature ventricular contractions. The VT has a pattern of left bundle-branch block in V_1 with an inferiorly directed axis. Ablation is performed at the area of earliest activation in the outflow tract, with successful elimination of tachycardia in more than 80% of patients. Occasionally idiopathic outflow tract VT originates from sites adjacent to the aortic annulus, the LV outflow tract, or in the epicardium.

The most common form of left-sided idiopathic VT originates from the LV apical septum. This arrhythmia is characterized on surface ECG by a pattern of right bundle-branch block in lead V_1, usually with a superiorly directed axis. It often responds to verapamil. It appears to be caused by reentry involving the Purkinje system. Ablation targeting characteristic electrograms in the reentry region is successful in more than 80% of patients.

【 】 SCAR-RELATED REENTRY CAUSING VENTRICULAR TACHYCARDIA

Sustained VT associated with structural heart disease is associated with a risk of sudden death. Most patients receive an implanted cardioverter defibrillator (ICD) that can terminate VT when it occurs. Catheter ablation is an important alternative to antiarrhythmic drug therapy for reducing the frequency of symptomatic VT and can be lifesaving if VT becomes incessant.

Any ventricular scar can cause reentry due to the anatomic barrier created by portions of the scar and slow conduction in areas with surviving myocytes dispersed in the scar. Myocardial infarction is the most common cause of scar, but idiopathic dilated cardiomyopathy, sarcoidosis, arrhythmogenic right ventricular dysplasia, and Chagas' disease can also result in VT substrate. Prior cardiac surgery with ventriculotomy or patch repairs is a common culprit. The ECG morphology of the VT suggests the location of the scar and the VT exit.

During mapping, areas of scar are identified and highlighted on 3D anatomic maps, allowing some VT that is hemodynamically unstable to be targeted. Pacing from the mapping catheter during sinus rhythm also helps identify the exit region. Ablation then targets conducting channels or the border of the scar region that contains the VT exit. Some epicardial VT can be approached by a subxiphoid percutaneous puncture into the pericardial space for mapping and ablation. Success rates are approximately 70% due to multiple potential reentry circuits. Procedure-related mortality is approximately 3%, some from uncontrollable VT when the procedure fails.

Bundle-branch reentry VT is a type of VT that is particularly susceptible to ablation, and is found in approximately 6% of patients with VT and structural heart disease. A diseased Purkinje system supports a reentry circuit revolving up one bundle branch and down the contralateral bundle branch. These patients often have intraventricular conduction delay or a pattern of left bundle-branch block during sinus rhythm and advanced ventricular dysfunction. Catheter ablation of the right bundle branch eliminates this VT, though other types of VT are often inducible.

【 】 ABLATION FOR ELECTRICAL STORM AND VENTRICULAR FIBRILLATION

Repetitive episodes of ventricular fibrillation causing *electrical storm* can be initiated by ectopic foci in the Purkinje system. Such cases are rare, but ablation targeting the initiating foci during periods of electrical storm with a strategy similar to that used for idiopathic VT can be lifesaving.

CONCLUSION

Ablation is a reasonable first-line therapy for most symptomatic supraventricular tachycardias caused by accessory pathways, atrial flutter, AV node reentrant tachycardia, and idiopathic VT. Its use for atrial fibrillation is increasing and further studies will continue to define the risks and benefits. Catheter ablation is an important adjunctive therapy to an implanted defibrillator for patients with recurrent VT associated with structural heart disease and can be lifesaving for patients with incessant VT or electrical storms.

SUGGESTED READING

Blomstrom-Lundqvist C, Scheinman MM, Aliot EM, et al. ACC/AHA/ESC guidelines for the management of patients with supraventricular arrhythmias—executive summary: a report of the American College of Cardiology/American Heart Association Task Force on Practice Guidelines and the European Society of Cardiology Committee for Practice Guidelines (Writing Committee to Develop Guidelines for the Management of Patients With Supraventricular Arrhythmias). *Circulation.* 2003;108:1871–1909.

Haissaguerre M, Extramiana F, Hocini M, et al. Mapping and ablation of ventricular fibrillation associated with long-QT and Brugada syndromes. *Circulation.* 2003;108:925–928.

Haissaguerre M, Jais P, Shah DC, et al. Spontaneous initiation of atrial fibrillation by ectopic beats originating in the pulmonary veins. *N Engl J Med.* 1998;339:659–666.

Joshi S, Wilber DJ. Ablation of idiopathic right ventricular outflow tract tachycardia: current perspectives. *J Cardiovasc Electrophysiol.* 2005;16(suppl 1):S52–S58.

Marchlinski FE, Callans DJ, Gottlieb CD, et al. Linear ablation lesions for control of unmappable ventricular tachycardia in patients with ischemic and nonischemic cardiomyopathy. *Circulation.* 2000;101:1288–1296.

Natale A, Newby KH, Pisano E, et al. Prospective randomized comparison of antiarrhythmic therapy versus first-line radiofrequency ablation in patients with atrial flutter. *J Am Coll Cardiol.* 2000;35:1898–1904.

Ouyang F, Cappato R, Ernst S, et al. Electroanatomic substrate of idiopathic left ventricular tachycardia: unidirectional block and macroreentry within the Purkinje network. *Circulation*. 2002;105:462–469.

Scheinman MM, Huang S. The 1998 NASPE prospective catheter ablation registry. *Pacing Clin Electrophysiol*. 2000;23:1020–1028.

Soejima K, Stevenson WG, Maisel WH, et al. Electrically unexcitable scar mapping based on pacing threshold for identification of the reentry circuit isthmus: feasibility for guiding ventricular tachycardia ablation. *Circulation*. 2002;106:1678–1683.

Tchou P, Jazayeri M, Denker S, et al. Transcatheter electrical ablation of right bundle branch. A method of treating macroreentrant ventricular tachycardia attributed to bundle branch reentry. *Circulation*. 1988;78:246–257.

CHAPTER 16

Indications and Techniques of Electrical Defibrillation and Cardioversion

Chirag M. Sandesara and Richard E. Kerber

HISTORY OF DEFIBRILLATION AND CARDIOVERSION

The deleterious effects of uncontrolled electrical current on cardiac rhythm were first recognized early in the 20th century. Concerned by accidental electrocutions of its line workers, the Consolidated Edison Company of New York supported research on the mechanisms and treatment of electrical accidents. Investigators at Johns Hopkins Hospital developed techniques of defibrillation—the termination of ventricular fibrillation—by an electrical shock in the 1930s. The first human defibrillation, in the operating room, was performed by Claude Beck in 1947. Transchest defibrillation using alternating current became a clinical reality when introduced by Paul Zoll in 1956, and direct current defibrillation was pioneered by Bernard Lown in 1962. The work of Zoll and Lown in combination with the description of closed-chest cardiac massage by Jude and colleagues in 1960 has formed the foundation of cardiopulmonary resuscitation from cardiac arrest for over 40 years.

Lown utilized a damped sinusoidal waveform, which—at the usually encountered human transthoracic impedance (70–80 Ω)—was effectively monophasic. In the Soviet Union, Gurvich described an underdamped sinusoidal waveform that was effectively biphasic; this waveform was not used in the West.

More recently, truncated exponential biphasic waveforms have now become the standard for transchest defibrillation; this is discussed further in this chapter.

In this chapter, the term *defibrillation* refers to the electrical termination of ventricular fibrillation (VF); *cardioversion* refers to the electrical termination of atrial fibrillation, atrial flutter, and supraventricular and ventricular tachycardias.

MECHANISMS OF DEFIBRILLATION AND CARDIOVERSION

How does an electric shock terminate a cardiac arrhythmia? There are three principal hypotheses. The critical mass hypothesis suggests that some proportion of the myocardium (not necessarily all) must be depolarized, so that the remaining muscle is inadequate to maintain the arrhythmia. The upper limit of vulnerability hypothesis argues that a sufficient current density throughout the ventricle must be achieved lest fibrillation be reinitiated by a subthreshold current density. Jones' group states that defibrillating shocks must prolong refractoriness in sufficient myocardium to terminate VF. These concepts are not mutually exclusive, and all three hypotheses may be applicable. Whether they also apply to the atrial myocardium for the termination of atrial fibrillation by electrical shock is not known. More organized arrhythmias, such as ventricular tachycardia and atrial flutter, terminate with lower energy than VF and atrial fibrillation, likely because only regional depolarization in the path of an advancing wavefront is required.

SHOULD DEFIBRILLATION BE PERFORMED IMMEDIATELY UPON DISCOVERY OF VF, OR SHOULD IT BE PRECEDED BY A PERIOD OF CPR?

Ventricular fibrillation is a lethal arrhythmia and demands instant termination as a lifesaving maneuver. The American Heart Association has encouraged immediate defibrillation of a victim of VF upon the availability of a defibrillator. However, two recent investigations by Cobb, Wik, and their coworkers have shown that if the initial application of shock is delayed (usually due to late arrival of rescuers at the scene of the cardiac arrest), a brief period of cardiopulmonary resuscitation (CPR) (ventilation, closed-chest compression) *prior* to the first shock will favorably enhance outcome. However, a third clinical trial, by Jacobs and associates, did not find that a period of CPR before defibrillation facilitates resuscitation. These observations led Weisfeldt and Becker to propose a three-phase model of VF-induced cardiac arrest: (1) the *electrical* phase consists of the first 4 minutes of VF. Shocks administered during this period have a high likelihood of achieving VF termination and resumption of spontaneous circulation. (2) The *circulatory* phase lasts from 4 to 10 minutes during VF. Shocks should be delayed in favor of a period of 1 to 3 minutes of CPR, including administration of epinephrine or vasopressin, to restore a more favorable milieu for defibrillation. (3) The *metabolic* phase begins after 10 minutes of VF. In this phase, changes in myocardial metabolism after prolonged VF require aggressive and invasive measures for reversal, such as cardiopulmonary bypass and/or hypothermia. Shocks given during this period without such preparatory measures are likely to result in pulseless electrical activity or asystole—conditions associated with a very low likelihood of survival.

The phases of VF/cardiac arrest outlined above are time-based. Could we achieve a more sophisticated insight into the myocardial milieu and thereby determine whether immediate electrical shock or preshock pharmacologic therapy or other resuscitative maneuvers should be employed in each particular case? Such insight might be afforded by a detailed analysis of the electrocardiographic VF signal itself. Experimental and clinical studies have shown that changes in VF frequency and amplitude occur over time. Such changes may be modulated pharmacologically, may correlate with coronary perfusion pressure (the difference between aortic and right atrial pressure during cardiac arrest), and may predict the response to a defibrillating shock. With better understanding of the VF signal and its relationship to the state of the myocardium, the optimal timing of the electrical shock could be guided by a microprocessor-based analysis of the VF signal integrated into the defibrillator, which would instantly instruct the operator whether to deliver a shock or employ other supportive measures, such as continuing CPR and administering vasopressors. Defibrillators employing such sophisticated techniques of VF analysis are now commercially available.

WHO SHOULD BE CARDIOVERTED FROM ATRIAL FIBRILLATION/ATRIAL FLUTTER, AND WHEN SHOULD THIS BE PERFORMED?

Sinus rhythm improves cardiac performance, especially in patients with mitral stenosis, left ventricular hypertrophy (aortic stenosis, hypertension, idiopathic hypertrophic subaortic stenosis), and/or diminished myocardial reserve (congestive heart failure, myocardial ischemia, and infarction). The coordinated atrial contraction of sinus rhythm improves ventricular filling and the associated cardiac rate is usually slower. Patients with these conditions are thus candidates for *elective* cardioversion. *Urgent* cardioversion may be required for patients with atrial or ventricular arrhythmias who have evidence of end-organ hypoperfusion and/or pulmonary edema.

In some cases, treatment of an underlying or causative condition may restore sinus rhythm without the necessity of electrical cardioversion. Common causes of atrial arrhythmias include hyperthyroidism, pulmonary embolism, congestive heart failure, and mitral stenosis. Postoperative cardiac patients frequently experience transient rhythm disturbances that may spontaneously revert to sinus rhythm.

Important factors that determine the immediate and long-term success of cardioversion of atrial arrhythmias include the duration of the arrhythmia, the extent of atrial fibrosis, and the size of the left atrium. High success rates have been reported for cardioversion of atrial fibrillation and atrial flutter, especially when the new biphasic waveforms are used. High transthoracic impedance (TTI)—the resistance of the chest to the flow of electrical current—will degrade current flow. Because current across the heart is what accomplishes the termination of the arrhythmia, high TTI may reduce the success of defibrillation or cardioversion, especially if the operator has selected a low shock energy.

THROMBOEMBOLISM

There is a significant risk of thromboembolism after cardioversion. Three factors contribute to this risk:

1. If there is a preexisting thrombus in the fibrillating atrium (especially likely in the left atrial appendage), the electrical shock and/or the resumption of atrial contraction may dislodge the thrombus.

2. The shock itself may have thrombogenic effects.

3. With prolonged atrial fibrillation an atrial myopathy develops, which results in a slow return to normal atrial contraction following cardioversion (see Chapter 10, which discusses this phenomenon in detail).

To prevent thromboembolism, therapeutic anticoagulation (INR 2.0–3.0) for 3 weeks prior to cardioversion and 4 weeks afterward is traditionally recommended.

The risk of thromboembolism associated with atrial fibrillation and cardioversion is higher in patients with mitral stenosis, a large left atrium from any cause, chronic atrial fibrillation, congestive heart failure, age greater than 75 years, previous thromboembolic events, diabetes, or hypertension. Although transthoracic echocardiography is able to image the left atrial cavity well, it is usually unsatisfactory for visualization of the left atrial appendage, the site of most atrial thrombi. However, transesophageal echocardiography (TEE) images the left atrial appendage well and is highly sensitive to the presence of thrombi. Manning and colleagues reported no embolic events during the cardioversion of atrial fibrillation when transesophageal echocardiography showed no thrombi were present in the atrial appendage and the patient received intravenous heparin for 2 days before cardioversion. This approach is known as TEE-guided cardioversion. If a thrombus in the left atrial appendage is seen by TEE, cardioversion should be delayed and anticoagulation for 3 weeks should be undertaken. Some clinicians repeat the TEE to ensure that the thrombus has lysed. Although thromboembolism after cardioversion of atrial flutter is less common, it has been reported, as have conditions associated with thromboembolism, such as left atrial "smoke" (spontaneous ultrasound contrast) on transesophageal echocardiography. Thus, anticoagulation before cardioversion of atrial flutter should be undertaken if persisting longer than 48 hours, similar to atrial fibrillation.

At present, TEE and cardioversion are generally carried out as two separate procedures, both requiring conscious sedation or anesthesia. Recently the two procedures have been combined by adding an electrode to the external surface of the transesophageal echo probe. Another electrode is placed on the anterior chest wall using a self-adhesive electrode pad. This allows a cardioverting direct current shock to be delivered, using the esophageal-chest pathway. Because the esophageal electrode is close to the heart and the pathway is shortened, less energy—typically 20 to 50 J—is required to terminate atrial fibrillation using this esophageal cardioversion technique. Initial clinical experience with this combined TEE/cardioversion approach has been reported and appears efficacious.

Whether the traditional or TEE-guided anticoagulation scheme is utilized, it is considered mandatory to maintain anticoagulation for at least 4 weeks after cardioversion, since in the absence of anticoagulation thrombi may form postcardioversion and embolism may occur despite a negative TEE precardioversion. Patients with paroxysmal atrial fibrillation, or those considered at high risk of recurrence of atrial fibrillation after cardioversion, may require permanent anticoagulation.

Antiarrhythmic drugs, such as amiodarone may facilitate cardioversion and maintenance of sinus rhythm after cardioversion. It is customary to withhold digitalis on the day of cardioversion (although this practice is not consistent with the long half-life of this drug). Digitalis-toxic rhythms should not be cardioverted, as the enhanced automaticity of such arrhythmias, combined with the shock, could result in ventricular fibrillation or bidirectional ventricular tachycardia.

TECHNIQUES OF CARDIOVERSION AND DEFIBRILLATION

【 】 ANESTHESIA

Because the electrical current passing across the thorax causes a painful tetanic contraction, elective cardioversion in these authors' opinion should be performed under general anesthesia; conscious sedation is often inadequate, with the patient experiencing and remembering severe discomfort. Bag-valve ventilation without endotracheal intubation is usually sufficient, but the presence of an anesthesiologist assures the ability to perform rapid endotracheal intubation if this becomes necessary.

【 】 SYNCHRONIZATION

It is essential to synchronize the electrical discharge on the R wave of the QRS complex; if the shock falls in the vulnerable period of the cardiac cycle, VF may be induced (Fig.16-1). This is the most frequent serious complication of elective cardioversion of atrial arrhythmias and usually results from the operator's failure to enable properly the synchronizing device or to verify that the R wave of the electrocardiogram (ECG) lead chosen is sufficiently tall to be recognized by the synchronizer. Recognition of the R wave of ventricular tachycardia is sometimes difficult owing to the morphology of the arrhythmia. If the patient is hemodynamically unstable owing to rapid ventricular tachycardia, unsynchronized shocks may be necessary.

【 】 ELECTRODES

Electrode placement on the chest is important to maximize current flow through the heart, which is what actually terminates the arrhythmia. Only a small proportion—as

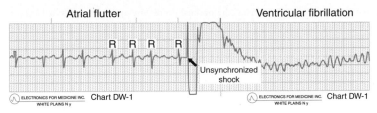

FIGURE 16-1. A complication of cardioversion: induction of ventricular fibrillation. The ventricular arrhythmia occurred because the operator failed to enable the synchronizer, resulting in inadvertent delivery of the shock on the vulnerable T wave instead of the intended delivery on the R wave. This complication is preventable by enabling the synchronizer and checking that it is properly functioning before shock delivery. (Reproduced with permission from Kerber RE. Transchest cardioversion: optimal techniques. In: Tacker WA, ed. *Defibrillation of the Heart: ICDs, AEDs and Manual.* St. Louis, MO: Mosby-Year Book; 1994. Chap. 7)

low as 4%—of the total transchest current flow actually traverses the heart. Numerous pathways have been used successfully, including apex–high right parasternal, anteroposterior, and apex–right infrascapular (Fig. 16-2). The apex–high right parasternal is most frequently used. Although it has been difficult to demonstrate the superiority of any one pathway over others in clinical studies, one pathway might prove superior in the individual patient. Thus, it is the authors' practice to move the electrodes to an alternate pathway when a patient whose atrial arrhythmia is expected to respond to elective cardioversion fails to convert with the initial shocks.

Electrodes should not be placed directly over the site of implanted pacemaker or defibrillator generators. Although manufacturers commonly mark electrodes to indicate the location of chest placement, electrode polarity does not seem to influence shock success, either for monophasic or biphasic waveforms.

Electrode size influences the impedance of the chest; larger electrodes yield lower impedance and thereby improve current flow, increasing the likelihood of arrhythmia

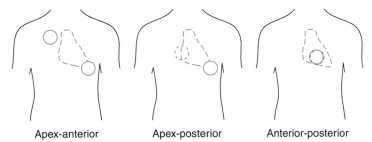

FIGURE 16-2. Electrode positions commonly used for transthoracic defibrillation and cardioversion. The apex-anterior position is most commonly used, but all are effective. If shocks given from one electrode pair position fail to terminate the arrhythmia, it is the authors' practice to quickly change to another position and repeat the shocks. (Reproduced with permission from Kerber RE. Transchest cardioversion: optimal techniques. In: Tacker WA, ed. *Defibrillation of the Heart: ICDs, AEDs and Manual.* St. Louis, MO: Mosby-Year Book; 1994. Chap. 7)

termination. For adult humans, the optimal paddle size appears to be 8 to 12 cm in diameter. The Association for the Advancement of Medical Instrumentation recommends a minimum electrode contact area of 50 cm^2 for each electrode. The total area of both electrodes should be at least 150 cm^2. Smaller pediatric paddles have been manufactured for children, but adult-size paddles should be used for children weighing more than 10 kg (approximately 1 year old). This minimizes transthoracic impedance.

Gels or pastes should not be smeared across the chest between paddle electrodes; the electrical current may follow the low-impedance pathway created by the paste, deflecting current away from the heart. In women, the apex electrode should be placed adjacent to or under the breast; placement on the breast results in a high transthoracic impedance and degrades current flow.

Cutaneous erythema after shocks is often noted at the location of the electrode placement. We have shown by skin biopsies that these are first-degree burns. Because there is preferential current flow at the edges of these electrodes, the erythema typically is most intense at the edges of the electrode location, outlining the electrode shape. Self-adhesive electrode pads constructed to have increased impedance at the pad edges allow more homogeneous current flow and may minimize these burns.

Self-adhesive electrode pads for defibrillation have other advantages. They allow continuous monitoring of cardiac rhythm before and after the shock as well as more physical separation of the generator from the patient (thus reducing the chance of the operator inadvertently receiving a shock); they also facilitate arrhythmia documentation. These pads are universally used in the new automated external defibrillators (AEDs), which are discussed later in this chapter.

NEW WAVEFORMS FOR DEFIBRILLATION AND CARDIOVERSION

For many years, truncated exponential biphasic waveforms have been used instead of damped sinusoidal monophasic waveforms for implantable cardioverter defibrillators. Their superiority for *transthoracic* defibrillation and cardioversion has been demonstrated, initially in the operating room and the electrophysiology laboratory, where VF is deliberately induced, and subsequently during out-of-hospital cardiac arrest. They are also superior for the electrical cardioversion of atrial arrhythmias. At any energy level, these biphasic waveforms yield higher rates of arrhythmia termination than damped sinusoidal monophasic waveforms. This has resulted in lower energy recommendations for biphasic defibrillation and cardioversion; however, clinical considerations (left atrial size, duration of arrhythmia) may suggest higher or lower energies. The American Heart Association has stated that biphasic waveform shocks ≤ 200 J are safe and effective for defibrillation, and similar biphasic shock energies are highly effective for cardioversion. Whether biphasic shocks > 200 J for defibrillation will be necessary for a significant number of VF patients is not known at present.

"Smart" biphasic waveform defibrillators incorporate technology to measure transthoracic impedance during the shock and instantaneously alter the waveform duration and/or voltage to compensate for impedance. Still other available defibrillators use a rectilinear near-rectangular fixed-pulse-duration waveform. Any of these biphasic waveform variants will be superior to the traditional damped sinusoidal monophasic waveform; whether any one biphasic waveform is superior to another for human defibrillation and cardioversion has yet to be established.

New waveforms for defibrillation have been investigated in animal models. These include sawtooth-shaped biphasic waveforms and multipulse multipathway shocks.

These have not yet been used for transthoracic defibrillation in humans. Triphasic and quadriphasic waveforms do not require additional capacitors or elaborate circuitry; these have shown superiority in animal studies.

MYOCARDIAL DAMAGE FROM DEFIBRILLATION AND CARDIOVERSION

Although a lifesaving technique, direct current shocks may cause myocardial damage, especially when repeated high-energy discharges are administered. Shocks cause mitochondrial dysfunction and free radical generation in the myocardium proportional to the energy used. Antioxidant strategies to minimize shock-induced cardiac damage have been investigated in experimental animals. Reducing shock energy/current as well as minimizing the number of shocks delivered will limit shock-induced myocardial damage. Some clinicians delay repeating a failed shock (for atrial fibrillation) for 1 or 2 minutes in the hope of preventing damage, but there is no convincing evidence for this approach; the authors' practice is to repeat shocks as necessary without delay. Biphasic waveforms seem to be less toxic, perhaps simply by requiring less energy to achieve defibrillation.

AUTOMATED EXTERNAL DEFIBRILLATORS AND PUBLIC ACCESS DEFIBRILLATION

In the 1980s, efforts to reduce the mortality associated with out-of-hospital cardiac arrest emphasized training of emergency medical technicians to recognize VF and to defibrillate using traditional manual defibrillators. Subsequently, automated external defibrillators (AEDs) were introduced; these small, light, and relatively inexpensive devices acquire an ECG via self-adhesive monitor-defibrillator pads applied to the cardiac arrest victim's thorax. A microprocessor in the defibrillator analyzes the ECG thus acquired; if the algorithm for VF is satisfied, the device sounds a warning and then delivers a shock. The ease of application and use of these devices make training requirements minimal, and biphasic waveforms in presently available units enhance the effectiveness of these AEDS. Requirements for AED algorithm performance and safety have been published. Initial experience with AEDs has been reported from aircraft, airports, and gambling casinos, and all reports have been highly favorable. Many communities are now equipping "first responders," such as police officers, firefighters, and security guards, with AEDs. Placement of AEDs in areas known to have a high rate of cardiac arrest—airports, prisons, gyms—is an appropriate and cost-effective strategy. Controlled trials of this strategy have shown its effectiveness. The American Heart Association strongly supports these efforts under the rubric of *public access defibrillation*.

AUTOMATIC IMPLANTABLE CARDIOVERTER DEFIBRILLATORS

Automatic implantable cardioverter defibrillators (ICDs) have revolutionized the treatment of patients at risk of life-threatening ventricular arrhythmias causing sudden cardiac death. ICD pulse generators are implanted in the right or left upper chest and in certain circumstances, they are implanted in the abdomen. Either a single chamber device is implanted as a right ventricular lead with shock coils placed in the right ventricular apex or septum. A dual-chamber system includes a right atrial lead placed in the atrial appendage in addition to a right ventricular lead. The Food and Drug Administration first approved the use of ICDs in 1985. Initial clinical research was tailored toward secondary prevention of sudden cardiac death. Several secondary prevention clinical trials were performed to assess the utility of ICDs in cardiac arrest survivors. The Antiarrhythmics versus Implantable Defibrillators (AVID) trial, Cardiac Arrest Study Hamburg (CASH) trial, and the Canadian Implantable Defibrillator Study (CIDS) all proved the usefulness of implantation of defibrillators in patients who already had a history of cardiac arrest or hemodynamically significant VT. Ad hoc analyses of these studies confirmed that patients with the lowest ejection fraction had the greatest benefit. Primary prevention studies including the Multicenter Automatic Defibrillator Implantation trial (MADIT), Multicenter Automatic Defibrillator Implantation trial II (MADIT II), Multicenter Unsustained Tachycardia trial (MUSTT), and the Sudden Cardiac Death in Heart Failure trial (SCD-HeFT) all demonstrated that ICDs can reduce mortality in patients at risk for sudden cardiac death due to ventricular arrhythmias. Based on these studies, ICDs are indicated for patients who present with VT and sudden cardiac death. They are also indicated for patients with NYHA class II and class III heart failure, ejection fraction < 35%, and have either ischemic or nonischemic cardiomyopathy (based on CMS guidelines derived from the SCD-HeFT trial).

ICDs are also indicated for patients presenting with a prior infarction, with an ejection fraction < 40%, who have spontaneous nonsustained VT and have also had an electrophysiology study showing inducible VT based on the MADIT and MUSTT studies. Patients who fulfill MADIT II criteria (at least 1 month post-infarction with EF ≤ 30%) are candidates for ICD implant. Several other patients at high risk for life-threatening ventricular arrhythmias due to long QT syndrome, Brugada syndrome, or hypertrophic obstructive cardiomyopathy and who usually have a normal ejection fraction may still benefit from ICD implantation.

HOME DEFIBRILLATORS

Although widespread placement of AEDs in public spaces will improve survival after cardiac arrest, it is known that over two-thirds of cardiac arrests occur at home. Should AEDs be placed in homes of patients with known heart disease who have an increased risk of cardiac arrest? (Patients at the highest risk—e.g., those with ischemic heart disease with ejection fractions less than 35%—should receive an implanted cardioverter defibrillator). For an AED to be effective when used to treat a cardiac arrest at home, the following must happen: (1) a spouse (or family member/friend) previously trained in AED use, must be at home; (2) the spouse must witness the arrest; (3) the spouse must retrieve the AED; (4) the spouse must correctly apply and turn on the AED; and (5) the AED must be in proper operating condition. These requirements are not trivial, and initial experience with AED use at home suggested that in an emergency, spouses, often elderly, may forget to retrieve their AED and/or be unable to apply and use it correctly.

One potential solution to this problem is the recent development of a wearable defibrillator. The patient wears a vest in which electrodes are incorporated and an ECG is fed to a defibrillator that is worn in a holster-like device (Fig. 16-3). The ECG is continuously analyzed; if the VF algorithm is satisfied, the device initially delivers an audible and tactile alarm. If VF is not actually present (e.g., if one of the ECG leads in the vest loses skin contact and the resultant artifact simulates VF), the patient has about 30 seconds to disable the device; if it is not disabled during the alert period, the defibrillator charges and then automatically delivers a biphasic shock. Initial clinical experience has been favorable.

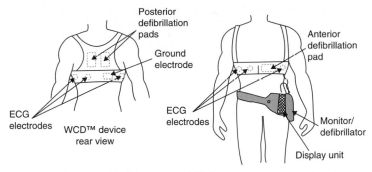

FIGURE 16-3. A wearable, fully automatic defibrillator. The patient wears electrodes in a vest; the ECG is continuously analyzed. If the algorithm for VF is satisfied, the device initiates an audible and tactile alarm; this allows the device to be disabled by the patient if the "arrhythmia" was artifactual (e.g., a loose or faulty lead). If the device is not disabled within 20 to 30 seconds, a shock is delivered automatically. (Reprinted from Aurrichio A, Klein H, Geller C, et al. Clinical efficacy of the wearable cardioverter defibrillator in acutely terminating episodes of ventricular fibrillation. *Am J Cardiol.* 1998;81:1253–1257, with permission from Excerpta Medica, Inc.)

HYPOTHERMIA

Two recent multicenter trials have shown that the deliberate induction of hypothermia by application of external cooling devices affords protection to the brains of patients who have been defibrillated and resuscitated from VF/VT but who remain comatose after resuscitation (i.e., anoxic encephalopathy). By cooling such patients to about 33°C for 24 to 36 hours, neurologic outcome improved. This strategy has been endorsed by the American Heart Association. Could hypothermia applied before or during VF/VT (intra-arrest hypothermia) facilitate defibrillation and resuscitation? Recent animal studies in mice and pigs have suggested this is so. A major challenge is to develop methods to lower core temperature in patients to about 33°C rapidly—within a few minutes—in order to render this a feasible strategy for intra-arrest application, because external cooling in patients requires several hours to reach 33°C. Experimental methods currently being evaluated include intravenous iced saline, chemical slurries, and intrapulmonary cold perfluorocarbons. This is a fertile field for future research.

CONCLUSION

As the professional baseball player and folk philosopher Yogi Berra may have said, "Predictions are difficult—especially about the future." Nevertheless, we offer some predictions of the state of the art of defibrillation and cardioversion in the next decade. The ECG signal of VF will be analyzed quickly and automatically and shock timing will be guided by information extracted from the ECG. Defibrillators in public places will become as common and accepted as fire extinguishers, and brief training in their use will be widespread, thanks largely to the Public Access Defibrillation program of the American Heart Association. Finally, defibrillators in the homes of patients with ischemic heart disease and/or a known propensity to arrhythmia (perhaps revealed by genetic analysis) will be an accepted part of cardiovascular therapy. These strategies hold great promise for combating the international epidemic of sudden cardiac death.

SUGGESTED READING

Abela BS, Zhao D, Alvarado T, et al. Intra-arrest cooling improves outcomes in a murine cardiac arrest model. *Circulation.* 2004;109:2786–2791.

American Heart Association. Guidelines 2005 for cardiopulmonary resuscitation and emergency cardiac care. *Circulation.* 2005;112:IV1–IV41.

Antiarrhythmics Versus Implantable Defibrillators (AVID) investigators. A comparison of antiarrhythmic-drug therapy with implantable defibrillators in patients resuscitated from near-fatal ventricular arrhythmias. *N Engl J Med.* 1997;337:1576–1583.

Arnold AZ, Mick MJ, Mazurek RP, et al. Role of prophylactic anticoagulation for direct current cardioversion in patients with atrial fibrillation or atrial flutter. *J Am Coll Cardiol.* 1992;19:851–855.

Barnard SA, Gray TW, Brist MD, et al. Treatment of comatose survivors of out-of-hospital cardiac arrest with induced hypothermia. *N Engl J Med.* 2002;346:557–563.

Black I, Hopkins AP, Lee CLL, et al. Evaluation of transesophageal echocardiography before cardioversion of atrial fibrillation and atrial flutter in nonanticoagulated patients. *Am Heart J.* 1993;126:375–381.

Boddicker K, Zhang Y, Zimmerman MB, et al. Hypothermia improves defibrillation success and resuscitation outcomes from ventricular fibrillation. *Circulation.* 2005;111:3195–3201.

Caffrey SL, Willoughy P, Pepe PE, et al. Public use of automated external defibrillators. *N Engl J Med.* 2002;347:1242–1247.

Callaway CW, Menegazzi JJ. Waveform analysis of ventricular fibrillation to predict defibrillation. *Curr Opin Crit Care.* 2005;11:192–199.

Caterine MR, Spencer KT, Pagan Carlo LA, et al. Direct current shocks to the heart generate free radicals: an electron paramagnetic resonance study. *J Am Coll Cardiol.* 1996;28:1598–1609.

Dendi R, Zhang Y, Brooks L, et al. Rapid cardiopulmonary intra-arrest hypothermia improves resuscitation outcomes from ventricular fibrillation cardiac arrest. *Circulation.*2005;112:II-323. Abstract.

Hooker DR, Kowenhoven WB, Langworth CR. The effect of alternating electrical currents on the heart. *Am J Physiol.* 1933;103:444–454.

Moss AJ, Zareba W, Hall WJ. Prophylactic implantation of a defibrillator in patients with myocardial infarction and reduced ejection fraction (MADIT II). *N Engl J Med.* 2002;346:877–883.

Scholten MF, Thornton AF, Jordaens LJ, et al. Usefulness of transesophageal echocardiography using a combined probe when converting atrial fibrillation to sinus rhythm. *Am J Cardiol.* 2005;94:470–473.

Valenzuela T, Roe DJ, Nichol G, et al. Outcomes of rapid defibrillation by security officers after cardiac arrest in casinos. *N Engl J Med.* 2000;343:1206–1209.

Weaver DL, Peberdy MA. Defibrillation in public places—one step closer to home. *N Engl J Med.* 2002;347:1223–1224.

Weisfeldt M, Becker L. Resuscitation after cardiac arrest: a three-phase time-sensitive model. *JAMA.* 2002;288:3035–3038.

Zhang Y, Ramabadran R, Boddicker K, et al. Triphasic shocks are superior to biphasic shocks for transthoracic defibrillation: experimental studies. *J Am Coll Cardiol*. 2003;42:568–575.

Zhang Y, Rhee B, Davis L, et al. Quadriphasic waveforms are superior to triphasic waveforms for transthoracic defibrillation in a cardiac arrest swine model with high impedance. *Resuscitation*. 2006;68:251–258.

CHAPTER (17)

Diagnosis and Management of Syncope

Judith A. Mackall and Mark D. Carlson

Syncope is a sudden loss of consciousness and postural tone caused by transient decreased cerebral blood flow and is associated with spontaneous recovery. Syncope can occur suddenly, without warning, or be preceded by light-headedness, dizziness, nausea, diaphoresis, and blurred vision. The incidence of syncope increases with age and its causes include cardiovascular disorders, disorders of vascular tone or blood volume, and cerebrovascular disorders. The cause is often multifactorial and cannot be determined in up to 50% of cases. Syncope caused by cardiovascular disorders is associated with the highest risk for mortality, approaching 50% over 5 years and 30% in the first year after diagnosis. Syncope that is not associated with cardiac disease or is of undetermined cause is associated with the lowest mortality risk (6–10% over 3 years and 24% over 5 years). It is important to distinguish syncope from other causes of loss of consciousness, including seizures, hypoglycemia, and trauma.

CARDIOVASCULAR DISORDERS

Cardiovascular disorders cause syncope due to severe obstruction or cardiac rhythm disturbances that decrease cardiac output (Table 17-1). Obstructive lesions and arrhythmias frequently coexist; one may accentuate the effects of the other. Loss of consciousness during or immediately after exertion is common and may be the presenting symptom in patients with obstructive lesions.

Both sinus node disease and atrioventricular conduction disorders may cause syncope. In the *bradycardia–tachycardia syndrome* (sick sinus syndrome accompanied by atrial tachyarrhythmias), syncope often occurs with asystole at the termination of tachycardia.

Supraventricular tachyarrhythmias rarely cause syncope unless other abnormalities are present (obstructive cardiovascular disease, neurocardiogenic reaction, or a rapid ventricular rate in patients with Wolff–Parkinson–White [WPW] syndrome who experience atrial fibrillation). Ventricular tachycardia is the most common arrhythmic cause of syncope and often occurs in the setting of structural heart disease torsade de pointes can cause syncope in patients with long QT syndrome. The most common causes of acquired long QT syndrome are antiarrhythmic drugs (types Ia and III) and electrolyte disorders (hypokalemia and hypomagnesemia).

DISORDERS OF VASCULAR CONTROL OR BLOOD VOLUME

Disorders of vascular control or blood volume that cause syncope include the reflex syncopes and a number of causes for orthostatic intolerance (Table 17-2).

TABLE 17-1

Cardiovascular Disorders Associated with Syncope

Obstructive

Aortic stenosis
Hypertrophic cardiomyopathy
Mitral stenosis
Prosthetic mitral or aortic valve malfunction
Atrial myxoma
Pulmonary embolism
Pulmonary hypertension
Tetralogy of Fallot
Cardiac tamponade

Arrhythmic

Sinoatrial disease
Atrioventricular block
Supraventricular tachyarrhythmias
Ventricular tachycardia
Pacemaker disorders

【 】 REFLEX SYNCOPE

Reflex syncopes are caused by sudden failure of the autonomic nervous system to maintain sufficient vascular tone resulting in hypotension (and sometimes bradycardia). The two most common causes are neurocardiogenic (vasodepressor or vasovagal) and the carotid sinus syndrome. The other forms are termed situational because they occur in association with specific activities or conditions (such as micturition, defecation, swallowing, coughing, or postprandial). Neurocardiogenic syncope is often provoked by standing, warm environments, emotional distress, and pain. It is usually preceded by nausea, sweating, light-headedness, or visual alterations but can occur suddenly. The reflexes responsible for neurocardiogenic syncope are normal. Gravity-mediated displacement of blood and venous pooling decreases venous return to the heart, resulting in increased myocardial contractility that activates ventricular mechanoreceptors. The increased afferent neural traffic mimics hypertension, paradoxically decreasing efferent sympathetic activity, resulting in hypotension (vasodepressor response), and in some cases, increasing vagal efferent activity resulting in bradycardia.

【 】 CAROTID SINUS HYPERSENSITIVITY

Carotid sinus hypersensitivity is most common in men ≥ 50 years old and is precipitated by pressure on the carotid sinus baroreceptors that leads to sinus arrest or arteriovenous (AV) block (cardioinhibitory response), vasodilatation (a vasodepressor response), or both (mixed response).

【 】 SYNDROMES OF ORTHOSTATIC INTOLERANCE

Orthostatic hypotension may occur due to hypovolemia or disturbances in vascular control. Primary autonomic disorders that affect vascular control are often idiopathic and may follow either an acute or chronic course. The secondary forms occur in conjunction with another illness (such as amyloidosis or diabetes), in the setting of a known biochemical or structural alteration, or following exposure to various drugs or toxins (heavy metals, alcohol, and some chemotherapeutic agents) (Table 17-3).

TABLE 17-2

Disorders of Vascular Control and Blood Volume

Reflex Syncope

   Neurocardiogenic
   Situational
   Carotid sinus hypersensitivity

Orthostatic Intolerance

   Autonomic nervous system disorders
      Primary autonomic failure
         Pure autonomic failure
         Multiple system atrophy
         Postural orthostatic tachycardia syndrome
            Peripheral or partial dysautonomia
            Hyperadrenergic
         Acute autonomic failure
      Secondary autonomic failure
         Amyloidosis
         Diabetes
         Sarcoidosis
         Renal failure
         Cancer
         Nerve growth factor deficiency
         Beta-hydroxylase deficiency
      Pharmacologic agents
      Certain heavy metals
         Mercury
         Lead
         Arsenic
         Iron

Intravascular Volume Depletion

   Anemia
   Blood loss
   Dehydration
   Diuretics

Venous Pooling/Vasodilation

   Prolonged bed rest
   Prolonged weightlessness
   Pregnancy
   Venous varicosities
   Pharmacologic agents
   Hyperbradykininism
   Mastocytosis
   Carcinoid syndrome

【　】 PRIMARY CAUSES OF AUTONOMIC FAILURE

Primary autonomic failure (PAF) and multiple system atrophy (MSA) are manifested by orthostatic hypotension, syncope, and varying degrees of autonomic nervous system dysfunction. MSA involves the somatic system as well. The syndromes affect twice as many men as women; symptoms usually begin between the fifth and sixth decades of

TABLE 17-3

Pharmacologic Agents that May Cause or Worsen Orthostatic Intolerance

Angiotensin-converting enzyme inhibitors
Alpha-receptor blockers
Calcium-channel blockers
Beta-blockers
Phenothiazines
Tricyclic antidepressants
Bromocriptine
Opiates
Diuretics
Hydralazine
Ganglionic-blocking agents
Nitrates
Sildenafil citrate
Monoamine oxidase inhibitors
Chemotherapeutic agents
    Vincristine
    Vinblastine

life. In the postural orthostatic tachycardia syndrome (POTS), heart rate increases excessively in response to upright posture. The more common type, peripheral (or partial) dysautonomia, is associated with inability to increase peripheral vascular resistance when upright, leading to blood pooling followed by tachycardia and enhanced myocardial contraction. The hyperadrenergic form is associated with tremor, hyperhidrosis, diarrhea, panic attacks, and severe migraine headaches. Although supine catecholamine levels are normal, upright levels are often elevated (over 600 mg/dL) in patients and the response to isoproterenol is excessive (> 30 bpm increase in response to 1 μg/min).

Acute autonomic failure is characterized by rapid widespread failure of both the parasympathetic and sympathetic, but not the somatic, nervous systems. Merely attempting to sit up in bed may cause syncope. Many patients suffer from anhidrosis and disturbances in bowel and bladder function that result in abdominal pain, cramping, bloating, nausea, and vomiting.

A variety of systemic disorders or environmental and pharmacologic agents may cause syncope by impacting blood volume or vascular control (Tables 17-2 and 17-3).

CEREBROVASCULAR DISORDERS

Patients with cerebrovascular occlusive disease may require higher-than-normal arterial blood pressure to maintain consciousness. Syncope can occur in patients with occluded brachiocephalic vessels, as occurs in pulseless disease (e.g., aortic arch syndrome and Takayasu arteritis). Syncope associated with changing positions of the head can occur due to narrowing of the vertebral arteries by skeletal deformities of the cervical spine in patients with Klippel–Feil deformity, cervical spondylosis, and cervical osteoarthritis. In patients with the *subclavian steal syndrome* syncope occurs during upper extremity exercise when blood flow is shunted retrograde, by the circle of Willis, to the distal subclavian artery. These patients exhibit diminished brachial arterial pressure on the affected side, a bruit that is maximal over the supraclavicular area adjacent to the origin of the vertebral artery, and symptoms during exercise of the involved extremity. Syncope can be a presenting symptom of cerebral emboli or atherosclerotic disease of the vertebrobasilar system.

【 】 APPROACH TO THE PATIENT

One of the most important goals is to determine if the patient has a cause for syncope that is life threatening. In addition, effective therapy often depends on a precise and accurate diagnosis.

HISTORY AND PHYSICAL EXAMINATION

The history and physical examination may alone diagnose the etiology or distinguish syncope from other causes of loss of consciousness. The history should include questions about the first event, how often and in what settings syncope occurred, observations of bystanders, prescription and nonprescription remedies, and family history of cardiovascular disease, neurologic disorders, and early sudden death.

Blood pressure and heart rate should be measured in the supine, sitting, and upright positions immediately and 3 to 5 minutes after standing. Orthostatic hypotension is present if systolic blood pressure falls by 20 mm Hg or diastolic blood pressure falls by 10 mm Hg during the first 2 minutes of standing. A Valsalva maneuver may reproduce cough syncope; hyperventilation for 2 to 3 minutes may reproduce episodes that are related to anxiety. Carotid sinus massage may induce bradycardia, but is not recommended for those who may have carotid atherosclerotic disease. A pause of longer than 3 seconds during massage suggests that carotid sinus hypersensitivity caused syncope.

Blood tests that contribute to diagnosis include a complete blood count, serum electrolytes, supine and upright serum catecholamine levels, and drug levels. Almost all patients should undergo a 12-lead surface electrocardiogram. A transthoracic echocardiogram should be performed whenever heart disease is suspected. Patients at risk for coronary artery disease should undergo a stress test. Continuous ECG monitoring (Holter monitor) is used for suspected arrhythmic syncope; an event recorder may prove efficacious, particularly if the episodes are infrequent. Patients with very infrequent episodes may benefit from an implantable loop recorder. When noninvasive testing does not diagnose arrhythmic causes, an electrophysiologic study may be indicated in high-risk patients including those with coronary artery disease and those with bundle-branch or bifascicular block.

Tilt-table testing is based on the principle that orthostatic stress provokes reflex syncope in susceptible individuals (Table 17-4). A positive test is one that provokes a hypotensive episode (or in the case of POTS, a tachycardic episode) that reproduces the patient's symptoms. The specificity of tilt-table testing is reported to be near 90% and the sensitivity between 20% and 74%.

TREATMENT

Patients should minimize exposure to factors that provoke syncope, situations in which they or others could be injured were they to lose consciousness, and should take measures to avoid syncope (lie down) should they experience prodromal symptoms. Unconsciousness individuals should be placed supine with the head turned to the side. Clothing that fits tightly around the neck or waist should be loosened.

【 】 SYNDROMES OF ORTHOSTATIC INTOLERANCE

Patients with orthostatic hypotension should be instructed to move their legs prior to rising slowly from the bed or a chair (Table 17-5). If possible, medications that aggravate the problem should be discontinued. Physical maneuvers and salt and water loading have benefited some patients. Biofeedback therapy has been useful when neurocardiogenic syncope is provoked by psychogenic stimuli. Beta-adrenoceptor

TABLE 17-4

Head-Up Tilt-Table Testing

Indications for Head-Up Tilt-Table Testing

1. Unexplained recurrent syncope or single syncopal episode associated with injury (or significant risk of injury) in absence of organic heart disease.
2. Unexplained recurrent syncopal episodes or single syncopal episode associated with injury (or significant risk of injury) in setting of organic heart disease after exclusion of potential cardiac cause of syncope.
3. After identification of a cause of recurrent syncope in situations in which determination of an increased predisposition to neurocardiogenic syncope could alter treatment.

Conditions in Which Tilt-Table Testing May Be Useful

1. Differentiating conclusive syncope from epilepsy.
2. Evaluation of recurrent near syncope or dizziness.
3. Evaluation of syncope in autonomic failure syndromes.
4. Exercise-induced or postexercise-induced syncope in absence of organic heart disease in patients in whom exercise stress testing cannot reproduce an episode.
5. Evaluation of recurrent unexplained falls.

antagonists were among the first drugs used to prevent neurocardiogenic syncope. Several vasoconstrictive agents, including the alpha-receptor stimulants dexedrine, methylphenidate, and midodrine, have been used. Midodrine is used to treat orthostatic hypotension and has been shown to prevent neurocardiogenic syncope in two randomized trials. The alpha-2-receptor agonist clonidine may be most useful in patients with both hypertensive and hypotensive episodes. Other vasoconstrictive substances, such as theophylline, ephedrine, and yohimbine, are reported to be effective; but tolerance of these agents is often poor. Bupropion tends to have fewer sexual side effects but may aggravate hypertension.

The acetylcholinesterase inhibitor pyridostigmine may be an effective agent for both orthostatic hypotension and POTS. The agent is safe and effective and seems to be able to prevent falls in blood pressure without exacerbating supine hypertension. The serotonin reuptake inhibitors have been shown to prevent recurrent neurocardiogenic syncope. In patients with orthostatic hypotension or autonomic failure syndromes who have anemia, erythropoietin not only raises red cell counts but has vasoconstrictive effects. Octreotide, a synthetic somatostatin analogue, causes splanchnic mesenteric vasoconstriction, thus enhancing venous return to the heart.

Patients with asystole during tilt testing or syncope and those with the cardioinhibitory or mixed forms of carotid sinus hypersensitivity may benefit from permanent pacing. Pacing reduces recurrent syncope and injuries in elderly patients with frequent falls and cardioinhibitory carotid sinus hypersensitivity. Pacing may prolong the duration of prodromal symptoms, allowing patients sufficient time to take evasive action and avoid syncope.

[ ] CEREBROVASCULAR DISORDERS

Anticoagulants and/or platelet antiaggregant agents are recommended for the prevention of embolic disease from the heart or central vessels. Endarterectomy or percutaneous dilatation should be considered in carotid arterial occlusive disease.

TABLE 17-5

Orthostatic Intolerance Syndrome Therapies

Treatment	Application	Form Effective in				Problems
		NCS	PD	HA	OH	
Reconditioning	Aerobic exercise 20 min 3 times/wk	X	X	X	X	If done too vigorously may worsen symptoms
Physical maneuvers (tilt training, etc.)	30 min 3 times/d	X	X		X	Noncompliance is common
Sleeping with head tilted upright	During sleep	X		X		
Hydration	2 L PO/d	X	X		X	Edema
Salt	2–4 g/d	X	X		X	Edema
Fludrocortisone	0.1–0.2 mg PO qd	X	X		X	Hypokalemia, hypomagnesemia, edema
Metoprolol	25–100 mg bid	X				Fatigue
Labetalol	100–200 mg PO bid			X		Fatigue
Midodrine	5–10 mg PO tid	X	X		X	Nausea, scalp itching, supine hypertension
Methylphenidate	5–10 mg PO tid	X	X	X		Anorexia, insomnia, dependency
Bupropion	150–300 mg XL/qd		X	X		Tremor, agitation, insomnia
Clonidine	0.1–0.3 mg PO bid / 0.1–0.3 mg patch qwk		X	X	X	Dry mouth, blurred vision
Pyridostigmine	30–60 mg PO/d		X		X	Nausea, diarrhea
SSRI-escitalopram	10 mg PO/d	X	X	X	X	Tremor, agitation, sexual problems
Erythropoietin	10,000–20,000 μg sq q/week	X	X		X	Pain at injection site, expensive
Octreotide	50–200 μg SC tid		X		X	Nausea, diarrhea, gallstone
Permanent pacing		X				

204

【 】 CARDIOVASCULAR DISORDERS

Cardiac surgery is often the treatment of choice for patients with syncope caused by obstructive heart disease. Patients with hypertrophic cardiomyopathy and syncope may respond well to pharmacologic therapy, but certain patients may benefit from AV sequential pacing, sugery, or an implantable cardioverter defibrillator. The treatment of arrhythmias that cause syncope is discussed in detail elsewhere (see Chapters 10–12). Bradyarrhythmias usually require the implantation of a permanent pacemaker but may respond to withdrawal of a drug. Implantable cardioverter-defibrillators are the first-line therapy for most ventricular tachycardias, although some patients may require antiarrhythmic drugs or catheter ablation to reduce symptoms or shocks from the ICD.

In patients with polymorphic ventricular tachycardia in the setting of a long QT interval (torsade de pointes), the potential offending drug(s) (usually an antiarrhythmic drug) should be stopped. Acute therapy includes intravenous magnesium and measures to increase the heart rate and shorten electrical diastole (e.g., cardiac pacing). Long-term therapy for congenital long QT syndrome may include beta-blockers, permanent pacing, an implantable defibrillator, and lifestyle changes.

Patients with syncope should be hospitalized with continuous ECG monitoring if it is reasonably likely that the episode resulted from a life-threatening abnormality or if recurrence with significant injury seems likely. Patients who are known to have a normal heart and for whom the history strongly suggests vasovagal or situational syncope may be treated as outpatients if the episodes are neither frequent nor severe. When the cause is unknown, treatment must be targeted to the most likely cause and to prolong life. Certain high-risk patients may benefit from a pacemaker or an implantable cardioverter defibrillator even when it is not clear that bradycardia or a ventricular arrhythmia caused syncope.

CONCLUSION

Syncope, transient loss of consciousness and postural tone as a result of decreased cerebral blood flow with spontaneous recovery, is common and can occur because of a number of underlying mechanisms and disorders, some of which may be normal or benign and do not require therapy (a single episode of neurocardiogenic syncope), and others that are life-threatening and require intervention (e.g., ventricular arrhythmias, aortic stenosis). Identifying the cause for syncope is important for establishing a prognosis and to guide therapy. In addition, syncope must be distinguished from other causes of loss of consciousness (e.g., seizures, trauma, metabolic abnormalities, and certain drugs). Syncope can be classified as cardiac, noncardiac, unknown origin, or multifactorial. The history, physical examination, and certain tests can be used to identify the likely cause and guide therapy in many cases. Yet in many cases, the cause may remain obscure, more than one explanation may exist, or syncope may have occurred as a result of more than one process. In these cases, clinical judgment and assessment of the risks and benefits of therapies are required for effective management.

SUGGESTED READING

Benditt D, Ferguson D, Grubb BP, et al. Tilt table testing for accessing syncope and its treatment: an American College of Cardiology consensus document. *J Am Coll Cardiol.* 1996;28:263–267.

Brignole M, Alboni P, Benditt D, et al. Guidelines on the management, diagnosis and treatment of syncope. *Eur Heart J.* 2001;22:1256–1306.

Grubb BP. Neurocardiogenic syncope and related disorders of orthostatic intolerance. *Circulation.* 2005;111:2997–3006.

Grubb BP, Kosinski D. Orthostatic hypotension: causes, classification and treatment. *Pacing Clin Electrophysiol.* 2003;26:892–901.

Grubb BP, Olshanski B. *Syncope: Mechanisms and Management.* Malden, MA: Blackwell-Futura, 2005.

Kapoor WN. Current evaluation and management of syncope. *Circulation.* 2002;106:1606–1609.

Low P, ed. *Clinical Autonomic Disorders.* 2nd ed. Philadelphia, PA: Lippincott-Raven; 1997.

Mathias C, Bannister R eds. *Autonomic Failure: A Textbook of Clinical Disorders of the Autonomic Nervous System.* 45th ed. Oxford: Oxford University Press; 1999:307–320.

Soteriades ES, Evans JC, Larson MG, et al. Incidence and prognosis of syncope. *N Engl J Med.* 2002;347:878.

Strickberger SA, Benson DW, Biaggioni I, et al. AHA/ACCF scientific statement on the evaluation of syncope. From the American Heart Association Councils on Clinical Cardiology, Cardiovascular Nursing, Cardiovascular Disease in the Young, and Stroke, and the Quality of Care and Outcomes Research Interdisciplinary Working Group; and the American College of Cardiology Foundation; in collaboration with the Heart Rhythm Society; endorsed by the American Autonomic Society. *Circulation.* 2006;113:316–327.

CHAPTER (18)

Sudden Cardiac Death

*Matthew R. Reynolds, Mintu Turakhia,
Duane S. Pinto, and Mark E. Josephson*

DEFINITION

Sudden cardiac death (SCD) is the unexpected natural death from a cardiac cause within a short time period from the onset of symptoms in a person without any prior condition that would appear lethal. SCD most commonly results from cardiac arrest due to a fatal arrhythmia and may or not occur in the background of structural heart disease or coronary artery disease (CAD).

EPIDEMIOLOGY

SCD accounts for almost half a million deaths each year in the United States, with exact totals depending on the definition used. Worldwide, SCD comprises 50% of overall cardiac mortality in developed countries. When the definition of SCD is restricted to death less than 2 hours from onset of symptoms, 12% of all natural deaths are sudden and 88% of these are a result of cardiac disease. SCD is also the most common and often the first manifestation of CAD. In autopsy-based studies, a cardiac etiology of sudden death has been reported in 60% to 70% of sudden death victims. Approximately 60% of SCDs occur outside the hospital setting. First-known arrhythmic events account for approximately 85% to 90% of SCDs, while the remaining 10% to 15% are due to recurrent events.

The incidence of SCD increases with age, largely in part to higher incidence and prevalence of coronary disease and left ventricular dysfunction. Among sudden natural deaths, the proportion with cardiac causes also increases with advancing age. Still, SCD accounts for approximately 20% of all sudden deaths in patients younger than age 20 years. Overall, SCD in infants, children, adolescents, and young adults is rare.

In parallel with higher incidence of CAD, SCD has a much higher incidence in men than in women. Seventy percent to ninety percent of SCDs occur in men. However, women are more likely than men to suffer SCD without prior evidence of coronary heart disease, and a greater percentage of sudden deaths occur outside of the hospital in women. Blacks have higher age-adjusted mortality rates for SCD than nonblacks.

RISK FACTORS

The major risk factors for SCD are established CAD or high risk for CAD, previous myocardial infarction (MI), decreased ejection fraction (EF), and a history of ventricular arrhythmias. These are potent risk factors that increase the *relative* risk of SCD, but the contribution of SCD in those with such risk factors to the cumulative rate of SCD is relatively low. Most cases of SCD occur in the general population without a known history of heart disease, followed by patients who are high risk for CAD or have established CAD. Despite the fact that numerous population-based studies have shown a strong relationship between risk factors for coronary heart disease (CHD) and SCD, no study has identified a single set of risk factors specific for SCD. Cigarette smoking is one of the few behavioral risk factors that is associated with a disproportionate number of sudden deaths. There are many reports linking stress, particularly emotional stress, to ventricular arrhythmias and SCD.

Twenty percent to thirty-five percent of sudden deaths in young adults occur in the absence of identifiable cardiac structural abnormalities. Among infants, up to 10% of cases of crib deaths or sudden infant death syndrome may be due to cardiac arrhythmias, including QT syndromes. Overall, sudden death is rare in young athletes, but in the United States, one-third of these cases have hypertrophic cardiomyopathy on autopsy.

PATHOPHYSIOLOGY

Ventricular tachycardia (VT) degenerating into ventricular fibrillation (VF) is the most common electrical sequence of events in SCD (Fig. 18-1). Polymorphic VT or torsades de pointes may be the initial arrhythmia in patients with acute ischemia or genetic syndromes. In advanced heart failure or in the elderly, bradyarrhythmias or electromechanical dissociation may be the primary electrical event. The bradyarrhythmias may be secondary to pump or hemodynamic failure. *Commotio cordis* is an extremely rare phenomenon where a critically timed mechanical blow to the chest results in VF.

In acute ischemia, rapid polymorphic VT and VF are the predominant malignant arrhythmias. Ventricular arrhythmias can also be a sign of reperfusion after thrombolysis, percutaneous revascularization, or spontaneous reperfusion. In the subacute phase of MI (within the first 3 days), SCD may occur, but the predominant arrhythmias are accelerated idioventricular rhythm and idioventricular tachycardia, which subside after 2 or 3 days and have no prognostic significance. In the late phases, when the infarction is healed, monomorphic VT is the predominant arrhythmia. Critical areas of the reentrant circuits are formed by surviving myocardial fibers in the border zone of a healed infarction. The transition from organized VT to VF or the development of primary VF is usually from simultaneous ventricular activation by multiple localized areas of microreentry circuits.

Atrial flutter (AFL) or atrial fibrillation (AF) with very rapid ventricular responses may also be the primary electrical event preceding VT/VF, particularly in patients with CAD or advanced heart disease. SCD can also occur in patients with the Wolf–Parkinson–White (WPW) syndrome, in which very rapid ventricular response in AF degenerates into VF due to rapidly conducting accessory pathways.

ETIOLOGY

Table 18-1 lists cardiac abnormalities associated with sudden cardiac death.

【 】 CORONARY ATHEROSCLEROSIS

CHD is present in 40% to 86% of SCD survivors, depending on age and gender. SCD can occur in the absence of infarction but usually happens in the presence of diffuse coronary disease. Although the majority of patients who suffer SCD have severe multivessel coronary disease, fewer than half of the patients resuscitated from VF

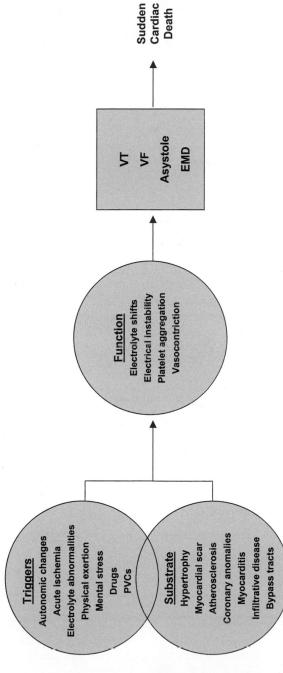

FIGURE 18-1. Interaction between structural cardiac abnormalities, functional changes, and triggering factors in the pathophysiology of SCD. The role of triggering factors, such as physical exertion or drugs, is being increasingly recognized. (PVCs, premature ventricular contractions; EMD, electromechanical dissociation; VF, ventricular fibrillation; VT, ventricular tachycardia.)

TABLE 18-1

Cardiac Abnormalities Associated with Sudden Cardiac Death

Ischemic Heart Disease

Coronary atherosclerosis
  Acute MI
  Chronic ischemic cardiomyopathy
Anomalous origin of coronary arteries
Hypoplastic coronary artery

Coronary artery spasm
Coronary artery dissection
Coronary arteritis
Small vessel disease

Nonischemic Heart Disease

Cardiomyopathies
  Idiopathic dilated cardiomyopathy

  Hypertrophic cardiomyopathy
  Hypertensive cardiomyopathy
  Arrhythmogenic right ventricular
    cardiomyopathy
Infiltrative and inflammatory heart disease
  Sarcoidosis
  Amyloidosis
  Hemochromatosis
  Myocarditis

Valvular heart disease
Aortic Stenosis
  Aortic regurgitation
  Mitral valve prolapse
  Infective endocarditis
  Congenital heart disease
Tetralogy of Fallot
  Transposition of the great vessels
    (post–Mustard-Senning)
  Ebstein anomaly
  Pulmonary vascular obstructive disease
  Congenital aortic stenosis
  Primary electrical abnormalities
  Long QT syndrome
  Short QT syndrome
  WPW syndrome
  Congenital atrioventricular block
  Idiopathic ventricular tachycardia
  Idiopathic ventricular fibrillation
    Syndrome of right bundle-branch
      block, ST elevation, and sudden
      death (Brugada syndrome)
    Catecholaminergic polymorphic
      ventricular tachycardia
Nocturnal death in Southeast Asian men

Drug-induced and other toxic agents
  Antiarrhythmic drugs (class Ia, Ic,
    and III)
  Erythromycin
  Clarithromycin
  Astemizole

  Terfenadine
  Pentamidine
  Ketoconazole
  Trimethoprim-sulfamethoxazole
  Psychotropic drugs (tricyclic
    antidepressants, haloperidol,
    phenothiazines, chloral hydrate)

  Probucol
  Cisapride
  Cocaine
  Chloroquine
  Alcohol
  Phosphodiesterase inhibitors
  Organophosphates

Electrolyte abnormalities
  Hypokalemia
  Hypomagnesemia
  Hypocalcemia
  Anorexia nervosa and bulimia
  Liquid protein dieting
  Diuretics

exhibit evidence of MI in the form of elevated cardiac enzymes, and less than 20% have Q-wave MI. Following recovery from acute MI, patients remain at chronically increased risk for SCD. Ejection fraction is the most important predictor of sudden death in this group.

【 】 NONATHEROSCLEROTIC DISEASE OF THE CORONARY ARTERIES

Congenital coronary artery anomalies, found in approximately 1% of all patients undergoing angiography and in 0.3% of those undergoing autopsy, can be complicated by SCD, often exercise-related, in up to 30% of patients. The highest-risk anomalies are origin of the left main coronary artery from the right aortic sinus or origin of the right coronary artery from the left coronary sinus. Life-threatening ventricular arrhythmias and SCD have been described in patients with coronary artery spasm.

Acquired and inherited disease of the connective tissue and blood vessels may also affect the coronary arteries, leading to ischemia and SCD, including Marfan's syndrome, after labor and delivery, and infections and inflammatory vasculitides. Myocardial bridges have been reported in association with SCD during exercise, but they are also an incidental finding at autopsy in up to 25% of patients dying of other causes.

【 】 CARDIOMYOPATHIES

Idiopathic Dilated Cardiomyopathy

Idiopathic dilated cardiomyopathy is the substrate for approximately 10% of SCDs in the adult population. Mortality in idiopathic dilated cardiomyopathy is high, reaching 10% to 50% annually, and seems most closely tied to the severity of pump dysfunction. SCD in idiopathic dilated cardiomyopathy is usually attributed to both polymorphic and monomorphic ventricular tachyarrhythmias. The terminal event can, however, also be asystole or electromechanical dissociation, especially in patients with advanced left ventricular dysfunction.

Hypertrophic Cardiomyopathy

The incidence of SCD in patients with *hypertrophic cardiomyopathy* (HCM) is 2% to 4% per year in adults and 4% to 6% per year in children and adolescents. There are few reliable predictors of SCD in patients with HCM. A clinical history of spontaneous, sustained monomorphic VT or sudden death in family members with HCM indicates a worse prognosis, as does onset of symptoms in childhood. The magnitude of outflow tract gradient does not appear to predict the risk of sudden death, but an association between extreme hypertrophy and SCD has been reported. Patients with wall thicknesses > 30 mm had a 20-year risk of sudden death approaching 40% in one series. Genotypic analysis is considered less reliable in risk assessment than family history. (See also Chapter 40.)

Hypertensive Cardiomyopathy

Left ventricular hypertrophy (LVH) has been identified as one of the strongest blood pressure–independent risk factors for sudden death. In the Framingham study, electrocardiogram (ECG) evidence of LVH doubled the risk of SCD. Hypertensive patients with LVH also have a significantly greater prevalence of premature ventricular contractions and complex ventricular arrhythmias than do patients without LVH or normotensive patients.

【 】 INFLAMMATORY OR INFILTRATIVE MYOCARDIAL DISEASE

Myocardial scar, regardless of etiology, may lead to ventricular arrhythmias and sudden death due to tissue electrical heterogeneity. Myocarditis, which can lead to minimal scarring, is responsible for 11% to 22% of SCD, according to one autopsy study. Primary amyloidosis may involve the heart in one-third of cases. Amyloid deposition in the ventricular myocardium leads to electrical heterogeneity and delayed activation, which are risk factors for sudden death. *Arrhythmogenic right ventricular dysplasia* (ARVD) is a rare, usually inherited cardiomyopathy characterized by fatty or fibrofatty replacement of myocardium associated with recurrent ventricular tachycardia with left bundle-branch block morphologies. In the early stages of the disease, VT is often precipitated by exercise. The course and prognosis of ARVD are highly variable.

【 】 CONGENITAL HEART DISEASE

An increased risk of SCD has been found predominantly in four congenital conditions: *tetralogy of Fallot, transposition of the great vessels, aortic stenosis,* and *pulmonary vascular obstruction.* Patients who have undergone reparative surgery for *tetralogy of Fallot* have a reported risk of sudden cardiac death of 6% before age 20. A QRS duration ≥180 ms has been found to be the most sensitive predictor of SCD, and ventricular tachyarrhythmias in adults after repair of tetralogy of Fallot and correlates with other parameters of right ventricular volume overload.

【 】 PRIMARY ELECTRICAL ABNORMALITIES

Long QT Syndrome

Sudden cardiac death is one of the hallmarks of the idiopathic long QT syndrome (LQTS), a group of genetically distinct disorders resulting from an ion channel or auxillary subunit mutation. Congenital LQTS accounts for 3,000 to 4,000 sudden childhood deaths per year in the United States.

The long QT interval reflects abnormal prolongation of repolarization. Other characteristics of this disorder, in addition to the prolonged (> 440 ms for males or > 460 ms for females, corrected for heart rate) QT interval, include abnormal T-wave contours, relative sinus bradycardia, a family history of early sudden death, and a propensity for recurrent syncope and SCD due to polymorphic VT (torsades de pointes) and VF. Mutations in seven genes have been identified so far. Most cases are caused by three mutations: LQT1 (42%), LQT2 (45%), and LQT3 (8%). The rare autosomal recessive Jervell–Lange–Nielsen syndrome is also associated with congenital deafness. Cases of SCD and abnormally short QT interval have also been recently described and attributed to a potassium channel mutation.

Over 90% of the congenital forms of LQTS have been linked to specific chromosomal defects, resulting in a genetically based classification (LQT1 through LQT6) with important functional and prognostic implications. The risk of sudden death in LQTS is influenced by the duration of the QT interval, corrected for heart rate (QTc), the specific genetic defect, gender, family history, and possibly other factors. Torsades de pointes can be triggered by different stimuli, typically involving high adrenergic states (e.g., exercise).

Brugada Syndrome

The syndrome of SCD associated with complete or incomplete right bundle-branch block and persistent ST-segment elevation in leads V_1 through V_3 in patients without demonstrable structural heart disease is known as the Brugada syndrome. Patients with this ECG pattern and prior cardiac arrest or syncope have high rates of sudden death during follow-up. Mutations in the sodium channel gene SCN5A have been implicated as the cause of Brugada syndrome in some families; different mutations of the same gene are also responsible for LQTS type 3. The significance of Brugada-type ECG findings in individuals with no personal or family history of arrhythmias remains unclear.

Idiopathic Ventricular Fibrillation

Several types of idiopathic polymorphic VT have been described that are associated with an unfavorable prognosis. These include idiopathic VF, torsades de pointes with a short coupling interval, and catecholaminergic polymorphic VT. They can occur in sporadic or familial forms and are frequently associated with catecholamine release during physical or emotional stress. In survivors of cardiac arrest, the diagnosis of idiopathic VF is made by exclusion. Catecholaminergic or familial polymorphic VT is an exceptionally rare form of bidirectional or polymorphic VT due to mutations in the cardiac ryanodine receptor (RyR2) and calsequestrin (CASQ2) genes.

【 】 DRUGS AND OTHER TOXIC AGENTS

Proarrhythmia

Class I and class III antiarrhythmic drugs exhibit a dose-dependent antiarrhythmic effect in structurally normal and abnormal hearts. Many other agents with diverse actions have been implicated in the induction of tachyarrhythmias, including erythromycin, terfenadine, pentamidine, and certain psychotropic drugs. Most of these drugs produce toxicity by prolonging repolarization and QTc, leading to torsades de pointes. In other patients, drug-induced LQTS may actually make a background mutation or polymorphism(s) in a congenital LQTS gene clinically apparent. The list of drugs implicated in LQTS is vast and rapidly expanding, and online sites such as www.torsades.org can provide comprehensive, timely information.

Cocaine

Cocaine can precipitate life-threatening cardiac events, including SCD. Cocaine causes coronary vasoconstriction, increases cardiac sympathetic effects, and precipitates cardiac arrhythmias irrespective of the amount ingested, prior use, or whether there is an underlying cardiac abnormality.

Electrolyte Abnormalities

There is an almost linear inverse relationship between serum potassium concentration and the probability of VT in patients with acute MI. *Hypokalemia* is often found in patients during and following resuscitation from a cardiac arrest. Many of the electrophysiologic effects of hypokalemia are similar to those caused by digitalis and catecholamine stimulation, explaining the high risk of ventricular arrhythmias when a combination of these factors is present. An association between *magnesium deficiency* and SCD has been reported in humans, especially as a cofactor in drug-induced torsades de pointes. Hypomagnesemia in humans is generally associated with CHF, digitalis use, chronic diuretic use, hypokalemia, and hypocalcemia, making it difficult to establish whether the hypomagnesemia alone precipitates arrhythmias. Acute administration of magnesium has been successfully used in the treatment of drug-induced torsades de pointes, although hypomagnesemia is not usually documented in this situation.

MANAGEMENT

【 】 ESTABLISHING THE UNDERLYING CARDIAC PATHOLOGY

After successful resuscitation from cardiac arrest and a period of hemodynamic and respiratory stabilization, every effort should be made to establish the cause of cardiac arrest and the likelihood of recurrence. It is important to determine if cardiac arrest was the result and not cause of acute circulatory or respiratory collapse.

Underlying cardiac disease should first be investigated. Myocardial ischemia and infarction should be excluded. Echocardiography can help determine left ventricular function, regional wall-motion abnormalities, valvular heart disease, or cardiomyopathies. Cardiac catheterization is often recommended to evaluate the coronary anatomy and hemodynamics. Other tests—such as radionuclide studies, magnetic resonance imaging, or cardiac biopsy—may be necessary in selected patients. An underlying cardiac disease can be found in most patients.

At the same time, every effort should be made to exclude potentially reversible causes of SCD, including transient ischemic episodes in patients who are candidates for complete revascularization and in whom the onset of the arrhythmia is clearly preceded by ischemic ECG changes or symptoms.

RISK STRATIFICATION FOR SUDDEN CARDIAC DEATH

Current parameters used to risk-stratify patients with CAD for SCD include medical history (presence of nonsustained VT, syncope), EF, ECG (QRS duration, QT interval, QT dispersion), signal-averaged electrocardiogram (SAECG), heart rate variability, and baroreflex sensitivity. Unfortunately, each of these individual parameters lacks very high sensitivity and specificity for identifying vulnerable patients. Measurement of microvolt T-wave alternans, which assess beat to beat changes in ventricular repolarization, has been shown to have strong negative predictive value in some select patient groups.

Even invasive electrophysiologic testing showed that patients with ischemic cardiomyopathy who had no inducible for ventricular tachyarrhythmias had essentially the same risk of SCD as those who had inducible ventricular arrythmias. Moreover, the positive predictive accuracy of inducibility of ventricular tachycardia has been relatively low in consecutive series of patients with recent MI. Therefore, at present, only LV dysfunction reliably defines "high-risk" for SCD in patients with ischemic cardiomyopathy.

Invasive electrophysiologic studies (EPS) may be useful in select patient groups. Electrode-tipped catheters are typically placed via the femoral or internal jugular veins to right atrium, right ventricle, and His bundle, and repeated programmed electrical stimulation is administered to pace the heart in an attempt to induce arrhythmias. Induction of sustained monomorphic VT is the generally accepted end point for programmed ventricular stimulation. Inducible VT on EPS has been demonstrated to strongly predict recurrent ventricular arrhythmias and sudden death. EP testing is also useful in patients with structural heart disease who present with unexplained syncope. VT is the most common abnormal finding in these patients, but demonstration of His–Purkinje conduction disease or hemodynamically unstable supraventricular tachycardia can also be important. In survivors of cardiac arrest due to VF, the value of electrophysiologic testing is less clear, but it may be of diagnostic utility in selected circumstances. However, EP testing is not used in selecting nonischemic patients for ICDs because of its poor sensitivity and specificity.

TREATMENT OPTIONS FOR PATIENTS AT RISK FOR SUDDEN CARDIAC DEATH

【　】 PHARMACOLOGIC THERAPY

Beta-Blockers

Of all the therapies currently available for the prevention of SCD, none is more established or effective in patients with CHD than beta-blockers. Large randomized studies have repeatedly and compellingly demonstrated marked reductions in total mortality and SCD by nonselective beta-blockers (propranolol) and cardioselective agents such as metoprolol. The benefits of beta-blockade are additive to standard treatment for CHF. Beta-blockers are effective in the setting of ventricular arrhythmias provoked by a high sympathetic tone, as in patients with congenital long-QT syndrome, arrhythmogenic right ventricular dysplasia, or CHF. Importantly, the beneficial effects of beta-blockers on cardiac mortality are most pronounced in patients who are at higher risk for SCD, such as those with CHF, atrial and ventricular arrhythmias, post-MI, and diabetes.

Angiotensin-Converting Enzyme Inhibitors

Although the mortality benefit from angiotensin-converting enzyme (ACE) inhibitors in heart failure patients is thought to stem primarily from a reduction in pump failure, a specific reduction in the incidence of sudden death may be present as well. Although data from individual trials have been conflicting on this issue, a meta-analysis of trials including over 15,000 post-MI patients reported a 20% reduction in SCD in ACE-inhibitor-treated subjects (HR 0.80; 95% confidence interval [CI] 0.70–0.92). Whether these results also pertain to angiotensin receptor blockers is not known.

Antiarrhythmic Drugs

The efficacy and safety of antiarrhythmic drugs in preventing sudden death has been disappointing. Amiodarone is widely considered the most effective antiarrhythmic agent for treating a variety of arrhythmias, including AF and VT. It is a class III antiarrhythmic agent with additional class I, II, and IV properties and has unusual pharmacokinetics, with a delayed onset of action and an elimination half-life of up to 53 days after chronic therapy

Amiodarone has been shown to reduce SCD rates significantly following MI in several placebo-controlled randomized studies, but its effects on total mortality are inconsistent. Intravenous amiodarone remains a powerful parenteral drug for the acute treatment of patients with life-threatening ventricular arrhythmias. The efficacy of intravenous amiodarone in patients with recurrent, hemodynamically unstable VT refractory to lidocaine, procainamide, and bretylium is approximately 40% in prospective studies, and about 80% of the arrhythmias are suppressed within the first 48 hours. For out of hospital cardiac arrest, intravenous amiodarone has been shown to be more effective than intravenous lidocaine.

【　】 NONPHARMACOLOGIC THERAPY

Implantable Cardioverter Defibrillators

In patients with ischemic cardiomyopathy, implantable cardioverter defibrillators (ICDs) have demonstrated remarkable effectiveness in prevention of SCD, with an overall 1-year survival rate of 92% in patients with documented life-threatening ventricular tachyarrhythmias. Three randomized, controlled trials have demonstrated ICDs to be superior to antiarrhythmic medications in the secondary prevention of SCD. Recent primary prevention studies have also demonstrated improved survival of *high-risk* patients with ischemic cardiomyopathy who have had ICDs implanted as compared to conventional drug therapy. ICDs are effective in detecting and terminating ventricular tachyarrhythmias and can prevent bradycardia with pacing. Because their mode of action is therapeutic rather than preventive, ICD therapy must often be combined with other antiarrhythmic strategies, such as drugs or catheter ablation, to prevent frequent recurrences of tachyarrhythmias.

Several ICD primary prevention trials in patients with nonischemic cardiomyopathy and heart failure have also been conducted, but the results have not been as consistently positive as in the post-MI population. The largest of these is the SCD-HeFT, in which the benefit of ICDs in the trial was highly statistically significant and appeared similar for the ischemic and nonischemic subgroups. The most compelling data may come from a pooled analysis of five primary prevention trials enrolling 1854 patients. ICD therapy led to a 31% relative risk reduction in mortality. The absolute risk reduction was estimated at 2% per year.

ICDs are also used in less common conditions associated with a high risk of sudden cardiac death, including hypertrophic cardiomyopathy, long QT syndrome, and the Brugada syndrome.

SUGGESTED READING

Bardy GH, Lee KL, Mark DB, et al. Amiodarone or an implantable cardioverter-defibrillator for congestive heart failure. *N Engl J Med.* 2005;352:225–237.

Ewy G. Cardiopulmonary and cardiocerebral resuscitation. in: Furter V, O'Rourke RA, Walsh RA, et al., eds. *Hurst's The Heart.* 12th ed. New York: McGraw-Hill; 2008:1187–1201.

Moss AJ, Hall WJ, Cannom DS, et al. Improved survival with an implanted defibrillator in patients with coronary disease at high risk for ventricular arrhythmia. Multicenter Automatic Defibrillator Implantation Trial investigators. *N Engl J Med.* 1996;335:1933–1940.

Moss AJ, Zareba W, Hall WJ, et al. Prophylactic implantation of a defibrillator in patients with myocardial infarction and reduced ejection fraction. *N Engl J Med.* 2002;346:877–883.

Priori SG, Schwartz PJ, Napolitano C, et al. Risk stratification in the long-QT syndrome. *N Engl J Med.* 2003;348:1866–1874.

Reynolds MR, Josephson ME. Sudden cardiac death. In: Fuster V, Alexander RW, O'Rourke RA, et al., eds. *Hurst's The Heart.* 11th ed. New York, NY: McGraw-Hill; 2004:1051–1078.

Solomon SD, Zelenkofske S, McMurray JJ, et al. Sudden death in patients with myocardial infarction and left ventricular dysfunction, heart failure, or both. *N Engl J Med.* 2005;352:2581–2588.

Turakhia M, Tseng ZH. Sudden cardiac death: epidemiology, mechanisms, and therapy. *Curr Probl Cardiol.* 2007;32:501–546.

Weaver EF, Robles de Medina EO. Sudden death in patients without structural heart disease. *J Am Coll Cardiol.* 2004;43:1137–1144.

Zipes DP, Camm AJ, Borggrefe M, et al. ACC/AHA/ESC 2006 guidelines for management of patients with ventricular arrhythmias and the prevention of sudden cardiac death: a report of the American College of Cardiology/American Heart Association Task Force and the European Society of Cardiology Committee for Practice Guidelines (Writing Committee to Develop Guidelines for Management of Patients with Ventricular Arrhythmias and the Prevention of Sudden Cardiac Death). *J Am Coll Cardiol.* 2006;48:e247–e346.

CHAPTER (19)

CPR and Post-Resuscitation Management

Jooby John and Gordon A. Ewy

Sudden death, primarily due to out-of-hospital cardiac arrest (OHCA), remains the single leading cause of death in the United States, with more than a thousand deaths daily. Cardiac arrest itself is the abrupt termination of organized cardiac activity resulting in circulatory collapse, due to either electrical or mechanical malfunction. Its consequences are immediate and devastating with rapid development of end-organ damage. Permanent neurologic damage sets in within 4 minutes of circulatory arrest. The gravest of these consequences include hypoxic encephalopathy, permanent neurologic damage, and death. Cardiac arrest is clinically suspected when sudden collapse occurs and is confirmed by the absence of a discernible pulse or cardiac sounds. An electrocardiogram (ECG), if performed, will show the patient to have a rhythm consistent with ventricular tachycardia (VT), ventricular fibrillation (VF), asystole, or an organized nonperfusing rhythm. The latter is referred to as *pulseless electrical activity* (PEA) or electromechanical dissociation (EMD).

This chapter summarizes our current state of knowledge regarding the pathophysiology, as well as recommendations for treatment, of this near-lethal disease. It will also serve to introduce the concept of cardiocerebral resuscitation (CCR), a new approach that has been shown to dramatically improve survival in patients with OHCA.

OHCA survival rates hover close to 1% to 7% in major cities in the United States, with in-hospital rates being around 10% to 15%. Despite five decades of guidelines advocating cardiopulmonary resuscitation (CPR) as a treatment for cardiac arrest, survival rates have remained stagnant. As it stands today, CPR is advocated for two distinct diseases, primary arrhythmogenic cardiac arrest (typically pulseless VT or VF), and respiratory arrest with consequent hypoxia and *secondary* precipitation of global cardiac ischemia and arrest (usually PEA or asystole).

PATHOPHYSIOLOGY OF CARDIAC ARREST

Cardiac arrest in adults secondary to VF is a consequence of uncoordinated myocardial activity. One minute into persistent VF, coronary blood flow declines to zero, and by 4 minutes carotid blood flow is also at zero. In the absence of resuscitative efforts, progressive equalization of arterial and venous pressures occurs, leading to circulatory standstill. The end result is a distension of the right ventricle and progressive impairment in left ventricular diastolic function and a final agonal contraction terminating in the "stone heart" (Fig. 19-1).

【 】 RESPIRATORY ARREST

Alternatively, respiratory arrest leads to a predictable drop in arterial oxygen tension, ensuing myocardial hypoxia, and secondary cardiac arrest. These usually present as PEA or asystole. Logically, the appropriate management of this disease would involve mitigation

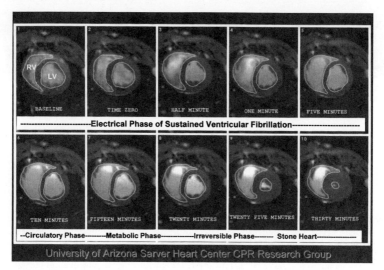

FIGURE 19-1. MRI depiction of changes in right ventricular (RV) and left ventricular (LV) volumes with untreated ventricular fibrillation in the swine VF model. Notice how initially LV and RV are both enlarged. However, with time, the LV undergoes agonal ischemic contracture leading to a "stone heart." (Reprinted with permission from Sorrell VL, Bhatt RD, Berg RA, et al. Cardiac magnetic resonance imaging investigation of sustained ventricular fibrillation in a swine model—with a focus on the electrical phase. *Resuscitation.* 2007; MAY;73(2):279–286. Copyright © Elsevier.)

of the precipitating cause. Examples of this form of cardiac arrest, in adults, include drug overdose, choking ("café coronary"), catastrophic neurologic events, suffocation, drowning, and carbon monoxide poisoning. A ready application of this doctrine, in the café coronary setting, is the utility of the Heimlich maneuver in relieving respiratory arrest secondary to choking.

Cardiac Arrest in the Pediatric Population

Respiratory arrests encompass the majority of cardiac arrests in children. This is an important subgroup to recognize, as children rarely have underlying primary cardiac or coronary artery disease (CAD). Consequently, they are far more likely to have had a respiratory arrest and secondary cardiac arrest, and in them the restoration of oxygenation and ventilatory function is of overriding importance. It is in this population that reestablishment of arterial oxygen tension is crucial for successful resuscitation and survival. Therefore, the emphasis in children has to be on the *reestablishment of alveolar gas exchange*, while simultaneously supporting circulation with chest compressions and vasoactive medications. Nonetheless, it is sobering to note that once cardiac arrest has set in for a prolonged period of time, it becomes the determining factor in the patient's survival. It is important to restore circulation while simultaneously working on correcting the primary etiology of the respiratory arrest.

Cardiac Arrest in Adults

Conversely in adults, most cardiac arrests are of primary cardiac origin with VF, as a consequence of myocardial ischemia secondary to CAD. In these patients, the pulmonary alveoli and the entire left heart, intrinsically untouched from the primary arrhythmogenic process, are flush with oxygenated blood and require no immediate replenishment. Moreover, these patients continue to breathe for a brief period of time, postarrest, as the medullary respiratory center is still active and continues to fire. This is responsible for the gasping and agonal breathing phenomenon seen in up to 40% of individuals with OHCA. They stop spontaneous respiratory efforts when the respiratory center finally succumbs to hypoxic injury and shuts down its phasic discharge activity. But the lack of blood flow ensures that the alveoli remain replete with oxygen. This is the essential logic behind *prioritizing circulatory support over respiratory support* in the case of adults with cardiac arrest.

Circulatory support is, of course, established by precordial chest compressions. Chest compressions halt the progression of circulatory arrest and its downstream consequences by providing phasic arterial blood flow. When chest compressions are accurately executed, pressure on the cardiac chambers during the "compression phase" ejects blood out of the left ventricle (LV) and into the peripheral circulation and from the right ventricle into the pulmonary capillary system. This physiology dominates in the early phase of cardiac arrest and is similar to the mechanism of open cardiac massage. However, there is also a "thoracic pump" mechanism that predominates in the later components of cardiac arrest. In this process, the chest compression causes passive inflow and outflow of blood from the thoracic cage with the heart acting as a flaccid conduit. This theory comes from the observation that patients in cardiac arrest were able to stay awake by repetitively coughing and thereby moving blood through the circulation simply based on their intrathoracic pressure fluctuations. Case reports in the cardiac catheterization laboratory have shown patients able to maintain hemodynamically significant blood pressures during malignant ventricular arrhythmias by coughing forcefully 30 to 60 times a minute. Obviously this is not a strategy that can be widely advocated because of its unpredictable outcome. The consensus opinion is that both mechanisms play a role in reestablishing circulatory flow, "cardiac compression" in the early phase and "thoracic pump" in the later phase. Nevertheless, it is sobering to remember that total coronary flow with precordial compressions is only around 20% to 40% of prearrest values. With the increasing duration of cardiac arrest, LV relaxation is first affected. The LV continues to progressively thicken. Magnetic resonance imaging (MRI) studies have shown that ischemic contracture finally sets in after about 20 to 30 minutes of untreated VF, the so called "stone heart." At this point, reversion to a perfusing rhythm is highly improbable.

【 】 CORONARY PERFUSION PRESSURE

Coronary perfusion pressure (CPP) is defined as the difference between the aortic and right atrial pressure during the release phase of external cardiac compression. It is the "driving pressure" that causes blood to flow into the coronary tree. This pressure is built up slowly with chest compressions, such that first compressions do not generate a significant CPP, but the last compressions (prior to stopping compressions for the rescue breaths) generate significant CPP (Figs. 19-2 and 19-3). The CPP has been shown to be the *central* determinant of survival in prolonged VF. When chest compressions are interrupted (for so-called rescue breathing, tracheal intubation, placement of an intravenous line, or even rhythm and pulse analysis), the CPP falls, and with it the chances for survival. This is the theoretical rationale for continuous chest compression (CCC), wherein the essential determinant for cardiac survival, the CPP, is constantly preserved. The same principle applies for cerebral perfusion where near-continuous chest compressions are essential for cerebral perfusion.

【 】 PHASES OF VENTRICULAR FIBRILLATION

Survival rates decrease by about 7% to 10% for every *1 minute* that a person remains in ventricular fibrillation. VF is a common arrhythmia associated with cardiac arrest in

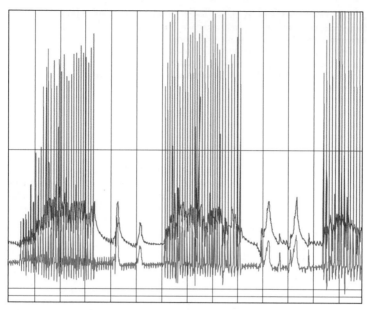

FIGURE 19-2. Coronary perfusion pressures with interrupted chest compressions (30:2 compression-to-breaths ratio). Aortic pressure is in dark blue and right atrial pressure is in light blue. The CPP is the difference between these two pressures. Notice how the coronary perfusion pressure takes time to build up. It drops once chest compressions are interrupted and has to be reestablished with the next round of chest compressions. (Reprinted with permission from Ewy GA, Zuercher M, Hilwig RW, et al. Improved neurological outcome with continuous chest compressions compared with 30:2 compressions-to-ventilations cardiopulmonary resuscitation in a realistic swine model of out-of-hospital cardiac arrest. *Circulation.* 2007; Nov 27;116(22):2525–2530. Copyright © Lippincott Williams & Wilkins.)

adults, and is the one associated with the best prognosis. The time-sensitive, three-phase concept for VF was put forth in 2002 by Weisfeldt and Becker. This elegant model divides VF into an electrical phase (0–5 minutes), circulatory/mechanical phase (5–15 minutes), and metabolic phase (after 15 minutes). The appropriate management for VF has to be tailored to the phase during which it will be delivered.

Electrical Phase (0–5 Minutes)

In the *electrical phase*, there is enough myocardial energy reserve that defibrillation alone (without chest compression) is sufficient to restore a perfusing rhythm. The most well-known application of this is the implantable cardiac defibrillators (ICDs) that deliver therapy within seconds of an unstable VT or VF, and are consequently highly effective. Automated external defibrillators (AEDs) are also extremely useful in this phase. Public access AEDs have demonstrated dramatic improvements in survival in patients who have collapsed in casinos or airports. These patients are defibrillated within minutes because of their proximity to an AED and, since they are in the electrical phase, do often return to a perfusing hemodynamically stable rhythm.

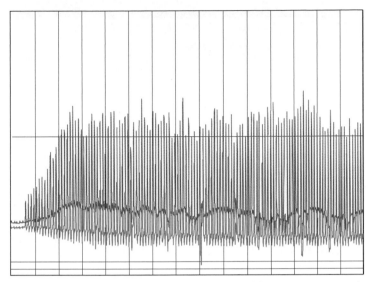

FIGURE 19-3. Coronary perfusion pressures with continuous chest compressions. Here the coronary perfusion pressures are established and secondary to the uninterrupted nature of the chest compressions, remain constant. (Reprinted with permission from Ewy GA, Zuercher M, Hilwig RW, et al. Improved neurological outcome with continuous chest compressions compared with 30:2 compressions-to-ventilations cardiopulmonary resuscitation in a realistic swine model of out-of-hospital cardiac arrest. *Circulation.* 2007; Nov 7;116(22):2525–2530. Copyright © Lippincott Williams & Wilkins.)

Circulatory/Mechanical Phase (5–15 Minutes)

In the *circulatory phase* of VF, the incessant myocardial contractions coupled with the now-prolonged lack of coronary blood flow will have resulted in depletion of myocardial high-energy phosphate stores as well as cellular acidosis. Electrocardiographically, this is manifested by the decreasing amplitude of the VF waveform with a transition to the "fine" fibrillatory waves on the ECG. Defibrillation in the absence of chest compressions is rarely successful in this phase, as even if the VF is terminated, the patient ends up in a PEA rhythm. Successful resuscitation here requires the restoration of myocardial energy stores. It is here that chest compressions play a pivotal role in restoring some degree of coronary (and cerebral) perfusion. Postcompression VF waveforms show an increase in amplitude, higher median frequency, and a "coarser" rhythm, and are associated with higher likelihood of successful defibrillation and neurologically intact survival.

Metabolic Phase (After 15 Minutes)

The third phase, the *metabolic phase*, is universally associated with diminishing odds of successful defibrillation. End-organ damage has already set in, with irreversible cellular impairment. Strategies that may delay the onset of this *phase of irremediable damage* are being investigated. Therapeutic hypothermia may be useful even in this late stage. However, very few patients survive following >15 minutes of untreated cardiac arrest.

PULSELESS ELECTRICAL ACTIVITY AND ASYSTOLE

PEA and asystole are important to recognize because they are not amenable to *electrical defibrillation therapy*. When VF is the initial rhythm, the chance of survival is significantly higher than when PEA or asystole is the presenting rhythm. Although VF in an adult is very strongly associated with CAD, PEA and asystole are usually not. The exception is when they are seen in the terminal phase of VF arrests. When VF is defibrillated in the circulatory/mechanical phase without predefibrillatory chest compressions, these postdefibrillation rhythms are usually PEA. Predefibrillatory *and* postdefibrillatory chest compressions have been shown to be effective in preventing the emergence of PEA.

One has to consider secondary causes of cardiac arrest when PEA is otherwise the primary rhythm; the **5 Hs** (**H**ypovolemia, **H**ypoxia, **H**ydrogen ion = acidosis, **H**yperkalemia or **H**ypokalemia, and **H**ypothermia) and the **5Ts** (**T**ension pneumothorax, **T**amponade, **T**ablets = drug overdose, **T**hrombosis coronary, and **T**hrombosis pulmonary). Identifying and remedying the underlying cause is of vital importance in the successful resuscitation of these patients.

Asystole is often a secondary and invariably terminal rhythm, and is the inevitable result of both nonintervened PEA and VF. Patients are often later in time and have consequently poorer prognosis. However, the same etiologies of PEA can also sometimes be present with asystole and should therefore be investigated, and treated if found. One of the pitfalls in diagnosing and treating asystole is when very fine VF is interpreted as asystole. In these cases, it would be prudent to make sure that the cables are connected and the gain is turned up, and to look at other ECG leads (especially perpendicular leads) to see if the VF pattern can be discerned. If the ECG leads are not available and fine VF is suspected, the defibrillatory paddles can be turned by 90 degrees to confirm that it is not VF. If fine VF is suspected, the arrhythmia should be defibrillated. There is no convincing evidence that a mistake here (i.e., defibrillation of asystole) adversely affects the patient's chances of survival.

It should be noted that in a recent North American prospective epidemiologic study, about 20% of adult cardiac arrest patients who initially presented as PEA/asystole had subsequent conversion to VF.

Recognition of life extinct (ROLE) guidelines in England deem 20 minutes of asystole, despite advanced resuscitative measures, as grounds for termination of resuscitative efforts.

GUIDELINES FOR CPR AND ECC

Evidence-based guidelines for CPR and emergency cardiac care (ECC) have been hampered by the relative paucity of controlled clinical trials in humans. CPR was first introduced as a treatment for cardiac arrest in 1960, when Kouwenhoven and coworkers developed the technique of external chest compression in the supine position. This practice was quickly adopted and standardized. Subsequently periodic guidelines have been published by the American Heart Association (AHA) in collaboration with the International Liaison Committee on Resuscitation (ILCOR), with an emphasis on CPR and ECC. The 2000 guidelines emphasized a 15:2 chest compression ratio and three stacked defibrillation shock attempts. Since then, emerging data have been credible showing that *both over-ventilation and interruptions in chest compressions* are independent predictors of adverse outcomes. The 2005 guidelines included significant changes in the delivery of CPR and ECC in an out-of-hospital setting (Table 19-1). The most noteworthy of these include a recommendation to increase the chest compression to ventilation ratio from the previous 15:1 to 30:2, a proposal intended to increase the duration for which continuous chest compression is delivered. Even so, it is important to realize that

TABLE 19-1

Major Differences Between the 2000 and 2005 Guidelines

		2000 Guidelines	2005 Guidelines
1	Alerting EMS (only children)	Phone first and then CPR	CPR for 2 min and then call
2	Unwitnessed adult	Shock first	200 CC then shock
3	Rescue breath	Take a deep breath	Take a normal breath
4	Rescue breath duration	1–2 s	Under 1 s
5	Ventilation rate	12–15/min	8–10/min
6	CC ratio	15:2	30:2
7	2-person CPR	Switch when fatigued	Every 2 min or 5 cycles (150 CC)
8	Defibrillation	3 shocks without CC	1 shock followed by CC
9	Defibrillation energy	3 monophasic stacked	360 J monophasic or 150–200 biphasic
10	Postdefibrillation	Pulse and rhythm analyses	Immediate CC
11	Intubated patients	Pause CPR to give breaths	Give breaths during CC
12	Drug delivery	Drug-CPR-shock	Drugs not to interrupt CC
13	High-dose epinephrine	May be used	Not recommended
14	Hypothermia	Not recommended	Recommended for VF arrest

CC, chest compression.

the 2005 guidelines were formulated on the basis of *consensus opinion* rather than concrete data.

CARDIOCEREBRAL RESUSCITATION

CCR is an innovative approach to the management of cardiac arrest that specifically capitalizes on the fact that the CPP is the most important determinant of survival in an adult cardiac arrest. Chest compression is the only realistic means by which coronary and cerebral perfusion pressures can be maintained in the presence of circulatory arrest. Thus, one may attempt continuous chest compressions (CCC) in cardiac arrest.

The AHA "chain of survival" has bystander-administered CPR as an integral link. However, various clinical studies have shown bystander CPR to be present in only about 20% to 30% of witnessed arrests. Anonymous surveys have indicated that bystanders are more likely to do chest compressions if they do not have to perform mouth-to-mouth rescue breathing. An option in the AHA guidelines indicates that "if a person is unwilling to perform mouth-to-mouth resuscitation, he or she should rapidly attempt resuscitation, omitting mouth-to-mouth ventilation." The other major hindrance is that, even when following guidelines, EMS (emergency medical services) providers are rarely able to deliver the *recommended 80 to 100 compressions a minute* because of the interruption for rescue breaths. Motivated basic life support (BLS) trained medical students at the University of Arizona were able to deliver only an average of 43 compressions a minute when following the old 15:2 AHA guidelines, as opposed to 133 compressions per minute while doing CCC. As a final point, CCC is easier to learn and teach and is much more likely to be implemented in an out-of-hospital witnessed cardiac arrest.

The effectiveness of CCC has now been tested in several clinical studies. A Belgian study in the 1980s and a telephone-dispatched Seattle experience published in 2000, showed that traditional CPR was not better than CCC in OHCA. More recently, the SOS-KANTO study demonstrated that OHCA survival was higher in those patients who got bystander chest compressions only versus those who received chest compressions and rescue breathing. A prospective study from Arizona of survival after OHCA showed that in patients with witnessed cardiac arrests and VF, survival increased from 4.7% to 17.6% after CCR training for EMS personnel was widely implemented. An additional 3-year observational analysis from Wisconsin showed that neurologically intact survival increased from 15% to 39% after the institution of CCR. One can safely surmise that CCR with CCC is easier to perform, more likely to be performed, and is as effective (if not more) than traditional CPR.

COMPONENTS OF CCR

CCR is a comprehensive approach to resuscitation with three vital interrelated components for each level of the disease (Fig. 19-4):

1. The bystander who witnesses the arrest.

2. Emergency medical services (EMS) personnel.

3. Post-resuscitation hospital care.

Bystanders respond after calling EMS with continuous chest compressions at an approximate rate of 100/min. They are then told to continue compression till EMS personnel arrive or until an AED is found and deployed.

EMS personnel are specifically instructed to defibrillate VF only if the patient has been receiving chest compressions by a bystander or if they have personally witnessed the arrest. If not, they are to give CCC for 2 minutes *before analysis* to determine if a patient has shockable rhythm. *Even if the patient is in a shockable VF/VT rhythm on arrival*, and there are no chest compressions performed, EMS personnel are instructed to give CCC for 2 minutes. If they witness the collapse, the patient is now in the electrical phase of VF and can safely be defibrillated first without initiating CCC. Even if they arrive in the electrical phase of an unwitnessed arrest, EMS personnel do no harm by initiating CCC prior to defibrillation. However, if the patient is in the circulatory phase, defibrillation without CCC can be detrimental to survival. Hence, the recommendation to deliver 200 CCC unless it is a witnessed arrest by the EMS personnel, or reliable data indicate that the patient received chest compressions from the time of initial collapse until the arrival of EMS personnel.

One of the aspects of CCR that has been incorporated into the 2005 guidelines is the approach to patients who revert back to a normal rhythm after defibrillation of VF. Despite restoration of a postdefibrillation organized electrical rhythm, these hearts are still mechanically sluggish, and thus will most likely present as PEA instead of a hemodynamically stable rhythm. Immediate postdefibrillation chest compressions will restore coronary flow, replenish high-energy myocardial phosphate stores, and ultimately increase the likelihood that these patients will reach neurologically intact hospital discharge end points.

【 】 VENTILATION

Notwithstanding these differences, the paradigm change in CCR as opposed to traditional CPR is the role of ventilation. The fundamental precept of ABC (airway, breathing, and circulation) is not applicable in the setting of cardiac arrest, for the simple reason that establishing an airway or breathing for the patient does not address the

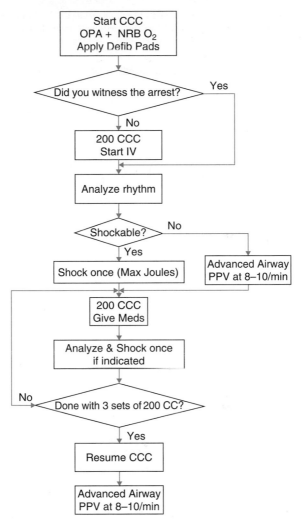

FIGURE 19-4. Cardiocerebral resuscitation improves neurologically intact survival of patients with witnessed out-of-hospital cardiac arrest and a shockable rhythm. (CCC, continuous chest compressions; OPA oropharyngeal airway; PPV positive pressure ventilation; NRB non rebreather.) (This figure is based on data presented in the publication by Kellum MJ, Kennedy KW, Barney R, et al. Cardiocerebral Resuscitation Improves Neurologically Intact Survival of Patients with Out-of-Hospital Cardiac Arrest. *Ann Emerg Med* 2008;52:244–252.)

primary reason for the collapse—that is, a malignant arrhythmia that has precipitated cardiac arrest. Focusing on the ABCs is fraught with actions that worsen survival by diminishing CPP: (1) interruption of chest compressions for intubation or even establishment of an airway; and (2) positive-pressure ventilation that increases intrathoracic pressures, decreases passive venous return, and in turn decreases an already feeble cardiac output. There are observational data that suggest that, in the primary cardiac arrest patient, ventilation can be deferred for up to 12 minutes while CCC is being performed. Part of this has to do with the fact that chest compressions cause some degree of passive ventilatory efforts secondary to the movement of the thoracic cage.

POST-RESUSCITATION CARE

The effectiveness of resuscitative efforts is not just linked to return of spontaneous circulation (ROSC). Neurologically intact survival is the ultimate goal of resuscitation treatment strategies and is reflected in the inclusion of "cerebral" in "cardiocerebral resuscitation." Even after successful ROSC, more than 60% of patients do not survive to hospital discharge. Following ROSC these patients are subject to a vicious and global reperfusion injury, mediated through lipolysis, proteolysis, inflammation, coagulation, and ultimately cellular death and apoptosis. Promising data suggest that by intermittently supplying blood flow at reduced rates, chest compression may condition organs (so-called ischemic preconditioning) to reperfusion injury and thus attenuate eventual cellular death and end-organ damage.

The 2005 International Consensus Conference on Cardiopulmonary Resuscitation and Emergency Cardiovascular Care Science with Treatment Recommendations recommended a goal-directed hemodynamic support strategy for post-cardiac arrest patients. However, this recommendation was largely derived from data gathered in patients with septic shock who were administered goal-directed therapy and found to have better outcomes. Resuscitated patients require close monitoring in an intensive care unit setting as they are prone to repeat hemodynamic instability as well as recurrent cardiac arrhythmias.

About 50% of adult patients with VF arrest have an acute myocardial infarction as the underlying etiology. If a myocardial infarction (confirmed by an ECG or cardiac biomarkers) is suspected, prompt revascularization of the target vessel by percutaneous techniques is usually the preferred therapy. More aggressive approaches envision routine cardiac catheterization for all patients who have had a cardiac arrest as significant CAD and occlusion have been demonstrated even in the absence of diagnostic ECG changes.

Post-resuscitation disease refers to the multisystem damage sustained as a result of ischemic and reperfusion organ injury. This permutation of post-resuscitation ischemic and reperfusion injury combined with a systemic inflammatory response and multiorgan dysfunction has been defined as the *post-cardiac arrest syndrome*. This manifests as hypoxic encephalopathy, myocardial dysfunction, aspiration pneumonia, ischemic gut injury, ischemic hepatopathy, renal dysfunction, and peripheral limb ischemia. Myocardial dysfunction manifests as depressed biventricular function immediately post-resuscitation that improves over the next few days (in the absence of significant myocardial infarction). Post-ischemic stunning as well as free radical endotoxin- and cytotoxin-mediated injury are thought to be instrumental in this usually transient myocardial depression.

One of the more exciting treatments for post-resuscitation care is therapeutic hypothermia. Early studies of moderate (28–32°C) and severe induced hypothermia (28°C) showed worse outcomes compared to standard treatment. However, *mild therapeutic induced hypothermia* (32–34°C for 12–24 hours) has been shown to be beneficial. The data come from three randomized controlled trials and a meta-analysis that all show improved outcomes with the use of *mild* therapeutic hypothermia. It is now a recommendation advocated by the 2005 AHA Guidelines and ILCOR for patients with VF arrest who have ROSC, but remain in a coma. However, rates of use remain low (30–40%) both in the United States and Europe. Another strategy that might possibly improve outcomes is the establishment of euglycemia, though the results from clinical studies were less compelling. Hyperventilation is preferably avoided as low P_{CO_2} levels in head-injury patient have been shown to be associated with worse outcomes.

Seizures/myoclonus, consequent to hypoxic brain injury, are seen in up to 40% of resuscitated patients and should be treated promptly with anticonvulsants. There is, however, no evidence that prophylactic anticonvulsants are useful.

Predictors of poor outcomes for OHCA include: (1) advanced age, (2) severe comorbidities including cancer or stroke, (3) preexisting cardiac disease and/or LV systolic dysfunction, (4) CPR greater than 5 minutes duration, (5) development of sepsis, (6) recurrence of arrhythmias, (7) PEA or asystole on presentation, (8) persistent coma, and (9) unwitnessed arrest and/or lack of bystander CPR. Most in-hospital deaths are secondary to noncardiac causes, usually respiratory complications or anoxic encephalopathy. Bilateral absence of cortical response *to median nerve somatosensory-* evoked potentials predicted poor outcome with 100% specificity when used in normothermic patients who were comatose for at least 72 hours after cardiac arrest. The best prognostic sign post-resuscitation recovery is the return of consciousness.

THE PHARMACOLOGY OF RESUSCITATION

The most significant determinant of drug effectiveness in cardiac arrest is the early use of the drug in the resuscitative efforts. No placebo-controlled clinical trials have ever been done testing the use of vasopressors in cardiac arrest. Their use is entirely based on animal studies, observational data, and consensus opinion. Epinephrine has stood the test of time as first-line agent for a cardiac arrest and is used in all forms of cardiac arrest. Epinephrine causes immediate peripheral vasoconstriction by its alpha-adrenergic effect, and thereby increases coronary and cerebral perfusion. Of lesser importance (and possibly harmful) are the positive cardiac inotropic and chronotropic effects secondary to its beta-adrenergic effects. *This has been demonstrated in studies that show adequate effectiveness of epinephrine in resuscitation, even when given with beta-blockers.* Epinephrine can cause resolution of asystole and make the VF waveform coarser and more susceptible to defibrillation. Epinephrine 0.5- to 1-mg IV is administered every 3 to 5 minutes till ROSC is achieved.

However, epinephrine and other vasoconstrictors are not entirely safe. *Epinephrine* increases myocardial oxygen demand, decreases VF generation thresholds, and possibly increases the incidence of post-resuscitation myocardial dysfunction. The quandary with epinephrine is that although epinephrine is more useful later on in cardiac arrest for facilitating ROSC, it is precisely in the later stages that it has its most deleterious effects. This lead to an early interest in the use of beta-blockers for cardiac arrest. There are several case reports describing the use of beta-blockers in VF/pulseless VT. Animal studies indicate that beta-blockers might improve myocardial oxygen requirements and attenuate ischemic myocardial damage. Nevertheless, concerns remain about their negative inotropic effects as well as iatrogenic hypotension. Because high-quality human clinical data are lacking, beta-blockers currently have no proven role in the acute management of cardiac arrest. However, they can be still considered if multiple doses of epinephrine have been given and the patient exhibits recurrent ventricular tachyarrhythmia.

Vasopressin, which causes peripheral vasoconstriction through AVPR1 receptors on vascular smooth muscle, is a more controversial drug. An earlier subgroup analysis showed vasopressin to be of benefit in patients presenting with asystole, but this finding has not been replicated in subsequent trials. *Moreover, those patients did not have improved neurologically intact survival.* Two large randomized trials subsequently have shown no benefit for vasopressin over epinephrine. *Since the half-life of vasopressin is 10 to 20 minutes,* it is administered as a one-time 40-U IV dose.

Amiodarone, developed originally as an antianginal agent in 1961, and to a lesser extent lidocaine, are antiarrhythmic drugs of choice for pulseless VT /VF, especially of presumed ischemic etiology. Amiodarone was superior to lidocaine in the ALIVE trial, and is the recommended first-line antiarrhythmic agent for VF/VT arrest. Amiodarone is administered as a single 300-mg IV push, followed if necessary by another 150-mg IV push. Lidocaine is given as a 1- to 1.5-mg/kg IV push up to a maximum of 3 mg/kg. Procainamide is no longer recommended as an antiarrhythmic agent.

Sodium bicarbonate (1 mEq/kg every 15 min) is currently *not recommended* in cardiac arrests. Even though cardiac arrest is associated with both metabolic and respiratory acidosis, exogenous bicarbonate has not been shown to improve outcomes. Furthermore, it has been associated with post-resuscitation hypernatremia, volume overload, worsened intracellular acidosis and cardiac contractility, and downstream metabolic alkalosis. Specific situations in which it might be useful include hyperkalemia and pre-arrest severe metabolic acidosis, as in aspirin or tricyclic antidepressant overdose.

Magnesium sulfate (1–4-mg IV) can be given in suspected cases of torsades de pointes and polymorphic VT with suspected hypomagenesmia. However, it is not recommended as a routine strategy for cardiac arrest.

Atropine (1-mg IV every 3–5 minutes) is helpful when PEA is secondary to severe bradycardia though infra-His and advanced heart blocks do not typically respond to atropine. Atropine has no role in VF/VT arrests. Severe bradycardia may also respond to *transcutaneous pacing* (TCP). However, asystole usually does not, and routine TCP is *not recommended for asystolic patients.*

Routine fibrinolysis in cardiac arrest patients was not associated with improved survival in clinical studies and is not at present recommended.

【 】 ROUTE OF ADMINISTRATION

As soon as feasible, IV access should be established in a patient with cardiac arrest (without interruption of chest compressions!). The upper extremity is preferred, as lower extremity circulation is feeble in the setting of a cardiac arrest. One particular advantage of epinephrine, vasopressin, atropine, naloxone, and lidocaine is their ability to be delivered through the endotracheal tube into the bronchial tree. The IV dose is typically diluted in 5 to 10 mL of water or normal saline and squirted deep into the bronchial tree. Endotracheal instillation should be followed sequentially by insufflations of the Ambu bag to facilitate drug delivery. The optimal endotracheal doses of these drugs are, however, unknown, and so the recommendation is to deliver them endotracheally only if IV access is not available and cannot be obtained in a timely manner. Lately in adults, direct intraosseus injections of these medications are frequently used by EMS personnel. *In animal studies, this route has been shown to be comparable to central venous administration.*

PROBLEMS WITH 2005 AHA GUIDELINES

Neurologically intact survival at hospital discharge, a relevant end point for clinical studies of cardiac arrest, has been very low (1–6%) and, more disquietingly, stagnant for many decades now. The most concerning aspect of the current guidelines has been their *emphasis on "rescue breathing."* There are several problems with mouth-to-mouth breathing as currently advocated.

The most compelling argument against it is the widespread bystander reluctance to deliver direct mouth-to-mouth breathing. Reported prevalence rates of bystander CPR in most U.S. cities range from 27% to 33%. This translates into fewer instances where any CPR is performed, despite strong data that suggest that CCC is far better than no CPR at all. Also rescue breathing, *even when performed correctly* by a single rescuer, takes time away from chest compression, which is the most significant generator of CPP. Moreover, positive-pressure ventilation diminishes venous return in what is already a precarious cardiac output generated by chest compression. Even short-term interruption in chest compressions is associated with decreased ROSC, reduced chances of successful defibrillation, myocardial stunning, and adverse outcomes in animal models.

This reasoning has been reflected in the 2005 guidelines, where the chest compression to rescue breathing ratio has been increased. Despite the increased emphasis on chest compression, there remains an interruption of chest compressions, and ultimately this will adversely impact CPP and downstream survival. A 2007 Japanese study showed only a 10% to 30% willingness to perform compressions plus rescue breathing as opposed to a 70% to 100% willingness to perform chest compression only. From a practical perspective, the bystander who will not give rescue breaths at a 15:2 ratio is unlikely to give rescue breaths at 30:2 or even 300:2! CCC is the only hope of getting more bystanders to commit to administering CCR in a timely and effective fashion. A recent swine study from the University of Arizona with 64 animals comparing CCC to the new 30:2 compression ratios showed significantly improved survival in the CCC group. Another 2007 study from the United Kingdom showed that even in a closely monitored environment, and with the new 30:2 compression ratios, there were excessive delays in initiating chest compressions, prolonged interruptions in chest compression, and excessive preshock pauses. The simplest and most elegant solution would be to expound CCC for all cardiac arrest patients. *This would reliably increase the frequency of bystander-initiated CPR and, very likely, survival rates across the board.*

2008 AHA SCIENCE ADVISORY

In April 2008, the AHA released a science advisory statement that recommended hands-only CCC for witnessed cardiac arrests, *omitting rescue breathing*, if either the bystander is not trained in CPR or is not confident in his or her ability to provide conventional 30:2 CPR. This was meant as an amendment to the 2005 AHA guidelines taking into account the more recent animal and human studies as well as the consensus opinion of the AHA ECC committee. Hence, the AHA guidelines now recommend with equal import, CCC and traditional CPR, and no longer consider traditional CPR to be superior to CCC. This advisory could not have been timelier in advocating for the cardinal principle of CCR. This paradigm change is expected to significantly boost the prevalence of bystander-initiated CPR. Nevertheless, this "call to action" still does *not* apply to unwitnessed adult cardiac arrests, and as expected, cardiac arrests in children.

Resuscitation science is a rapidly expanding field with exciting results from multiple clinical studies emerging over the last few years. Bystander-initiated CPR remains a crucial predictor of survival, and if we are to aim for a widespread improvement in OHCA survival rates, we will have to enlist and educate the layperson to administer CCR. Revised guidelines will be published in 2010 by the ILCOR and the AHA when all the available evidence will be reevaluated. Observational analyses over the next few years should confirm whether CCC has genuinely succeeded in increasing the prevalence of bystander-initiated CPR. The expectation is that, with the then-extensive availability of human data, and the demonstration of the utility and superiority of CCR over traditional CPR, cardiocerebral resuscitation will come to represent the face of the discipline in the 21st century.

SUGGESTED READING

American Heart Association. 2005 Guidelines for Cardiopulmonary Resuscitation and Emergency Cardiovascular Care. *Circulation*. 2005;112:IV1–203.

Berg RA, Kern KB, Sanders AB, et al. Bystander cardiopulmonary resuscitation. Is ventilation necessary? *Circulation*. 1993;88:1907–1915.

Bobrow BJ, Clark LL, Ewy GA, et al. Minimally interrupted cardiac resuscitation by emergency medical services for out-of-hospital cardiac arrest. *JAMA*. 2008;299: 1158–1165.

Ewy GA. Cardiocerebral resuscitation: the new cardiopulmonary resuscitation. *Circulation.* 2005;111:2134–2142.

Ewy GA. Cardiology patient page. New concepts of cardiopulmonary resuscitation for the lay public: continuous-chest-compression CPR. *Circulation.* 2007;116:e566–e568.

Ewy GA. Continuous-chest-compression cardiopulmonary resuscitation for cardiac arrest. *Circulation.* 2007;116:2894–2896.

Ewy GA, Zuercher M, Hilwig RW, et al. Improved neurological outcome with continuous chest compressions compared with 30:2 compressions-to-ventilations cardiopulmonary resuscitation in a realistic swine model of out-of-hospital cardiac arrest. *Circulation.* 2007;116:2525–2530.

Sanders AB, Kern KB, Atlas M, et al. Importance of the duration of inadequate coronary perfusion pressure on resuscitation from cardiac arrest. *J Am Coll Cardiol.* 1985;6:113–118.

Sayre MR, Berg RA, Cave DM, et al. Hands-only (compression-only) cardiopulmonary resuscitation: a call to action for bystander response to adults who experience out-of-hospital sudden cardiac arrest. A science advisory for the public from the American Heart Association Emergency Cardiovascular Care Committee. *Circulation.* 2008;117:2162–2167.

Weisfeldt ML, Becker LB. Resuscitation after cardiac arrest: a 3-phase time-sensitive model. *JAMA.* 2002;288:3035–3038.

CHAPTER 20

Diagnosis and Management of Heart Failure

Robert McCray and Gary S. Francis

Chronic heart failure is a complex clinical syndrome that has multiple causes and etiologies. The core lesion involves structural and functional changes in the heart and peripheral vasculature that lead to impaired systolic and diastolic function. The resultant clinical manifestations are variable, but the most common symptoms include exertional dypsnea, orthopnea, and nocturnal dypsnea. Other common signs and symptoms include edema, fatigue, and chest congestion.

PATHOPHYSIOLOGY

In heart failure there is always an index event that occurs in the heart leading to structural and functional changes. The index event may be clinically obvious, such as an acute myocardial infarction, or it may be more insidious, such as genetic mutations that over time lead to structural and functional abnormalities. When there is left ventricular (LV) damage or perverse loading conditions, the myocardium responds with chronic myocyte hypertrophic and fibrotic adaptation. The LV diameter can enlarge, thereby temporarily maintaining stroke volume. LV performance can remain adequate in the face of a low stroke volume to meet metabolic needs, and symptoms can be minimal. However, with progressive dilation of the LV, the capacity of the heart to eject blood is impaired and LV filling pressure rises, leading to dypsnea, fatigue, and tissue congestion. In the late stages of systolic heart failure, further dilation of the LV and left atrial chambers leads to mitral regurgitation and replacement of normal myocardial architecture with elongated myocytes and extensive fibrosis.

Systolic heart failure can be due to many causes, including hypertension, valvular heart disease, coronary artery disease, chemotherapy, myocarditis, infiltrative processes, and endocrine disorders. In every patient, a specific etiology should be sought out and treated according to etiology when possible. The central feature of systolic heart failure is a large heart with a dilated LV chamber and impaired ejection of blood. The process of LV remodeling or dilation can take years to occur. In many cases, the progression can be attenuated, eliminated, or even reversed with appropriate medical therapy. The term "cure," however, is rarely applied.

Diastolic heart failure or heart failure with a preserved ejection fraction (EF) often coincides with systolic heart failure. However, certain features of diastolic heart failure are distinct, including impaired ventricular filling, increased chamber stiffness, and increased LV end-diastolic pressure relative to end-diastolic volume. The LV chamber is often small with hypertrophy of the LV myocardium being common but not invariable. The epidemiology of heart failure with preserved EF and the natural history of this syndrome are also somewhat different than what is observed with systolic heart failure. Diastolic heart failure tends to occur in older patients, particularly women, and there are no well-established guidelines for treatment. However, once a patient is hospitalized with overt heart failure and a preserved EF, the prognosis is equally severe as that of

TABLE 20-1

RAAS Blocking Drugs Commonly Used to Treat Heart Failure in the United States

Generic	Brand	Dose
ACE Inhibitors		
Captopril	Capoten	6.25–150 mg tid
Enalapril	Vasotec	2.5–20 mg bid
Fosinopril	Monopril	10–80 mg qd
Lisinopril	Prinvil, Zestril	5–20 mg qd
Quinapril	Accupril	5–20 mg bid
Ramipril	Altace	2.5–20 mg qd
ARBs		
Candesartan	Atacand	8–32 mg qd/bid
Losartan[a]	Cozaar	50–100 mg qd/bid
Valsartan	Diovan	80–320 mg qd
Irbesartan[a]	Avapro	150–300 mg qd
Telmisartan[a]	Micardis	40–80 mg qd
Olmesartan[a]	Benicar	20–40 mg qd
Aldosterone Antagonists		
Spironolactone	Aldactone	25–50 mg qd
Eplerenone[b]	Inspra	25–50 mg qd

[a]Currently not approved by the U.S. Food and Drug Administration for heart failure.
[b]Approved for post-myocardial infarction.

systolic heart failure. Dyspnea, tissue congestion, and renal insufficiency occur similarly in diastolic and systolic heart failure.

Heart failure is characterized by neurohormonal activation, presumably in an attempt to maintain perfusion pressure. However, excessive chronic activation of the sympathetic nervous system and the renin–angiotensin–aldosterone system (RAAS) eventually facilitates LV remodeling at the cellular level, thus contributing to the progression of the syndrome. Other neurohormones and cytokines also contribute to the pathophysiology, promoting fibrosis, hypertrophy, and impaired LV function. Specific molecular abnormalities can be identified in the myocytes of the failing heart. The recognition that neurohormonal activation leads to a progression of heart failure has laid the framework for drugs designed to block the sympathetic nervous system (beta-adrenergic blockers) and the RAAS (angiotensin-converting enzyme [ACE] inhibitors, angiotensin receptor blockers [ARBs], and aldosterone receptor blockers) (Tables 20-1 and 20-2).

TABLE 20-2

Beta-Blockers Commonly Used to Treat Heart Failure in the United States

Generic	Brand	Dose
Carvedilol	Coreg	3.125–25 mg bid
Metoprolol succinate	Toprol XL	25–200 mg qd
Bisoprolol[a]	Zebeta	1.25–10 mg qd

[a]Currently not approved by the U.S. Food and Drug Administration for heart failure.

DIAGNOSIS

The diagnosis of heart failure is made by performing a careful history and physical examination. It should be verified by imaging of the heart, typically echocardiography. In acute heart failure when there is doubt about the diagnosis, plasma B-type natriuretic peptide (BNP or NT-proBNP) levels are helpful for verification. In patients with advanced heart failure, there is often increased jugular venous pressure and pulmonary rales, and in some cases ascites and peripheral edema. A murmur of mitral and tricuspid regurgitation may be evident and an S_3 gallop can sometimes be heard at the apex of the heart. The severity of the symptoms does not always parallel the magnitude of LV dysfunction as reflected by the LV EF. The target of therapy depends on the extent of symptoms. For example, lung congestion, worsening shortness of breath, and edema are most responsive to loop diuretics. Progressive remodeling is most responsive to long-term beta-blockers and drugs designed to block the RAAS.

MANAGEMENT OF HEART FAILURE

【 】 STAGE I: AT RISK FOR HEART FAILURE

Stage I does not represent true heart failure, but rather indicates the presence of risk factors that are known to precede the onset of heart failure. Structural changes in the heart have not yet developed, and cardiac function is normal. However, conditions such as hypertension, diabetes mellitus, and hyperlipidemia need to be vigorously treated to prevent heart failure.

【 】 STAGE II: STRUCTURAL ABNORMALITIES PRESENT IN THE ABSENCE OF SIGNS AND SYMPTOMS OF HEART FAILURE

Patients with stage II heart failure have demonstrable cardiac pathology, such as left ventricular hypertrophy (LVH), coronary disease, or valvular heart disease, but signs and symptoms of heart failure are absent. A low EF in the absence of heart failure symptoms is not uncommon. As with stage I, in the absence of symptoms there is no heart failure, but the patient is at even greater risk to develop heart failure than in stage I, and now has underlying structural heart disease. Such patients should be aggressively treated. Blood pressure must be well-controlled, and ACE inhibitors or ARBs along with beta-blockers are indicated. Therapy with beta-blockers and RAAS blockers can slow the progression of LV remodeling, including LVH and LV dilation. Loop diuretics to relieve congestion may not always be necessary, but thiazides to control high blood pressure might be employed. Concomitant risk factors, such as diabetes mellitus, obstructive sleep apnea, and hyperlipidemia should be vigorously controlled.

【 】 STAGE III: SIGNS AND SYMPTOMS OF HEART FAILURE WITH DEMONSTRABLE STRUCTURAL HEART DISEASE

These patients make up the bulk of the heart failure population. They are often stable and ambulatory, but may be hospitalized with acute decompensation. Nearly all of these patients will benefit from a loop diuretic, though perhaps not on a daily basis. They must be followed with careful monitoring of their volume status and have their therapy adjusted accordingly. Beta-blockers, ACE inhibitors, or ARBs—and in advanced cases spironolactone or eplerenone—should be used to control progressive LV remodeling. Intolerance of beta-blockers and/or RAAS blockers is predictive of a very poor prognosis. The need for hospitalization also predicts a much worse prognosis. A low-sodium diet is usually necessary, typically less than 2 g/day. Moderate exercise is encouraged for ambulatory patients.

【 】 STAGE IV: HIGHLY SYMPTOMATIC HEART FAILURE

The highly symptomatic heart failure of stage IV requires special measures, such as hospitalization for intra-aortic balloon pump (IABP), left ventricular assist devices (LVAD), ultrafiltration or dialysis, heart transplantation, heart failure surgery, or palliative care.

These patients are said to have "end-stage heart failure," and have special needs that are sometimes uniquely available at large academic health centers. They are often cared for by teams of heart failure specialists experienced in the complex care of critically ill patients.

【 】 RAAS BLOCKERS

ACE inhibitors or ARBs are almost always indicated in patients with symptomatic heart failure, and are also indicated in pre-heart failure (stage II). These drugs should be titrated slowly over days to weeks to maximal doses used in the large clinical trials. Patients who are intolerant of ACE inhibitors should be given a trial of ARBs. In some cases, ACE inhibitors and ARBs are used together, but hypotension, hyperkalemia, and renal insufficiency are more frequent. Patients with antecedent renal insufficiency and diabetes mellitus must be monitored very carefully when using RAAS blockers to avoid serious hyperkalemia and worsening renal function. It is not unexpected that some patients will have about a 20% increase in serum creatinine and/or develop modest, asymptomatic hypotension while taking RAAS blockers, but these changes are not typically an indication to stop the RAAS inhibitor. Aldosterone receptor blockers (spironolactone) are usually initiated for patients with New York Heart Association (NYHA) class IV heart failure, or patients who were class IV but have become class III. When symptomatic hypotension occurs with RAAS blockers, it may be related to volume depletion from loop diuretics. Temporarily withdrawing loop diuretics and resuming them at lower doses often alleviates symptomatic hypotension. Intolerance to RAAS blockers is associated with a very poor prognosis.

【 】 BETA-ADRENERGIC BLOCKERS

As with RAAS blockers, patients should be started on a beta-blocker if LV dilation or reduced LV EF is detected by echocardiogram, even in the absence of signs and symptoms of heart failure. These drugs should be continued indefinitely, along with RAAS blockers, even if LV dilation and EF return to normal following treatment. There are few contraindications to beta-blockers in patients with heart failure, but these might include high-grade AV block, severe hypotension or shock, or severe decompensated heart failure with a very low cardiac index (i.e., less than 2.0 L/min/m²). When patients are hospitalized with acute heart failure, beta-blockers are often temporarily discontinued, but can usually be restarted in the hospital prior to discharge when the patient is hemodynamically stable. Thus severe but stable NYHA class IV heart failure is not a contraindication for beta-blockers; tolerability remains very high in patients with advanced heart failure. Patients who do not tolerate beta-blockers usually have a very poor prognosis.

【 】 DIURETICS

Most patients with stage III and IV heart failure will require loop diuretics. Patients hospitalized with volume overload will usually require intravenous loop diuretics, often given as a continuous drip. The aim of therapy in acute heart failure is to afford a diuresis with a weight loss of 3 to 5 Ib/day. Low blood pressure is not usually a contraindication to use of loop diuretics in patients with overt pulmonary congestion. Often, potassium must be replenished in order to maintain a serum potassium level of at least 4 mEq/L. For hospitalized patients who are refractory to intravenous loop diuretics, oral metolazone, and in some cases intravenous thiazide, should be added. In the absence of pulmonary congestion, especially when there is a poor diuretic response, there may be no compelling need for high-dose diuretics, and one might consider stopping the medication or lowering the dose.

【 】 DIGITALIS GLYCOSIDES

Digitalis is sometimes symptomatically helpful in patients with NYHA class III and class IV heart failure with persistent signs and symptoms. Smaller doses are recommended with an aim toward serum digoxin levels around 1 ng/mL. Digitalis reduces sympathetic tone, increases parasympathetic activity, and is useful in controlling heart rate when atrial fibrillation is present. There is only modest improvement in inotropic state. Current trials indicate that use of digoxin in patients with symptomatic heart failure reduces the severity of symptoms and the frequency of hospitalization for decompensated heart failure. However, there are no data indicating a significant survival benefit.

【 】 SPECIAL CONSIDERATIONS

In many patients, drug and dietary noncompliance are an important cause of acute heart failure exacerbations. Patients with heart failure tend to be older and have multiple comorbidities. Therapy should be continuous with all comorbidities considered while treating the patient. Uncontrolled hypertension, myocardial ischemia, rapid atrial fibrillation, nonsteroidal anti-inflammatory drugs, chemotherapy, and thiazolidinediones can each precipitate decompensation of stable heart failure. Infection and uncontrolled diabetes should be vigorously treated.

【 】 HEART TRANSPLANT AND ASSIST DEVICES

Patients who are stage IV or late stage III are potentially candidates for heart transplantation. The primary indication for heart transplantation is severe, very symptomatic heart failure despite optimal medical therapy when there are no alternative options or contraindications. It is expected that following heart transplantation the patient will be able to lead a full life, have excellent psychological and social support systems, and that other organs will remain in good working order. The decision to do heart transplantation is very complex and beyond the scope of this synopsis. Because of severe organ shortages, heart transplantation is essentially rationed to those patients who have the greatest chance of durable benefit. The follow-up of patients is also complex, and is usually carried out by teams of health care workers with expertise and experience in this area. In general, patients are referred to a heart transplant center for complete evaluation.

When it is likely the patient will die within 24 to 48 hours without a new heart, various strategies have been devised to temporarily sustain cardiac function using a left ventricular assist device (LVAD) until a new heart becomes available. Right ventricular, biventricular, and total artificial hearts are also available, depending on need. The new specialty of device therapy is rapidly changing, and busy heart transplant centers now have teams of health care workers who are expert in formulating the decision to implant a mechanical device, choosing which device to implant, the actual implantation of the device itself (which can entail open heart surgery), and the postop care of device patients. Cardiologists and heart transplant surgeons usually work closely together. An LVAD may be used as a "bridge to transplant" until a new heart becomes available, usually for 1 to 3 months, or even as "destination therapy" where there is no intent to ever do heart transplantation, but the goal is to basically alleviate signs and symptoms of heart failure and extend life if possible. The destination therapy strategy is under intensive study, and device therapy in general is now being carefully monitored. Data are being systematically collected and entered into a national registry so we can learn more about these evolving treatments. Device therapy and heart transplantation are expensive, labor intensive, and aimed at a relatively narrow spectrum or patients with severe heart failure. Only through the systematic collection and analysis of longitudinal data can we learn how to use these emerging tools.

【　】 UNRESOLVED ISSUES

There are several vexing problems regarding the treatment of patients with heart failure:

1. So-called diastolic heart failure or heart failure with preserved LV systolic function is poorly defined and proper treatment is unclear. There are currently no large clinical trials to guide therapy. As with systolic heart failure, beta-blockers, RAAS blockers, and diuretics are commonly used.

2. The treatment of acute decompensated heart failure is an area of intense research, but proof of a survival benefit with commonly used therapies has been elusive. Treatment is largely empirical. As with diastolic heart failure, there are no large clinical trials to guide therapy. Positive inotropic agents tend to increase mortality, but they may have some role in patients that are in a state of low cardiac output with a systolic blood pressure less than 90 mm Hg. Intravenous diuretics are commonly used to relieve acute congestion. Intravenous vasodilators such as nitroglycerin and nitroprusside can be employed to reduce congestion and improve forward flow, provided that the mean BP is greater than 65 mm Hg.

3. Selecting patients who will most likely benefit from an implantable cardiodefibrillator (ICD) has been a difficult problem, as sudden cardiac death is not a clearly predictable event in an individual patient. Moreover, NYHA class II patients have a somewhat greater chance of sudden cardiac death, but have fewer symptoms and often a more preserved EF. There is an inverse relationship between the EF and incidence of sudden death, so that patients with an EF less than or equal to 30% are more likely to benefit from an ICD. However, the implanted ICD is unlikely to be used to terminate ventricular tachycardia and/or ventricular fibrillation in many patients with a low EF, leading to a tendency to over-prescribe ICDs, an expensive form of treatment that is not without inherent risk. Better predictors of which patient will benefit from ICD placement are needed.

SUGGESTED READINGS

Francis GS, Tang WHW. Angiotensin converting enzyme inhibitors, angiotensin II receptor blockers and aldosterone receptor blockers. In: Manson JA, Buring J, Ridker P, et al., eds. *Clinical Trials in Heart Disease. A Companion to Braunwald's Heart Disease*. Philadelphia, PA: Saunders; 2004:227–241.

Francis GS, Tang WHW. Clinical evaluation of heart failure. In: Mann D, ed. *Heart Failure: A Companion to Braunwald's Heart Disease*. Philadelphia, PA: Saunders; 2004: 507–526.

Francis GS, Tang WHW, Poole-Wilson PA, et al. Pathophysiology of heart failure. In: Fuster V, ed. *Hurst's The Heart*. 12th ed. New York, NY: McGraw-Hill; 2008:691–712.

Hunt SA, Abraham WT, Chin MH, et al. ACC/AHA 2005 guideline update for the diagnosis and management of chronic heart failure in the adult: summary article. *J Am Coll Cardiol*. 2005;46:1116–1143.

CHAPTER (21)

Dyslipidemia and Other Cardiac Risk Factors

Robert L. Huang, David J. Maron, Paul M. Ridker, Scott M. Grundy, and Thomas A. Pearson

Prevention of coronary heart disease (CHD) requires identification and treatment of risk factors. *Primary prevention* refers to strategies to prevent clinical manifestation of disease in asymptomatic individuals. *Secondary prevention* refers to efforts to prevent recurrent clinical events in patients with established disease. *Risk factor management prevents and treats coronary atherosclerosis, and should be included as an integral part of any management plan for the many acute and chronic manifestations of this disease.* The intensity of preventive interventions should correspond to the patient's level of absolute risk.

RISK ASSESSMENT AND RISK FACTOR EVALUATION

【 】 CATEGORIES OF ABSOLUTE RISK

Most risk algorithms divide absolute risk into three categories: high, intermediate, and low. Patients at high risk deserve the most intense risk-reduction therapy. Those at intermediate risk are candidates for preventive interventions to the extent that therapy is safe, efficacious, and cost-effective. Finally, low-risk patients should follow public health recommendations for primary prevention of CHD and may benefit from risk-reducing drug therapy.

Each category of absolute risk can be expressed quantitatively (Table 21-1). Patients without CHD whose absolute 10-year risk for CHD equals that of patients who already manifest clinical CHD (such as those with diabetes mellitus) are said to have a *CHD risk equivalent*. It is recognized that there are limitations to this approach, as these risk estimates are highly dependent on age. Lifetime risk may be more appropriate than 10-year risk in several prevention settings.

【 】 IDENTIFICATION OF VERY-HIGH-RISK PATIENTS

An update to the National Cholesterol Education Program (NCEP) Adult Treatment Panel III (ATP III) guidelines proposed a new classification of patients as very high risk who deserve especially aggressive low-density lipoprotein cholesterol (LDL-C) lowering. These individuals are those with established CHD plus (1) multiple major risk factors (especially diabetes), (2) severe and poorly controlled risk factors (especially continued cigarette smoking), (3) the metabolic syndrome (especially triglycerides ≥ 200 mg/dL, plus non–high-density lipoprotein cholesterol ≥ 130 mg/dL with high-density lipoprotein cholesterol [HDL-C] < 40 mg/dL), and (4) patients with acute coronary syndromes. Patients with established CHD and elevated levels of C-reactive protein (CRP) also are classified as a very-high-risk group.

TABLE 21-1

Risk Categories

Risk Category	10-Year Absolute Risk for Myocardial Infarction (%) (Nonfatal + Fatal)
High	> 20
Intermediate	10–20
Low	< 10

Adapted from *Third Report of the National Cholesterol Education Program (NCEP) Expert Panel on Detection, Evaluation, and Treatment of High Blood Cholesterol in Adults (Adult Treatment Panel III). Final Report.* National Heart, Lung, and Blood Institute National Institutes of Health NIH pub. no. 02-5215 September 2002, or http://www.nhlbi.nih.gov/guidelines/cholesterol/atp3full.pdf. Accessed March 3, 2008.

【 】 IDENTIFICATION OF HIGH-RISK PATIENTS WITH CORONARY HEART DISEASE RISK EQUIVALENTS

Clinical Coronary Heart Disease

Included in the category of clinical CHD are patients with a history of acute coronary syndromes, stable angina, and coronary revascularization procedures. Patients with a prior history of myocardial infarction (MI) have a 10-year risk for recurrent nonfatal or fatal MI of about 26%. Stable angina pectoris confers a 10-year risk for acute MI of approximately 20%.

Noncoronary Atherosclerosis

Patients in this group include those with peripheral arterial disease, abdominal aortic aneurysm, and symptomatic carotid artery disease or asymptomatic disease with > 50% stenosis. The absolute risk for MI in patients with noncoronary atherosclerosis is equal to recurrent MI in patients with established CHD.

Diabetes

Patients with diabetes, particularly middle-age and older patients with type 2 diabetes, who do not manifest CHD, carry a risk for major coronary events equivalent to that of nondiabetic patients with established CHD. Moreover, many patients with type 2 diabetes have had a silent MI, and many others have silent ischemia. Thus, patients with diabetes are at high risk, and ATP III has designated *diabetes as a CHD equivalent.*

【 】 MULTIPLE RISK FACTORS WITHOUT CLINICAL CORONARY HEART DISEASE

Patients without known atherosclerosis often have multiple risk factors (Table 21-2) that contribute to CHD risk. Absolute risk for development of CHD over the next decade can be estimated by Framingham risk tables (Tables 21-3 and 21-4). These tables calculate absolute risk for the development of *hard CHD* (nonfatal and fatal MI) over the next 10 years but exclude *soft CHD* (stable and unstable angina). Using this method, asymptomatic patients with multiple risk factors can be stratified into high-risk and intermediate-risk categories. *A CHD risk equivalent is defined when the absolute 10-year risk for hard CHD events exceeds 20%.*

TABLE 21-2

Major Risk Factors Other than LDL Cholesterol[a]

Cigarette smoking
Hypertension (blood pressure ≥ 140/90 mm Hg or on antihypertensive medication)
Low HDL cholesterol (< 40 mg/dL)
Family history of premature CHD (CHD in male first-degree relative < 55 y; CHD in female first-degree relative < 65 y)
Age (men ≥45 y; women ≥55 y)

[a]Diabetes is regarded as a CHD risk equivalent.

Adapted from *Third Report of the National Cholesterol Education Program (NCEP) Expert Panel on Detection, Evaluation, and Treatment of High Blood Cholesterol in Adults (Adult Treatment Panel III). Final Report.* National Heart, Lung, and Blood Institute National Institutes of Health NIH pub. no. 02-5215 September 2002, or http://www.nhlbi.nih.gov/ guidelines/cholesterol/atp3full.pdf. Accessed March 3, 2008.

TABLE 21-3

Estimate of 10-Year Risk for Men (Framingham Point Scores)

Age (y)	Points
20–34	−9
35–39	−4
40–44	0
45–49	3
50–54	6
55–59	8
60–64	10
65–69	11
70–74	12
75–79	13

Total Cholesterol (mg/dL)	Points				
	Age 20–39 y	Age 40–49 y	Age 50–59 y	Age 60–69 y	Age 70–79 y
< 160	0	0	0	0	0
160–199	4	3	2	1	0
200–239	7	5	3	1	0
240–279	9	6	4	2	1
≥ 280	11	8	5	3	1

	Points				
	Age 20–39 y	Age 40–49 y	Age 50–59 y	Age 60–69 y	Age 70–79 y
smoker	0	0	0	0	0
er	8	5	3	1	1

g/dL)	Points
	−1
	0
	1
	2

TABLE 21-3

Estimate of 10-Year Risk for Men (Framingham Point Scores) (*Continued*)

Systolic BP (mm Hg)	If Untreated	If Treated
< 120	0	0
120–129	0	1
130–139	1	2
140–159	1	2
≥ 160	2	3

Point Total	10-Year Risk (%)
< 0	< 1
0	1
1	1
2	1
3	1
4	1
5	2
6	2
7	3
8	4
9	5
10	6
11	8
12	10
13	12
14	16
15	20
16	25
≥17	≥30

Adapted from *Third Report of the National Cholesterol Education Program (NCEP) Expert Panel on Detection, Evaluation, and Treatment of High Blood Cholesterol in Adults (Adult Treatment Panel III). Final Report.* National Heart, Lung, and Blood Institute National Institutes of Health NIH pub. no. 02-5215 September 2002, or http://www.nhlbi.nih.gov/guidelines/cholesterol/atp3full.pdf. Accessed March 3, 2008.

TABLE 21-4

Estimate of 10-Year Risk for Women (Framingham Point Scores)

Age (y)	Points
20–34	−7
35–39	−3
40–44	0
45–49	3
50–54	6
55–59	8
60–64	10
65–69	12
70–74	14
75–79	16

TABLE 21-4

Estimate of 10-Year Risk for Women (Framingham Point Scores) (*Continued*)

Total Cholesterol (mg/dL)	Points				
	Age 20–39 y	Age 40–49 y	Age 50–59 y	Age 60–69 y	Age 70–79 y
< 160	0	0	0	0	0
160–199	4	3	2	1	1
200–239	8	6	4	2	1
240–279	11	8	5	3	2
≥ 280	13	10	7	4	2

	Points				
	Age 20–39 y	Age 40–49 y	Age 50–59 y	Age 60–69 y	Age 70–79 y
Nonsmoker	0	0	0	0	0
Smoker	9	7	4	2	1

HDL (mg/dL)	Points
≥60	−1
50–59	0
40–49	1
< 40	2

Systolic BP (mm Hg)	If Untreated	If Treated
< 120	0	0
120–129	1	3
130–139	2	4
140–159	3	5
≥ 160	4	6

Point Total	10-Year Risk, %
< 9	< 1
9	1
10	1
11	1
12	1
13	2
14	2
15	3
16	4
17	5
18	6
19	8
20	11
21	14
22	17
23	22
24	27
≥ 25	≥ 30

Adapted from *Third Report of the National Cholesterol Education Program (NCEP) Expert Panel on Detection, Evaluation, and Treatment of High Blood Cholesterol in Adults (Adult Treatment Panel III). Final Report.* National Heart, Lung, and Blood Institute National Institutes of Health NIH pub. no. 02-5215 September 2002, or http://www.nhlbi.nih.gov/guidelines/cholesterol/atp3full.pdf. Accessed March 3, 2008.

High-Risk Patients Identified by Major Risk Factors Plus Emerging Risk Factors

Some intermediate-risk patients (10-year CHD risk of 10–20%) determined by the Framingham risk score are at higher risk because of advanced subclinical coronary atherosclerosis. These individuals can be identified by screening for "emerging risk factors" defined by the NCEP ATP III guidelines (see Table 21-5). *Noninvasive testing in asymptomatic patients should be used for risk assessment (prognosis) and not for diagnosis of coronary artery disease.* Noninvasive tests with the most evidence to improve risk prediction beyond the Framingham risk score include high-sensitivity CRP, coronary artery calcium scanning, exercise treadmill testing, and carotid ultrasound. Currently, the American Heart Association (AHA) and Centers for Disease Control and Prevention (CDC) recommend the optional use of CRP in intermediate-risk patients to direct further evaluation and therapy.

【 】 IDENTIFICATION OF INTERMEDIATE-RISK AND LOW-RISK PATIENTS

Patients at intermediate risk are those without known atherosclerosis but with two or more conventional risk factors whose 10-year risk for CHD is 10% to 20%. Patients with no more than one risk factor are low risk and have a 10-year risk for CHD of less than 10%.

TABLE 21-5

Emerging Risk Factors

Lipid
- Triglycerides
- Lipoprotein remnant particles
- Lipoprotein(a)
- Small LDL particles
- HDL subspecies
- Apolipoprotein B
- Apolipoprotein AI
- Total cholesterol/HDL cholesterol ratio

Nonlipid
- Homocysteine
- Thrombogenic/hemostatic factors
- Inflammatory markers
- Impaired fasting glucose

Detection of Subclinical Atherosclerosis
- Ankle brachial index
- Tests for myocardial ischemia
- Tests for atherosclerotic plaque burden (e.g., coronary calcium scanning, carotid sonography)

HDL, high-density lipoprotein; LDL, low-density lipoprotein.

Adapted from *Third Report of the National Cholesterol Education Program (NCEP) Expert Panel on Detection, Evaluation, and Treatment of High Blood Cholesterol in Adults (Adult Treatment Panel III). Final Report.* National Heart, Lung, and Blood Institute National Institutes of Health NIH pub. no. 02-5215 September 2002, or http://www.nhlbi.nih.gov/guidelines/cholesterol/atp3full.pdf. Accessed March 3, 2008.

An important question is how to manage patients who have a single, treatable categorical risk factor but are otherwise at low risk. A fundamental principle of primary prevention is that *all categorical risk factors must be treated, regardless of absolute risk*. Although a person with only one risk factor—such as hypertension, smoking, or hypercholesterolemia—has less than a 10% 10-year risk of CHD, the presence of a single major risk factor at 50 years of age is associated with a substantially increased lifetime risk for CHD and markedly shorter survival. Therefore, patients with even one single categorical risk factor should not be ignored even if found to have a low absolute risk by Framingham scoring (Tables 21-3 and 21-4).

PRACTICE RECOMMENDATIONS

The remainder of this chapter provides specific practice recommendations in accordance with national guidelines for primary and secondary prevention of CHD (see Tables 21-6 and 21-7).

【 】 LOWERING LOW-DENSITY LIPOPROTEIN CHOLESTEROL

Table 21-8 shows the LDL cholesterol goals and cutpoints for therapy classified by risk category. For patients at very high risk, it is < 70 mg/dL. LDL lowering can be achieved with nondrug and drug therapies. *The importance of nondrug therapies must not be minimized.* Reducing the intake of cholesterol-raising fatty acids (saturated and *trans* fatty acids) and dietary cholesterol is a key component of nondrug therapy. Major sources of dietary saturated fatty acids are dairy fats (e.g., milk, butter, cream, cheese, and ice cream) and animal fats (e.g., fatty cuts of meat [especially hamburger], fatty processed meats, lard, and tallow). *Trans* fatty acids are present in shortening and hard margarine, and often in processed foods. Rich sources of dietary cholesterol are eggs, dairy fats, and other animal products. For patients on cholesterol-lowering therapies, their daily intake of cholesterol-raising fatty acids should be less than 7% of total calories. Dietary cholesterol intake should be lowered to less than 200 mg/d.

LDL-C may also be lowered by the addition of certain foods. A daily intake of 2 to 3 g/day of plant stanols or sterol esters can reduce LDL-cholesterol by 6% to 15%. High intakes (5–10 g) of viscous dietary fiber can decrease LDL levels another 3% to 5%. Monounsaturated and polyunsaturated fatty acids will lower LDL and may reduce global risk for CHD via other mechanisms. When combined with a low-saturated-fat, low-*trans*-fat diet, the addition of plant sterols, viscous fibers, and nuts can reduce LDL-C comparable to the effect of a low-dose statin.

Table 21-9 shows drugs used for lipid therapy. Statins are the most effective LDL-lowering drugs. Most patients tolerate statins with few side effects. Occasional patients (0.5–2%) may have a mild rise in liver transaminases, but this change is not believed to be an indication of hepatotoxicity. Statin-induced myopathy, defined as a serum creatinine kinase level of more than 10 times the upper limit of normal, has been observed in 0.1% to 0.5% of patients treated with statins during randomized controlled trials. Some patients have biopsy-proven myopathy but normal creatinine kinase levels; thus, normal creatinine kinase levels do not rule out myopathy. Table 21-10 lists risk factors for severe myopathy.

For every doubling of the dose of a statin, the LDL level will fall by about 6%. A more efficacious way to enhance LDL lowering is to combine statins with ezetimibe or bile acid sequestrants.

【 】 IDENTIFICATION AND TREATMENT OF METABOLIC SYNDROME

Patients with the metabolic syndrome should be counseled to make intensive lifestyle changes, especially weight reduction and increased physical activity.

TABLE 21-6

Guide to Primary Prevention of Cardiovascular Disease

Risk Intervention and Goals	Recommendations
Smoking: Goal: Complete cessation. No exposure to environmental tobacco smoke	Ask about tobacco use status at every visit. In a clear, strong, and personalized manner, advise every tobacco user to quit. Assess the tobacco user's willingness to quit. Assist by counseling and developing a plan for quitting. Arrange follow-up, referral to special programs, or pharmacotherapy. Urge avoidance of exposure to second-hand smoke at work or home.
BP control Goal: < 140/90 mm Hg; < 130/85 mm Hg if renal insufficiency or heart failure is present; or < 130/80 mm Hg if diabetes is present	Promote healthy lifestyle modification. Advocate weight reduction; reduction of sodium intake; consumption of fruits, vegetables, and low-fat dairy products; moderation of alcohol intake; and physical activity in persons with BP ≥ 130 mm Hg systolic or 80 mm Hg diastolic. For persons with renal insufficiency or heart failure, initiate drug therapy if BP ≥ 130 mm Hg systolic or 85 mm Hg diastolic (≥ 80 mm Hg diastolic for patients with diabetes). Initiate drug therapy for those with BP $\geq 140/90$ mm Hg if 6 to 12 months of lifestyle modification is not effective, depending on the number of risk factors present. Add BP medications, individualized to other patient requirements and characteristics (e.g., age, race, need for drugs with specific benefits).
Dietary intake Goal: An overall healthy eating pattern	Advocate consumption of a variety of fruits, vegetables, grains, low-fat or nonfat dairy products, fish, legumes, poultry, and lean meats. Match energy intake with energy needs and make appropriate changes to achieve weight loss when indicated. Modify food choices to reduce saturated fats (< 10% of calories), cholesterol (< 300 mg/dl), and *trans*-fatty acids by substituting grains and unsaturated fatty acids from fish, vegetables, legumes, and nuts. Limit salt intake to < 6 g/d. Limit alcohol intake (≤ 2 drinks/d in men, ≤ 1 drink/d in women) among those who drink.
Aspirin Goal: low-dose aspirin in persons at higher CHD risk (especially those with 10-y risk of CHD $\geq 10\%$)	Do not recommend for patients with aspirin intolerance. Low-dose aspirin increases risk for gastrointestinal bleeding and hemorrhagic stroke. Do not use in persons at increased risk for these diseases. Benefits of cardiovascular risk reduction outweigh these risks in most patients at higher coronary risk. Doses of 75–160 mg/d are as effective as higher doses. Therefore, consider 75–160 mg aspirin per day for persons at higher risk (especially those with 10-y risk of CHD $\geq 10\%$).

Blood lipid management

Primary goal: LDL-C < 160 mg/dL. If ≤ 1 risk factor is present, LDL-C < 130 mg/dL; if ≥ 2 risk factors are present and 10-y CHD risk is < 20%; or LDL-C < 100 mg/dL if ≥ 2 risk factors are present and 10-y CHD risk is ≥ 20% or if patient has diabetes

Secondary goals (if LDL-C is at goal range): If triglycerides > 200 mg/dL, then use non-HDL-C as a secondary goal:
non-HDL-C < 190 mg/dL for ≤ 1 risk factor;
non-HDL-C < 160 mg/dL for ≥ 2 risk factors and 10-y CHD risk ≤ 20%;
non-HDL-C < 130 mg/dL for diabetics or for ≥ 2 risk factors and 10-y CHD risk >20%

Other targets for therapy:
Triglycerides > 150 mg/dL;
HDL-C < 40 mg/dL in men and < 50 mg/dL in women

If LDL-C is above goal range, initiate additional therapeutic lifestyle changes consisting of dietary modifications to lower LDL-C: < 7% of calories from saturated fat, cholesterol < 200 mg/d, and, if further LDL-C lowering is required, dietary options (plant stanols/sterols not to exceed 2 g/d and/or increased viscous [soluble] fiber [10–25 g/d]), and additional emphasis on weight reduction and physical activity. If LDL-C is above goal range, rule out secondary causes (liver function test, thyroid-stimulating hormone level, urinalysis). After 12 weeks of therapeutic lifestyle change, consider LDL-lowering drug therapy if ≥ 2 risk factors are present, 10-y risk > 10%, and LDL-C ≥ 130 mg/dL; ≥ 2 risk factors are present, 10-y risk < 10%, and LDL-C ≥160 mg/dL; or ≤ 1 risk factor is present and LDL-C is ≥ 190 mg/dL. Start drugs and advance dose to bring LDL-C to goal range, usually a statin but also consider bile acid–binding resin or niacin. If LDL-C goal not achieved, consider combination therapy (statin + resin, statin + niacin). After LDL-C goal has been reached, consider triglyceride level: if 150–199 mg/dL, treat with therapeutic lifestyle changes. If 200–499 mg/dL, treat elevated non-HDL-C with therapeutic lifestyle changes and, if necessary, consider higher doses of statin or adding niacin or fibrate. If >500 mg/dL, treat with fibrate or niacin to reduce risk of pancreatitis. If HDL-C < 40 mg/dL in men and < 50 mg/dL in women, initiate or intensify therapeutic lifestyle changes. For higher-risk patients, consider drugs that raise HDL-C (e.g., niacin, fibrates, statins).

TABLE 21-6

Guide to Primary Prevention of Cardiovascular Disease (*Continued*)

Risk Intervention and Goals	Recommendations
Physical activity Goal: At least 30 min of moderate-intensity physical activity on most (and preferably all) days of the week	If cardiovascular, respiratory, metabolic, orthopedic, or neurologic disorders are suspected, or if patient is middle-aged or older and is sedentary, consult physician before initiating vigorous exercise program. Moderate-intensity activities (40%–60% of maximum capacity) are equivalent to a brisk walk (15–20 min/mile). Additional benefits are gained from vigorous-intensity activity (> 60% of maximum capacity) for 20–40 min on 3–5 d/wk. Recommend resistance training with 8–10 different exercises 1–2 sets per exercise, and 10–15 repetitions at moderate intensity ≥ 2 d/wk. Flexibility training and an increase in daily lifestyle activities should complement this regimen.
Weight management Goal: Achieve and maintain desirable weight (body mass index 18.5–24.9 kg/m²). When body mass index is ≥ 25 kg/m², waist circumference at iliac crest level ≤ 40 in. in men, ≤ 35 in. in women	Initiate weight-management program through caloric restriction and increased caloric expenditure as appropriate. For overweight/obese persons, reduce body weight by 10% in first year of therapy.
Diabetes management Goals: Normal fasting plasma glucose (< 110 mg/dl) and near normal HbA$_{1c}$ (< 7%)	Initiate appropriate hypoglycemic therapy to achieve near-normal fasting plasma glucose or as indicated by near-normal HbA$_{1c}$. First step is diet and exercise. Second-step therapy is usually oral hypoglycemic drugs: sulfonylureas and/or metformin with ancillary use of acarbose and thiazolidinediones. Third-step therapy is insulin. Treat other risk factors more aggressively (e.g., change BP goal to < 130/80 mm Hg and LDL-C goal to < 100 mg/dl).

BP, blood pressure; CHD, coronary heart disease; LDL-C, low-density lipoprotein cholesterol; HDL-C, high-density lipoprotein cholesterol; INR, international normalized ratio.

Reproduced with permission from Pearson TA, Blair SN, Daniels SR, et al. AHA guidelines for primary prevention of cardiovascular disease and stroke: 2002 update. Consensus panel guide to comprehensive risk reduction for adult patients without coronary or other atherosclerotic vascular diseases. *Circulation*. 2002;106:388–391.

TABLE 21-7

Secondary Prevention for Patients with Coronary and Other Vascular Disease[a] (See Chapter 59 for ACC/AHA Classification)

Goals	Intervention Recommendations and Level of Evidence
Smoking Goal Complete cessation; no exposure to environmental tobacco smoke	<ul><li>Ask about tobacco use status at every visit. I (3)</li><li>Advise every tobacco user to quit. I (B)</li><li>Assess the tobacco user's willingness to quit. I (B)</li><li>Assist by counseling and developing a plan for quitting. I (B)</li><li>Arrange follow-up, referral to special programs, or pharmacotherapy (including nicotine replacement and bupropion). I (B)</li><li>Urge avoidance of exposure to environmental tobacco smoke at work and home. I (B)</li></ul>
Blood Pressure Control Goal < 140/90 mm Hg Or < 130/80 mm Hg if patient has diabetes or chronic kidney disease	**For All Patients** <ul><li>Initiate or maintain lifestyle modification—weight control; increased physical activity; alcohol moderation; sodium reduction; and emphasis on increased consumption of fresh fruits, vegetables, and low-fat dairy products. I (B)</li></ul> **For Patients with Blood Pressure >140/90 mm Hg (or >130/80 mm Hg for Individuals with Chronic Kidney Disease or Diabetes)** <ul><li>As tolerated, add blood pressure medication, treating initially with beta-blockers and/or ACE inhibitors, with addition of other drugs such as thiazides as needed to achieve goal blood pressure. I (A)</li></ul> (For compelling indications for individual drug classes in specific vascular diseases, see Seventh Report of the Joint National Committee on Prevention, Detection, Evaluation, and Treatment of High Blood Pressure [JNC 7].)
Lipid Management Goal LDL-C < 100 mg/dl If triglycerides are ≥ 200 mg/dL, non-HDL-C should be < 130 mg/dl[b]	**For All Patients** <ul><li>Start dietary therapy. Reduce intake of saturated fats (to < 7% of total calories), *trans*-fatty acids, and cholesterol (to < 200 mg/dl). I (B)</li><li>Adding plant stanol/sterols (2 g/d) and viscous fiber (>10 g/d) will further lower LDL-C.</li><li>Promote daily physical activity and weight management. I (B)</li><li>Encourage increased consumption of omega-3 fatty acids in the form of fish[c] or in capsule form (1 g/d) for risk reduction. IIb (B)</li><li>For treatment of elevated triglycerides, higher doses are usually necessary for risk reduction.</li></ul>

247

TABLE 21-7

Secondary Prevention for Patients with Coronary and Other Vascular Disease[a] *(Continued)*

Goals	Intervention Recommendations and Level of Evidence
	For Lipid Management
	Assess fasting lipid profile in all patients, and within 24 hours of hospitalization for those with an acute cardiovascular or coronary event. For hospitalized patients, initiate lipid lowering medication as recommended below before discharge according to the following schedule:
	• LDL-C should be < 100 mg/dl **I (A)**, and
	• Further reduction of LDL-C to < 70 mg/dl is reasonable. **IIa (A)**
	• If baseline LDL-C is ≥ 100 mg/dL, initiate LDL-lowering drug therapy.[d] **I (A)**
	• If on-treatment LDL-C ≥ 100 mg/dL, intensify LDL-lowering drug therapy (may require LDL-lowering drug combination[e]). **I (A)**
	• If baseline LDL-C is 70–100 mg/dL, it is reasonable to treat to LDL-C < 70 mg/dL. **IIa (B)**
	• If triglycerides are 200–499 mg/dL, non–HDL-C should be < 130 mg/dL. **I (B)**, and
	• Further reduction of non–HDL-C to < 100 mg/dL is reasonable. **IIa (B)**
	• Therapeutic options to reduce non–HDL-C are:
	• More intense LDL-C-lowering therapy **I (B)**, or
	• Niacin[f] (after LDL-C-lowering therapy) **IIa (B)**, or
	• Fibrate therapy[g] (after LDL-C-lowering therapy) **IIa (B)**
	• If triglycerides ≥ 500 mg/dL,[g] therapeutic options to prevent pancreatitis are fibrate[f] or niacin[f] before LDL-lowering therapy; and treat LDL-C to goal after triglyceride-lowering therapy. Achieve non–HDL-C ≤ 130 mg/dL if possible. **I (C)**
Physical Activity Goal 30 minutes, 7 days per week (minimum 5 days per week)	• For all patients, assess risk with a physical activity history and/or an exercise test, to guide prescription. **I (B)**
	• For all patients, encourage 30 to 60 minutes of moderate-intensity aerobic activity, such as brisk walking, on most, preferably all, days of the week, supplemented by an increase in daily lifestyle activities (e.g., walking breaks at work, gardening, household work). **I (B)**

- Encourage resistance training 2 d/wk. IIb (C)
- Advise medically supervised programs for high-risk patients (e.g., recent acute coronary syndrome or revascularization, heart failure). I (B)
- Encourage resistance training 2 d/wk. IIb (C)
- Advise medically supervised programs for high-risk patients (e.g., recent acute coronary syndrome or revascularization, heart failure). I (B)

Weight Management Goal Body mass index: 18.5 to 24.9 kg/m^2 Waist circumference: men < 40 inches, women < 35 inches	- Assess body mass index and/or waist circumference on each visit and consistently encourage weight maintenance/reduction through an appropriate balance of physical activity, caloric intake, and formal behavioral programs when indicated to maintain/achieve a body mass index between 18.5 and 24.9 kg/m^2. I (B) - If waist circumference (measured horizontally at the iliac crest) is ≥ 35 inches in women and ≥ 40 inches in men, initiate lifestyle changes and consider treatment strategies for metabolic syndrome as indicated. I (B) - The initial goal of weight loss therapy should be to reduce body weight by approximately 10% from baseline. With success, further weight loss can be attempted if indicated through further assessment. I (B)
Diabetes Management Goal HbA$_{1c}$ < 7%	- Initiate lifestyle and pharmacotherapy to achieve near-normal HbA$_{1c}$. I (B) - Begin vigorous modification of other risk factors (e.g., physical activity, weight management, blood pressure control, and cholesterol management as recommended above). I (B) - Coordinate diabetic care with patient's primary care physician or endocrinologist. I (C)
Antiplatelet Agents/ Anticoagulants	- Start aspirin 75–162 mg/d and continue indefinitely in all patients unless contraindicated. I (A) - For patients undergoing coronary artery bypass grafting, aspirin should be started within 48 hours after surgery to reduce saphenous vein graft closure. Dosing regimens ranging from 100–325 mg/d appear to be efficacious. Doses higher than 162 mg/d can be continued for up to 1 year. I (B) - Start and continue clopidogrel 75 mg/c in combination with aspirin for up to 12 months in patients after acute coronary syndrome or percutaneous coronary intervention with stent placement (≥ 1 month for bare metal stent, ≥ 3 months for sirolimus-eluting stent, and ≥ 6 months for paclitaxel-eluting stent). I (B) - Patients who have undergone percutaneous coronary intervention with stent placement should initially receive higher-dose aspirin at 325 mg/d for 1 month for bare metal stent, 3 months for sirolimus-eluting stent, and 6 months for paclitaxel-eluting stent. I (B)

TABLE 21-7

Secondary Prevention for Patients with Coronary and Other Vascular Disease*a* (Continued)

Goals	Intervention Recommendations and Level of Evidence
	• Manage warfarin to international normalized ratio = 2.0–3.0 for paroxysmal or chronic atrial fibrillation or flutter, and in post-MI patients when clinically indicated (e.g., atrial fibrillation, left ventricular thrombus). I (A) • Use of warfarin in conjunction with aspirin and/or clopidogrel is associated with increased risk of bleeding and should be monitored closely. I (B)
Renin–Angiotensin– Aldosterone System Blockers	**ACE Inhibitors** • Start and continue indefinitely in all patients with left ventricular ejection fraction ≤40% and in those with hypertension, diabetes, or chronic kidney disease, unless contraindicated. I (A) • Consider for all other patients. I (B) • Among lower-risk patients with normal left ventricular ejection fraction in whom cardiovascular risk factors are well controlled and revascularization has been performed, use of ACE inhibitors may be considered optional. IIa (B) **Angiotensin Receptor Blockers** • Use in patients who are intolerant of ACE inhibitors and have heart failure or have had a MI with left ventricular ejection fraction ≤ 40%. I (A) • Consider in other patients who are ACE inhibitor intolerant. I (B) • Consider use in combination with ACE inhibitors in systolic-dysfunction heart failure. IIb (B) **Aldosterone Blockade** • Use in post-MI patients, without significant renal dysfunction*b* or hyperkalemia,*c* who are already receiving therapeutic doses of an ACE inhibitor and beta-blocker, have a left ventricular ejection fraction ≤ 40%, and have either diabetes or heart failure. I (A)

Beta-Blockers	• Start and continue indefinitely in all patients who have had MI, acute coronary syndrome, or left ventricular dysfunction with or without heart failure symptoms, unless contraindicated. I (A)
	• Consider chronic therapy for all other patients with coronary or other vascular disease or diabetes unless contraindicated. IIa (C)
Influenza Vaccination	• Patients with cardiovascular disease should have an influenza vaccination. I (B)

BP, blood pressure; TG, triglycerides; BMI, body mass index; HbA$_{1c}$, major fraction of adult hemoglobin; MI, myocardial infarction; CHF, congestive heart failure; ACE, angiotensin-converting enzyme.

[a]Patients covered by these guidelines include those with established coronary and other atherosclerotic vascular disease, including peripheral arterial disease, atherosclerotic aortic disease, and carotid artery disease. Treatment of patients whose only manifestation of cardiovascular risk is diabetes will be the topic of a separate AHA scientific statement.

[b]Non–HDL-C total cholesterol minus HDL-C.

[c]Pregnant and lactating women should limit their intake of fish to minimize exposure to methylmercury.

[d]When LDL-lowering medications are used, obtain at least a 30–40% reduction in LDL-C levels. If LDL-C < 70 mg/dl is the chosen target, consider drug titration to achieve this level to minimize side effects and cost. When LDL-C < 70 mg/dl is not achievable because of high baseline LDL-C levels, it generally is possible to achieve reductions > 50% in LDL-C levels by either statins or LDL-C-lowering drug combinations.

[e]Standard dose of statin with ezetimibe, bile acid sequestrant, or niacin.

[f]The combination of high-dose statin and fibrate can increase risk for severe myopathy. Statin doses should be kept relatively low with this combination. Dietary supplement niacin must not be used as a substitute for prescription niacin.

[g]Patients with very high triglycerides should not consume alcohol. The use of bile acid sequestrant is relatively contraindicated when triglycerides > 200 mg/dL

[h]Creatinine should be < 2.5 mg/dl in men and < 2.0 mg/dl in women.

[i]Potassium should be < 5.0 mEq/L.

Reproduced with permission from Smith SC, Allen J, Blair SN, et al. AHA/ACC guidelines for secondary prevention for patients with coronary and other atherosclerotic disease: 2006 update. *J Am Coll Cardiol.* 2006;47:2130–2139.

> TABLE 21-8

LDL Cholesterol Goals and Cutpoints for Initiating Therapy Classified by Risk Category

Risk Category	LDL Goal (mg/dL)	LDL Level at Which to Initiate Therapeutic Lifestyle Changes (mg/dL)	LDL Level at Which to Consider Drug Therapy (mg/dL)
CHD or CHD risk equivalents (10-year risk > 20%)	< 100	≥ 100	≥ 130 (100–129: drug optional)
2 + risk factors (10-year risk 20%)	< 130	≥ 130	10-year risk 10–20%: ≥ 130 10-year risk < 10%: ≥ 160
0–1 risk factor	< 160	≥ 160	≥ 190 (160–189: LDL-lowering drug optional)

Adapted from *Third Report of the National Cholesterol Education Program (NCEP) Expert Panel on Detection, Evaluation, and Treatment of High Blood Cholesterol in Adults (Adult Treatment Panel III). Final Report.* National Heart, Lung, and Blood Institute National Institutes of Health NIH pub. no. 02-5215 September 2002, or http://www.nhlbi.nih.gov/guidelines/cholesterol/atp3full.pdf. Accessed March 3, 2008.

Furthermore, in higher-risk patients with the metabolic syndrome, drug therapies directed toward metabolic risk factors are indicated, such as lipid-lowering drugs, antihypertensives, and low-dose aspirin. Insulin-sensitizing agents may be helpful; however, there is insufficient evidence from controlled clinical trials that they will reduce risk. See Chapter 48 for a discussion of the metabolic syndrome.

【 】 ATHEROGENIC DYSLIPIDEMIA: HYPERTRIGLYCERIDEMIA, LOW HIGH-DENSITY LIPOPROTEIN, AND SMALL, DENSE LOW-DENSITY LIPOPROTEIN

Although high LDL-C is the primary lipid risk factor, other lipid parameters increase the risk of CHD in persons with or without an elevated LDL-C. Specifically, the combination of elevated concentrations of triglycerides, small, dense LDL-C, and low levels of HDL-C is referred to as *atherogenic dyslipidemia*. This is a complex dyslipidemia that usually results from a generalized metabolic disorder related to *insulin resistance*. Patients with insulin resistance often have the metabolic syndrome. Atherogenic dyslipidemia is an increasingly common contributor to CHD because of the growing prevalence of obesity, diabetes, and the metabolic syndrome. Patients with atherogenic dyslipidemia often have concomitant abnormalities of inflammation (elevated CRP) and hypofibrinolysis (elevated plasminogen activator inhibitor-1).

The drugs that most effectively modify atherogenic dyslipidemia are fibrates and niacin. Several trials with fibrates have shown a significant reduction of major coronary events. The role of fibrates as add-on therapy to statins is being evaluated in ongoing clinical trials. The risk for severe myopathy is increased in patients treated with statins

TABLE 21-9

Drugs Used for Lipid Therapy

Drug Class	Agents and Daily Doses	Lipid/Lipoprotein Effects		Side Effects	Contraindications
Statins	Lovastatin (20–80 mg) Pravastatin (20–80 mg) Simvastatin (20–80 mg) Fluvastatin (20–80 mg) Atorvastatin (10–80 mg) Rosuvastatin (5–40 mg)	LDL-C HDL-C TG	↓18–63% ↑5–15% ↓7–30%	Myopathy Increased liver enzymes	Absolute: Active or chronic liver disease Relative: Concomitant use of certain drugs (see Table 21-10)
Cholesterol absorption inhibitors	Ezetimibe (10 mg)	LDL-C HDL-C TG	↓18% ↑1–2% ↓7–9%	Rare increase in liver enzymes	None established; statin should not be added to ezetimibe in patients with active or chronic liver disease
Bile acid sequestrants	Cholestyramine (4–16 g) Colestipol (5–20 g) Colesevelam (2.6–3.8 g)	LDL-C HDL-C TG	↓15–30% ↑3–5% No change or increase	GI distress Constipation Decreased absorption of other drugs	Absolute: Dysbetalipoproteinemia TG > 400 mg/dL Relative: TG > 200 mg/dL
Nicotinic acid	Immediate-release nicotinic acid (1.5–3 g), extended release nicotinic acid (1–2 g), sustained-release nicotinic acid (1–2 g)	LDL-C HDL-C TG	↓5–25% ↑15–35% ↓20–50%	Flushing Hyperglycemia Hyperuricemia (or gout) Upper GI distress Hepatotoxicity	Absolute: Chronic liver disease Severe gout Relative: Diabetes Hyperuricemia Peptic ulcer disease

253

TABLE 21-9

Drugs Used for Lipid Therapy (Continued)

Drug Class	Agents and Daily Doses	Lipid/Lipoprotein Effects		Side Effects	Contraindications
Fibric acids	Gemfibrozil (600 mg bid) Fenofibrate (160 mg)	LDL-C (may increase in patients with high TG)	↓5–20%	Dyspepsia Gallstones Myopathy	Absolute: Severe renal disease Severe hepatic disease
		HDL-C TG	↑10–20% ↓20–50%		

^aLDL reduction is as great as 25% when combined with a statin.

Adapted from *Third Report of the National Cholesterol Education Program (NCEP) Expert Panel on Detection, Evaluation, and Treatment of High Blood Cholesterol in Adults (Adult Treatment Panel III). Final Report.* National Heart, Lung, and Blood Institute National Institutes of Health NIH pub. no. 02-5215 September 2002, or http://www.nhlbi.nih.gov/guidelines/cholesterol/atp3full.pdf. Accessed March 3, 2008.

TABLE 21-10

Risk Factors for Severe Myopathy from Statin Therapy

- Age > 80 y
- Small body frame and frailty
- Multisystem disease (e.g., chronic renal insufficiency, especially as a result of diabetes)
- Multiple medications
- Specific concomitant medications or consumptions (with various statins, check package insert for warnings)
  - Fibrates (especially gemfibrozil, but other fibrates too)
  - Nicotinic acid (rarely)
  - Cyclosporine
  - Azole antifungals
  - Itraconazole and ketoconazole
  - Macrolide antibiotics
  - Erythromycin and clarithromycin
  - HIV protease inhibitors
  - Nefazodone (antidepressant)
  - Verapamil
  - Large quantities of grapefruit juice (>1 quart per day)
  - Alcohol abuse (independently predisposes to myopathy)
- Perioperative periods[a]
- Acute illnesses[a].

[a]In most patients admitted to the hospital for acute illnesses or surgery, statin therapy should be temporarily discontinued.

Adapted with permission from Pasternak RC, Smith SC Jr, Bairey-Merz CN, et al. ACC/AHA/NHLBI clinical advisory on the use and safety of statins. *Circulation.* 2002;106;1024–1028.

and fibrates, hence it is prudent to limit the use of a statin and fibrate combination to higher-risk patients. Niacin lowers the concentration of triglycerides and small, dense LDL particles, and raises HDL-C. Niacin has more side effects than fibrates. Omega-3 fatty acids (fish oil) in doses of 2 to 4 g are effective in reducing triglycerides by 20% to 30% associated with small increases in HDL-C and LDL-C. Novel therapies for raising HDL-C are under development. Pharmacologic inhibition of cholesteryl ester transfer protein is capable of raising HDL-C by 50% to 100%; however, their efficacy in decreasing CHD outcomes has recently come into question.

【 】 CIGARETTE SMOKING

Patients and their family members may be especially receptive to a smoking cessation intervention after an acute event (i.e., a teachable moment). The goal is *complete cessation and no exposure to environmental tobacco smoke.*

Intervention for smoking cessation includes asking about tobacco use status at every visit; advising to quit smoking; assessing willingness to quit; assisting by counseling and developing a plan to quit; and arranging follow-up, referral to special programs, or pharmacotherapy (nicotine replacement, buproprion, or varenicline). Even brief interventions may be effective and should, at a minimum, be provided to every patient who uses tobacco (Table 21-11). In primary prevention of CHD events, *a previous smoker's relative risk declines nearly to that of a nonsmoker in a year or less.* In patients with CHD,

TABLE 21-11

Strategies for Successful Cessation of Cigarette Smoking: The Five A's

Ask	Systematically identify all tobacco users at every visit (e.g., include tobacco as a vital sign).
	Determine exposure to environmental tobacco smoke at home or at work.
Advise	Provide a clear, strong, and personalized message, urging every tobacco user to quit.
	Review benefits of quitting and risk of continuing.
Assess	Assess patient's willingness to quit at each visit.
Assist	Have the patient develop a quit plan, including setting a quit date, identifying sources of support for cessation for family and friends, removing tobacco and other cues from the home and work environment.
	Provide counseling, information materials, and other behavioral interventions.
	Recommend use of pharmacotherapy, including varenicline, bupropion SR, nicotine gum, nicotine inhaler, nicotine nasal spray, or nicotine patch.
Arrange	Provide a reminder on the quit date.
	See the patient shortly after the quit date to assess success.
	If unsuccessful, identify barriers and solutions to their removal.

Adapted from Fiore MC. *Treating Tobacco Use and Dependence.* Rockville, MD: U.S. Department of Health and Human Services, Public Health Service; 2000; or http://www.ncbi.nlm.nih.gov/books/bv.fcgi?rid=hstat2.section.7741. Accessed March 18, 2008.

achieving complete abstinence from smoking compares favorably with the health benefits of any intervention in modern cardiology.

[ ] HYPERTENSION

Normal blood pressure is < 120/80 mm Hg. The Joint National Committee (JNC) on Detection, Evaluation, and Treatment of High Blood Pressure recommends a treatment goal of < 140/90 mm Hg. Lower goals are recommended for patients with renal insufficiency, heart failure, or diabetes (Tables 21-6 and 21-7). The reader is referred to Chapter 29 for a discussion of the treatment of hypertension.

[ ] DIABETES

Diabetes mellitus is an independent risk factor for CHD, increasing risk for type 1 as well as type 2 patients by two to four times. At least 65% of people with diabetes die from cardiovascular disease. Approximately 25% of MI survivors have diabetes. *Diabetic patients without a history of MI have as high a risk of coronary mortality as do nondiabetic patients with a history of MI.* Once patients with type 2 diabetes suffer an MI, their prognosis for recurrent MI and survival is much worse than that for CHD patients without diabetes. See Chapter 49 for a complete discussion of diabetes and CHD.

Diabetes abolishes the usual protection from CHD afforded a premenopausal woman. Diabetic women have twice the risk of recurrent MI compared with diabetic men.

Weight loss and exercise are key lifestyle modifications because they improve the constellation of metabolic abnormalities that accompany diabetes. Although the optimal proportion of dietary fat and carbohydrate is controversial, calorie restriction for obesity and avoidance of sugar and saturated fat are recommended. *Beta-blockers should not be withheld from diabetic patients following MI unless strong contraindications exist, because diabetic MI survivors have fewer deaths if treated with beta-blockers. Although there is no consistent evidence to support intensive glycemic control as a strategy to reduce macrovascular complications, aggressive lipid and blood pressure management in patients with diabetes lowers CHD risk.* Hemoglobin A_{1C} of < 7% is the treatment goal for patients with diabetes.

【 】 PHYSICAL INACTIVITY

Physical inactivity is an independent risk factor for CHD and roughly doubles the risk. There is an inverse dose-response relation between the amount of exercise performed weekly, from 700 to 2000 kcal of energy, and death from cardiovascular disease and all causes. Walking 1 mile burns approximately 100 kcal. For primary and secondary prevention, 30 minutes or more of moderate-intensity physical activity on most, and preferably all, days is recommended. Only about 20% of U.S. adults meet this goal. Exercise testing should be recommended to apparently healthy men over 45 and women over 55 who are sedentary, as well as to younger adults with coronary risk factors, before starting a *vigorous* physical activity program (intensity > 60% individual maximum oxygen consumption). For secondary prevention, exercise testing is recommended to guide exercise prescription, and high-risk patients should exercise in a medically supervised setting.

【 】 OBESITY

Body mass index (BMI) should be calculated for all patients, and waist circumference measured in patients with a BMI ≥ 25. *Overweight* is defined as a BMI of 25 to 29.9, and *obesity* as BMI ≥ 30. In adults with BMI ≥ 25, increased relative risk is indicated with a waist circumference >102 cm (> 40 in) in men and > 88 cm (> 35 in) in women. See Chapter 53 for a discussion on obesity.

Treatment should focus on diet and exercise to prevent weight gain and to produce moderate weight loss over years. Lost weight is usually regained unless a program consisting of dietary therapy, physical activity, and behavior therapy is continued indefinitely. There is no effective pharmacologic therapy for long-term weight loss.

RISK FACTORS FOR WHICH INTERVENTIONS HAVE NOT BEEN SHOWN TO LOWER RISK OF CORONARY HEART DISEASE

【 】 LIPOPROTEIN(A)

Several retrospective case-control studies support the view that lipoprotein(a), or Lp(a), is an independent risk factor for thromboembolic disease. However, results of the major prospective studies evaluating baseline Lp(a) concentration and future risks of MI and stroke are inconsistent. It is unclear whether Lp(a) provides information incremental to the conventional lipid profile, and no recommendation for screening can be made. If elevated levels prove to increase risk among hypercholesterolemic individuals, it may be prudent to lower levels of LDL-C even more aggressively in such individuals than the current guidelines dictate. Knowledge of Lp(a) levels may also be useful in the selection of agents to lower LDL-C (e.g., niacin) and may identify a possible treatable cause in the occasional patient with CHD and none of the major risk factors.

【　】 HYPERHOMOCYSTEINEMIA

Hyperhomocysteinemia is an independent marker for cardiovascular disease in several groups of high-risk subjects. Hyperhomocysteinemia may be classified as moderate (16–30 µmol/L), intermediate (31–100 µmol/L), or severe (> 100 µmol/L). The most important factor affecting plasma concentration is dietary intake of folate and vitamins B_6 and B_{12}. Lowering homocysteine has not been shown to be effective in reducing CHD risk; therefore its routine measurement and treatment is not recommended.

【　】 OXIDATIVE STRESS

Evidence from randomized controlled trials indicates that supplementation with beta-carotene, vitamin C, and vitamin E offers no benefit for CHD prevention. Observational evidence supports the consumption of diets rich in fruits and vegetables.

UNMODIFIABLE RISK FACTORS

【　】 AGE AND SEX AS RISK FACTORS FOR ATHEROSCLEROTIC DISEASE

The incidence and prevalence of CHD increase sharply with age, so that age might be considered one of the most potent cardiovascular risk factors. CHD incidence rates in men are similar to those in women 10 years older. Persons at an advanced age (e.g., 75+ years) should have the risks and benefits of preventive cardiology interventions weighed on an individual basis, but typically derive the greatest benefit because they have the highest risk.

【　】 POSTMENOPAUSAL STATUS

Postmenopausal women with or without CHD who have not been on estrogen replacement therapy should not be started on hormonal therapy for the purpose of primary or secondary prevention. The decision to continue or discontinue hormone therapy should be based on established noncardiovascular benefits and risks, and on patient preference. In chronic users of hormone therapy, medication should be discontinued, at least temporarily, if a woman develops an acute coronary syndrome or is immobilized. Oral estrogen therapy is contraindicated in women with moderately severe hypertriglyceridemia (e.g., serum triglycerides > 400 mg/dL), but in such women transdermal estrogen might be an appropriate substitute for noncardiovascular indications.

【　】 FAMILY HISTORY OF EARLY-ONSET CHD

More than 35 case-control and prospective studies have consistently identified an association between CHD and a history of first-degree relatives with early onset CHD. Although CHD in a male relative with onset at age 55 years or less, or in a female relative with onset at age 65 years or less, is defined as a positive family history, the larger the number of relatives with early-onset CHD or the younger the age of CHD onset in the relative, the stronger is the predictive value. *Although considered a nonmodifiable risk factor, a positive family history should result in the careful screening of individual risk factors known to aggregate in families. Such familial aggregations may represent monogenic factors with known phenotypic expressions and inheritance patterns, polygenic factors with less clear modes of expression and inheritance, or shared environments.* Thus, family members of patients with CHD at a younger age represent fruitful targets for risk factor assessment. *Risk factor screening should extend to the siblings and children of early-CHD patients.*

OTHER PHARMACOLOGIC THERAPY

【 】 ANTIPLATELET AND ANTICOAGULANT THERAPY

Low-dose aspirin, 75 to 160 mg/d, is recommended for primary and secondary prevention among individuals with a 10-year risk of CHD ≥10%. Treatment should be continued indefinitely. If aspirin is contraindicated in a CHD patient, clopidogrel 75 mg daily is recommended. If neither antiplatelet agent can be taken, warfarin (international normalized ratio [INR] goal of 2.0–3.0) is recommended for secondary prevention.

【 】 BETA-BLOCKERS

For primary prevention, beta-blockers are recommended as first-line therapy for hypertension. For secondary prevention, beta-blockers are recommended for all patients who have had MI, an acute coronary syndrome, or left ventricular dysfunction with or without heart failure symptoms, and continued indefinitely unless contraindicated. Beta-blockers should be considered as chronic therapy for all patients with CHD, other vascular disease, or diabetes unless contraindicated.

【 】 RENIN–ANGIOTENSIN–ALDOSTERONE SYSTEM BLOCKERS

Angiotensin-converting enzyme (ACE) inhibitors are at least as effective as diuretics in the primary prevention of CHD death or nonfatal MI, although national guidelines continue to recommend diuretics as first-line agents for the treatment of hypertension. ACE inhibitors are appropriate first-line antihypertensive therapy in patients with diabetes, and they are an excellent second step after diuretic therapy in most hypertensive patients. For secondary prevention, ACE inhibitors should be prescribed indefinitely to all patients following MI and to patients with clinical evidence of congestive heart failure. ACE inhibitors should be considered as chronic therapy for all other patients with coronary or other atherosclerotic vascular disease.

Angiotensin-receptor blockers (ARBs) should be prescribed for patients who are intolerant of ACE inhibitors and have heart failure or have had an MI with left ventricular ejection fraction ≤ 40%. ARBs should be considered in other patients with CHD or other atherosclerotic disease who are ACE inhibitor intolerant.

THE PRACTICE OF PREVENTIVE CARDIOLOGY

【 】 IMPLEMENTATION OF PREVENTIVE CARDIOLOGY SERVICES

Improved application of proven interventions for prevention requires a variety of strategies targeted to patients, health care providers, inpatient care settings, ambulatory care settings, and health systems. *Professional societies strongly recommend that risk-factor management be part of the optimal care of patients at high risk for cardiovascular disease, and therefore the responsibility of all health care providers.*

SUGGESTED READING

Maron DJ, Grundy SM, Ridker PM, et al. Preventive strategies for coronary heart disease. In: Fuster V, O'Rourke R, Alexander RW, et al., eds. *Hurst's The Heart*. 12th ed. New York, NY: McGraw-Hill; 2007:1204–1227.

Pearson TA, Blair SN, Daniels SR, et al. AHA guidelines for primary prevention of cardiovascular disease and stroke: 2002 update. Consensus panel guide to comprehensive risk reduction for adult patients without coronary or other atherosclerotic vascular diseases. *Circulation.* 2002;106:388–391.

Smith SC, Allen J, Blair SN, et al. AHA/ACC guidelines for secondary prevention for patients with coronary and other atherosclerotic disease: 2006 update. Endorsed by the National Heart, Lung, and Blood Institute. *J Am Coll Cardiol.* 2006;47: 2130–2139.

Third Report of the National Cholesterol Education Program (NCEP) Expert Panel on Detection, Evaluation, and Treatment of High Blood Cholesterol in Adults (Adult Treatment Panel III). Final Report. National Heart, Lung, and Blood Institute National Institutes of Health NIH pub. no. 02-5215 September 2002, or http://www.nhlbi.nih.gov/guidelines/cholesterol/atp3full.pdf. Accessed March 3, 2008.

CHAPTER 22

Management of Patients with Chronic Ischemic Heart Disease

Robert A. O'Rourke

Chronic stable angina is the first presentation of ischemic heart disease in about 50% of patients. The number of patients with stable angina in the United States approximates 17 million people, excluding patients who do not seek medical attention for their chest pain or who are shown to have a noncardiac cause of chest discomfort. Angina pectoris is a clinical syndrome that consists of recurrent discomfort or pain in the chest, jaw, shoulder, back, or arm associated with myocardial ischemia, but without myocardial necrosis. It is typically precipitated or aggravated by exertion or emotional stress and relieved by nitroglycerin. Angina usually occurs in patients with coronary artery disease (CAD) affecting one or more large epicardial arteries. However, angina often is present in individuals with valvular heart disease, hypertrophic cardiomyopathy, and uncontrolled hypertension. It also occurs in patients with normal coronary arteries and myocardial ischemia due to coronary artery spasm or endothelial dysfunction. The symptom of "angina" is often observed in patients with noncardiac disorders affecting the esophagus, chest wall, or lungs.

ETIOLOGY

Coronary atherosclerosis is the cause of angina pectoris in most patients. Other causes include congenital artery abnormalities, coronary artery spasm, coronary thromboembolism, coronary vasculitis, aortic stenosis, mitral stenosis with resulting severe right ventricular hypertension, severe pulmonary hypertension, pulmonic stenosis, hypertrophic cardiomyopathy, and systemic arterial hypertension. Disorders in which angina occurs less frequently include aortic regurgitation, idiopathic dilated cardiomyopathy, and syphilitic heart disease. Mitral valve prolapse rarely causes true angina pectoris. Certain conditions may alter the balance between myocardial oxygen supply and demand and precipitate or aggravate angina pectoris, including severe anemia, tachycardia, fever, and hyperthyroidism.

CLASSIFICATION

The Canadian Cardiovascular Society Grading Scale (Table 22-1) is commonly used to classify the severity of angina pectoris, with the most severe symptoms occurring at rest and the least severe only with excessive exercise.

TABLE 22-1

Canadian Cardiovascular Society Functional Classification of Angina Pectoris[a]

I.   Ordinary physical activity, such as walking and climbing stairs, does not cause angina. Angina results from strenuous or rapid or prolonged exertion at work or recreation.
II. Slight limitation of ordinary activity. Walking or climbing stairs rapidly, walking uphill, walking or stair climbing when under emotional stress. Walking more than two blocks on level ground and climbing more than one flight of ordinary stairs at a normal pace.
III. Marked limitation of ordinary physical activity. Walking one to two blocks on level ground and climbing more than one flight of stairs under normal conditions.
IV. Inability to carry on any physical activity without discomfort—anginal symptoms may be present at rest.

[a]See also Chapter 1.

Modified with permission from Campeau L. Letter: Grading of angina pectoris. Circulation. Sep 1, 1976;54(3):522–523.

DIAGNOSIS OF ANGINA PECTORIS

HISTORY AND PHYSICAL EXAMINATION

After a description of the chest discomfort is obtained, the physician makes an integrated assessment of the location, quality, and duration of discomfort; inciting factors; and factors relieving the pain. The most commonly used classification scheme for chest pain divides patients into three groups: *typical angina, atypical angina,* and *noncardiac chest pain* (Table 22-2). Angina is further labeled as *stable* when its characteristics have been unchanged over the preceding 60 days. The presence of unstable angina predicts a much higher short-term risk of an acute coronary event. *Unstable angina* is defined as angina that presents in one of three major ways: rest angina, severe new-onset angina, or prior angina increasing in severity (see Chapter 23).

Usually, the discomfort of chronic stable angina pectoris is precipitated by physical activity, emotions, eating, or cold weather. Certain patients are able to describe accurately the extent and type of exercise at which they reproducibly experience their chest pain. Emotions—particularly anger, excitement, and frustration—often precipitate angina in patients with coronary CAD. Cigarette smoking induces chest discomfort or lowers the exertion threshold for angina in some patients. In most patients, anginal discomfort has a characteristic crescendo nature. It develops and increases to a plateau over 10 to 30 seconds and disappears within minutes if the exertion is discontinued. The discomfort usually lasts only a few minutes, occasionally 10 to 15 minutes. Very rarely, it may last up to 30 minutes. The discomfort of angina is most often located substernally or just to the left of the sternum. In describing the discomfort, some patients clench their fists over their upper sternum (Levine's sign), a sign of high diagnostic accuracy. Radiation of the pain down the left arm or to the neck or jaw is common. The pain often radiates down the arms or to the neck, jaw, teeth, shoulders, or back. In addition to exertion, drugs that increase heart rate and blood pressure can precipitate angina, as can cocaine.

Patients with stable angina may have many asymptomatic or silent episodes of myocardial ischemia. Also, myocardial ischemia may result in symptoms from either systolic or diastolic left ventricular (LV) dysfunction without the characteristic chest discomfort. Exertional dyspnea and fatigue are two common manifestations equivalent to angina that are usually also relieved with rest and nitroglycerin.

TABLE 22-2

Clinical Classification of Angina

Typical angina (definite)
(1) Substernal chest discomfort with a characteristic quality and duration that is
    (2) provoked by exertion or emotional stress and (3) relieved by rest or NTG.
Atypical angina (probable)
    Meets two of the above characteristics.
Noncardiac chest pain
    Meets one or none of the typical anginal characteristics.

Data complied from Diamond GA, Staniloff HM, Forrester JS, et al. Computer-assisted diagnosis in the noninvasive evaluation of patients with suspected coronary disease. *J Am Coll Cardiol.* 1983;1:444–455.

During an anginal attack, many patients appear pale and quiet. Diaphoresis and alterations in blood pressure and heart rate are common. A fourth (most common) or third heart sound, mitral regurgitant systolic murmur, bibasilar pulmonary rates, or palpable systolic impulse at the apex may be present. Evidence of noncoronary atherosclerotic disease such as a carotid bruit, diminished pedal pulse, or abdominal aneurysm increases the likelihood of CAD.

【 】 CLINICAL EVALUATION OF THE LIKELIHOOD OF CORONARY ARTERY DISEASE

Clinicopathologic studies have demonstrated that it is possible to predict the probability of CAD on the basis of the history and the physical examination. The most powerful predictors of the probability of CAD are pain type, age, and sex (Table 22-3).

 TABLE 22-3

Pretest Likelihood of Cad in Symptomatic Patients According to Age and Sex[a]

Age (years)	Nonanginal Chest Pain		Atypical Angina		Typical Angina	
	Men	Women	Men	Women	Men	Women
30–39	4	2	34	12	76	26
40–49	13	3	51	22	87	55
50–59	20	7	65	31	93	73
60–69	27	14	72	51	94	86

[a]Each value represents the percent with significant CAD on catheterization.

Reproduced with permission from Gibbons RJ, Balady GJ, Beasley JW, et al. ACC/AHA Guidelines for Exercise Testing. A report of the American College of Cardiology/American Heart Association Task Force on Practice Guidelines (Committee on Exercise Testing). *J Am Coll Cardiol.* 1997;30(1):260–311.

TABLE 22-4

Invasive Testing—Coronary Angiography Recommendations for Coronary Angiography to Establish a Diagnosis in Patients with Suspected Angina, Including Those with Known CAD Who have a Significant Change in Anginal Symptoms

Class I[a]

1. Patients with known or possible angina pectoris who have survived sudden cardiac death.

Class IIa[b]

1. Patients with an uncertain diagnosis after noninvasive testing in whom the benefit of a more certain diagnosis outweighs the risk and cost of coronary angiography.
2. Patients who cannot undergo noninvasive testing due to disability, illness, or morbid obesity.
3. Patients with an occupational requirement for a definitive diagnosis.
4. Patients who by virtue of young age at onset of symptoms, noninvasive imaging, or other clinical parameters are suspected of having a nonatherosclerotic cause of myocardial ischemia (coronary artery anomaly, Kawasaki disease, primary coronary artery dissection, radiation-induced vasculoplasty).
5. Patients in whom coronary artery spasm is suspected and provocative testing may be necessary.
6. Patients with a high pretest probability of left main or three-vessel CAD.

Class IIb

1. Patients with recurrent hospitalization for chest pain in whom a definite diagnosis is judged necessary.
2. Patients with an overriding desire for a definitive diagnosis and a greater than low probability of CAD.

Class III[c]

1. Patients with significant comorbidity in whom the risk of coronary arteriography outweighs the benefits of the procedure.
2. Patients with an overriding personal desire for a definitive diagnosis and a low probability of CAD.

[a]*Class I:* Conditions for which there is evidence and/or general agreement that a given procedure or treatment is useful and effective.

[b]*Class II:* Conditions for which there is conflicting evidence and/or a divergence of opinion about the usefulness/efficacy of a procedure or treatment.

IIa: Weight of evidence/opinion is in favor of usefulness/efficacy.

IIb: Usefulness/efficacy is less well established by evidence/opinion.

[c]*Class III:* Conditions for which there is evidence and/or general agreement that the procedure/treatment is not useful and in some cases may be harmful.

Data compiled from Gibbons RJ, Abrams J, Chatterjee K, et al., Guidelines for the management of patients with chronic stable angina: a report of the ACC/AHA Task Force on Practice Guidelines. *J Am Coll Cardiol.* 2007;50(23):2264–2274.

[ ] DIAGNOSTIC TESTS

For further information on diagnostic tests, see Chapter 4.

Electrocardiogram and Chest Roentgenogram

A resting 12-lead electrocardiogram (ECG) should be recorded in all patients with symptoms suggestive of angina; however, it will be normal in 50% of patients with chronic angina. Evidence of prior Q-wave myocardial infarction (MI) on the ECG makes CAD very likely. Patients with a completely normal resting ECG *rarely have significant LV systolic dysfunction.* An ECG obtained during chest pain is abnormal in about 50% of patients with angina and a normal resting ECG. ST-segment elevation or depression establishes a high likelihood of angina and indicates ischemia at a low workload, suggesting an unfavorable prognosis. The chest roentgenogram is often normal in patients with stable angina pectoris and is more useful in diagnosing noncardiac causes of chest pain.

Electrocardiographic Exercise Stress Testing

The ECG exercise stress test is the test that is most frequently used to obtain objective evidence of myocardial ischemia as well as prognostic information in patients with known CAD (see also Chapter 4). Although wide variations are seen, the mean sensitivity is 68% and the mean specificity about 77%. The modest sensitivity of the exercise ECG is generally lower than that of imaging procedures. The diagnostic value of the test is significantly decreased by the presence of abnormalities such as bundle-branch block, ST-T-wave changes, or left ventricular hypertrophy (LVH) on the resting ECG. Diagnostic testing is most valuable when the pretest probability of obstructive CAD is intermediate. In these conditions, the test result has the largest effect on the posttest probability of disease and thus on clinical decisions.

Rest Echocardiography

Assessment of global systolic function and the presence of regional systolic wall-motion abnormalities may help establish the diagnosis of chronic ischemic heart disease. The extent and severity of regional and global abnormalities are important considerations in choosing appropriate medical or surgical therapy. However, most patients undergoing a diagnostic evaluation for angina do not need a resting echocardiogram.

Myocardial Perfusion Imaging

Patients who should undergo cardiac stress testing with imaging, as opposed to exercise ECG alone, for the diagnosis of CAD include those in the following categories: (1) complete left bundle-branch block (LBBB), electronically paced ventricular rhythm, and preexcitation syndromes; (2) patients who have >1 mm of resting ST-segment depression, including those with LVH or who are taking drugs such as digitalis; (3) patients who are unable to exercise to a level high enough to give meaningful results on routine stress ECG (pharmacologic stress imaging should be considered); and (4) patients with angina who have undergone prior revascularization, in whom localization of ischemia, establishing the functional significance of lesions, and demonstrating myocardial viability are important considerations. Several methods can be used to induce stress, including (1) exercise (treadmill or bicycle) and (2) pharmacologic techniques (dipyridamole, adenosine, or dobutamine). When the patient can exercise to an appropriate level of cardiovascular stress for 6 to 12 minutes, exercise stress testing generally is preferred to pharmacologic stress. Myocardial perfusion imaging (MPI) is more expensive than exercise ECG testing, but it provides higher sensitivity and specificity. MPI plays a major role in risk stratification of patients with CAD. A normal perfusion scan in patients with CAD indicates a rate of cardiac death and MI of 0.9%

per year, nearly as low as that of the general population. Incremental prognostic information will be gained from the number, size, and location of perfusion defects in combination with the amount of thallium 201 lung uptake on poststress images (see also Chapter 4).

Stress Echocardiography

Stress echocardiography relies on imaging LV segmental wall motion and thickening during stress compared with baseline. It has a reported sensitivity and specificity similar to those of MPI (see also Chapter 4). If a patient is unable to exercise, pharmacologic stress is achieved most commonly by using dobutamine. To help enhance endocardial border definition, intravenous (IV) contrast agents are frequently used. The choice of stress echocardiography or MPI depends on the available facilities, local expertise, and considerations of cost-effectiveness.

Coronary Angiography

Coronary angiography (also discussed in Chapter 7) is considered the "gold standard" for the diagnosis of CAD, although it is invasive and moderately expensive. Direct referral for diagnostic coronary angiography in patients with chest pain possibly due to myocardial ischemia is appropriate when noninvasive tests are contraindicated or likely to be inadequate. Patients with noninvasive tests that are abnormal but not clearly diagnostic often require clarification of an uncertain diagnosis by coronary angiography. In certain cases a second noninvasive test (imaging modality) may be recommended for a patient with a low likelihood of CAD but an intermediate-risk exercise treadmill result. Coronary angiography is likely to be most appropriate for patients with typical anginal symptoms and a high clinical probability of severe CAD or for individuals with *high-risk noninvasive tests*. In diabetic patients, the diagnosis of chronic stable angina can be particularly difficult because of the absence of characteristic symptoms of myocardial ischemia as a result of autonomic and sensory neuropathy. Thus, a lower threshold for coronary angiography is appropriate. The American College of Cardiology/American Heart Association (ACC/AHA) recommendations concerning the value of coronary angiography are listed in Table 22-4. Coronary luminal contrast angiography may underestimate coronary artery stenosis because of coronary artery remodeling in areas of atheroma, which demonstrate much more disease by intravascular ultrasound.

Electron beam computed tomography (EBCT) is being used with increasing frequency. However, the specificity of a positive result may be as low as 49%, and the predictive accuracy is less than 70%. The role of EBCT in CAD diagnosis and risk stratification has been controversial. A consensus report of an ACC/AHA expert consensus writing group does not recommend EBCT for routine screening of asymptomatic patients for CAD or its use in most patients with chest pain. (However, EBCT scores that are greatly increased [> 400 units] will likely lead to a very aggressive approach in patients at intermediate risk.) See also Chapter 59.

【 】 DIFFERENTIAL DIAGNOSIS

Table 22-5 lists the differential diagnosis of angina pectoris. Usually the distinction is clear if an accurate history is obtained and a complete physical examination is properly performed.

【 】 PATHOPHYSIOLOGY

A disparity between the supply of coronary blood flow (CBF) and the metabolic demands of the myocardium (MVO_2) is the primary factor in ischemic heart disease. This imbalance may result in clinical manifestations of ischemia when myocardial demand exceeds the capacity of the coronary arteries to deliver an adequate supply of

TABLE 22-5

Differential Diagnosis of Chest Pain

1. Angina pectoris/myocardial infarction
2. Other cardiovascular causes
   a. Likely ischemic in origin
      (1) Aortic stenosis
      (2) Hypertrophic cardiomyopathy
      (3) Severe systemic hypertension
      (4) Severe right ventricular hypertension
      (5) Aortic regurgitation
      (6) Severe anemia/hypoxia
   b. Nonischemic in origin
      (1) Aortic dissection
      (2) Pericarditis
      (3) Mitral valve prolapse
3. Gastrointestinal
   a. Esophageal spasm
   b. Esophageal reflux
   c. Esophageal rupture
   d. Peptic ulcer disease
4. Psychogenic
   a. Anxiety
   b. Depression
   c. Cardiac psychosis
   d. Self-gain
5. Neuromusculoskeletal
   a. Thoracic outlet syndrome
   b. Degenerative joint disease of cervical/thoracic spine
   c. Costochondritis (Tietze's syndrome)
   d. Herpes zoster
   e. Chest wall pain and tenderness
6. Pulmonary
   a. Pulmonary embolus with or without pulmonary infarction
   b. Pneumothorax
   c. Pneumonia with pleural involvement
7. Pleurisy

oxygen. In normal hearts there is an excess CBF reserve, so that ischemia does not occur even with very vigorous exercise. Atherosclerosis in the epicardial coronary arteries or in the coronary microvasculature may cause an imbalance between supply and demand at even modest levels of exercise. Heart rate, myocardial contractility, and systolic wall tension—which is related to LV systolic pressure and volume—are the major determinants of myocardial oxygen demand. Oxygen supply to the myocardium is dependent upon the oxygen-carrying capacity of blood and the CBF. Narrowing of the large coronary arteries transiently by vasospasm or permanently by obstructive lesions may increase the coronary resistance sufficiently to reduce CBF. Patients with coronary atherosclerosis also have endothelial dysfunction, which may manifest itself by a failure of the coronary vasculature to dilate in response to normal vasodilatory stimuli such as increased flow, exercise, tachycardia, acetylcholine, or cold pressor testing. Most patients with angina pectoris due to coronary atherosclerosis have *myocardial ischemia caused by both epicardial coronary obstruction and endothelial dysfunction* of both large and small vessels.

【 】 CIRCADIAN RHYTHM OF MYOCARDIAL ISCHEMIA

The prevalence of MI, unstable angina, variant angina, and silent ischemia is greatest in the morning, during the first few hours after awakening; the threshold for precipitating anginal attacks in patients with stable angina also appears to be lowest in the morning. The diurnal variation in ischemic threshold is attributed to the endogenous rhythms of catecholamine secretion and to the sensitivity to coronary vasoconstrictors, both of which appear to be highest in the morning. The increase in sympathetic nervous system activity is associated with increases in heart rate, blood pressure, contractility, and MVO_2. The lowered morning anginal threshold and the higher morning systolic blood pressure mandate early-morning use of antianginal and antihypertensive medications.

RISK STRATIFICATION OF PATIENTS WITH CHRONIC ISCHEMIC HEART DISEASE

The prognosis for the patient with chronic artery disease is usually related to four patient factors. First, LV performance is the strongest predictor of long-term survival in patients with CAD, and the ejection fraction (EF) is the most often used measure of the presence and the degree of LV dysfunction. The second predictive factor is the anatomic extent and severity of atherosclerotic involvement of the coronary arteries. The number of stenosed coronary arteries is the most common measure of this factor. The third patient factor affecting prognosis is evidence of a recent coronary plaque rupture, indicating a much higher short-term risk for cardiac death or nonfatal MI. Worsening clinical symptoms with unstable features is an important clinical marker of a complicated plaque. The fourth prognostic factor is the patient's general health and noncoronary comorbidity. Risk stratification of patients with chronic stable angina by stress testing with exercise or pharmacologic agents has been shown to permit identification of groups of patients with low, intermediate, or high risk for subsequent cardiac events. Noninvasive test findings that identify high-risk patients are listed in Table 22-6. Patients identified as high risk are generally referred for coronary arteriography independent of their symptomatic status. The ACC/AHA Guidelines for Risk Stratification using Coronary Angiography in Patients with Stable Angina are listed in Table 22-7.

TREATMENT OF CHRONIC STABLE ANGINA

There are two major purposes in the treatment of stable angina. The first is to prevent MI and death and thereby *increase the quantity of life*. The second is to reduce symptoms of angina and the frequency and severity of ischemia, which should *improve the quality of life*. The choice of therapy often depends on the clinical response to initial medical therapy, although some patients (and many physicians) prefer coronary revascularization in situations where either may be successful. Patient education, cost-effectiveness, and patient preference are important components in this decision-making process.

【 】 GENERAL

Patients with angina pectoris due to coronary atherosclerosis should be evaluated for risk factors for coronary disease; whenever possible, these risk factors should be corrected. Tobacco in all forms should be avoided. Hypertension and diabetes should be well controlled. Ideal body weight should be achieved. A low-fat, low-cholesterol diet should be instituted, and a lipid profile determined.

TABLE 22-6

Noninvasive Risk Stratification

High risk (greater than 3% annual mortality rate)

1. Severe resting left ventricular dysfunction (LVEF < 35%).
2. High-risk treadmill score (score ≤ 11).[a]
3. Severe exercise left ventricular dysfunction (exercise LVEF < 35%).
4. Stress-induced large perfusion defects (particularly if anterior).
5. Stress-induced multiple perfusion defects of moderate size.
6. Large, fixed perfusion defect with LV dilation or increased lung uptake (thallium 201).
7. Stress-induced moderate perfusion defect with LV dilation or increased lung uptake (thallium 201).
8. Echocardiographic wall-motion abnormality (involving more than two segments) developing at low dose of dobutamine (≤ 10 mg/kg/min) or at a low heart rate (< 120 beats per minute).
9. Stress echocardiographic evidence of extensive ischemia.

Intermediate risk (1–3% annual mortality rate)

1. Mild/moderate resting left ventricular dysfunction (LVEF = 35–49%).
2. Intermediate-risk treadmill score (−11 < score < 5).
3. Stress-induced moderate perfusion defect without LV dilation or increased lung intake (thallium 201).
4. Limited stress echocardiographic ischemia with a wall motion abnormality only at higher doses of dobutamine involving less than or equal to two segments.

Low risk (less than 1% annual mortality rate)

1. Low-risk treadmill score (score ≥ 5).
2. Normal or small myocardial perfusion defect at rest or with stress.
3. Normal stress echocardiographic wall motion or no change of limited resting wall-motion abnormalities during stress.

---

[a]Duke Treadmill Score.
Data compiled from Gibbons RJ, Abrams J, Chatterjee K, et al., Guidelines for the management of patients with chronic stable angina: a report of the ACC/AHA Task Force on Practice Guidelines. *J Am Coll Cardiol.* 2007;50(23):2264–2274.

【 】 ANTIPLATELET AGENTS

Aspirin, 80 to 325 mg/day, should be used routinely by all patients with acute and chronic ischemic heart disease with and without clinical symptoms in the absence of contraindications. In those unable to take aspirin, clopidogrel may be used. The efficacy of newer antiplatelet agents, such as glycoprotein IIb/IIIa inhibitors in the management of chronic stable angina has not been established.

【 】 LIPID-LOWERING AGENTS

Recent clinical studies have conveniently demonstrated that lowering of low-density-lipoprotein (LDL) cholesterol with HMG-CoA reductase inhibitors (statins) can decrease the risk of adverse ischemic events in patients with established CAD. Thus, lipid-lowering therapy should be recommended even in the presence of mild to moderate elevations of LDL cholesterol in patients with chronic stable angina. Patients with ischemic heart disease should have LDL cholesterol levels below 100 mg/dL (2.6 mmol/L). It is now known that the statins have many favorable effects on endothelial function beyond decreasing LDL cholesterol levels and may reverse the endothelial response to chemical or physical stresses causing coronary vasoconstriction. Lowering of LDL cholesterol with statins has been shown by intravascular ultrasound to cause regression of atherosclerotic plaques in many coronary stenotic lesions.

TABLE 22-7

Recommendations for Coronary Angiography for Risk Stratification in Patients with Chronic Stable Angin[a]

Class I

1. Patients with disabling (Canadian Cardiovascular Society [CCS] classes III and V) chronic stable angina despite medical therapy.
2. Patients with high-risk criteria on noninvasive testing regardless of anginal severity.
3. Patients with angina who have survived sudden cardiac death or serious ventricular arrhythmia.
4. Patients with angina and symptoms and signs of congestive heart failure.
5. Patients with clinical characteristics that indicate a high likelihood of severe CAD.

Class IIa

1. Patients with significant LV dysfunction (EF < 45%), CCS class I or II angina, and demonstrable ischemia but less than high-risk criteria on noninvasive testing.
2. Patients with inadequate prognostic information after noninvasive testing.

Class IIb

1. Patients with disabling CCS class I or II angina, preserved LV function (EF > 45%), and less than high-risk criteria on noninvasive testing.

Class III

1. Patients with disabling CCS classes I or II angina who respond to medical therapy and have no evidence of ischemia on nonivasive testing.
2. Patients who prefer to avoid revascularization.

See classes I to III as described in Table 22-4.

Data compiled from Gibbons RJ, Abrams J, Chatterjee K, et al., Guidelines for the management of patients with chronic stable angina: a report of the ACC/AHA Task Force on Practice Guidelines. *J Am Coll Cardiol.* 2007;50(23):2264–2274.

【 】 NITROGLYCERIN AND NITRATES

The standard first-line therapy of angina remains sublingual nitroglycerin (NTG), which usually relieves the symptoms within 1 to 5 minutes NTG may be taken acutely either as a sublingual tablet (0.3–0.6 mg) or as an oral spray, each puff of which is calculated to deliver 0.4 mg. Monotherapy with sublingual or oral spray NTG is usually not satisfactory unless the episodes are rare.

The American College of Cardiology/AHA–ASIM Guidelines for chronic stable angina recommend long-acting beta-blockers and/or calcium antagonists in preference to long-acting nitrates in patients with recurrent angina (see Chapter 59). Nevertheless, long-acting nitrates are used prophylactically in many patients who have frequent episodes of angina. The many forms of nitrates include a slowly absorbed buccal capsule, a transdermal ointment or patch, and sublingual or oral forms that are absorbed more slowly. In general, it is important to start with a low dosage and to increase the dose progressively. The most common side effects are headache, dizziness, and postural hypotension. It should also be noted that the coadministration of long-acting nitrates and sildenafil (Viagra) significantly increases the risk of potentially life-threatening hypotension.

The *major problem* with long-term use of nitroglycerin and long-acting nitrates is the development of *nitrate tolerance*. For practical purposes, the administration of nitrates with an adequate nitrate-free interval (8–12 hours) appears to be the most effective method of preventing nitrate tolerance. For many patients, this can be from about 9 PM to 7 AM. Nitroglycerin ointments should be removed about 8 or 9 PM. Isosorbide dinitrate (ISDN; 10–60 mg) can be given orally in doses of 30 mg twice a day at 8 AM and 5 PM or three times a day at 8 AM, 1 PM, and 5 PM. Isosorbide mononitrate (ISMO), a metabolite of ISDN, is administered orally in 20-mg doses at 7 AM and 2 PM. An extended-release form of isosorbide mononitrate (IMDUR) can be taken orally as a single 60-mg dose at 7 or 8 AM. Patients who have angina at night may need either to plan the nitrate-free period for another time or to use a beta-blocker or calcium-channel blocker concurrently.

Patients should be instructed that if an anginal episode persists for more than 10 minutes despite their having taken three sublingual NTG tablets or an equivalent dose of NTG spray, they should report promptly to the nearest medical facility for further evaluation and management.

【 】 BETA-BLOCKERS

Beta-adrenergic blocking agents, which reduce heart rate and myocardial contractility both at rest and during exertion, are very effective in the management of patients with angina pectoris. Many beta-blockers are available. In general, long-acting cardioselective agents (e.g., metoprolol) are preferred in patients who have a history of bronchospastic disease, diabetes mellitus, or peripheral vascular disease. However, it should be noted that even cardioselective beta-blockers can produce bronchospasm in some patients. All beta-blockers can worsen heart block or depress LV function and worsen heart failure. Fatigue, inability to perform exercise, lethargy, insomnia, nightmares, worsening claudication, and erectile dysfunction are other possible side effects.

In treating stable angina, it is essential that the dose of beta-blockers be adjusted to *lower the resting heart rate to 55 to 60* beats per minute. If discontinued, beta-blockers should be tapered over 3 to 10 days, when possible, to avoid a rebound worsening of angina pectoris.

【 】 CALCIUM ANTAGONISTS

Calcium-channel blockers decrease myocardial oxygen requirements by producing arterial dilation and often by reducing myocardial contractility. In addition, calcium-channel blockers produce coronary vasodilation and prevent coronary artery spasm. Drugs, such as verapamil and diltiazem also tend to reduce heart rate. Clinical trials comparing calcium antagonists and beta-blockers have demonstrated that calcium antagonists are as effective as beta-blockers in relieving angina and improving exercise time to onset of angina or ischemia. The calcium antagonists are also effective in reducing the incidence of angina in patients with vasospastic angina. In the International Multicenter Angina Exercises (Image Trial), combination therapy with metoprolol and nifedipine increased the exercise time to ischemia compared to either drug alone.

Thus, long-acting calcium antagonists, including slow-release and long-acting dihydropyridines (nifedipine and amlodipine) and nondihydropyridines (verapamil and diltiazem), should be used in combination with beta-blockers when initial treatment with beta-blockers is not successful or as a substitute for beta-blockers when initial treatment leads to unacceptable side effects. Calcium-channel blockers are the preferred agents in patients with a history of asthma, chronic obstructive pulmonary disease, or severe peripheral vascular disease. Combined therapy with a long-acting cardioselective beta-blocker and a long-acting dihydropyridine calcium-channel blocker is particularly beneficial. Some patients may benefit from triple therapy with a long-acting nitrate, a beta-blocker, and a calcium-channel blocker.

【 】 ANGIOTENSIN-CONVERTING ENZYME INHIBITORS

The potential cardiovascular protective effects of angiotensin-converting enzyme (ACE) inhibitors have been suspected for some time. As early as 1990, results from the Survival and Ventricular Enlargement (SAVE) and Studies of Left Ventricular Dysfunction (SOLVD) trials showed that ACE inhibitors reduced the incidence of recurrent MI and that this effect could not be attributed to the effect on blood pressure alone. At the same time, Alderman demonstrated that a high plasma renin level was associated with a significantly higher incidence of death from MI in patients with moderate hypertension and that this effect was independent of blood pressure level.

The results of the Heart Outcomes Prevention Evaluation (HOPE) trial now confirm that the use of the ACE inhibitor ramipril (10 mg/day) reduced cardiovascular death, MI, and stroke in patients who were at high risk for, or had, vascular disease in the absence of heart failure. The primary outcome in HOPE was a composite of cardiovascular death, MI, and stroke. However, the results of HOPE were so definitive that each of the components of the primary outcome by itself also showed statistical significance.

The Microalbuminuria, Cardiovascular, and Renal Outcomes (MICRO)-HOPE, a substudy of the HOPE study, has provided new clinical data on the cardiorenal therapeutic benefits of ACE inhibitor intervention in a broad range of middle-aged patients with diabetes mellitus who are at high risk for cardiovascular events.

ACE inhibitors should be used as routine secondary prevention for patients with known CAD, particularly in diabetics without severe renal disease.

【　】 POTENTIAL NEW ANTIANGINAL THERAPIES

Ranolazine is the first member of a new class of drugs believed to reduce angina by partially inhibiting fatty acid oxidation, thereby increasing glucose oxidation and generating more adenosine triphosphate (ATP) per molecule of oxygen consumed. In the Monotherapy Assessment of Ranolazine, a well-designed, well-conducted clinical trial in which patients were randomized to receive one of two doses of ranolazine or placebo showed that both doses of ranolazine were more effective than placebo at reducing symptoms and improving exercise capacity when added to conventional doses of atenolol, diltiazem, or amlodipine. This drug has been approved by the U.S. Food and Drug Administration for the treatment of angina refractory to other medical therapy.

MYOCARDIAL REVASCULARIZATION

Some patients with stable angina pectoris are candidates for revascularization, either with coronary artery bypass graft (CABG) surgery or with percutaneous coronary intervention (PCI). The two general indications for revascularization are (1) the presence of symptoms that are not acceptable to the patient, either because of restriction of physical activity and lifestyle or because of side effects from medications; or (2) the presence of coronary arteriographic findings indicating clearly that the patient would have a significantly better prognosis with revascularization than with medical therapy. In general, patients with stable angina should have objective evidence of myocardial ischemia prior to revascularization. Additional major considerations include the age of the patient, presence of other comorbid conditions, grade or class of angina experienced by the patient on maximal therapy, extent and severity of myocardial ischemia on noninvasive testing, degree of LV dysfunction, and distribution and severity of CAD.

In a recent clinical trial using revascularization and aggressive drug evaluation, which randomized 2,287 patients to optimal medical therapy (OMT) versus OMT and PCI and which followed patients 4.6 years on average, there was no difference in the primary end point of MI, death, and stroke in these patients with moderate angina in these two treatment arms. These patients had stable angina, abnormal coronary arteriography, and rest- or stress-induced myocardial ischemia. They *did not* have acute coronary syndrome. Thus, patients with stable angina can be treated initially with modifiable risk factor reduction and antianginal medication for up to 3 years following OMT alone and later if necessary; about 30% will eventually require revascularization.

CABG provides good symptomatic relief for most patients who have suitable vessels. It is the treatment of choice for patients with severe CAD, including greater than 50% left main stenosis or three-vessel disease with impaired LV function. It is also indicated in severely symptomatic patients with two-vessel disease that includes a high-grade stenosis of the proximal left anterior descending artery and in patients in whom revascularization is indicated, but who have a lesion that is not amenable to PCI. Vein grafts have a failure rate that approaches 50% at 10 years. In contrast, internal mammary grafts have a superior patency and thus should be used whenever possible during the CABG.

With the proliferation of various new debulking techniques, intracoronary stents, and drug-eluting stents, PCI can be successfully performed on a wide variety of native vessel and graft lesions. The advantages of PCI for the treatment of CAD include a low level of procedure-related morbidity and mortality, a short hospital stay, early return to activity, and the feasibility of multiple procedures. However, PCI is not possible for all patients; it is accompanied by a significant incidence of restenoses; and there is an occasional need for emergency CABG surgery. The recommendations of the ACC/AHA/ACP–ASIM Chronic Stable Angina Guidelines for revascularization with PCI or CABG in patients with stable angina are listed in Table 22-8.

TABLE 22-8

Revascularization for Chronic Stable Angina[a]

Class I

1. CABG for patients with significant left main coronary disease.
2. CABG for patients with three-vessel disease. The survival benefit is greater in patients with abnormal LV function (EF < 50%).
3. CABG for patients with two-vessel disease with significant proximal left anterior descending CAD and either abnormal LV function (EF < 50%) or demonstrable ischemia on noninvasive testing.
4. PCI for patients with two- or three-vessel disease with significant proximal left anterior descending CAD, who have anatomy suitable for catheter-based therapy, normal LV function, and no treated diabetes.
5. PCI or CABG for patients with one- or two-vessel disease CAD without significant proximal left anterior descending CAD but with a large area of viable myocardium and high-risk criteria on noninvasive testing.
6. CABG for patients with one- or two-vessel CAD without significant proximal left anterior descending CAD who have survived sudden cardiac death or sustained ventricular tachycardia.
7. In patients with prior PCI, CABG, or PCI for recurrent stenosis associated with a large area of viable myocardium or high-risk criteria on noninvasive testing.
8. PTCA[b] or CABG for patients who have not been successfully treated by medical therapy and can undergo revascularization with acceptable risk.

Class IIa

1. Repeat CABG for patients with multiple saphenous vein graft stenoses; especially when there is significant stenosis of a graft supplying the LAD, it may be appropriate to use PTCA for local saphenous vein graft lesions or multiple stenoses in poor candidates for reoperative surgery.
2. Use of PCI or CABG for patients with one- or two-vessel CAD without significant proximal LAD disease but with a moderate area of viable myocardium and demonstrable ischemia on noninvasive testing.
3. Use of PCI or CABG for patients with one-vessel disease with significant proximal LAD disease.

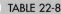

TABLE 22-8

Revascularization for Chronic Stable Angina*a* (*Continued*)

Class IIb

1. Compared with CABG, PCI for patients with two- or three-vessel disease with significant proximal left anterior descending CAD, who have anatomy suitable for catheter-based therapy, and who have treated diabetes or abnormal LV function.
2. Use of PCI for patients with significant left main coronary disease who are not candidates for CABG.
3. PCI for patients with one- or two-vessel disease CAD without significant proximal left anterior descending CAD who have survived sudden cardiac death or sustained ventricular tachycardia.

Class III

1. Use of PCI or CABG for patients with one- or two-vessel CAD without significant proximal left anterior descending CAD, who have mild symptoms that are unlikely due to myocardial ischemia or who have not received an adequate trial of medical therapy and (a) have only a small area of viable myocardium or (b) have no demonstrable ischemia on noninvasive testing.
2. Use of PCI or CABG for patients with borderline coronary stenoses (50–60% diameter in locations other than the left main coronary artery) and no demonstrable ischemia on noninvasive testing.
3. Use of PCI or CABG for patients with insignificant coronary stenosis (< 50% diameter).
4. Use of PCI in patients with significant left main coronary disease who are candidates for CABG.

See classes I to III as described at bottom of Table 22-4 and Chapter 59.

CABG, coronary artery bypass graft; CAD, coronary artery disease; EF, ejection fraction; LAD, left anterior descending (coronary artery); LV, left ventricular; PCI, percutaneous coronary intervention; PTCA, percutaneous transluminal coronary angioplasty.

*a*Recommendations for revascularization with PTCA (or other catheter-based techniques) and CABG in patients with stable angina.
*b*PTCA is used in these recommendations to indicate PTCA or other catheter-based techniques, such as stents, atherectomy, and laser therapy.

It is important to remember that most patients with chronic angina have not been shown to have an increased survival rate with invasive treatment, but require invasive treatment mainly to control their symptoms.

OTHER THERAPIES IN PATIENTS WITH REFRACTORY ANGINA

Evidence has emerged regarding the relative efficacy, or lack thereof, of a number of techniques for the management of refractory chronic angina pectoris. These techniques should be used only in patients who cannot be managed adequately by medical therapy and who are not candidates for revascularization (interventional and/or surgical) (see *Hurst's The Heart*, 12th edition, 2008).

SUGGESTED READING

Cheiltin MD, Hutter AM, Brindis RG, et al. ACC/AHA expert consensus documents: use of sildenafil (Viagra) in patients with cardiovascular disease. *J Am Coll Cardiol.* 1999;33:273–282.

Comparison of coronary artery bypass surgery with angioplasty in patients with multivessel disease: the Bypass Angioplasty Revascularization Investigation (BARI) investigators. *N Engl J Med.* 1996;335:217–225. Erratum appears in *N Engl J Med.*1997;336:147.

Eagle KA, Guyton RA, Davidoff R, et al. ACC/AHA 2004 guideline update for coronary artery bypass graft surgery: a report of the American College of Cardiology/American Heart Association Task Force on Practice Guidelines (Committee to Update the 1999 Guidelines for Coronary Artery Bypass Graft Surgery). *J Am Coll Cardiol.* In press.

Gibbons RJ, Chatterjee K, Daley J, et al. American College of Cardiology/American Heart Association, American College of Physicians–American Society of Internal Medicine (ACC/AHA/ACP–ASIM) guidelines for the management of patients with chronic stable angina: a report of the ACC/AHA Task Force on Practice Guidelines (Committee on the Management of Patients with Chronic Stable Angina). *J Am Coll Cardiol.* 2003;41:160–168.

King SB, III, Smith SC, Hirshfeld JW, Jr, et al. 2007 Focused update of the ACC/AHA/SCAI 2005 guideline update for percutaneous coronary intervention: a report of the American College of Cardiology/American Heart Association Task Force on Practice Guidelines. *J Am Coll Cardiol.* 2008;51:172–209.

Mark DB, Shaw L, Harrell FE, et al. Prognostic value of a treadmill exercise score in outpatients with suspected coronary artery disease. *N Engl J Med.* 1991;325:849–853.

O'Rourke RA: Optimal medical management of patients with chronic ischemic heart disease. *Curr Probl Cardiol.* 2001;26:195–244.

O'Rourke RA, O'Gara P, Douglas JS Jr. Diagnosis and management of patients with chronic ischemic heart disease. In: Fuster V, O'Rourke RA, Walsh RA, et al., eds. *Hurst's The Heart.* 12th ed. New York, NY: McGraw-Hill; 2008:1474–1503.

CHAPTER 23

Definitions and Pathogenesis of Acute Coronary Syndromes

Joseph M. Sweeny and Valentin Fuster

Atherosclerosis represents a systemic disease involving the intima of large- and medium-sized arteries including the aorta, carotid, coronary, and peripheral arterial systems. Now considered a chronic immunoinflammatory, fibroproliferative, lipid-driven, progressive process, atherosclerosis is the leading underlying mechanism for coronary heart disease (CHD). Widely accepted as the most common cause of death and disability in the United States, it is estimated that 40 million individuals live with CHD in the world today. CHD represents a continuum of disease pathologies and has been classified as chronic CHD, acute coronary syndromes, and sudden cardiac death. Acute coronary syndromes are a spectrum of ischemic myocardial events that range from unstable angina (UA) to non-ST elevation myocardial infarction (NSTEMI) and ST-elevation myocardial infarction (STEMI). Although distinct in clinical presentation, they all share a similar pathophysiologic mechanism of vulnerable atherosclerotic plaque disruption with superimposed thrombus formation and subsequent degrees of antegrade coronary blood flow cessation with reduced myocardial oxygen supply. The thrombotic sequelae underlying this response are mainly the consequences of a multifactorial disease process triggered by endothelial injury followed then by a cascade of events that include a complex interplay of inflammation, cell signaling, immunomodulation, cellular proliferation, angiogenesis, vasoconstriction, and cell death. A comprehensive understanding of the pathogenesis of atherosclerosis and thrombosis as well as the clinical manifestations of acute coronary syndromes will ultimately assist the clinician in preventing, diagnosing, and treating this common and potentially fatal disease.

PATHOGENESIS OF ATHEROTHROMBOSIS AND ACUTE CORONARY SYNDROMES

【 】 INFLAMMATION

Studies have indicated that there are certain vascular sites of predilection for atherosclerosis. These sites are classically characterized by areas of low sheer stress frequently found in arterial branches, bifurcations, and curvatures that predispose to turbulent blood flow. Interestingly, these changes in blood flow dynamics have been shown to locally upregulate the genetic expression of specific cellular adhesion molecules such as intercellular adhesion molecule (ICAM-1) and vascular cell adhesion molecule (VCAM-1) on the endothelium and circulating leukocytes. This process leads to the adherence, migration, and accumulation of monocytes and T cells to the endothelium. Chemoattractants, such as monocyte chemotactic protein-1 (MCP-1), osteopontin, and modified low-density lipoprotein (LDL) are produced by the endothelium as well as monocytes and vascular smooth muscle cells and attract monocytes, macrophages, and T cells into the endothelium,

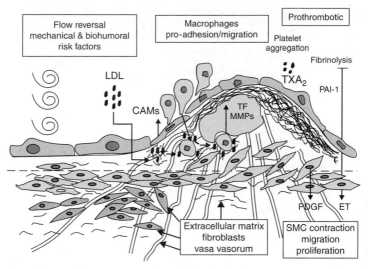

FIGURE 23-1. Schematic representation of atherosclerotic lesion progression. Initial blood flow dynamics in vulnerable areas of circulation promote up-regulation of genes that promote cell adhesion. Endothelial activation by inflammatory cell response mediates LDL cholesterol migration through a more permeable endothelial surface. Macrophage foam cells and activated T cells release proteolytic enzymes, which soften the lipid core and increase the vulnerability for rupture. (CAM, cell adhesion molecules; ET, endothelin; LDL, low density lipoprotein; MMP, metalloproteinase; PAI-1, plasminogen activator inhibitor-1; SMC, smooth muscle cells; TF, tissue factor; TXA2, thromboxane A2.) (Reproduced with permission from Fuster V, Moreno PR, Fayad ZA, et al. Atherothrombosis and high-risk plaque. pt1: evolving concepts. *J Am Coll Cardiol.* 2005;46:937–954. Figure 7. Elsevier, Inc.)

which migrate through to the vessel wall. Further upregulation of cell adhesion molecules and receptors facilitates subendothelial recruitment of mononuclear cells within the arterial wall, which eventually helps to delineate a focal region of inflammation (Fig. 23-1).

【 】 ENDOTHELIAL ACTIVATION AND INFLAMMATION

Endothelial activation refers to a specific change in endothelial phenotype, characterized by an increase in endothelial–leukocyte-platelet adhesiveness and interactions, increased cell–cell permeability, a shift from an anticoagulant to a procoagulant milieu, and a change from a growth-inhibiting state to a growth-promoting state mediated through an elaborate cytokine release. An increasing body of evidence indicates an important role for reactive oxygen species (ROS)-mediated modulation of signal-transduction pathways in many of the processes involved in endothelial activation, and various factors have been found to contribute to ROS formation and endothelial activation including many well-described cardiovascular risk factors (Table 23-1). Specifically, elevated LDL cholesterol, elevated very-low-density lipoprotein (VLDL), low concentrations of high-density lipoprotein (HDL), and reactive oxygen species caused by hypertension, cigarette smoking, diabetes mellitus, estrogen deficiency, and advancing age, have all been linked to endothelial activation and injury.

In a nonathrogenic state, locally produced nitric oxide (NO) normally acts as a local vasodilator through the vascular smooth muscle cells (VSMC) and can additionally inhibit platelet aggregation. However, in the setting of endothelial dysfunction, a paradoxical

TABLE 23-1

Endothelial Activation/Dysfunction in Atherosclerosis

Phenotypic features
1. Reduced vasodilator and increased vasoconstrictor capacity
2. Enhanced oxidant stress with increased inactivation of nitric oxide
3. Increased expression of endothelin
Enhanced leukocyte molecule expression (ICAM, VCAM)
Increased chemotactic molecule expression (MCP-11, IL-8)
Increased prothrombotic and reduced fibrinolytic phenotype
Increased growth-promoting phenotype
Factors contributing to endothelial activation/dysfunction
1. Dyslipidemia and atherogenic lipoprotein modification, elevated LDL, VLDL, Lp(a)
2. LDL modification (oxidation, glycation)
3. Reduced HDL
4. Increased angiotensin II and hypertension
5. Insulin resistance
6. Estrogen deficiency
7. Smoking
8. Hyperhomocysteninemia
9. Advancing age
10. Infection

response to NO is observed in large vessels and the microcirculation, leading instead to a vasoconstrictive response. This paradoxical response, and an actual reduction in NO release and prostaglandin (PGI2) synthesis, together act to facilitate the permeability of lipids into subendothelial spaces.

Oxidized LDL cholesterol is a major contributor to endothelial dysfunction. Influx and retention of these and other athrogenic lipoproteins in the arterial intima constitutes the central pathogenic process in atherogenesis. Once LDL cholesterol becomes internalized through the activated vascular endothelium and into the vessel wall, it is taken up by resident macrophages and activated foam cells. Modified LDL cholesterol is also chemotactic for other monocytes through a monocyte-derived chemotactic protein (MCP-1), thereby expanding the inflammatory response and precipitating proliferation of smooth muscle cells and fibroblasts—a process that results in thickening of the arterial wall.

By continually multiplying in the focal lesion, monocyte-derived activated macrophages and lymphocytes release proteolytic enzymes, metalloproteinases, hydrolytic enzymes, cytokines, and growth factors that can cause focal necrosis, thereby slowly creating an enlarging necrotic lipid core surrounded by a fibrous cap. T cell activation that follows antigen presentation by macrophages further enhances the inflammatory response by releasing interferon-gama and TNF-alpha and -beta. It has been suggested that the intricate inflammatory regulation and maladaptive functions of the resident macrophages in atheromatous plaques is orchestrated by CD40 ligand that is expressed on macrophages, T cells, endothelial cells, and smooth muscle cells. In fact, the central role of CD40 ligand in atherosclerosis is further supported by the observation of antiathrogenic effects CD40-blocking antibodies have in murine models of atherosclerosis.

Angiogenesis or neovascularization also plays a pivotal role in the atheroma-forming process and may further contribute to plaque progression. By providing a direct conduit and source for inflammatory cell recruitment into the vessel wall, extracellular cholesterol deposits into the lipid core and a potential source for intraplaque hemorrhage, neovascularization contributes to plaque destabilization increased vulnerability.

【 】 PLAQUE RUPTURE AND THROMBOSIS

Uneven thinning, weakening, and rupture of the fibrous cap usually occurs at the shoulder regions of lesions, as this is an area that is the site of T cell and macrophage accumulation, activation, and apoptosis. The release of matrix-degrading proteinases such as the matrix metalloproteinases (MMPs) weakens the vulnerable, already thinned fibrous cap. This in combination with apoptosis of vascular smooth muscle cells eventually exposes tissue factor (TF) that is abundant in the atheroma in macrophages to circulating blood. Upon contact of TF with the circulating blood, the extrinsic coagulation cascade is initiated and the formation of prothrombin (factor II) and thrombin (factor IIa) ensues. A potent platelet activator, thrombin formation along with fibrin create the obstruction that ultimately diminishes antegrade blood flow (Fig. 23-2).

【 】 CELLULAR MECHANISMS OF THROMBUS FORMATION

As a consequence of plaque rupture, platelets progress through a sequence of stages leading to adhesion, activation, and aggregation all in a fashion to contain the damaged endothelium via a platelet plug. Platelets adhere to the ruptured plaque core through interactions with exposed TF. TF, in turn, has a potent effect on further activating platelets. The circulating von Willebrand factor (vWF) is capable of binding exposed collagen in the plaque and glycoprotein (GP) receptors in the platelet membrane. Platelet activation results from the action of numerous agonists that bind to the platelet

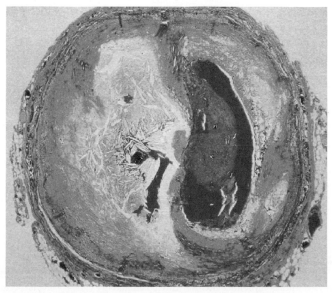

FIGURE 23-2. Plaque rupture. Cross-section of a coronary artery delineating atherosclerotic plaque rupture with a nonocclusive intracoronary thrombus.

membrane and initiate intracellular signaling. These platelet agonists include 5-hydroxytryptamine (5-HT), epinephrine, adenosine diphosphate (ADP), and arachadonic acid (AA). Once activated, platelets continue to secrete agonists from dense granules, prompting further activation of platelets and culminating in the formation of a platelet plug that provides a surface for coagulation cascades. At the same time, activated platelets synthesize thromboxane (TXA2), which is a potent platelet activator and vasoconstrictor. These processes occur in the environment of the atherosclerotic plaque lesion as a developing thrombus if formed.

The efficiency of the platelet response and recruitment is largely dependent upon both local as well as systemic factors that mediate the magnitude of thrombus formation. Local factors include the severity of the arterial wall damage. It is believed that when the initial injury is limited, the thrombogenic response is limited when compared to a deep ulcerated plaque rupture that precipitates a more robust thrombus formation. In addition, the platelet response depends in part on the geometric changes the ruptured plaque assumes.

Systemic influences associated with an increased blood thrombogenicity include cardiovascular risk factors (diabetes mellitus, smoking, catecholamines, elevated LDL, decreased HDL). This is supported by the observation that in approximately one-third of cases of acute coronary syndrome (ACS), there is no disruption of lipid-rich plaque, but only superficial erosion of small nonstenosis plaque. It is interesting to note that these plaques usually go undetected by standard angiography.

In addition to platelet aggregation on the injured endothelium, the clotting mechanism is similarly activated by expose of the plaque components to flowing blood. Through various pathways, the coagulation cascade generates thrombin, which catalyzes the formation of fibrin from fibrinogen. As well as possessing potent platelet agonist properties, fibrin acts to stabilize the platelet thrombus by forming a mesh network across the injured area.

Increased knowledge of both the complex platelet activation and aggregation pathways as well as the coagulation cascades have created numerous targets for potential pharmacologic therapies aimed at diminishing or eliminating the response to endothelial injury. These therapies are categorized as fibrinolytic agents, intrinsic coagulation cascade inhibitors (warfarin, direct thrombin inhibitors), and antiplatelet agents (aspirin and clopidogrel).

DEFINITIONS OF ACUTE CORONARY SYNDROMES

The clinical manifestation of a platelet-rich thrombus in a coronary artery is the development of an acute coronary syndrome (ACS). Acute coronary syndromes have a common end result: acute myocardial ischemia that has been shown to be associated with an increased risk of cardiac death and myonecrosis. The term ACS encompasses acute myocardial infarction with resultant ST-segment elevation or non–ST-segment elevation and unstable angina (Fig. 23-3). Efficient and timely triage of patients with ACS is essential given the life-threatening nature of the disease processes and the proven benefit that both medical and mechanical therapies provide. In the setting of more sensitive and specific serologic markers, imaging techniques, and pathologic characteristics, the European Society of Cardiology (ESC) and the American College of Cardiology (ACC) in 2000 reexamined the definition of myocardial infarction to provide for a more universal definition. A recently published revision in 2008 further qualified infarct size, circumstances leading up to the infarct, and the timing of the necrosis relative to the time of the observation (Table 23-2).

【 】 UNSTABLE ANGINA

Unstable angina (UA) characteristically originates from a nonocclusive thrombus without any evidence of myocardial necrosis. Given the subjective nature of angina pectoris, many classification schemes have been developed for unstable angina. For example, the Canadian Cardiovascular Society (CCS) rates anginal symptoms with level of activity.

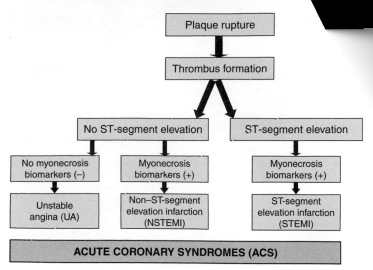

FIGURE 23-3. The development of atherosclerotic plaque rupture and the consequent clinical manifestations of acute coronary syndromes (ACS).

TABLE 23-2

Clinical Classification of Different Types of Myocardial Infarction

Type 1
Spontaneous myocardial infarction related to ischemia due to a primary coronary event such as plaque erosion and/or rupture, fissuring, or dissection.

Type 2
Myocardial infarction secondary to ischemia due to either increased oxygen demand or decreased supply—e.g., coronary spasm, coronary embolism, anemia, arrhythmias, hypertension, or hypotension.

Type 3
Sudden unexpected cardiac death, including cardiac arrest, often with symptoms suggestive of myocardial ischemia, accompanied by presumably new ST elevation, or new LBBB, or evidence of fresh thrombus in a coronary artery by angiography and/or autopsy, but death occurring before blood samples could be obtained, or at a time before the appearance of cardiac biomarkers in the blood.

Type 4a
Myocardial infarction associated with PCI.

Type 4b
Myocardial infarction associated with stent thrombosis as documented by angiography at autopsy.

Type 5
Myocardial infarction associated with CABG.

Adapted from ESC/ACCF/AHA/WHF Expert Consensus Document. Reproduced with permission from Thygesen K, Alpert J, White HD. Universal definition of myocardial infarction. *J Am Coll Cardiol.* 2007;50:2173–2195.

egorizing the severity and clinical circumstances in which angina occurs, Braunwald er classified unstable angina in 1989 as a means of providing a more uniform working nition of the syndrome in addition to obtaining valuable prognostic and diagnostic formation of this common and potentially fatal symptom.

Braunwald's classification of angina has been linked to risk of death or myocardial infarction at 1 year. The Agency for Health Care Policy and Research (AHCPR) has published guidelines that assess short-term risks of death or nonfatal myocardial infarction in patients with unstable angina.

There are other causes that may lead to acute coronary ischemia. For example, dynamic obstruction of Printzmetal's angina occurs in epicardial arteries commonly in the setting of endothelial dysfunction with an imbalance of vasoconstrictive properties. Coronary restenosis after percutaneous coronary intervention is also a mechanism of myocardial ischemia. This process is largely due to cellular proliferation and does not involve thrombus formation or spasm. Lastly, any condition that worsens cardiac myocardial oxygen supply in the setting of high demands such as fever or anemia in a patient with chronic coronary artery disease can also be a mechanism of myocardial ischemia.

【 】 NON–ST-SEGMENT ELEVATION MYOCARDIAL INFARCTION

Those patients with acute ischemic chest pain without electrocardiographic evidence of ST-segment elevation or Q waves, but with ischemia severe enough to cause significant myocardial damage by evidence of myocardial necrosis, represent non–ST-segment elevation myocardial infarction. Current markers for myocardial injury include creatinine kinase (CK), CK-MB isoforms, and troponin (Fig. 23-4). CK is very sensitive for detecting myocardial damage and has been shown to be related to the degree of infracted

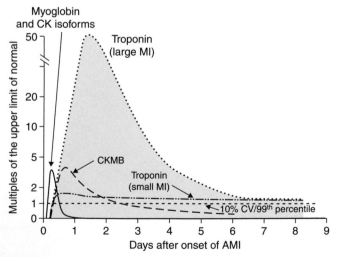

FIGURE 23-4. Timing and release of various biomarkers after acute ischemic myocardial infarction. (ACC/AHA 2007 Guidelines for the Management of Patients with Unstable Angina/Non-ST-Elevation Myocardial Infarction.) (Reproduced with permission from Anderson JL, et al. *Circulation.* 2007;116:803–877. Fig 4. Lippincott Williams & Wilkins. (http://lww.com))

myocardium. Initially elevated 4 to 8 hours after myocardial insult, CK measurement provides a valuable tool for assessing acute or subacute angina. However, noncardiac elevation of CK precludes the sole utilization of this enzyme.

Methods to increase the specificity of CK include measurements of CK-MB levels by immunoassay. CK-MB isoforms exist as only one form in cardiac muscle (CK-MB2), but do exist as different forms in the blood (CK-MB1). A ratio of CK-MB2 to CK-MB1 of greater then 2.5 has significantly improved the sensitivity of detecting myonecrosis within 6 hours.

The troponin complex consists of three subunits (TnI, TnT, and TnC) that act to regulate cardiac muscle contraction. Monoclonal antibody-based immunoassays have been developed to specifically detect cardiac TnT and TnI. As a consequence of the heightened sensitivity and specificity of cardiac troponins when compared to CK, it has been shown that up to 30% of patients with negative CK-MB levels are reclassified as having a NSTEMI with a positive troponin.

The level of troponin release has been linked to prognosis, and the higher the level, the higher risk for death or nonfatal myocardial infarction at 30 days. Regardless of the cause of elevation, it has been shown that troponin elevation represents an increased risk of death when compared to those patients without troponin elevation.

Troponin measurement early in the evaluation of a patient with angina is essential as there is evidence from randomized controlled trials showing the benefit of administration of glycoprotein IIb/IIIa inhibition to those patients with elevated troponin levels. Furthermore, early angiography with mechanical revascularization has been shown to be superior to medical therapy in patients with NSTEMI and troponin release. Within the first 6 hours of symptom onset, CK-MB isoforms and myoglobin were the most efficient for the diagnosis of NSTEMI, and troponin elevation was most useful for the late diagnosis of myocardial infarction as troponin levels remain elevated for 7 days.

【 】 ST-SEGMENT ELEVATION MYOCARDIAL INFARCTION

Considered the form of ACS with the highest mortality, ST-elevation myocardial infarction is manifested as an occlusive atherothrombosis followed by complete cessation of antegrade myocardial blood flow with subsequent ST-segment elevation on the surface electrocardiogram (ECG). Approximately 500,000 STEMIs occur each year in the United States, but there has been a steady decline in the mortality rates of this disease largely due to decreased a fatality with early reperfusion. The accurate diagnosis of STEMI is important, as its presence mandates immediate consideration for reperfusion therapy via thrombolytic agents or mechanically with percutaneous intervention. The World Health Organization criteria for an acute myocardial infarction require that two of the following three elements be present: (1) a history suggestive of coronary ischemia for a prolonged period of time (> 30 minutes), (2) evolutionary changes on serial ECGs suggestive of myocardial infarction, and (3) a rise and fall in serum cardiac markers that is consistent with myonecrosis. The 2004 ACC/AHA STEMI guidelines emphasize the importance of establishing regionalization of STEMI care facilities in an effort to reduce both the mortality and morbidity of this disease.

CONCLUSION

Atherosclerosis is a systemic disease that is initiated by endothelial injury by various mechanisms that produce a cascade of localized inflammation, lipid influx, and cellular proliferation that culminates in weakening of the atherosclerotic plaque. Platelet adherence, activation, and aggregation begin the process of localized hemostasis, but this soon develops into a maladaptive response with the formation of intraluminal thrombus and obstruction of coronary blood flow. ACS is the clinical manifestation of a platelet-rich thrombus developing in a coronary artery. By accurately diagnosing each patient as having unstable angina, NSTEMI, or STEMI with clinical acumen, ECG, and serum biomarkers, clinicians are now able to rapidly treat this potentially fatal disease.

SUGGESTED READING

Braunwald E. Application of current guidelines to the management of unstable angina and non-ST-elevation myocardial infarction. *Circulation.* 2003;108(suppl 1):III28–III37.

Fuster V, Badimon L, Badimon JJ, et al. The pathogenesis of coronary artery disease and the acute coronary syndromes. Part 1. *N Engl J Med.* 1992:326;242–250

Fuster V, Moreno PR, Fayad ZA, et al. Atherothrombosis and high-risk plaque. Part 1: evolving concepts. *J Am Coll Cardiol.* 2005;46:937–954.

Kim M, Kini A, Fuster V. Definitions of acute coronary syndromes. In: Fuster V, Alexander RW, O'Rourke RA, et al., eds. *Hurst's The Heart.* 12th ed. New York, NY: McGraw-Hill; 2008:2311–1319.

Libby P. Inflammation in atherosclerosis. *Nature.* 2002;420:868–874.

Shah PK, Falk E, Fuster V. Atherothrombosis: role of inflammation. In: Fuster V, Alexander RW, O'Rourke RA, et al., eds. *Hurst's The Heart.* 12th ed. New York, NY: McGraw-Hill; 2008:1235–1244.

Thygesen K, Alpert J, White HD. Universal definition of myocardial infarction. *J Am Coll Cardiol.* 2007;50:2173–2195.

CHAPTER 24

Diagnosis and Management of Patients with ST-Segment Elevation Myocardial Infarction

Eric H. Yang and Bernard J. Gersh

EPIDEMIOLOGY

Approximately 865,000 Americans suffer from an acute myocardial infarction (AMI) per year, one-third of which are caused by an acute ST-segment elevation myocardial infarction (STEMI). The incidence of AMI declined from 244 per 100,000 population in 1975 to 184 per 100,000 population in 1995. The in-hospital mortality rate also declined from 18% in 1975 to 12% in 1995. Nonetheless, AMI continues to be a serious public health problem. It has been estimated that 14.2 years of life are lost secondary to an AMI, and the cost to American society (both direct and indirect) is $142.5 billion per year.

DIAGNOSIS

【 】 SYMPTOMS

The classic symptom of AMI is precordial or retrosternal discomfort that is commonly described as a pressure, crushing, aching, or burning sensation. Radiation of the discomfort to the neck, back, or arms frequently occurs, and the pain is usually persistent. The discomfort typically achieves maximum intensity over several minutes and can be associated with nausea, diaphoresis, generalized weakness, and a fear of impending death. Some patients, particular the elderly, may also present with syncope, unexplained nausea and vomiting, acute confusion, agitation, or palpitations.

Approximately 20% of AMI patients are asymptomatic or have atypical symptoms. Painless myocardial infarction (MI) occurs more frequently in the elderly, women, diabetics, and postoperative patients. These patients tend to present with dyspnea or frank congestive heart failure as their initial symptom.

【 】 PHYSICAL EXAM

Patients can appear anxious and uncomfortable. Those with substantial left ventricular (LV) dysfunction at presentation may have tachycardia, pulmonary rales, tachypnea, and a third heart sound. The presence of a mitral regurgitant murmur suggests ischemic dysfunction of the mitral valve apparatus, rupture, or ventricular remodeling.

In patients with right ventricular infarction, increased jugular venous pressure, Kussmaul's sign, and a right ventricular third sound may be present. Such patients virtually always have inferior infarctions, usually without evidence of left-heart failure, and may have exquisite blood pressure sensitivity to nitrates or hypovolemia. In patients with extensive left ventricular dysfunction, shock is indicated by hypotension, diaphoresis, cool skin and extremities, pallor, oliguria, and possible confusion.

【 　】 ELECTROCARDIOGRAM

All patients presenting with chest pain should have an electrocardiogram (ECG) performed within 10 minutes of arrival to the emergency department. The classic initial ECG manifestations of STEMI, discussed in Chapter 2, involve an increase in the amplitude of the T wave (peaking), followed within minutes by ST-segment elevation. The R wave may initially increase in height but soon decreases, and often Q waves form. If the jeopardized myocardium is reperfused, the ST segment may promptly revert to normal, although T waves can remain inverted, and Q waves may or may not regress. Persistent ST-segment elevation after restoration of flow in the epicardial coronary artery is a marker of failed myocardial perfusion and associated with an adverse prognosis. In the absence of reperfusion, the ST segment gradually returns to baseline in several hours to days, and T waves become symmetrically inverted. Failure of the T wave to invert in 24 to 48 hours suggest regional pericarditis.

New-onset left bundle-branch block (LBBB) in the setting of chest pain is considered STEMI. The diagnosis of STEMI in the setting of old LBBB can be difficult. Findings suggesting STEMI include (1) ST-segment elevation ≥ 1 mm concordant with the QRS complex; (2) ST-segment depression ≥ 1 mm in leads V_1, V_2, or V_3; and (3) ST-segment elevation ≥ 5 mm discordant with the QRS.

The ECG has several limitations (Chapter 2), which relate to specificity and sensitivity.

【 　】 LABORATORY STUDIES

Myoglobin

Myoglobin is a 17.8-kd protein that is released from injured myocardial cells. As shown in Fig. 24-1, myoglobin release occurs within hours after the onset of infarction, reaches peak levels at 1 to 4 hours, and remains elevated for about 24 hours. Although the rapid rise allows for its use as an early marker for STEMI, myoglobin is not specific to myocardial cells and should not be used in isolation as a method for diagnosing MI.

【 　】 CK-MB

The MB isoenzyme of creatine kinase is present in the largest concentration in the myocardium, although small amounts (1%–2%) can be found in skeletal muscle, tongue, small intestine, and diaphragm. Creatinine kinase-MB (CK-MB) appears in serum within 3 hours after the onset of infarction, reaches peak levels at 12 to 24 hours, and has a mean duration of activity of 1 to 3 days. Other cardiac but non-AMI etiologies of increased CK-MB levels can occur after cardioversion, cardiac surgery, myopericarditis, percutaneous coronary intervention (PCI), and occasionally after rapid tachycardia. Noncardiac causes of increased CK-MB levels may occur with hypothyroidism, extensive skeletal muscle trauma, rhabdomyolysis, and muscular dystrophy.

Occasionally, the concentration of Creatinine kinase- MB (CK-MB) isoenzyme may be increased in the presence of normal total levels of CK enzyme. This finding usually indicates a small amount of myocardial necrosis in a patient whose baseline total CK enzyme level is at the low-normal end of the range (see Chapter 25).

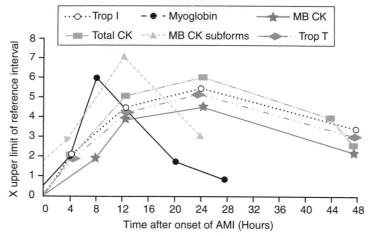

FIGURE 24-1. Temporal profile of the diagnostic biomarkers used for detecting MI. The plasma temporal profile for early detection is illustrated for myoglobin and CK-MB subforms. The markers CK-MB, total CK, and cardiac troponins I and T are all released with a similar initial time profile. However, troponins I and T remain elevated for 10 to 14 days and thus are better markers for late diagnosis than CK-MB.

Troponins

The cardiac troponins regulate the interaction of actin and myosin and are more cardiac specific than CK-MB. There are two isoforms of cardiac troponin: T and I. Their levels start to rise 3 to 12 hours after the onset of ischemia, peak at 12 to 24 hours, and may remain elevated for 8 to 21 days (troponin T) or 7 to 14 days (troponin I). Elevated troponin levels correlate with pathologically proven myocardial necrosis and indicate poor prognosis in patients with suspected acute coronary syndromes (see Chapter 25).

INITIAL MANAGEMENT

【 】 EVALUATION IN THE EMERGENCY DEPARTMENT

The cornerstone of STEMI therapy is a rapid and accurate evaluation in the emergency department. All patients presenting with complaints of chest discomfort should be rapidly triaged and allowed to bypass the emergency department waiting room. *An ECG should be obtained within the first 10 minutes of arrival and a focused history and physical examination assessing the symptoms and signs described in the diagnosis section of this chapter should be quickly performed.*

The physical examination also provides a method for the risk stratification of STEMI patients. As shown in Table 24-1, the Killip classification can be used as method to stratify patients and predict clinical outcomes.

【 】 INITIAL THERAPY

The initial management of patients in the emergency department includes the use of oxygen, aspirin, beta-blockers, analgesia, nitroglycerin, and anticoagulation with heparin (Table 24-2).

TABLE 24-1

Killip Classification for Patients with STEMI

Killip Class	Hospital Mortality (%)
I. No CHF	6
II. Mild CHF, rales, S_3, congestion on chest radiograph	17
III. Pulmonary edema	38
IV. Cardiogenic shock	81[a]

CHF, congestive heart failure.

[a]Has improved to about 60% with current therapy.

Oxygen

Although routine use of supplemental oxygen is common practice, hard evidence supporting its use is lacking. Low-flow oxygen therapy delivered by nasal cannula should be routinely given during the first 24 to 48 hours in most STEMI patients. Mild hypoxemia is not uncommon, even in the absence of apparent pulmonary congestion. Additionally, some patients may have dyspnea related to acute changes in left ventricular compliance and secondarily increased pulmonary interstitial fluid.

Aspirin

Aspirin is an antiplatelet agent that has been shown to decrease mortality in AMI patients by about 20%. It should be administered as early as possible and continued

TABLE 24-2

Initial Management of STEMI

Treatment	Dose	Notes
Oxygen	1–2 L	Use for first 24–48 h
Aspirin	160–325 mg chewable	If aspirin allergy exists, use clopidogrel 300 mg
Beta-blockers	Metoprolol 5 mg IV every 5 minutes for max 15 mg, then oral	Do not use if there are signs of heart failure of cardiogenic shock
Morphine	1–2 mg IV	Do not over-sedate patient
Nitroglycerin	Start drip at 5–10 μg/min and titrate to pain and blood pressure	Do not use in patients with recent use of a phosphodi esterase type 5 inhibitor (Viagara, etc.) or suspected RV infarct
Heparin	Unfractionated: 60 U/kg IV bolus (4000 U max) followed by 12 U/kg/h drip (max 100 U/h) Low molecular weight: enoxaparin 30 mg IV bolus then 1 mg/kg SQ every 12 h	Unfractionated heparin should be favored in patients undergoing primary PCI and those with severe renal dysfunction

indefinitely in patients with acute coronary syndromes. Chewable aspirin 160 to 325 mg should be given to patients at presentation, with a subsequent dose of 75 to 325 mg daily. For those with a history of a documented significant adverse reaction to aspirin, 300 mg of clopidogrel can be used as an alternative.

Beta-Blockers

The efficacy of beta-blockers in acute coronary syndromes has been documented with a decrease in early and late mortality. In pooled data from 28 trials of beta-blockers, the average mortality decrease was 28% at 1 week, with the majority of benefit occurring in the first 48 hours. Specifically, reinfarction was reduced by 18% and cardiac arrest by 15%. The long-term effects of beta-blockade for the secondary prevention of death after MI have also been established by large-scale randomized trials.

Traditionally, metoprolol has been the agent of choice and is initially administered intravenously as 5-mg boluses at 10-minute intervals for three doses followed by an oral dose. However, in patients with clinical evidence of heart failure, there is a 30% relative increase in the risk of cardiogenic shock. *Therefore, the use of beta-blockade in patients with evidence of hemodynamic instability should be delayed until the patients become stable.* Also, the routine initial intravenous dose should be reconsidered as standard therapy. Finally, the benefits of beta-blockade in patients undergoing primary PCI remain unclear and there have been no randomized prospective studies.

Analgesia

Morphine is frequently used for pain relief and is best administered intravenously in boluses of 1 to 2 mg, to a maximum of 10 to 15 mg for a normal adult. Respiratory depression can occur and care must be taken not to over-sedate patients. Morphine should be used with caution in patients with hemodynamic instability because of its effects on reducing cardiac preload.

Nitrates

Nitroglycerin causes a non–endothelium-dependent coronary vasodilatation, systemic venodilatation, reduced cardiac preload, and enhanced perfusion of ischemic myocardial zones. Intravenous nitroglycerin is effective in relieving chest pain and should be initiated at 5 to 10 μg/min and gradually increased with a goal of a 10% to 30% reduction in systolic blood pressure and symptomatic pain relief. In most patients, use of this agent will be tapered within 24 to 36 hours. Nitrates should not be administered to patients with recent sildenafil use. In addition, nitrates should be used with caution in RV infarct patients in order to avoid profound hypotension.

Heparin

Anticoagulation with heparin is essential in the management of STEMI. Currently two forms of heparin are utilized: unfractionated heparin and low molecular weight heparin (LMWH).

Unfractionated heparin, when bound to antithrombin III, inactivates factor Xa and thrombin. Its use has been widely studied and unfractionated heparin is considered a class I (see Chapter 59) indication for patients with STEMI undergoing primary PCI or receiving fibrin-specific thrombolytic agents. An initial bolus of 60 U/kg (4,000 U maximum) followed by a 12 U/kg/h (1,000 U/h maximum) infusion should be administered promptly. A goal aPTT of 1.5 to 2.0 times normal should be achieved. The LMWHs are glycosaminoglycans consisting of chains of alternating residues of D-glucosamine and uronic acid. When compared to unfractionated heparin, they have a more predictable anticoagulation effect due to a longer half-life, better bioavailability, and dose-independent clearance. The LMWHs have a greater activity against Xa than thrombin and their anticoagulation effect cannot be measured with standard laboratory tests.

The use of the LMWH enoxaparin in conjunction with thrombolysis has been studied in the ASSENT 3 (Assessment of the Safety and Efficacy of a New Thrombolytic regimen) and TIMI-25 EXTRACT (Enoxaparin and Thrombolysis Reperfusion for Acute Myocardial Infarction Treatment) trials. In the ASSENT 3 trial, patients treated with enoxaparin plus tenecteplase had a lower combined end point of 30-day mortality, in-hospital reinfarction, and in-hospital refractory ischemia than those treated with unfractionated heparin plus tenecteplase (11.4% versus 15.4 %, p = 0.0002). The TIMI 25 EXTRACT trial randomized 20,506 patients undergoing thrombolytic therapy for STEMI to anticoagulation with enoxaparin through the entire index hospitalization or unfractionated heparin for the initial 48 hours. The combined primary end point of death or recurrent MI at 30 days occurred in 9.9% of patients in the enoxaparin group and in 12% of those in the heparin group (p < 0.001).

Because of the delay in the onset of action of subcutaneous administration, an initial intravenous loading dose of 30 mg of enoxaparin followed by the traditional 1 mg/kg subcutaneous dose every 12 hours was used in both trials for patients less than 75 years of age.

Direct Thrombin Inhibitors

Direct thrombin inhibitors bind directly to thrombin and should be used as an alternative to heparin in patients with known or suspected heparin-induced thrombocytopenia. A recent meta-analysis of 11 randomized trials demonstrated that compared with heparin, direct thrombin inhibitors were associated with a lower risk of death or MI both at the end of treatment (4.3% versus 5.1%, p = 0.001) and at 30 days (7.4% versus 8.2%, p = 0.02). This difference was due primarily to a reduction in the incidence of reinfarction (2.8% versus 3.5%, p < 0.001) with *no difference in mortality* . There was no excess in intracranial hemorrhage with any direct thrombin inhibitor.

REPERFUSION STRATEGIES

Rapid reperfusion of ischemic myocardium is the main goal of STEMI management. Currently, the three main reperfusion strategies for STEMI are thrombolytic therapy, primary percutaneous coronary intervention (PCI), and thrombolytic facilitated PCI.

【 】 THROMBOLYTICS

Thrombolytic therapy for STEMI has been shown to be effective in reducing mortality in numerous randomized trials involving over 100,000 patients. It is widely available, easily administered, and is relatively inexpensive. However, only approximately 50% of STEMI patients are eligible for thrombolytic therapy (Table 24-3), and only 50% to 60% of patients treated with thrombolytics will achieve complete reperfusion. In addition, 10% to 20% of patients will experience reocclusion and 1% will suffer from a stroke caused by intracranial hemorrhage. Thrombolytic therapy is most effective when given within 3 hours from onset of chest pain.

Although streptokinase is still widely used around the world, fibrin-specific agents are almost exclusively used in the United States. Clinical trials of these agents have shown TIMI-3 flow rates in excess of 60%; however, there was no significant reduction in mortality or in the incidence of stroke when compared to non–fibrin-specific agents.

【 】 PRIMARY PCI

Approximately 95% of patients treated with primary PCI obtain complete reperfusion versus 50% to 60% of patients treated with thrombolytics. Primary PCI is also associated with a lower risk of stroke, and diagnostic angiography quickly defines coronary anatomy, LV function, and mechanical complications. However, invasive cardiovascular

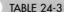

TABLE 24-3

Absolute and Relative Contraindications for Thrombolytic Therapy in Patients with ST-Segment Elevation Myocardial Infarction

Absolute Contraindications

Any prior intracranial hemorrhage
Known structural cerebral vascular lesion
Known intracranial neoplasm
Ischemic stroke within the past 3 months (except for acute stroke within 3 hours)
Suspected aortic dissection
Active bleeding or bleeding diathesis (excluding menses)
Significant closed-head or facial trauma within 3 months

Relative Contraindications

History of chronic, sever, poorly controlled hypertension
Systolic pressure >180 mm Hg or diastolic 110 mm Hg
History of prior ischemic stroke > 3 months previously, dementia, or known
   intracranial pathology not covered in absolute contraindications
Recent (within 2–4 weeks) internal bleeding
Noncompressible vascular punctures
Pregnancy
Active peptic ulcer
Current use of anticoagulants: the higher the INR, the higher the risk of bleeding
For streptokinase / anistreplase: prior exposure (more than 5 days previously) or
   prior allergic reaction to these agents

services are only available at < 20% of hospitals in the United States and require a significant investment in infrastructure, personnel, and training as well as maintenance in case volume and expertise.

A meta-analysis by Keeley and colleagues of 23 trials including 3,872 patients treated with primary PCI and 3,867 patients treated with thrombolytics showed that PCI was superior to thrombolytic therapy. Primary PCI was associated with a lower mortality rate (7% versus 9%, $p = 0.0002$), less reinfarction (3% versus 7%, $p = 0.0001$), and fewer strokes (1% versus 2%, $p = 0.0004$) at 30 days when compared to thrombolysis. PCI capability, however, is only available at < 20% of hospitals in the United States, and each 30-minute delay from symptom onset to balloon inflation during primary PCI is associated with a 7.5% relative increase in mortality at 1 year. In addition, a meta-analysis of data from 23 trials containing 7,739 patients comparing thrombolytic therapy to primary PCI by Nallamothu and Bates demonstrated that the mortality advantage of primary PCI is lost if the door-to-balloon time is 60 minutes greater than the door-to-needle time for thrombolytic therapy.

Three large-scale randomized trials have compared thrombolysis to transfer for primary PCI in STEMI patients. The combined end point of death, reinfarction, and disabling stroke at 30 days was significantly lower in the patients treated with primary PCI. Although transfer for primary PCI appears to be the treatment of choice, two important points need emphasizing. First, the transport time in these trials was extremely short (median time in the DANAMI2 trial was 32 minutes), and these times may not be achievable outside of a clinical trial and in areas in which longer distances and weather may play a substantial role in transit time. Second, thrombolytic therapy still has a critically important role during the "golden hour" of MI or when there is a delay in transfer. The mortality rates and infarct size in patients treated with thrombolytic therapy within the first 60 to 90 minutes of symptoms are extremely low, suggesting that thromblytic therapy still plays a vital role in the management of patients presenting to hospitals without primary PCI capability.

【 】 THROMBOLYTIC FACILITATED PCI

Thrombolytic-facilitated PCI refers to the pretreatment with thrombolytics in STEMI patients as a bridge to immediate PCI. This pretreatment has been proposed as a method to initiate earlier reperfusion and reduce ischemic time and infarct size in patients who experience a delay before the onset of PCI. Thrombolytic-facilitated therapy, however, can also expose patients to a higher risk of bleeding. Thrombolytic-facilitated PCI showed no survival benefit compared to primary PCI. In addition, thrombolytic-facilitated PCI is associated with a higher risk of major and minor bleeding compared to primary PCI. *Thus, thrombolytic-facilitated PCI should not be considered as a first-line reperfusion strategy for STEMI patients.*

【 】 SELECTION OF THE OPTIMAL REPERFUSION STRATEGY

STEMI patients presenting to a hospital with PCI capabilities should undergo primary PCI. Selection of a reperfusion strategy in patients who present to a hospital without PCI facilities is more complex. Patients who are not eligible for thrombolytic therapy should be immediately transferred to a tertiary care hospital for primary PCI. For those who are eligible for thrombolytic therapy, the clinician must consider two important factors: duration from onset of symptoms ("fixed" ischemia time) and transport time to the nearest PCI facility ("incurred" ischemia time). These two factors can be incorporated into a 2 × 3 table to select a reperfusion strategy (Fig. 24-2).

Patients facing a transport time < 30 minutes should be transferred for primary PCI. Thrombolytic-eligible patients who present < 2 to 3 hours from onset of symptoms and have > 60 minutes transport time should receive thrombolytic therapy. Patients presenting > 2 to 3 hours after the onset of chest pain and have a transport time of 60 minutes or less should be promptly transported for primary PCI. If the anticipated transport time is > 60 minutes

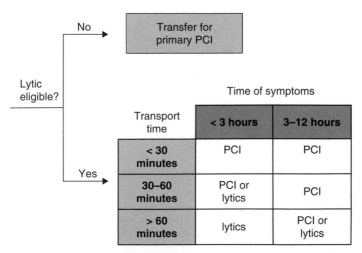

FIGURE 24-2. Reperfussion strategy for STEMI patients who present to hospitals without primary PCI. (Lytics, thrombolysis and transfer; PCI, transfer for percutaneous coronary intervention.)

for a patient presenting > 3 hours from the onset of chest pain, either thrombolytic therapy or primary PCI can be considered. The choice of using thrombolytic therapy should always be considered along with the risk of bleeding in each individual patient.

All patients receiving thrombolytic therapy should also be transferred to a PCI facility for potential failure to reperfuse (ongoing chest pain or < 50% resolution of ST-segment elevation at 90 minutes) and rescue PCI. Recent randomized data suggest that all STEMI patients treated with thrombolytic therapy benefited from routine coronary angiography during the index hospitalization.

ADJUVANT ANTIPLATELET THERAPY

【 】 CLOPIDOGREL

Clopidogrel is an oral thienopyridine pro-drug whose active metabolite inhibits the activation of platelets by adenosine diphosphate. Its antiplatelet effects are more potent than aspirin and less potent than the glycoprotein IIb/IIIa inhibitors.

Use with Thrombolytic Therapy

Clopidogrel, in combination with thrombolytic therapy, has been studied in the CLARITY-TIMI 28 trial. A total of 3,491 STEMI patients 75 years of age or younger treated with thrombolytics were randomized to therapy with aspirin plus placebo or aspirin plus clopidogrel. Clopidogrel was given as a 300-mg loading dose within minutes of thrombolysis and 75 mg daily thereafter. The composite primary end point of death, reinfarction prior to angiography, or occluded infarct-related artery at angiography occurred in 15% of patients in the clopidogrel group and 22% of patients in the placebo group ($p < 0.001$). The use of clopidogrel was not associated with a higher rate of major or minor bleeding.

Patients older than 75 years of age were included in COMMIT (Randomized, Placebo-Controlled trial of adding clopidogrel to aspirin in 46,000 AMI patients), which randomized 45,849 STEMI patients treated with thrombolysis to therapy with aspirin plus placebo or aspirin plus clopidogrel. In this trial, patients randomized to the clopidogrel arm received 75 mg of clopidogrel at the time of thrombolysis and then 75 mg daily for the duration of hospitalization. Patients in the clopidogrel arm had a lower rate of the composite end point of death, reinfarction, or stroke (9.3% versus 10.1%, $p = 0.002$) and no increase in major or minor bleeding.

The data from these two trials suggest that patients treated with thrombolytics should receive clopidogrel. For patients older than 75 years of age, 75 mg of clopidogrel without a loading dose should be used. In patients 75 years of age or younger, the current data suggest that a 300-mg loading dose followed by 75 mg daily of clopidogrel is beneficial and safe.

Use with Primary PCI

The benefit of aspirin plus clopidogrel in the setting of primary PCI for STEMI is unknown. No studies have compared early administration of clopidogrel to the early use of glycoprotein IIb/IIIa inhibitors in STEMI patients. *Therefore, clopidogrel should not be used in STEMI patients prior to visualization of the coronary anatomy at the time of coronary angiography.*

【 】 GLYCOPROTEIN IIB/IIIA INHIBITORS

Glycoprotein IIb/IIIa inhibitors are potent agents that inhibit the final common pathway for platelet aggregation. There are currently three intravenous agents available in the United States: abciximab, tirofiban, and eptifibatide.

Use with Thrombolytic Therapy

Thrombolysis has been shown to be a potent activator of platelets and the concomitant use of aspirin along with thrombolysis has been shown to be of benefit. Two dose-finding studies have shown that the glycoprotein IIb/IIIa inhibitor abciximab, when used in combination with half-dose thromboblytics, improves coronary artery blood flow in STEMI patients. Three subsequent randomized trials have investigated combination therapy with a glycoprotein IIb/IIIa inhibitor and half-dose thrombolytic therapy. These studies showed that combination therapy increases risk of bleeding and does not improve mortality. *Thus, glycoprotein IIb/IIIa inhibitors should not be used in combination with thrombolytic therapy.*

Use with Primary PCI

The early (prior to arrival in the catherization laboratory) versus delayed (at the time of catherization) use of glycoprotein IIb/IIIa inhibitors in STEMI patients has been investigated in eight randomized trials involving abciximab, tirofiban, and eptifibatide. A meta-analysis of six of these trials by Montalescot and colleagues showed that early administration of glycoprotein IIb/IIIa inhibitors in STEMI patients was associated with a greater prevalence of TIMI 2 or 3 flow (41.7 % versus 29.8 %, $p < 0.001$) in the infarct-related artery prior to PCI. Since prior studies have shown that better coronary artery flow after PCI is associated with fewer in-hospital and 1-year adverse outcomes, early administration of glycoprotein IIb/IIIa inhibitors should be *considered* in STEMI patients undergoing primary PCI.

PHARMACOTHERAPY AFTER REPERFUSION

【　】 ANGIOTENSIN-CONVERTING ENZYME (ACE) INHIBITORS

Treatment with ACE inhibitors within the first 24 hours of reperfusion is reasonable as long as no contraindications exist and the patient is hemodynamically stable. Patients with an ejection fraction of more than 45% and no clinical evidence of heart failure, significant mitral regurgitation, or hypertension can have therapy discontinued after determination of risk status while still hospitalized. Since captopril has the shortest half-life, overdosing and inadvertent hypotension may be most easily correctable with the use of this agent. In addition, the short half-life allows for more rapid titration. Intravenous administration is unnecessary unless the patient is unable to take oral medication. Duration of treatment is uncertain; however, many patients will be treated indefinitely.

【　】 BETA-BLOCKERS

Initiation of beta-blockade therapy in the CCU is essential in the management of STEMI patients. *Beta-blockers* have been shown to have both *acute and long-term benefits in STEMI patients* treated with either lysis or primary PCI. Short acting beta-blockade with metoprolol should be initiated as early as possible and rapidly titrated to the maximally tolerated dose. In patients who present with shock or heart failure, the initiation of beta-blockers should be delayed until patients become hemodynamically stable.

【　】 ASPIRIN

The use of aspirin in the initial management of STEMI patients was previously discussed. Once initiated, patients should remain on aspirin indefinitely. A dose between 75 and 162 mg a day is recommended. Patients who are allergic to aspirin should be given 75 mg of clopidogrel daily.

【 】 THIENOPYRIDINES

A thienopyridine, ticlopidine or clopidogrel, should be given in addition to aspirin to patients receiving *coronary artery stenting*. The minimal duration of therapy depends of the type of stent implanted. Patients with bare metal stents should be treated for a minimum of 30 days, while those with a drug-eluting stent should receive at least 1 year of therapy.

【 】 STATINS

Several trials have demonstrated that statins should be used in the secondary prevention of patients with coronary artery disease. In addition to lowering LDL cholesterol, statins have also been demonstrated to improve endothelial function, have antiplatelet effects, and reduce inflammation.

SECONDARY PREVENTION

Aggressive secondary prevention measures should be instituted during the initial hospitalization. These include smoking cessation, weight reduction, dietary modifications, glucose control, and enrollment in a cardiac rehab program.

SUGGESTED READING

Antman EM, Anbe DT, Armstrong PW, et al. ACC/AHA guidelines for the management of patients with ST-elevation myocardial infarction: a report of the American College of Cardiology/American Heart Association Task Force on Practice Guidelines (Committee to Revise the 1999 Guidelines for the Management of Patients with Acute Myocardial Infarction). *J Am Coll Cardiol.* 2004;44:e1–e211.

Ting H, Yang EH, Rihal CS. Reperfusion strategies for ST-segment elevation myocardial infarction. *Ann Intern Med.* 2006;145:610–617.

CHAPTER (25)

Diagnosis and Management of Patients with Unstable Angina and Non–ST-Segment Elevation Myocardial Infarction

Susan A. Matulevicius, Anand Rohatgi,
and James A. de Lemos

Unstable angina (UA) and non–ST-elevation myocardial infarction (NSTEMI) are two related forms of acute coronary syndrome (ACS) caused by rupture or erosion of an atherosclerotic plaque with platelet-thrombus formation and subsequent obstruction to coronary artery blood flow. They are differentiated from ST-elevation MI (STEMI; see Chapter 24) by the absence of ST elevation or a new left bundle-branch block on the presenting electrocardiogram (ECG). NSTEMI is further differentiated from UA by the detection of bloodstream markers of myocardial injury, including troponin I, troponin T, or creatinine kinase myocardial band (CK-MB). In 2004, the National Center for Health Statistics reported 1,565,000 discharges for ACS, of which 896,000 were for MI (both ST-EMI and NSTEMI), and 669,000 were for UA. Treatment of UA and NSTEMI is essentially identical, depending on level of risk.

Serum biomarkers, such as troponins I and T, C-reactive protein (CRP), brain natriuretic peptide (BNP), and N-terminal pro-BNP (NT pro-BNP) aid in more accurate risk stratification in patients with ACS. Newer therapies, including low-molecular-weight heparins (LMWH), factor Xa inhibitors and direct anti-thrombins, platelet glycoprotein (GP) IIb/IIIa receptor antagonists, thienopyridines (clopidogrel), early use of high-dose statins, and percutaneous revascularization with drug-eluting stents for *higher-risk* patients have improved outcomes in patients with UA/NSTEMI.

DEFINITION AND CLASSIFICATION

UA/NSTEMI is a clinical syndrome usually caused by atherosclerotic plaque rupture and thrombosis within a coronary artery, resulting in an imbalance in myocardial oxygen supply and demand, and associated with an increased risk of subsequent cardiac death and new or recurrent myocardial infarction. UA is defined as angina that is new-onset or abruptly increased in intensity, duration, or frequency within the past 60 days. NSTEMI is identified by clinical symptoms as UA plus myocardial injury as evidenced by elevated serum cardiac biomarkers.

ETIOLOGY

There are several potential causes for the imbalance between myocardial oxygen supply and demand seen in UA/NSTEMI, including:

1. Coronary artery luminal narrowing due to a nonocclusive thrombus that develops following rupture or erosion of an atherothrombotic plaque.

2. Severe coronary artery narrowing without spasm or thrombosis, which typically occurs in patients with progressive atherosclerosis or with restenosis within 6 months after percutaneous coronary intervention (PCI).

3. Intense focal spasm of a segment of an epicardial coronary artery (Prinzmetal or variant angina) causing dynamic obstruction of the coronary artery lumen.

4. Coronary artery dissection (a cause of ACS in women in the peripartum period).

5. Precipitating factors extrinsic to the coronary arterial bed that limit myocardial perfusion, including sudden increases in myocardial oxygen demand (sepsis, fever, tachycardia), reductions in coronary blood flow (hypotension), or decreased myocardial oxygen delivery (hypoxia, severe anemia).

DIAGNOSIS AND RISK STRATIFICATION

Expeditious evaluation of ACS patients is paramount to providing timely and appropriate therapies (Fig. 25-1). Initial evaluation of chest pain should triage patients into one of four categories: (1) noncardiac chest pain, (2) chronic stable angina, (3) possible ACS, or (4) definite ACS. Patients with symptoms suggesting ACS should be referred to a facility that can perform a thorough history and physical, ECG, and biomarker determination. Any chest pain lasting longer than 20 minutes, hemodynamic instability, or recent syncope or presyncope should be referred to a hospital emergency department and ideally should be transported by emergency medical services. Once it has been determined that a patient has a probable cardiac source of their symptoms, risk stratification into low-, intermediate-, or high-risk categories should be performed.

The American College of Cardiology/American Heart Association (ACC/AHA) 2007 Guideline Update for the Management of Patients with UA and NSTEMI uses features of the clinical history (advanced age, accelerating angina in last 48 hours, prior MI, Coronary artery bypass grafting [CABG] cerebrovascular or peripheral arterial disease, aspirin use); pain characteristics (intensity, duration, provocation of angina); clinical findings (pulmonary edema or other signs of heart failure); ECG findings; and levels of cardiac biomarkers to determine an individual's risk (Table 25-1). Transient ST-segment changes (> 0.05 mV) during a symptomatic episode at rest that resolve when the patient becomes asymptomatic strongly suggest acute ischemia and a high likelihood of underlying severe coronary artery disease (CAD). This early risk assessment is critical, as it establishes the intensity of future therapies. A patient with a low risk may be discharged home with aspirin and beta-blockers, often with an early outpatient stress test (within 72 hours of admission). High-risk patients may be admitted to a coronary care unit, treated with multiple drugs, and undergo coronary angiography and revascularization urgently. The risk assessment should be updated during hospitalization if a patient's clinical status, ECG, or cardiac biomarkers change, and as new data become available. Clinical risk predictor models, such as the TIMI and GRACE prediction tools, can help determine an individual's short-term and long-term risk and the need for aggressive therapy (Fig. 25-2).

[ ] INITIAL EVALUATION

UA/NSTEMI may present as rest angina, new-onset severe angina, or increasing angina as graded by the Canadian Cardiovascular Society Classifications. In patients with known underlying CAD, symptoms similar to prior episodes of angina or MI suggest ischemia and should be managed aggressively. Patients with known CABG may have atherothrombosis of venous bypass grafts and patients with PCI within the past 6 months may have restenosis and benefit from an early invasive treatment strategy.

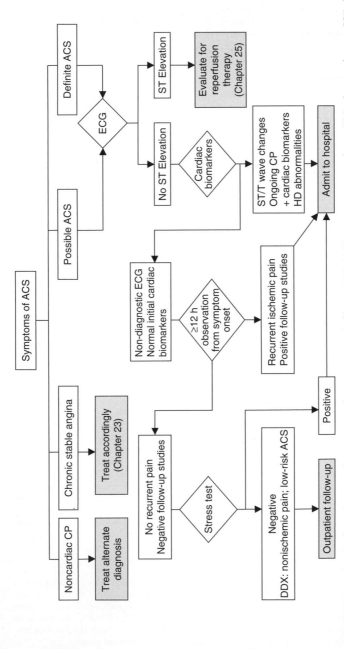

FIGURE 25-1. Algorithm for evaluation and management of patients suspected of having ACS. (ACS, acute coronary syndrome; ECG, electrocardiogram; DDX, differential diagnosis.) (Adapted from ACC/AHA guidelines.)

TABLE 25-1

Short-Term Risk of Death or Nonfatal Myocardial Infarction in Patients with UA/NSTEMI[a]

Feature	High Risk (≥ 2 Features)	Intermediate Risk (No High-Risk Features, ≥1 of the Following Features)	Low Risk (No High- or Intermediate-Risk Features, but Following Features May Be Present)
History	↑ Ischemic symptoms over last 48 h	Prior MI, PVD, CVD, disease, or CABG; prior ASA use	
Character of pain	> 20 min of ongoing rest pain	> 20 min rest pain, now resolved, with moderate or high likelihood of CAD	New-onset chest pain within 2 weeks to 2 months
		Rest pain relieved with rest or SL NTG or lasting < 20 min	
		Nighttime chest pain	
		New or progressive CCS class II or IV chest pain in the past 2 weeks without > 20 min of rest pain with moderate or high likelihood of CAD	
Clinical findings	Age > 75 y Pulmonary edema, rales New or worsening MR murmur, S_3 ↓BP, ↓ HR, ↑ HR	Age > 70 y	
ECG findings	Rest pain with transient ST-segment changes > 0.05 mV New bundle-branch block Sustained VT	T-wave changes Pathologic Q waves Resting ST depressions < 1 mm in multiple leads	Normal or unchanged ECG
Cardiac markers	TnT or TnI > 0.1 ng/mL	0.01 ng/mL < TnT < 0.1 ng/mL	Normal

ASA, aspirin; CABG, coronary artery bypass grafting; CAD, coronary artery disease; CCS, Canadian Cardiovascular Society; CVD, cerebrovascular disease; ECG, electrocardiogram; MR, mitral regurgitation; PVD, peripheral vascular disease; SL NTG, sublingual nitroglycerin; TnT, troponin T; TnI, troponin I.

[a]Estimation of the short-term risk of death and nonfatal cardiac ischemic events in UA is a complex multivariable problem that cannot be fully specified in a table; therefore, this table is meant to offer general guidance and illustration rather than rigid algorithms.

Adapted from Braunwald E, Mark CB, Jones RH, et al. *AHCPR Clinical Practice Guideline no. 10. Unstable Angina: Diagnosis and Management.* Rockville, MD: Agency for Health Care Policy and Research and the National Heart, Lung, and Blood Institute, U.S. Public Health Service, U.S. Department of Health and Human Services; 1994; AHCPR pub. no. 94-0602.

GRACE Risk Predictors:		Points	GRACE Risk Predictors:		Points
Age (y):	≤39	0	SBP (mm/Hg):	≤79.9	24
	40–49	18		80–99.9	22
	50–59	36		100–119.9	18
	60–69	55		120–139.9	14
	70–79	78		140–159.9	10
	80–89	91		160–199.9	4
	≥90	100		≥200	0
Positive CHF Hx		24	ST segment depression		11
Positive MI Hx		12	Cr (mg/dL):	≤0.39	1
Rest HR (bpm):	≤49.9	0		0.4–0.79	3
	50–69.9	3		0.8–1.19	5
	70–89.9	9		1.2–1.59	7
	90–109.9	14		1.6–1.99	9
	110–149.9	23		2–3.99	15
	150–199.9	35		≥4.0	20
	≥200	43	Positive cardiac markers		15
			No in–house PCI		14

TOTAL SCORE:

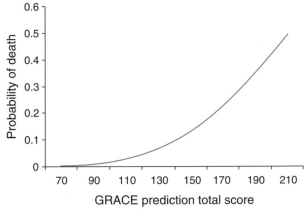

FIGURE 25-2. Clinical risk prediction tools. The GRACE scorecard and nomogram predict mortality 6 months postdischarge, and the TIMI risk score predicts risk of death, MI, or recurrent ischemia within 14 days of randomization. (Data complied from Antman EM, Cohen M, Bernink PJ, et al. The TIMI risk score for unstable angina/non-ST elevation MI: a method of prognostication and therapeutic decision making. *JAMA.* 2000;284:835–842; and Eagle KA, Lim MJ, Dabbous OH, et al. A validated prediction model for all forms of acute coronary syndrome: estimating the risk of 6-month post-discharge death in an international registry. *JAMA.* 2004;291:2727–2733.)

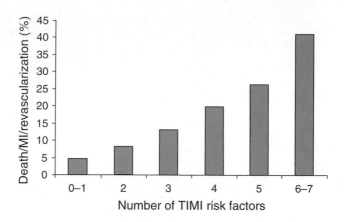

TIMI Risk Predictors

- Age ≥65 yr
- ≥3 CAD risk factors
  (hypertension, diabetes, high
  cholesterol, family history,
  smoking)
- Prior coronary stenosis ≥50%
- ST deviation
- ≥2 anginal events in 24 hr
- Elevated troponin or CK-MB
- ASA use within last 7 days

FIGURE 25-2. (*Continued*)

"Atypical" symptoms such as acute dyspnea, indigestion, unusual locations of pain, agitation, altered mental status, profound weakness, or syncope may be the presenting manifestations of ACS particularly in women, the elderly, and patients with long-standing diabetes mellitus. Atypical symptoms, especially within these patient subgroups, are associated with a higher risk of death and major complications.

【 】 HISTORY AND PHYSICAL EXAMINATION

Myocardial ischemia is commonly experienced as a pressure-like sensation in the retrosternal area; however, "anginal equivalents" may present as epigatric, arm, jaw, or back discomfort. Patients may describe the discomfort as *burning, squeezing, pressure-like*, or *heavy*, but less commonly *sharp, jabbing*, or *knife-like*. However, atypical features do not reliably exclude the possibility of UA/NSTEMI.

In a patient younger than 50 years of age who presents with symptoms of UA/NSTEMI, cocaine use should be considered as a potential trigger.

Once a complete history and physical have been performed, the physician caring for the patient with suspected UA/NSTEMI should classify the likelihood of the patient's symptoms being due to myocardial ischemia as being high, intermediate, or low. The history should take into account the nature of the anginal symptoms, prior CAD history, age, sex, and the number of traditional risk factors for CAD.

【　】 THE ELECTROCARDIOGRAM

A 12-lead ECG should be performed and shown to a physician within 10 minutes of arrival to the emergency room or other facility for all patients presenting with symptoms suggesting UA/NSTEMI. If the initial ECG is not diagnostic but there is a high clinical suspicion for ACS, serial ECGs should be performed to detect the development of ST depressions or elevations over the next 24 to 48 hours. A normal ECG during an episode of chest pain does not rule out ACS. Transient ST-segment depressions of at least 0.5 mm during chest discomfort that disappear with relief of the chest pain provide objective evidence of transient myocardial ischemia. Persistent T-wave inversions over the involved territory are common in patients with UA. Deep, symmetric T-wave inversions across the precordial leads suggest proximal, severe left anterior descending (LAD) coronary artery stenosis. An ECG with Q waves from a previous infarction or an old left bundle-branch block, signifying prior LV damage, may be seen in patients with UA/NSTEMI and is associated with a higher risk.

【　】 CARDIAC BIOMARKERS

Cardiac biomarkers are both diagnostic and prognostic in UA/NSTEMI. Traditionally, elevated serum levels of creatinine kinase (CK) or CK-MB were used to distinguish between UA and NSTEMI. However, the widespread use of the more sensitive cardiac biomarker, troponin, has improved the ability to diagnosis lesser degrees of myocardial necrosis. As a result, the proportion of patients classified as NSTEMI has increased markedly in recent years. Elevated levels of troponin T or I are independent predictors of adverse events in patients with clinical symptoms consistent with ACS, even when levels of CK and CK-MB are normal (see also Chapter 59 in *Hurst's The Heart*, 12th ed.). Patients with elevated troponin have a NSTEMI by definition and should be treated as being at high risk compared with UA patients with normal troponin levels. Patients with symptoms consistent with ACS and an initial set of enzymes that are negative within 6 hours of onset of symptoms should have serial enzymes drawn 8 to 12 hours after symptom onset to ensure that no myocardial damage has occurred.

Other biomarkers that provide important risk information in patients with UA/NSTEMI include BNP and NT-proBNP. Even when troponin levels are normal and no evidence of heart failure is present, higher levels of these neurohormones identify patients at increased risk for death and heart failure after an ACS presentation. Unlike the troponins, however, the therapeutic implications of BNP or NT-proBNP elevation in ACS are not entirely clear. Thus, it is recommended that these tests be ordered selectively rather than routinely in ACS.

【　】 ACUTE MYOCARDIAL PERFUSION IMAGING

In patients with normal cardiac biomarkers and nondiagnostic ECGs but a high suspicion of UA, acute rest myocardial perfusion imaging with technetium 99 sestamibi can be beneficial in diagnosing myocardial ischemia. Since imaging can be delayed for several hours after injection, sestamibi is more useful than thallium for rest myocardial imaging. ECG-gated imaging provides an assessment of myocardial wall motion in addition to perfusion information (Chapter 4). The sensitivity and negative predictive value of acute rest perfusion imaging are extremely high if sestamibi is injected during an episode of acute chest pain. The sensitivity decreases if the injection is done after the chest pain has resolved.

FOLLOW-UP TESTING

【　】 STRESS TESTING

Stress testing is often used for risk assessment in low- to intermediate-risk patients with UA/NSTEMI. If the purpose of the stress test is risk assessment in a patient with confirmed ACS, the testing should be performed with the patient on appropriate precautionary pharmacotherapy (aspirin, beta-blocker). However, in low-risk patients in whom the suspicion of ACS is low and the purpose is to *diagnose* CAD, it is reasonable to withhold beta-blockers to improve the diagnostic yield.

If the stress test shows high-risk findings, such as ST-segment depression at low exercise levels or large reversible perfusion defects on perfusion imaging, the patient should be referred urgently for coronary angiography since high-risk stress test abnormalities are correlated with higher event rates and more commonly with three-vessel CAD. If the stress test is negative or has low-risk results, the patient can be treated medically. In patients with baseline ECG abnormalities, exercise stress testing should be performed in conjunction with echocardiographic or nuclear imaging. In patients who are unable to exercise, pharmacologic stress testing should be performed with adenosine, dipyridamole, or dobutamine and nuclear or echocardiographic imaging.

【　】 CORONARY CT ANGIOGRAPHY

The ACC/AHA 2007 Guideline Update for the Management of Patients with UA and NSTEMI (Chapter 59) now states that noninvasive coronary CT imaging is a reasonable alternative to stress testing in low-risk to intermediate-risk patients (level of evidence B, class IIa). Since coronary CT angiography provides only diagnostic information, patients with *high-risk clinical features should not undergo coronary CT angiography* but should instead proceed to traditional coronary angiography and potential revascularization.

【　】 CORONARY ANGIOGRAPHY

In chronic CAD patients the risk of future cardiovascular events is proportional to the number of vessels with > 50% diameter stenosis and the presence and severity of left ventricular (LV) systolic dysfunction. However, the risk of short-term events in UA/NSTEMI is dominated by features of the *culprit lesion* (ECG changes, troponin elevation).

Among patients with UA/NSTEMI who undergo coronary angiography, approximately 85% will have significant CAD. CABG confers a survival benefit in patients with ≥ 50% left main stenosis or three-vessel disease with LV dysfunction. Importantly, patients with *no* significant lesions at angiography benefit from a reorientation of their management. Alternative causes of chest pain should be considered in patients with no significant coronary lesions on angiography, including pulmonary embolism, "syndrome X," and variant angina. If the coronaries are completely normal, antithrombotic and antiplatelet drugs can often be discontinued, and the need for antianginal medication reassessed. Symptomatic patients with "normal" coronary arteries may have significant atherosclerosis by intravascular ultrasound secondary to coronary artery remodeling.

PROGNOSIS

Prognosis in UA/NSTEMI depends on the morbidity and mortality expected from the extent of coronary disease, LV systolic function, and the short-term risk associated with the stability of the culprit lesion. Short-term risk is highest soon after the onset of symptoms due to risk from MI and its complications and the recurrence of ACS. Long-term risk is more difficult to quantify. However, the Global Registry of Acute Coronary

Events (GRACE) study, a multinational observational study of 5209 NSTEMI patients and 6149 UA patients, found a 6-month mortality rate of 6.2% in patients with NSTEMI and 3.6% in those with UA.

TREATMENT

The goals of therapy for UA/NSTEMI patients are threefold: (1) control/alleviate symptoms; (2) improve ischemia; and (3) prevent death, MI, or reinfarction.

【　】 IN-HOSPITAL TREATMENT

Suspected ACS patients should be treated with an aspirin (ASA), clopidogrel or a GP IIb/IIIa inhibitor, and either unfractionated heparin (UFH) or low-molecular-weight heparin (LMWH). If a patient has recurrent ischemia on ASA and clopidogrel, a GP IIb/IIIa inhibitor should be added prior to proceeding to coronary angiography. Statins and beta-blockers should be administered orally within the first 24 hours provided that the patient does not have any contraindications. Bed rest for the early phase of hospitalization and supplemental oxygen to keep arterial oxygen saturation > 90% should be ordered. All nonsteroidal anti-inflammatory drugs should be discontinued.

【　】 EARLY INVASIVE VERSUS EARLY CONSERVATIVE INITIAL MANAGEMENT

The ACC/AHA 2007 UA/NSTEMI Guideline Update (see Chapter 59) advocates two main strategies with regard to early catheterization and revascularization, "early invasive" and "early conservative" (Fig. 25-3). Low-risk patients or patients who prefer to avoid angiography and do not have high-risk features can be managed with intensive medical therapy in the early conservative strategy. These patients will only undergo coronary angiography if they experience recurrent ischemia (angina or ST-segment changes at rest or with minimal activity) or heart failure, or have a strongly positive stress test following completion of 48 to 72 hours of antithrombotic therapy. This strategy is better termed a "selective invasive" strategy, as 30% to 50% of patients managed with this strategy will cross over and undergo catheterization during or shortly following admission. In the early invasive strategy, patients who have no contraindications to cardiac catheterization undergo coronary angiography within 24 to 48 hours and PCI or surgical revascularization if suitable coronary anatomy is present.

A meta-analysis of the seven large, prospective, randomized trials that have evaluated the risks and benefits of each approach found that the relative risk (RR) of all-cause mortality (RR 0.75, 95% CI 0.63–0.90), nonfatal MI (RR 0.83, 95% CI 0.72–0.96), and recurrent UA (RR 0.69, 95% CI 0.65–0.74) were all reduced with an early invasive strategy. However, one of these seven trials, the Invasive versus Conservative Treatment in Unstable coronary Syndromes (ICTUS) trial, found no difference in the composite ischemic end point of MI and unstable angina requiring revascularization in the early conservative versus early invasive strategies at 1 year and 3 year follow-up in 1200 UA/NSTEMI patients who were troponin positive. Because of this trial, the ACC/AHA 2007 Guideline Update for the Management of Patients with UA and NSTEMI recognizes that an early invasive strategy may be an appropriate strategy for *some* cases of UA/NSTEMI.

The 2007 Guideline update recognizes important interactions between patient risk and the benefit of the invasive treatment strategy. The benefits of the early invasive approach are accentuated in high-risk patient prediction tools (see Table 25-1 and Fig. 25-2). In contrast, no benefit of a routine invasive approach is observed in low-risk UA patients.

Additional advantages of the early invasive strategy include earlier and more definitive risk stratification with early identification of the 10% to 15% of patients with no significant coronary stenoses and the approximately 20% of patients with three-vessel or left main CAD. This strategy reduces the need for antianginal medications and

TABLE 25-2

Anti-Ischemic and Antithrombotic Drugs in UA/NSTEMI

Medications	Route	Dose
NTG and nitrates		
NTG	Sublingual tablets	0.3–0.6 mg, up to 1.5 mg
	Spray	0.4 mg as needed
	Transdermal	0.2–0.8 mg/h every 12 h
	Intravenous	5–200 μg/min
Isosorbide dinitrate	Oral	5–80 mg 2 or 3 times daily
	Oral, slow release	40 mg 1 or 2 times daily
Isosorbide mononitrate	Oral	20 mg twice daily
	Oral, slow release	60–240 mg once daily
Beta-blockers		
Metoprolol	Oral	25–100 mg twice daily
Atenolol	Oral	25–100 mg once daily
Esmolol	Intravenous	50–200 μg/kg/min
Calcium-channel blockers[a]		
Diltiazem	Oral	30–90 mg 4 times daily
Verapamil	Oral	80–120 mg 3 times daily
Amlodipine	Oral	2.5–10 mg once daily
Nisoldipine	Oral	10–60 mg once daily
Felodipine	Oral	2.5–10 mg once daily
ACE inhibitors[b]		
Ramipril	Oral	2.5–5 mg twice daily
Captopril	Oral	25–100 mg 2 or 3 times daily
Enalapril	Oral	5–20 mg 2 twice daily
Perindopril	Oral	4–8 mg once daily
Angiotensin receptor blockers		
Candesartan	Oral	4–32 mg once daily
Losartan	Oral	25–100 mg once or twice daily
Valsartan	Oral	40–160 mg twice daily
Aldosterone receptor blockers		
Eplerenone	Oral	25–50 mg once daily
Spironolactone	Oral	25 mg once daily
Antiplatelets		
Aspirin	Oral	Initial dose of 325 mg followed by 81–325 mg daily
Clopidogrel	Oral	Initial dose of 300–600 mg followed by 75 mg daily
Anticoagulant therapy		
UFH	Intravenous	Initial dose 60 U/kg (max 4000 U) bolus then 12 U/kg/h (max 1000 U/h) for goal aPTT 50–70 s
Enoxaparin	Subcutaneous/intravenous	1 mg/kg twice a day (first dose may be preceded by 30-mg U IV bolus); if CrCl < 30 mL/min then 1 mg/kg once daily
Bivalirudin[c]	Intravenous	0.1 mg/kg bolus followed by infusion of 0.25 mg/kg/h

TABLE 25-2

Anti-Ischemic And Antithrombotic Drugs In UA/NSTEMI (*Continued*)

Medications	Route	Dose
Fondaparinux [d,e] Glycoprotein IIb/ IIIa inhibitors [f]	Subcutaneous	2.5 mg, once daily
Abciximab,[g]	Intravenous	0.25 mg/kg bolus followed by infusion of 0.125 µg/kg/min (maximum 10 µg/min) for 12–24 h
Eptifibatide	Intravenous	180 µg/kg bolus × 2 (10 min apart) followed by infusion of 2.0 µg/kg/min for 72–96 h
Tirofiban	Intravenous	0.4 µg/kg/min for 30 min followed by infusion of 0.1 µg/kg/min for 48–96 h

UFH, unfractionated heparin; CrCl, creatinine clearance; aPTT, activated partial thromboplastin time.

[a]If beta-blockers are not tolerated or are contraindicated.
[b]If blood pressure is not controlled with beta-blockers or in the presence of LV systolic dysfunction. May use other long-acting agents after titration.
[c]If used during PCI, must be used with a GP IIb/IIa inhibitor or clopidogrel.
[d]If used during PCI, must be used with concurrent UFH.

rehospitalization for myocardial ischemia among those who can have PCI performed on their culprit lesion.

Advantages of the early conservative strategy are the avoidance of the potential risks of invasive procedures, such as catheterization and the identification of high-risk patients with noninvasive stress testing.

【 】 ANTI-ISCHEMIC DRUGS

An overview of anti-ischemic and antithrombotic drugs is given in Table 25-2.

Nitrates

Nitroglycerin (NTG) reduces myocardial oxygen demand while enhancing myocardial oxygen delivery by vasodilating coronary vascular beds. PV decreases preload via venous pooling, thereby decreasing LV wall tension and decreasing myocardial oxygen demand. Epicardial and collateral coronary vasodilation by NTG can improve the redistribution of blood flow to ischemic myocardial regions.

Patients whose symptoms are not relieved with three 0.4-mg sublingual NTG tablets or sprays taken 5 minutes apart may benefit from intravenous NTG. The use of sildenafil (Viagra) within the previous 24 hours, tadalafil (Cialis) within the previous 48 hours, or the presence of hypotension (SBP < 90 mm Hg or > 30 mm Hg below baseline) are contraindications to NTG administration. The time between nitrate use and use of vardenafil (Levitra) has not been studied; therefore until further data are available, vardenafil should not be prescribed to patients who may need nitrate therapy.

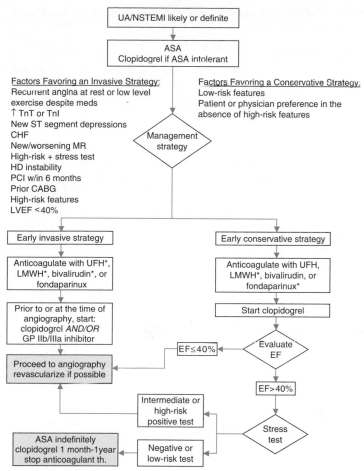

FIGURE 25-3. The ACC/AHA 2007 Guideline Update for the Management of Patients with UA and NSTEMI describes two different treatment strategies, termed "early conservative" and "early invasive." (*Preferred anticoagulant therapy.) (UA/NSTEMI, unstable angina/non-ST elevation myocardial infarction; ASA, aspirin; TnT, troponin-T; TnI, troponin-I; CHF, congestive heart failure; MR, mitral regurgitation; HD, hemodynamic; PCI, percutaneous coronary intervention; CABG, coronary artery bypass grafting; LVEF, left ventricular ejection fraction; UFH, unfractionated heparin; LMWH, low molecular weight heparin; GP IIb/IIIa inhibitor, glycoprotein IIb/IIIa inhibitor.) (Data complied from ACC/AHA 2007 guidelines.)

Intravenous NTG may be initiated at a rate of 10 μg/min as a continuous infusion and increased by 10 μg/min every 3 to 5 minutes until symptom relief or blood pressure response is noted. IV NTG can be administered as needed for the first 48 hours after UA/NSTEMI for persistent ischemia, heart failure, or hypertension as long as it does not preclude the use of other evidence-based cardioprotective medicines such as angiotensin-converting enzyme (ACE) inhibitors or beta-blockers. An upper limit of

200 µg/min of IV NTG is commonly used. After 48 hours, the patient should be transitioned to oral nitrate therapy for medical management of residual angina.

Morphine Sulfate

Morphine sulfate relieves pain through the opioid pain receptor as well as by diminishing the sympathetic nervous system's pain response, thereby decreasing catecholamine secretion and oxygen demand. Morphine also is a venodilator and decreases preload. Morphine sulfate is recommended (1–5 mg IV) for patients whose symptoms are not relieved despite NTG therapy.

Beta-Adrenergic Blockers

Beta-blockers reduce myocardial oxygen demand by slowing the heart rate, decreasing myocardial contractility, decreasing afterload, and prolonging the duration of diastole, thereby improving coronary and collateral blood flow. In the absence of contraindications, beta-blockers should be started *orally* within the first 24 hours of UA/NSTEMI. *Routine early intravenous beta-blocker therapy is no longer recommended.* Intravenous use should be reserved for specific indications such as hypertension or atrial arrhythmias and should not be administered to hemodynamically unstable patients or patients with signs of heart failure or a low output state.

Patients with significant sinus bradycardia (heart rate < 50 bpm) or hypotension (SBP < 90 mm Hg) generally should not receive beta-blockers until these issues are resolved. Short-acting cardioselective beta-blockers should be used in patients with reactive airways disease and up-titrated to obtain a heart rate of *50 to 60 bpm* as tolerated.

Calcium-Channel Blockers

Calcium-channel blockers inhibit both myocardial and vascular smooth muscle contraction, thereby reducing myocardial oxygen demand and improving myocardial blood flow. Nifedipine and amlodipine have the greatest peripheral arterial dilatory effect but little chronotropic effect, whereas verapamil and diltiazem have chronotropic and inotropic as well as some peripheral arterial dilatory effects.

Calcium-channel blockers may be useful for ongoing or recurring angina in patients receiving adequate doses of nitrates and beta-blockers, in those who are intolerant to either or both of these agents, or in patients with variant angina. Rapid-release short-acting dihydropyridines (e.g., nifedipine) must be avoided in ACS because of risk for adverse outcomes. Verapamil and diltiazem should be avoided in patient with pulmonary edema or severe LV systolic dysfunction and should be used with caution when combined with beta-blockers.

Angiotensin-Converting Enzyme Inhibitors/Angiotensin Receptor Blockers

ACE inhibitors reduce mortality and CV events in patients with MI and LV systolic dysfunction (LVEF < 40%), in patients with diabetes and CAD, and in patients with high-risk chronic CAD despite normal LV systolic function. Accordingly, ACE inhibitors should be used in most patients following UA/NSTEMI, unless contraindicated or blood pressure is borderline. Angiotensin receptor blockers (ARBs) may be useful in patients post-MI or with ischemic heart failure (HF) who are intolerant to ACE inhibitors.

Aldosterone Receptor Blockers

Eplerenone, a selective aldosterone receptor blocker, has been shown to have a mortality and morbidity benefit in patients who have had an MI with LV systolic dysfunction

(LVEF < 40%) and HF or diabetes. Spironolactone has been shown to have a mortality and morbidity benefit in both ischemic and nonischemic severe HF patients (NHYA class III and IV). Aldosterone receptor blockers should be administered to patients with HF or diabetes and an EF less than or equal to 40% who do not have significant renal dysfunction or hyperkalemia and are already on a therapeutic dose of an ACE inhibitor.

【 】 ANTIPLATELET THERAPY

Aspirin

ASA irreversibly inhibits cyclooxygenase-1 within the platelet, preventing the formation of thromboxane A_2 and thereby diminishing platelet aggregation, a critical contributor to thrombus formation after plaque rupture. In UA/NSTEMI patients, ASA therapy should be initiated immediately at a dose of 162 to 325 mg. The first dose should be chewed, and preferably a nonenteric coated ASA because it has faster buccal absorption. Subsequent doses may be swallowed. Thereafter, daily doses of 75 to 325 mg are prescribed. In patients who undergo PCI, higher initial dosages of 162 to 325 mg daily of ASA for 1 month after a bare-metal stent and 3 to 6 months after DES are recommended, which can then be decreased to 81 mg daily indefinitely (level of evidence A, class I recommendation [Chapter 59]). For patients not undergoing stenting, the patient may be discharged on an 81-mg daily dose.

Adenosine Diphosphate Receptor Antagonists

Ticlopidine and clopidogrel are thienopyridine derivatives that block the binding of ADP to the P_2Y_{12} receptor on the platelet surface, inhibiting ADP-mediated platelet activation. Because of potential safety concerns with ticlopidine (neutropenia, thrombotic thrombocytopenia [TTP]), clopidogrel has replaced ticlopidine for essentially all indications. The Clopidogrel versus Aspirin in Patients at Risk of Ischaemic Events (CAPRIE) trial compared 325 mg of ASA to 75 mg of clopidogrel and found that there was a slight reduction in the composite end point of ischemic stroke, MI, or symptomatic peripheral arterial disease in the clopidogrel arm in 1 to 3 years of follow-up. Because of the excess expense of clopidogrel and the lack of substantial improvement in risk, *clopidogrel monotherapy is indicated only for patients with a true allergy or serious intolerance to ASA*; otherwise ASA is the first-line antiplatelet medicine in patients with ACS.

The Clopidogrel in Unstable Angina to Prevent Recurrent Ischemic Events (CURE) trial evaluated the effects of combination therapy with ASA and clopidogrel versus ASA alone in UA/NSTEMI, since the drugs inhibit platelet aggregation through different pathways. The composite end point of CV death, MI, or stroke was significantly reduced from 11.5% of patients assigned to ASA alone to 9.3% of patients assigned to clopidogrel and ASA therapy; this difference persisted in both medical therapy and revascularization patients. *This is why dual antiplatelet therapy with both clopidogrel and ASA is recommended for at least 1 month and up to 1 year after UA/NSTEMI in medically treated patients.* Because of the risk of late in-stent thrombosis with drug-eluting stents (DES), clopidogrel is recommended for at least 1 year in patients who undergo PCI with DES. *For patients undergoing PCI with bare-metal stents, the preferred duration of clopidogrel therapy is 1 year.*

Excess bleeding was seen in the clopidogrel and ASA groups in clinical trials; however this mostly occurred in patients who underwent CABG within 5 days of receiving clopidogrel. Therefore administering a loading dose of clopidogrel (300–600 mg) prior to catheterization presents logistic challenges because a given patient may require CABG and would likely have surgery delayed if he or she had received clopidogrel. Many hospitals will delay clopidogrel loading until the need for CABG has been ruled out after angiography and then give a loading dose (300–600 mg) on the catheterization table if PCI is to be carried out immediately.

Platelet Glycoprotein IIb/IIIa Receptor Inhibitors

The GP IIb/IIIa receptor is a platelet surface receptor that undergoes a configurational change when activated that results in the binding of fibrinogen to platelet receptors, leading to platelet aggregation. The platelet GP IIb/IIIa receptor antagonists occupy these receptor sites and inhibit fibrinogen binding.

The GP IIb/IIIa receptor inhibitors are IV agents that are monoclonal antibodies to the beta-3 integrin of the IIb/IIIa receptor (abciximab) or synthetic molecules that mimic the fibrinogen receptor glycoprotein-binding sequence, either as peptidomimetics (eptifibatide) or as small inhibitory molecules (tirofiban).

There are two broad strategies for GP IIb/IIIa inhibitor use in ACS: (1) an "upstream" strategy in which either eptifibatide or tirofiban is administered in the emergency department or hospital for medical stabilization, usually in anticipation of an early invasive approach to PCI; or (2) use of eptifibatide or abciximab as adjunctive therapy in the cardiac catheterization laboratory immediately prior to PCI.

Because of cost and because cardiac catheterization is increasingly performed early after presentation, GP IIb/IIIa inhibitor administration may be deferred until the time of PCI. In the c7E3 Fab Anti-Platelet Therapy in Unstable Refractory Angina (CAPTURE) study, abciximab was associated with a 68% relative risk reduction in death or MI in troponin-positive patients but had no observable benefit in troponin-negative patients. The Intracoronary Stenting and Anti-thrombotic Regimen: Rapid Early Action for Coronary Treatment (ISAR-REACT)-2 study found that in UA/NSTEMI patients treated with ASA and clopidogrel, abciximab reduced the primary end point of death or MI by 25% in patients who were troponin-positive, but was ineffective in troponin-negative patients.

In general, antiplatelet therapy with ASA and antithrombotic therapy with either unfractionated heparin (UFH) or LMWH (see below) are administered to all patients with UA/NSTEMI. Additional antiplatelet therapy with clopidogrel is usually given (300–600 mg loading dose, then 75 mg daily) prior to or at the time of PCI. The GP IIb/IIIa inhibitors are usually reserved for high-risk patients who are likely to undergo early PCI and may be administered either upstream or at the time of PCI.

【 】 ANTITHROMBIN THERAPY

Indirect Thrombin Inhibitors: UFH and LMWH

UFH is a heterogeneous mixture of polysaccharides that inactivates factor IIa (thrombin), factor IXa, and factor Xa by accelerating the action of circulating antithrombin and preventing thrombus generation. LMWH is a mixture of smaller molecular weight chains of heparin that more preferentially inactivate factor Xa. Both UFH and LMWH help to prevent thrombus generation but do not lyse clot-bound thrombin.

Several trials have shown benefit to using UFH over placebo in ACS. In a meta-analysis of six trials comparing UFH and ASA therapy to ASA therapy alone, death, nonfatal MI, and recurrent angina were reduced by 33% in UFH-treated patients ($p = 0.06$).

UFH has poor bioavailability, with marked variability in anticoagulation response. UFH anticoagulant effects must be closely monitored by the activated partial thromboplastin time (aPTT). Dosing should be adjusted for weight (Table 25-2) and the aPTT should be measured every 6 hours until it has stabilized between 60 and 80 seconds and then every 12 to 24 hours to ensure stability of the anticoagulant effects. Heparin-induced thrombocytopenia (HIT) is a potential adverse effect of heparin (incidence, 1%–5%), and therefore requires serial platelet monitoring. There are two forms of HIT: (1) a mild form in which there is a slight decrease in platelet counts (rarely < 100,000/μL) that occurs early (1 to 4 days) after initiation of therapy, reverses quickly after discontinuation of heparin, and is of little clinical consequence; and (2) a more severe form that is an immune-mediated thrombocytopenia that typically occurs more than 5 days from therapy in heparin-naïve patients (earlier in patients that have received heparin within the previous 3 to 4 months), which can lead to thrombosis and significant morbidity and mortality. Heparin should be discontinued immediately when HIT is suspected, the patient's blood should be screened for antiplatelet antibodies, and direct thrombin inhibitors should be initiated for anticoagulation.

Compared to UFH, LMWH offers the advantages of more predictable anticoagulation, no need for routine laboratory monitoring, and once or twice daily subcutaneous dosing due to LMWH decreased nonspecific binding. LMWH also has a lower incidence of HIT than UFH.

Nine large randomized trials have directly compared LMWH with UFH. In five of six trials that used enoxaparin, enoxaparin versus UFH was associated with a pooled odds ratio of 0.91 (95% CI 0.83–0.99) for the composite end point of death, MI, or recurrent angina. However, three other trials evaluating two other LMWHs, nadroparin and dalteparin, showed no significant difference in death or nonfatal MI compared to UFH-treated patients. Enoxaparin has been shown to be superior to UFH in trials utilizing an early conservative strategy but not when an early invasive strategy was employed. Both UFH and enoxaparin have class I recommendations for use in UA/NSTEMI according to the ACC/AHA 2007 Guideline Update (Chapter 59).

Direct Thrombin Inhibitors

Two direct thrombin inhibitors, hirudin and bivalirudin, have been tested in patients with UA/NSTEMI. Only bivalirudin has adequate data to support a class I (Chapter 59) recommendation in the updated guideline. Lepirudin, the recombinant form of hirudin, is only indicated to treat patients with HIT.

Two studies have compared bivalirudin, a semisynthetic direct thrombin inhibitor, to heparin-based therapy. Bivalirudin offered no advantage to heparin in terms of 30-day rates of ischemia, major bleeding, and clinical outcomes. Given its higher cost, bivalirudin is not an attractive option for patients receiving GP IIb/IIIa inhibitors. In contrast, bivalirudin alone was comparable to heparin and a GP IIb/IIIa inhibitor with regard to efficacy and was associated with lower bleeding in patients who had received a thienopyridine prior to catheterization, but inferior to heparin and a GP IIb/IIIa if no thienopyridine had been administered.

Factor Xa Inhibitors

Factor Xa inhibitors act early in the coagulation cascade in order to prevent downstream reactions that promote thrombin generation. Fondaparinux is a pentasaccharide factor Xa inhibitor with a dose-independent clearance, a longer half-life than UFH, and less protein and endothelial binding, leading to predictable anticoagulation that only requires once-daily subcutaneous administration.

The Organization to Assess Strategies for Ischemic Syndromes (OASIS)-5 study evaluated fondaparinux versus LMWH in the treatment of UA/NSTEMI patients and found that compared to LMWH, fondaparinux was associated with identical short-term efficacy but less major bleeding at 9 days; moreover, rates of death, MI, and stroke at 6 months were reduced compared to UFH (11.3% versus 12.5%, $p < 0.001$). There was, however, an increased incidence of catheter-associated thrombus in the fondaparinux group, leading the ACC/AHA to recommend that supplemental UFH would be needed during angiography/PCI in patients treated with fondaparinux. Because of its long half-life, lack of reversibility, and the potential risk for catheter-associated thrombi, fondaparinux *is not* an attractive agent for invasively managed patients.

【 】 FIBRINOLYTIC THERAPY

Fibrinolytics are contraindicated for the treatment of UA/NSTEMI because of an increased risk of MI and bleeding with their use.

【 】 INTRA-AORTIC BALLOON PUMP

Although randomized data are limited evaluating the use of intra-aortic counterpulsation for the treatment of refractory ischemia, it has been used effectively to improve myocardial blood flow by increasing coronary filling during diastole and to reduce myocardial oxygen demand by decreasing afterload in early systole. Balloon pumps are particularly useful when UA/NSTEMI is complicated by cardiogenic shock.

【 】 LIPID-LOWERING THERAPY

The major clinical trials of lipid management post-ACS have supported aggressive LDL lowering. In the Myocardial Ischemia Reduction with Aggressive Cholesterol Lowering (MIRACL) study, atorvastatin 80 mg/d versus placebo started 24 to 96 hours after ACS was associated with an absolute risk reduction of 2.6% percent in the primary end point of death, MI, resuscitated cardiac arrest, or recurrent myocardial ischemia ($p = 0.048$) 16 weeks after therapy initiation.

The Zocor (Z) phase of the A to Z trial compared an early intensive statin regimen (simvastatin 40 mg followed by 80 mg) with a delayed and less-intensive regimen (placebo for 4 months followed by simvastatin 20 mg) for up to 24 months in patients with ACS. The primary end point of cardiovascular death, MI, readmission for ACS, or stroke was reduced in the early intensive statin arm compared to the delayed, less-intensive arm (HR 0.89; 95% CI 0.76–1.04); and cardiovascular death was reduced by 25% in the early intensive statin arm ($p = 0.05$).

In the Pravastatin or Atorvastatin Evaluation and Infection Therapy (PROVE IT)-TIMI 22 trial an intensive statin regimen of atorvastatin 80 mg was compared with a standard statin regimen of pravastatin 40 mg/d among 4162 patients with ACS. The atorvastatin arm achieved an average LDL cholesterol of 62 mg/dL versus an average of 95 mg/dL in the pravastatin arm. The primary end point of death, MI, UA, or revascularization after 30 days was reduced by 16% in the atorvastatin arm ($p < 0.0001$).

The ACC/AHA 2007 Guideline Update for the Management of Patients with UA and NSTEMI (Chapter 59) recommends that all UA/NSTEMI patients have a fasting lipid profile drawn within 24 hours of hospitalization and that statins be given to all UA/NSTEMI patients, regardless of baseline LDL-C. LDL-C should be reduced to at least less than 100 mg/dL and ideally to less than 70 mg/dL, as endorsed by the National Cholesterol Education Panel.

【 】 CORONARY REVASCULARIZATION

Coronary angiography is useful for defining the coronary artery anatomy in patients with UA/NSTEMI as well as identifying the subset of high-risk patients who will benefit from early revascularization. The goals of revascularization (surgical or percutaneous) are fourfold: (1) to improve prognosis, (2) to relieve symptoms, (3) to prevent ischemic complications, and (4) to improve functional capacity. The decision to revascularize a given lesion is based on the coronary anatomy, quantity of myocardium at risk, LV systolic function, and individual patient characteristics (comorbidities, life expectancy, symptom severity, functional status). The decision to perform revascularization must take all of these issues into account (Fig. 25-4).

【 】 PERCUTANEOUS CORONARY INTERVENTION

Given continued technical advances, widespread antiplatelet and anticoagulant therapy, as well as the use of stents, PCI provides a safe and durable option for revascularization in UA/NSTEMI. Stenting has reduced the incidence of both acute vessel closure and late restenosis. The use of DES has improved the restenosis rates but has modestly increased the risk of late coronary thrombosis. In select patients who have a high

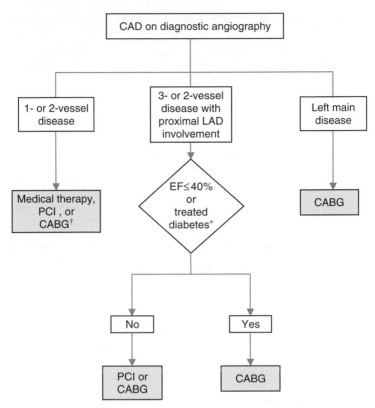

FIGURE 25-4. Revascularization strategy in UA/NSTEMI. (*There is conflicting information about these patients; most consider CABG to be preferable to PCI.) (†Therapeutic decision based on patient and lesion characteristics including comorbid conditions, severity of symptoms, lesion amenability to PCI, patient and physician preference.) (CAD, coronary artery disease; LAD, left anterior descending artery; PCI, percutaneous intervention; CABG, coronary artery bypass grafting.) (Data complied from ACC/AHA 2007 guidelines.)

surgical risk and amenable coronary anatomy, multivessel PCI can offer complete revascularization without surgical intervention.

Given recent concerns about late stent thrombosis with DES, particularly when ASA or clopidogrel are prematurely discontinued, it is imperative to ensure that a patient will be able to take ASA and clopidogrel uninterrupted for at least 1 year before placing a DES in a patient with UA/NSTEMI. Alternatives for patients at risk for premature antiplatelet therapy discontinuation—including those who are noncompliant, at increased bleeding risk, or who have upcoming surgery—include bare-metal stents, PTCA alone, CABG (if anatomy is suitable), or medical therapy.

【 】 SURGICAL REVASCULARIZATION

Because of dramatic changes in surgical, medical, and percutaneous therapy, there are very few data from trials using current PCI and surgical techniques to guide selection between PCI and CABG in patients with ACS and multivessel CAD (see Chapter 26).

CABG should be considered in high-risk patients with LV systolic dysfunction, patients with diabetes mellitus and multivessel CAD, and patients with two-vessel disease with severe proximal left anterior descending artery involvement, severe three-vessel CAD, or left main disease. In patients with multivessel disease and normal systolic function, multivessel PCI may be performed if the coronary lesion anatomy is amenable to PCI, the likelihood of complete revascularization with PCI is high, and the patient prefers a nonsurgical approach to revascularization.

SUGGESTED READING

Anderson J, Adams C, Antman E, et al. ACC/AHA 2007 guidelines for the management of patients with unstable angina/non-ST-elevation myocardial infarction: a report of the American College of Cardiology/American Heart Association Task Force on Practice Guidelines (Writing Committee to Revise the 2002 Guidelines for the Management of Patients with Unstable Angina/Non-ST-Elevation Myocardial Infarction) developed in collaboration with the American College of Emergency Physicians, the Society for Cardiovascular Angiography and Interventions, and the Society of Thoracic Surgeons endorsed by the American Association of Cardiovascular and Pulmonary Rehabilitation and the Society for Academic Emergency Medicine. *J Am Coll Cardiol.* 2007;50:e1–e157.

Antman EM, Cohen M, Bernink PJ, et al. The TIMI risk score for unstable angina/non-ST elevation MI: a method of prognostication and therapeutic decision making. *JAMA.* 2000;284: 835–842.

Bavry AA, Kumbhani DJ, Rassi AN, et al. Benefit of early invasive therapy in acute coronary syndromes a meta-analysis of contemporary randomized clinical trials. *J Am Coll Cardiol.* 2006;48:1319–1325.

Boersma, E, Harrington RA, Moliterno DJ, et al. Platelet glycoprotein IIb/IIIa inhibitors in acute coronary syndromes: a meta-analysis of all major randomized clinical trials. *Lancet.* 2002;359:189–198.

de Lemos JA, O'Rourke RA. Unstable angina and non-ST segment elevation myocardial infarction. In: Fuster V, Walsh RA, O'Rourke RA, et al., eds. *Hurst's The Heart.* 12th ed. New York, NY: McGraw-Hill; 2008:1351–1374.

Eagle KA, Lim MJ, Dabbous OH, et al. A validated prediction model for all forms of acute coronary syndrome: estimating the risk of 6-month post-discharge death in an international registry. *JAMA.* 2004;291:2727–2733.

Hayden M, Pignone M, Phillips C, et al. Aspirin for the primary prevention of cardiovascular events: a summary of the evidence for the U.S. Preventive Service Task Force. *Ann Intern Med.* 2002;136:161–172.

Hirsh J, Raschke R. Heparin and low-molecular-weight heparin: the seventh ACCP conference on antithrombotic and thrombolytic therapy. *Chest.* 2004;126:188S–203S.

Lichtenstein AH, Appel LJ, Brands M, et al. Diet and lifestyle recommendations revision 2006: a scientific statement from the American Heart Association Nutrition Committee. *Circulation.* 2006;114:82–96.

Shapiro BP, Jaffe AS. Cardiac biomarkers. In: Murphy JG, Lloyd MA, eds. *Mayo Clinic Cardiology: Concise Textbook.* 3rd ed. Rochester, MN: Mayo Clinic Scientific Press; 2007:773–780.

CHAPTER (26)

Percutaneous Coronary Intervention

Habib Samady, John S. Douglas Jr.,
and Spencer B. King III

DEVELOPMENT OF BALLOON ANGIOPLASTY

Percutaneous transluminal coronary angioplasty (PTCA) was conceived and shepherded into worldwide acceptance and application by Andreas R. Gruentzig; this technique has now eclipsed coronary bypass surgery as the most frequently performed revascularization procedure. Initially, coronary balloon angioplasty was performed for discrete, proximal, noncalcified subtotal lesions located in one coronary artery. A 10-year follow-up of Gruentzig's early Zurich series revealed an overall survival rate of 90%, and of 95% for those with single-vessel disease. Reintervention rates for patients undergoing percutaneous coronary intervention (PCI) have fallen steadily from the PTCA period to the stent period, and are now even lower with the drug-eluting stent (DES). Although PCI for stable angina does not impact myocardial infarction (MI) or death, PCI reduces these end points in high-risk acute coronary syndromes (ACS).

RANDOMIZED TRIALS OF PERCUTANEOUS CORONARY INTERVENTION

The Angioplasty Compared to Medical Therapy Evaluation (ACME), involving 212 patients with single-vessel disease and abnormal stress tests, revealed greater freedom from angina in the angioplasty group at 6 months, but there was no difference in rates of death or MI. The second Randomized Intervention Treatment of Angina (RITA-2) trial randomized 1,018 patients with stable angina and predominantly single-vessel disease to PTCA or medical therapy. Angina relief and treadmill performance were significantly better in the PTCA patients, but survival was not different after 7 years of follow-up. The Clinical Outcomes Utilizing Revascularization and Aggressive Drug Evaluation (COURAGE) trial randomized 2,287 patients with stable angina and one-, two-, or three-vessel disease to PCI (predominantly using bare-metal stents) or aggressive medical therapy. There was no reduction in death or MI in the PCI arm; however, there was greater improvement in angina at 1 year, which was not sustained over 5 years. A similar improvement in symptoms but not death or MI was found with revascularization compared with medical therapy in the Atorvastatin Versus Revascularization Treatment (AVERT) trial and the Medicine, Angioplasty, or Surgery Studies (MASS) I and II. Taken together, these data indicate that for patients with stable coronary syndromes, PCI reduces anginal symptoms but does not reduce death or MI rates.

In contrast, patients with ACS derive both symptomatic benefit and a reduction in death and recurrent MI with PCI compared with medical therapy. The Fast Revascularization During Instability in Coronary Disease (FRISC II) study strongly supported an invasive approach in patients with ACS randomized after 5 days of dalteparin

TABLE 26-1

Early Invasive Strategy Recommended in Unstable Angina
or Non–ST-Elevation Myocardial Infarction

Class I Indication
Any of the high-risk indications:
- Recurrent angina at rest or minimal activity despite therapy
- Elevated troponin
- New ST-segment depression
- Recurrent angina/ischemia with symptoms or signs of congestive heart failure or new or worsening mitral regurgitation
- Positive stress test
- Ejection fraction < 40%
- Hemodynamic instability
- Sustained ventricular tachycardia
- Percutaneous coronary intervention within 6 months or prior coronary artery bypass grafting
- Depressed LV systolic function
- High-risk score (e.g., TIMI, GRACE)

Reproduced with permission from King SB, Smith SC Jr, et al. 2007 focused update of the ACC/AHA/SCAI 2005 guideline update for percutaneous coronary intervention: a report of the American College of Cardiology/American Heart Association Task Force on Practice guidelines, *J Am Coll Cardiol.* Jan15;2008;51(2):172–209.

(Fragmin) therapy. Among men, the invasive strategy in FRISC II resulted in a 34% reduction in death or MI at 6 months and a 52% reduction in mortality. The invasive approach to ACS was further supported by the results of the Treat Angina with Aggrastat and Determine Cost of Therapy with Invasive and Conservative Strategy (TACTICS-TIMI 18) and has been incorporated as a class I recommendation in the ACC/AHA Guideline (Table 26-1).

PERCUTANEOUS CORONARY INTERVENTION VERSUS CORONARY ARTERY BYPASS GRAFTING

Two trials of patients with multivessel coronary artery disease were sponsored by the National Heart, Lung, and Blood Institute and performed in the United States. The first, the Emory Angioplasty versus Surgery Trial (EAST), was a single-center study; while the larger Bypass Angioplasty Revascularization Investigation (BARI) involved 18 centers. In-hospital mortality was similar for angioplasty and bypass surgery. Survival for 7 to 8 years was similar in both studies. The difference favoring surgery is completely explained by a striking advantage of surgery for the diabetic patients. The Arterial Revascularization Therapy Study (ARTS), Stent or Surgery (SOS) study, and Argentine Randomized Study of Stents Versus CABG in Multivessel Disease (ERACI-2) have shown reduced reintervention rates with stents but have not established that PCI is comparable to surgery in multivessel diabetic patients. ARTS II was a comparison of patients with multivessel disease treated with DES with the surgical and bare-metal stent arm of ARTS I. At 1 year, 89.5% of DES-treated patients with MACE-free had a better outcome than ARTS I CABG patients. However, repeat intervention was performed in 8.5% of ARTS II DES patients compared with 4.1% of ARTS I CABG patients, showing a narrowing of the reintervention gap of PCI versus CABG. The New York state registry allowed comparison of 59,314 patients treated for multivessel disease with bare-metal stents and CABG. After adjusting for baseline differences between groups, the CABG patients had significantly better outcomes at 3 years. The two ongoing trials—FREEDOM

(Future Revascularization Evaluation of Patients with Diabetes Mellitus: Optimal Management of Multivessel Disease) and SYNTAX (Synergy Between Percutaneous Coronary Intervention with Taxus and Cardiac Surgery)—comparing DES to CABG in multivessel disease will provide further guidance for future decision-making in this population.

DEVICES AND STRATEGIES FOR CORONARY INTERVENTION

Directional atherectomy, rotational ablation, cutting balloons, and intravascular laser therapy have been used for debulking coronary lesions. Although each has niche applications, their use has declined in recent years. Directional atherectomy is sometimes used in bulky bifurcation lesions, laser therapy, and cutting balloons for in-stent restenosis, and rotational atherectomy for heavily calcified lesions.

【 】 STENTS: THE DOMINANT STRATEGY

Stents were developed for two indications: to reduce restenosis and to solve acute vessel closure after angioplasty; they were first implanted in 1986. Stents were approved in 1994 for the elective treatment of de novo lesions in native coronary arteries. Stenting became firmly established when it was found that antiplatelet therapy with thienopyridines and aspirin was effective in preventing stent thrombosis.

【 】 DRUG-ELUTING STENTING

Prevention of restenosis postintervention was first documented with endovascular brachytherapy for in-stent restenosis. The inhibition of cell division by radiation has now been replicated with drugs delivered locally from a polymer coating on stents. Rapamycin (sirolimus)- and paclitaxel-eluting stents have been shown to reduce angiographic restenosis from 20% to 30% with the control stents to 5% to 10% with the drug-eluting stents. The Sirolimus-Eluting Balloon Expandable Stent in the Treatment of Patients with de Novo Native Coronary Artery Lesions (SIRIUS) and Paclitaxel Eluting Stent (TAXUS) trials showed marked inhibition of neointima formation over the stents and therefore a reduction in angiographic restenosis. Recently, a third DES, the Medtronic AVE ABT-578 eluting Driver stent, was approved by the Food and Drug Administration (FDA) for clinical use in the United States based on the ENDEAVOR 1, 2, and 3 trials demonstrating safety and efficacy. Preliminary data from SPIRIT II comparing the everolimus-eluting stent with the Taxus stent revealed similar late lumen loss, restenosis, and MACE. The Xience everolimus-eluting stent is currently under consideration by the FDA for approval. It should be noted that *the trial results overestimate the restenosis impact because of the routine angiograms required. In real-world practice, where routine angiograms are not performed in asymptomatic patients, the impact on reintervention has been less and a reduction in MI or death rates has not yet been demonstrated.*

The cost effectiveness of DES compared with bare-metal stents is a balance between their higher up-front costs and the avoidance of repeat revascularization. Subgroups in which DES are most likely to be cost effective compared with bare-metal stents include diabetics, long lesions, small vessels, perhaps left main or proximal left anterior descending (LAD) locations, saphenous vein grafts, or other lesions with high restenosis rates with bare-metal stents.

Emerging Concerns with Drug-Eluting Stents

Although drug-eluting stents have clearly become the dominant PCI strategy in the United States, recent reports of coronary endothelial dysfunction, coronary vasospasm, hypersensitivity reactions, delayed vessel healing, delayed endothelialization, and late-stent thrombosis have emerged. The clinical presentation of stent thrombosis is often ST-elevation MI, with mortality rates of 30% to 50%. The data regarding the incidence of late stent thrombosis with DES compared with bare-metal stents are conflicting. Some studies suggest nonsignificantly higher rates of late stent thrombosis with DES (Fig. 26-1), while other studies suggest that when stenting is performed in "off-label" locations (e.g., bifurcation disease, left main disease, ostial or diffuse disease) there may be a mortality advantage of DES over bare-metal stenting (NHLBI Dynamic Registry). What is clear is that there is consensus on the need for adequate patient counseling against the premature discontinuation of dual antiplatelet therapy and the need for its prolonged use in patients receiving DES. Risk factors for stent thrombosis include performance of complex PCI, inadequate stent expansion or strut apposition, and premature discontinuation of dual antiplatelet therapy.

ADJUNCTIVE STRATEGIES

【 　】 THIENOPYRIDINES

Clopidogrel inhibits platelet activation by irreversibly blocking the ADP (P2Y12) receptor. In stable angina and troponin-negative ACS patients, a 600-mg clopidogrel loading dose administered 2 hours prior to PCI is as effective as clopidogrel plus abciximab. However, in troponin-positive patients the combination of clopidogrel and abciximab is superior to clopidogrel alone. Recent guidelines recommend (1) for patients receiving bare-metal stents, at least 4 weeks of dual antiplatelet therapy and ideally up to 12 months unless patients are at increased risk of bleeding, in which case it should be given for 2 weeks; and (2) for patients receiving DES, at least 12 months of dual antiplatelet therapy with DES implantation, if patients are not at high risk of bleeding. Dual antiplatelet therapy long-term (beyond 12 months) may be considered for patients receiving DES. Patients taking daily aspirin prior to PCI should take 75 to 325 mg before PCI is performed. For patients not previously on aspirin, 300 to 325 mg should be taken at least 2 hours prior to PCI. After PCI, 162 to 325 mg of aspirin should be given for at least 1 month in patients receiving bare-metal stents, 3 months for patients receiving sirulo-mus-eluting stents, and 6 months for patients receiving pacletaxil-eluting stents, after which all patients should receive 75 to 162 mg of aspirin daily lifelong. Reports of 10% to 15% of aspirin resistance and up to 25% clopidogrel resistance potentially contributing to higher stent thrombosis risk have emerged. The use of reliable, standardized, simple tests of platelet activity would facilitate the diagnosis of aspirin and clopidogrel resistance.

【 　】 IIb/IIIa PLATELET RECEPTOR INHIBITORS

These platelet receptor blockers have been used as an adjunct to coronary intervention. The antibody fragment, abciximab; the peptide, eptifibatide; and the nonpeptide small-molecule agent, tirofiban, have each reduced periprocedural events, most commonly CK-MB elevation. Meta-analysis has suggested a small survival benefit. Other studies have shown no benefit on cardiac events in stable patients who have been given high-dose clopidogrel several hours before the procedure. These agents are recommended for PCI in the ACC/AHA unstable angina and non–ST-segment elevation MI guidelines.

【 　】 THROMBIN INHIBITORS

Unfarctionated heparin has been the primary thrombin inhibitor used during PCI over the last two decades. An activated clotting time of 300 seconds is targeted (or 200–250 seconds with concomitant IIb/IIIa inhibitor use). Low-molecular-weight heparin (LMWH) has advantages over unfractionated heparin (UFH) in being more bioavailable; being less inhibited by platelet factor 4; causing less thrombocytopenia; and having more predictable anticoagulant effects, eliminating the need for activated clotting

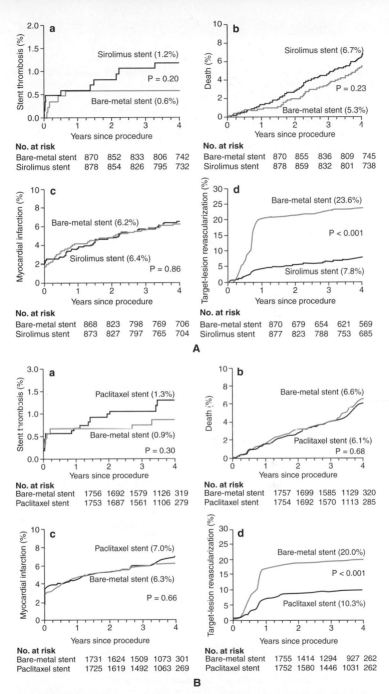

FIGURE 26-1. A. Analysis of randomized trials of sirolimus versus bare-metal stents on stent thrombosis, death, myocardial infarction, and target lesion revascularization. **B.** Analysis of randomized trials of paclitaxel versus bare-metal stents on stent thrombosis, death, myocardial infarction, and target lesion revascularization.

319

time monitoring in the cath lab. Therefore, LMWH use for PCI is currently a class IIa indication. Achieving a factor Xa level > 0.5 IU/mL has been a suggested target that was achieved by an 0.5-mg/kg bolus of intravenous enoxaparin. In the absence of factor Xa level monitoring, if PCI is performed within 8 hours of LMWH, no further LMWH is recommended. If the PCI is performed between 8 and 12 hours, a 0.3-mg/kg bolus of enoxaparin is recommended intravenously. The direct thrombin inhibitor Hirulog (bivalirudin) is also FDA approved for use during PCI. Advantages of these agents for PCI include the ease of monitoring their action with ACT measurement, their ability to inactivate clot-bound thrombin, and a favorable safety profile. In the latest guideline statement, bivalirudin has a class IIa indication for use in low-risk patients who are undergoing elective PCI. It has been suggested that optimal antithrombin therapy for PCI in certain complex patient subgroups, such as those with a high risk of bleeding, renal failure, and heparin-induced thrombocytopenia, is perhaps best accomplished with a direct thrombin inhibitor, whereas those with troponin positivity, diabetes, thrombus-containing lesions, and ST-elevation infarction are probably best managed with an indirect thrombin inhibitor and IIb/IIIa platelet receptor inhibitor.

【 】 INTRAVASCULAR ULTRASOUND

Although coronary angiography is the reference standard for the diagnosis of coronary artery disease, it has major limitations. Assessment of the significance of intermediate or indeterminant lesions, plaque characterization, recognition of diffuse intimal thickening, and accurate assessment of vessel dimensions and lesion extent are important pre-PCI determinations in which intravascular ultrasound (IVUS) greatly surpasses angiography. A minimal lumen cross-sectional area 3.0 to 4.0 mm^2 in major epicardial vessels and a left main minimal lumen diameter of 2.8 mm or minimal lumen area of 5.9 mm^2 indicates physiologic significance. Unopposed stent struts and stent underexpansion are thought to contribute to DES thrombosis and restenosis. It has been suggested that routine IVUS imaging during DES implantation is indicated in a number of high-risk patient subsets (renal failure, limitations to dual anti-platelet use, diabetes, poor LV function) and in high-risk lesion subsets (left main, bifurcations, ostial site, small vessels, long lesions, in-stent restenoses). Newly developed virtual histology IVUS, permitting plaque characterization into one of four phenotypes (fibrous, fibrofatty, necrotic core, or calcium) is a potentially useful addition to the diagnostic armamentarium of the interventionalist and is currently being studied.

【 】 FRACTIONAL FLOW RESERVE

Even experienced angiographers cannot adequately assess the physiologic significance of moderate coronary lesions. Fractional flow reserve (FFR) has emerged as a simple, reliable, and reproducible guidewire-based physiologic assessment of lesion severity and is defined as the ratio of distal coronary and aortic pressure during maximal hyperemia. An FFR < 0.75 has been shown to be accurate in predicting ischemia, and it is safe to defer PCI when FFR is ≥ 0.75. When microvascular disease is suspected, an FFR value of < 0.80 is indicative of ischemia. This adjunctive tool, which can be safely performed in a few minutes, brings substantial value to the patient and is cost effective in many applications.

【 】 EMBOLIC PROTECTION AND THROMBECTOMY DEVICES

A variety of occlusion–aspiration and filter-based strategies have evolved for embolic protection during saphenous vein graft interventions, which reduce atheroembolic MI by approximately 50% and constitute a class I indication in PCI guidelines. There has been limited application of embolic protection in native vessel PCI. A rheolytic thrombectomy device known as the AngioJet (POSSIS Medical, Minneapolis, MN) has become available for treatment of intracoronary thrombus, and it has proved useful in the setting of ACS associated with large thrombi and in treatment of stent thrombosis. The Export (Medtronic-AVE, Santa Rosa, CA) and PRONTO (Vascular Solutions, Minneapolis, MN) catheters are much simpler aspiration catheters that have proved useful in removing intracoronary thrombus.

HYBRID REVASCULARIZATION

The hybrid approach incorporates DES implantation and minimally invasive coronary surgery, the combination of these adjunctive strategies permitting complete revascularization. Most commonly the left internal mammary artery (LIMA) is used to bypass the LAD coronary artery, and non-LAD coronary artery targets are stented. This approach is thought to be ideal for patients with complex LAD coronary artery disease (ostial, bifurcation, or diffuse proximal involvement), significant but noncritical left main disease, and diabetes where LIMA-to-LAD coronary artery may have a mortality advantage. Avoidance of a sternotomy and cardiopulmonary bypass shortens hospitalization and hastens recovery. However, specialized surgical skills are necessary and long-term follow-up is not yet available.

HEMODYNAMICALLY SUPPORTED PCI

Intra-aortic balloon pump counterpulsation is widely available for hemodynamic support of high-risk PCI but provides limited support. The Tandem Heart Percutaneous Ventricular Assist device (CardiacAssist, Pittsburgh, PA) is a relatively simple centrifugal pump that provides sufficient hemodynamic support (up to 5.5 L/min) to sustain patients who are transiently without cardiac output, and has been used to provide circulatory protection during high-risk PCI or bridging to another therapy such as cardiac surgery, a left ventricular assist device, or transplantation. Complications such as bleeding, infection, thrombocytopenia, and anemia have been described with this device.

CLOSURE DEVICES

A variety of devices are currently available to close common femoral artery access sites following PCI. They permit earlier ambulation, enhance patient comfort, increase costs, and do not significantly alter overall access site complication rates. Rarely, infection or vascular compromise may occur and necessitate surgery.

INDICATIONS FOR CORONARY INTERVENTION

In general, when one is selecting PCI, there should be assurance that the operator can treat, with a high probability of success, the coronary lesion(s) accounting for the symptoms or signs of myocardial ischemia. Further, the associated risk and durability of the revascularization should be acceptable—as compared with bypass surgery or medical therapy—during both early and long-term follow-up. The latter estimate requires consideration of the likelihood and consequences of acute, subacute, late, and very late stent thrombosis, restenosis, and incomplete revascularization. Additional factors to be considered include the use of DES versus bare-metal stents, and the tolerability, cost, and risks associated with long-term dual antiplatelet therapy. The American College of Cardiology/American Heart Association Guidelines for Percutaneous Transluminal Coronary Angioplasty and Coronary Bypass Surgery provide a detailed analysis of many

TABLE 26-2

Recommendations for PCI Adopted from the ACC/ AHA/SCAI 2005 Guideline Update in Patients with Asymptomatic Ischemia or Class I to III Angina

Class IIa	One or more lesions in one or more vessels with high likelihood of success and low risk; vessels subtend large area of viable myocardium or produce moderate to severe ischemia (*level of evidence: B*); or a recurrent stenosis following PCI (*level of evidence: C*); or left main stenosis > 50% in CABG-ineligible patient (*level of evidence: B*); or SVG lesions in poor candidate for reoperation (*level of evidence: C*).
Class IIb	Efficacy of PCI in multivessel disease patients with proximal LAD stenosis and diabetes or an abnormal left ventricle is less well established (*level of evidence: B*); PCI may be considered in non-LAD sites producing ischemia (*level of evidence: C*).
Class III	Small amount of myocardium at risk, absence of ischemia, low PCI success, mild symptoms unlikely to be ischemia, increased PCI risk, left main stenosis and eligible for CABG, < 50% stenosis (*level of evidence: C*).

ACC, American College of Cardiology; AHA, American Heart Association; CABG, coronary artery bypass grafting; LAD, left anterior descending artery; PCI, percutaneous coronary intervention; SCAI, Society of Cardiac Angiography and Intervention; SVG, saphenous vein graft.

of these issues. Table 26-2 summarizes the Guideline recommendations for patients with asymptomatic ischemia or classes I to III angina.

SELECTION OF PATIENTS

【 】 SINGLE-VESSEL DISEASE

Percutaneous revascularization is an attractive option for many symptomatic patients who fail medical therapy and who have anatomically suitable lesions. For patients with complex bifurcation proximal LAD disease, consideration should be given to surgical revascularization. In experienced hands, endoscopic LIMA to LAD may be an attractive approach. It is important, however, to remember that there is no survival benefit of angioplasty compared with medical therapy.

【 】 MULTIVESSEL DISEASE

Rational selection of patients requires a careful analysis of multiple issues, including a risk-benefit assessment of each ischemia-producing lesion, a projection of the possible completeness and durability of the physiologic revascularization, and an estimate of resource consumption compared with surgery and medical therapy. In the experience of the Emory Angioplasty Versus Surgery Trial (EAST), 71% of index segments were revascularized in PTCA patients; while in the Bypass Angioplasty Revascularization Investigation (BARI 2D), 90% of the segments were revascularized by PCI or CABG. Culprit-lesion angioplasty is clearly an accepted strategy, but care must be taken to avoid significant residual ischemia after intervention. A strategy of physiologic (FFR)-guided PCI for multivessel disease may assure complete revascularization of ischemic territories without subjecting patients to the short- and long-term risk of unnecessary revascularization of angiographically stenotic but nonischemic lesions. Retrospective analyses have shown that compared to the standard angiographic guided approach, this strategy results in fewer stents deployed, lower costs, and improved outcomes. A randomized trial of physiologic (FFR) versus angiographic guided revascularization in multivessel disease is currently underway. The risks of PCI are increased in the presence of unstable angina, advanced age, poor left ventricular function, extensive coronary disease, comorbid conditions, and female gender.

SELECTION OF LESIONS

【 】 LESION CHARACTERISTICS

In the ACC/AHA/SCAI *2005 Guideline Update for PCI*, six high-risk lesion characteristics (type C) were recognized as important in the stent era. Four lesion classifications were suggested by considering the presence or absence of a type-C lesion and whether the vessel was patent or occluded (Table 26-3). This classification was shown to provide improved prediction of success and complications compared to the old ACC/AHA lesion classification. Interestingly, thrombus, bifurcation, and left main lesions do not appear, but remain important predictors of adverse outcome in the experience of the authors (see "Left Main Coronary Lesions" and "Bifurcation Lesions" below).

TABLE 26-3

Society of Cardiac Angiography and Intervention Lesion Classification System: Characteristics of Class I to IV Lesions[a]

Type I lesions (highest success expected, lowest risk)
(1) Does not meet criteria for C lesion
(2) Patent vessel
Type II lesions
(1) Meets any of these criteria for ACC/AHA C lesion:diffuse (greater than 2-cm length); excessive tortuosity of proximal segment; extremely angulated segments, greater than 90 degrees; inability to protect major side branches; degenerated vein grafts with friable lesions
(2) Patent vessel
Type III lesions
(1) Does not meet criteria for C lesion
(2) Occluded vessel
Type IV lesions
(1) Meets any of these criteria for ACC/AHA C lesion: diffuse (greater than 2-cm length); excessive tortuosity of proximal segment; extremely angulated segments, greater than 90 degrees; inability to protect major side branches; degenerated vein grafts with friable lesions; occluded for more than 3 months
(2) Occluded vessel

[a]See Chapter 59.

ACC, American College of Cardiology; AHA, American Heart Association.

Adapted from Krone RJ, Shaw RE, Klein LW, et al. Evaluation of the American College of Cardiology/American Heart Association and the Society for Coronary Angiography and Interventions lesion classification system in the current "stent era" of coronary interventions (from the ACC-National Cardiovascular Data Registry). *Am J Cardiol* 2003;92:389–394.

【 】 LEFT MAIN CORONARY LESIONS

The early experience with PTCA of left main lesions was unfavorable. Although acute results were more favorable with bare-metal stents, late outcomes remained poor (restenosis rate of 21%, late death 7.4%). With DES, 6- to 12-month mortality of left main PCI is approximately 2% to 4% in experienced hands. This is comparable to in-hospital mortality for CABG. Angiographic restenosis for the ostial and mid left main coronary artery is ≤ 5%, but much higher for distal left main stenosis, particularly when it involves the bifurcation. With two-stent approaches, there is an approximately 2% stent thrombosis rate and a 20% to 40% restenosis rate. This mandates angiographic surveillance at 3 months, and probably at 9 months, in order to detect and treat restenosis. Even for ostial or mid left main disease, longer-term follow-up will be required before this strategy is recommendable to all comers. The ACC/AHA/SCAI Guidelines recommend CABG for patients with left main disease who are surgical candidates. However, for patients who are not candidates for CABG, PCI is an option, but prolonged dual antiplatelet therapy and angiographic surveillance should be mandated.

【 】 CHRONIC TOTAL OCCLUSIONS

Chronic total occlusions (CTO) are found in up to 30% of diagnostic angiograms, but accounted for only 5.7% of coronary interventions in the NHLBI Dynamic Registry in 2004. Unrevascularized CTOs in multivessel disease patients may portend worse prognosis at 3 year follow-up. However, PCI of CTOs remains technically challenging and has lower success rates (50%–70%) even with experienced operators. Stiffer guidewires, the Safe Cross guidewire (IntraLuminal Therapeutics, Carlsbad, CA), coupling guidance with radiofrequency energy, and a helical screw-in microcatheter are examples of new technology to assist the PCI operator in successfully crossing the CTO. Drug-eluting stent implantation significantly improves outcomes compared with bare-metal stents.

【 】 BIFURCATION LESIONS

Bifurcation lesions remain difficult to treat effectively in the cath lab. Compared to nonbifurcation lesions, bifurcations were found to be more complex (angulated, eccentric, ostial, tortuous) and have a higher need for repeat intervention. To protect the side branch, many bifurcation techniques were developed (T-stenting, modified T-stenting, provisional T-stenting, Y- and V-stenting, culotte stenting, and crush stenting). None, however, proved superior to a single stent if side-branch patency was achieved with balloon dilation. The simple approach of stenting the main branch and provisional stenting of the side branch is currently recommended for most situations. If there is uncertainty regarding the need to stent the side branch, measurement of FFR is both safe and feasible. Koo and associates found that no side branch with < 75% stenosis had FFR < 0.75, and of 73 lesions with ≥75% stenosis, only 27% were functionally significant. Dedicated bifurcation stents are under development.

【 】 IN-STENT RESTENOSIS

The clinical presentation of in-stent restenosis includes exertional angina (64%), unstable angina (26%), and acute MI in 10% of 1,186 cases. The treatment options included balloon angioplasty, cutting balloon angioplasty, rotational atherectomy, and repeat bare-metal stent deployment. The use of intracoronary brachytherapy was shown to reduce restenosis, but brachytherapy was cumbersome, resulted in delayed healing, and raised concerns regarding late stent thrombosis and aneurysm formation . Drug-eluting stents have become the dominant strategy for treatment of bare-metal stent restenosis. When DES restenosis occurs, performing IVUS may be particularly important to rule out stent underexpansion or strut malapposition, both of which could be treated with high-pressure inflations. If the stent appears well deployed, repeat DES placement, medical therapy, or surgical revascularization should be considered, although there are very few data to guide therapy in this situation.

【 　】 AORTOCORONARY GRAFT LESIONS

PCI of distal anastomotic stenoses of saphenous vein grafts (SVGs) and LIMA grafts occurring within 1 year of CABG is safe and effective. Proximal SVG anastomotic and midgraft lesions have high restenosis rates, especially when long lesions are present. Atheromatous SVG lesions begin to appear about 3 years after CABG, and PCI is frequently associated with periprocedural MI caused by atheroembolization, a complication *not* prevented by IIb/IIIa platelet receptor inhibitors. Stent implantation is more effective than balloon angioplasty in SVG PCI. Distal and proximal embolic protection devices result in approximately 50% reduction in 30-day MACE. Proximal embolic protection are used when there is insufficient room beyond the target lesion for distal protection. Use of embolic protection during PCI of de novo SVG lesions is a class I indication in the ACC/AHA Guideline Statement and is cost-effective. Treatment of no-reflow after stenting includes aspiration of the stagnant dye column, hemodynamic support if needed, and administration of microvascular dilators distally (nitroprusside, calcium-channel blocker, or adenosine). Drug-eluting stents yield superior outcomes to bare-metal stents for SVG PCI. A high late cardiac event rate following SVG PCI relates largely to progression of atherosclerosis outside the stented segments. Consideration of native vessel intervention, including CTO recanalization whenever possible, careful surveillance, and aggressive risk factor modification, is warranted for these patients.

LESION CHARACTERISTICS

The importance of coronary stenosis angiographic morphology in predicting the outcome of coronary angioplasty is reflected in the ACC/AHA PTCA Guidelines. In an effort to update this classification based on the results of contemporary coronary intervention using stents and IIb/IIIa platelet inhibitors, Ellis and colleagues analyzed results from 10,907 lesions and proposed a new classification scheme for risk stratification (see Table 26-4). Nine preintervention variables were independently correlated with adverse outcome. Recent predictive models have been developed in the New York State Registry, in the Northern New England Registry, and at the Cleveland Clinic.

SELECTION OF DEVICES

Table 26-5 outlines the various technologies compared with balloon dilatation.

In the United States, stents are selected for primary treatment of almost all lesions in vessels ≥ 2.5 mm in diameter in patients who can tolerate at least short-term dual antiplatelet therapy. However, balloon angioplasty remains a useful option in persistently symptomatic patients with critical lesions in vessels < 2.5 mm or in selected patients who cannot tolerate dual antiplatelet therapy. Rotational atherectomy or cutting balloon angioplasty is reserved for heavily calcified lesions and for debulking in-stent restenosis. Suitable lesions for directional atherectomy are generally ostial or bifurcation lesions in vessels ≥ 3 mm in diameter.

PERFORMANCE OF CORONARY INTERVENTION

Current guidelines recommend that cardiologists who wish to become competent in coronary intervention receive special training in diagnostic and therapeutic catheterization during an additional year after the standard fellowship training program, and maintain skills

TABLE 26-4

New Risk-Assessment Schema[a]

Strongest correlates	Nonchronic total occlusion
	Degenerated saphenous vein graft (SVG)
Moderately strong correlates	Length ≥ 10 mm
	Lumen irregularity
	Large filling defect
	Calcium + angle ≥ 45 degrees
	Eccentric
	Severe calcification
	SVG age ≥ 10 years
Highest risk	Either of strongest correlates
High risk	≥ 3 moderate correlates and the absence of strong correlates
Moderate risk	1–2 moderate correlates and the absence of strong correlates
Low risk	No risk factors

[a]Based on analysis of 10,907 lesions treated in the stent and IIb/IIIa era.

Adapted from Ellis SG, Guetta V, Miller D, et al. Relation between lesion characteristics and risk with percutaneous intervention in the stent and glycoprotein IIb/IIIa era: an analysis of results from 10,907 lesions and proposal for new classification scheme. *Circulation.*1999;100: 1971–1976.

by performance of a minimum of 75 procedures per year. Ideally, operators with an annual procedural volume < 75 should only work at active centers (> 600 procedures per year) with on-site cardiac surgery. The Accreditation Council for Graduate Medical Education (ACGME) has defined the curriculum for the fourth year of training in interventional cardiology, and the American Board of Internal Medicine (ABIM) has established a subspecialty cardiac exam to certify properly trained cardiologists in interventional cardiology. Laboratory procedural volume is important and inversely related to adverse procedural outcomes.

【 】 CORONARY INTERVENTIONAL PROCEDURE

Prior to coronary intervention, patients receive an explanation of the procedure, including the operator's estimate of success, possible complications, risks, and benefits. Antiplatelet therapy is used routinely. The therapy most widely used is aspirin, 160 to 325 mg daily. Patients in whom stenting is planned also receive clopidogrel, usually in a 300- to 600-mg loading dose, unless pretreatment for several days has been performed. The platelet glycoprotein (GP) IIb/IIIa receptor blockers are frequently used in patients with a high risk of thrombotic events.

【 】 RESULTS OF CORONARY INTERVENTION

The technical performance of balloon angioplasty, atherectomy, and stenting is beyond the scope of this manual. Experienced interventional cardiologists should offer the best insight into the performance of the procedure and should be valuable consultants in the process of determining which patients are expected to benefit from interventions. Experienced operators should achieve primary success rates in excess of 95% in ideal proximal lesions, compared with a reduced success rate in recent (< 3 months) total occlusions or in attempts to treat fibrotic, calcified, eccentric stenoses located distally in tortuous coronary arteries. In all techniques, including stenting, lesion characteristics are

TABLE 26-5

New Coronary Interventional Strategies Compared with Balloon Angioplasty

Technique	Indications	Contraindications	Advantages and Limitations
Balloon angioplasty	Focal stenosis	Insignificant narrowing, no ischemia, unimportant artery	Broad applicability, lower cost; poor outcome in thrombotic, calcified lesions; significant restenosis
Stents	Focal stenosis	Heavy calcification or thrombus, vessel diameter < 2.5 mm	Reduced emergency CABG and restenosis; more expensive, rare stent thrombosis
Directional atherectomy	Focal noncalcified	Diffuse disease, severe tortuosity or bend	Debulks, reduced restenosis; more expensive, frequent non–Q-wave MI, more expensive, technically diffcult
Rotational atherectomy	Focal calcified stenosis, ostial site	Thrombus, large plaque burden, severe tortuosity or bend	Effective in calcified lesions, reduced elastic recoil; more expensive, similar restenosis, transient left ventricular dysfunction
Laser	Ostial lesion, SVG, in-stent restenosis	Severe calcification, tortuosity or bend	Debulks effectively; increased cost, similar restenosis
Transluminal extraction atherectomy	Thrombotic lesion, bulky SVG lesion	Severe tortuosity or bend, calcification	Thrombus and plaque removed; high complication rate in native vessels, distal embolization
Rheolytic thrombectomy	Thrombus	No thrombus	Effective thrombus removal; no plaque removal

SVG, saphenous vein graft; CABG, coronary artery bypass grafting; MI, myocardial infarction.

a major determinant of the outcome of the procedure. Selection for interventional procedures should always consider the expected long-term as well as the acute outcomes.

【　】 COMPLICATIONS

Patients undergoing PCI are subject to the same complications encountered with the performance of coronary arteriography. In addition, because instrumentation of the atherosclerotic lesion takes place, coronary artery dissection, perforation, thrombus formation, and coronary artery spasm may occur, leading to acute occlusion of the coronary artery or of side branches arising from it. Atheroembolism may occur and lead to MI in an otherwise successful procedure. Occlusion of the treated artery is the most common serious complication of coronary angioplasty and accounts for most of the morbidity and mortality related to the procedure.

The use of stents has significantly reduced the risk of urgent bypass surgery and Q-wave MI. New complications specifically related to the use of nonballoon devices include coronary perforation, distal atheroembolization, arterial access complications increased by the use of GP IIb/IIIa blockers, and "domino stenting" (additional stents to treat end-of-stent dissections). The progression of disease at sites that are not treated should also be considered a late complication of PCI. Aggressive lipid management in the Lescol Intervention Prevention Study (LIPS) trial has been shown to reduce post-PCI events. Other prevention measures are critical and must be part of the management of all patients undergoing interventional procedures (see also Chapter 21).

FUTURE DIRECTIONS

The future of coronary intervention is bright indeed. Restenosis is becoming a small, manageable problem; however, progression of disease remains a challenge that is currently being addressed on multiple fronts, with good prospects for meaningful solutions.

SUGGESTED READING

Braunwald E, Antman EM, Beasley JW, et al. ACC/AHA 2002 Guidelines for the Management of Patients with Unstable Angina and Non–ST-Segment Elevation Myocardial Infarction. *J Am Coll Cardiol*. 2002;40:1366–1374.

Douglas JS Jr, King SB III. Percutaneous coronary intervention. In: Fuster V, Alexander RW, O'Rourke RA, et al., eds. *Hurst's The Heart*. 12th ed. New York, NY: McGraw-Hill; 2007:1427–1449.

Gruentzig A. Transluminal dilatation of coronary artery stenosis. *Lancet*. 1978;1:263.

Hannan EL, Racz MJ, McCallister BD, et al. A comparison of three-year survival after coronary artery bypass graft surgery and percutaneous transluminal coronary angioplasty. *J Am Coll Cardiol*. 1999;33:63–72.

Holmes DR, Hirshfeld J, Faxon D, et al. ACC expert consensus document on coronary artery stents: document of the American College of Cardiology. *J Am Coll Cardiol*. 1998;32:1471–1482.

King SB III, Smith SC Jr., Hirshfeld JW Jr., et al. 2007 Focused Update of the ACC/AHA/SCAI 2005 Guideline Update for Percutaneous Coronary Intervention. *J Am Coll Cardiol*. 2008;51:172–209.

Marroquin OC, Selzer F, Mulukutla SR et al. A comparison of bare-metal and drug-eluting stents for off-label indications. *N Engl J Med*. 2008;358:342–352.

Moses JW, Leon MB, Popma JJ, et al. Drug-eluting stent trials. A multicenter randomized clinical study of the sirolimus-eluting stent in native coronary lesions: clinical outcomes. *Circulation*. 2002;106:II-392.

Stone GW, Moses JW, Ellis SE, et al. Safety and efficacy of sirolimus- and paclitaxel-eluting coronary. *N Engl J Med*. 2007;356:998–1008.

CHAPTER 27

Mechanical Interventions in Acute Myocardial Infarction

Anwar Tandar and William E. Boden

There are more than 800,000 cases of new or recurrent ST-segment elevation acute myocardial infarction (STEMI) in the United States annually. Despite profound improvements in care during the last 20 years, and dramatic reductions in in-hospital mortality from approximately 13% to 15% with conventional care to current levels of 3% to 6% with primary percutaneous coronary intervention (PCI) and fibrinolytic therapy, respectively, up to one-third of patients presenting with STEMI within 12 hours of symptom onset still receive no reperfusion therapy. Primary PCI, when performed rapidly by experienced operators at high-volume centers in a timely fashion, has become established as the preferred reperfusion approach for patients with STEMI, although fibrinolysis may be more suitable for some patients and in some circumstances. The development of new catheter-based treatment approaches and devices, more robust and effective adjunctive antiplatelet and antithrombin therapies, and improvements of system-based treatment pathways, including national quality improvement initiatives to enhance clinical outcomes, have armed interventional cardiologists with the needed tools to achieve optimal care of the STEMI patient.

PRIMARY PERCUTANEOUS CORONARY INTERVENTION IN STEMI

The ACC/AHA STEMI guidelines recommend PCI as the initial approach to management of STEMI, contingent upon treatment at centers with a skilled PCI laboratory and rapid initiation (within 90 minutes of first medical contact) (Fig. 27-1). This is based on multiple, randomized clinical trials demonstrating superiority of rapid primary PCI over fibrinolysis in STEMI, although ACC/AHA guidelines also state that there is no strong preference between PCI and fibrinolysis as the choice of initial reperfusion therapy in patients who present within 3 hours after symptom onset. In the setting within which the ACC/AHA guidelines recommend primary PCI, it offers several important potential advantages over pharmacologic reperfusion: it is suitable for ≥ 90% of patients, establishes initial thrombolysis in myocardial infarction (TIMI) grade 3 flow in 70% to 90% of patients, nearly eliminates the risk of intracranial hemorrhage, and may be particularly beneficial in high-risk patients, such as those with cardiogenic shock, severe congestive heart failure, or hemodynamic or electrical instability. If resource and logistical constraints did not limit more broad-based adoption of primary PCI, this would likely become the universal "dominant default strategy" for prompt early reperfusion.

In a previous meta-analysis of 23 randomized STEMI trials comparing primary PCI with fibrinolytic therapy (Fig. 27-2), there were significant reductions in short-term mortality, nonfatal MI, and stroke. Additionally, based on the 5 studies (Table 27-1) that compared emergent hospital transfer for primary PCI (with additional transfer-related delay averaging 39 minutes) with on-site fibrinolysis, PCI was still associated with significantly better outcomes; however, the difference was mainly driven by less reinfarction in the setting of low rates of rescue and early angiography. As noted above, the greatest absolute

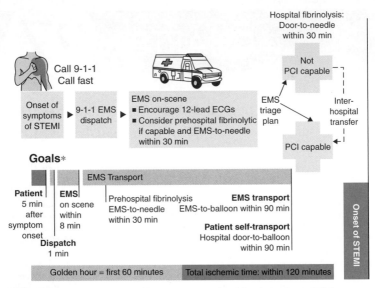

FIGURE 27-1. Transport scheme for STEMI. (Reproduced from ACC/AHA STEMI Guidelines 2004.)

benefit of primary PCI occurs among patients at highest risk, as reported in several randomized trials. The Should We Emergently Revascularize Occluded Coronaries for Cardiogenic Shock (SHOCK) trial randomized 302 patients with cardiogenic shock to emergency revascularization versus medical stabilization, and showed that mortality at 6 months was 50% versus 63%, respectively ($p = 0.03$). This important observation has been corroborated in other smaller studies of STEMI patients presenting in cardiogenic shock.

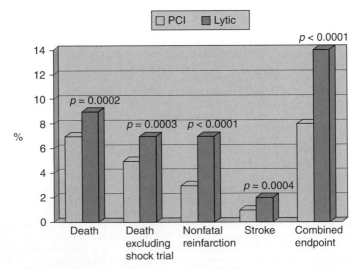

FIGURE 27-2. Meta-analysis of 23 randomized trials of PCI versus lysis ($n = 7,739$).

TABLE 27-1

Randomized Trials Comparing 30-day Outcomes in Patients Transferred for Primary PCI Versus Fibrinolytic

	Death	Reinfarction	Stroke	Composite	p-value	Delay (minutes)
Vermeer (n = 150)						
PCI	6.7	1.3	2.7	10.7	0.25	90
Alteplase	6.7	9.3	2.7	18.7		
PRAGUE-1 (n = 200)						
PCI	6.9	1.0	0	7.9	0.005	88
Alteplase	14.1	10.1	1.0	23.2		
AIR PAMI (n = 137)						
PCI	8.4	1.4	0	8.5	0.33	104
Alteplase	12.1	0	4.5	13.6		
DANAMI-2 (n = 1,572)						
PCI	6.6	1.6	1.1	8.0	0.0004	61
Alteplase	7.5	6.3	2.0	13.5		
PRAGUE-2 (n = 850)						
PCI	6.8	NA	NA	8.4	0.003	92
Streptokinase	10.0			15.2		

BENEFITS OF EARLY REPERFUSION: THE EARLY OPEN ARTERY THEORY

The early-open-artery theory suggests that benefits of reperfusion in patients with STEMI are directly related to the speed and completeness with which patency of the infarct-related coronary artery is reestablished, and may be more important than whether pharmacologic or mechanical intervention is used. Mortality is lower among patients in whom TIMI grade 2 to 3 flow, compared with TIMI grade 0 to 1 flow, was achieved within 90 minutes after acute MI. This is strongly supported by clinical studies confirming the important relationship between achieving prompt antegrade coronary flow of the infarct artery and improved clinical outcomes, both for primary PCI and fibrinolysis. An analysis by Boersma and associates indicated that the 35-day mortality benefit associated with early treatment equated to 1.6 lives per 1,000 patients per hour of delay from symptom onset to treatment, with even more of an impact of time in the early hours (Fig. 27-3). Achieving normal (TIMI-3) antegrade flow in the infarct artery is critical to optimizing clinical outcomes with both thrombolytic therapy and primary PCI. Primary PCI typically achieves TIMI-3 flow in 90% to 95% of patients, versus 50% to 55% in patients treated with new-generation thrombolytic agents. ACC guidelines recommend a target door-to-balloon time < 90 minutes. Newer combination therapy with low-dose thrombolytic and platelet glycoprotein IIb/IIIa inhibitors may further improve TIMI-3 flow rate (to 70%–75%), but this is still well below the TIMI-3 flow rates achieved with primary PCI.

MECHANICAL REPERFUSION AND ADJUNCTIVE THERAPIES

【 】 STENTS AND ADJUNCTIVE MECHANICAL DEVICES

The continued evolution in the development and use of stents—particularly over the last decade—has revolutionized the treatment of coronary artery disease (CAD) and has proven to diminish mortality and immediately alleviate anginal symptoms in STEMI patients.

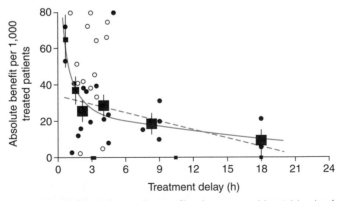

FIGURE 27-3. Absolute 35-day mortality versus fibrinolytic treatment delay. *Solid circle*, information from trials included in Fibrinolytic Therapy Trialists' Collaborative Group Analysis. *Open circles*, information from additional trials. *Small squares*, data beyond scales of x/y cross. The linear and nonlinear regression lines are fitted within these data, weighted by inverse of the variance of the absolute benefit in each data point. *Solid squares*, average effects in six time-to-treat groups (areas of squares inversely proportional to variance of absolute benefit described). (Reproduced with permission from Boersma E, Maas AC, Deckers JW, et al. Early thrombolytic treatment in acute myocardial infarction: reappraisal of the golden hour. *Lancet*. 1996;348:771–775.)

Studies have established the superiority of the drug-eluting stent (DES) in the reduction of target vessel revascularization (TVR) and restenosis when compared to the bare-metal stent (BMS) (Taxus IV, SIRIUS, and RAVEL trials). There are only a handful of noteworthy randomized clinical trials directly evaluating the efficacy of DES in acute MI to date. These studies include the Paclitaxel Eluting Stent Versus Conventional Stent in Myocardial Infarction with ST-segment Elevation (PASSION) trial, the Trial to Assess the Use of the Cypher Stent in Acute Myocardial Infarction Treated with Balloon Angioplasty (TYPHOON), the Sirolimus Eluting Stent Versus Bare Metal Stent in Acute Myocardial Infarction (SESAMI) trial, and the Comparison of Angioplasty with Infusion of Tirofiban or Abciximab and with Implantation of Sirolimus Eluting or Uncoated Stents for Acute Myocardial Infarction (MULTISTRATEGY) trial. These trials are summarized in Table 27-2. Despite the many differences in trial design and primary study end points, these trial data generally support the safety of using DES in patients with acute MI. It has been consistently observed that DES significantly reduce restenosis without major short-term risk, as compared with BMS implantation. These findings are important, as there was historical concern regarding the increased risk of subacute stent thrombosis in acute MI due to significant thrombus burden.

A meta-analysis from seven pivotal randomized trials evaluating DES versus BMS in STEMI concluded that DES significantly reduces the need for revascularization in patients with acute MI, without changes in incidence of subsequent death or MI (Fig. 27-4).

【 】 INTRACORONARY ASPIRATION/THROMBECTOMY DEVICES

Significant clot burden may complicate acute STEMI management. Prospective clinical studies have shown that intracoronary thrombectomy and thrombus aspiration may improve TIMI 3 flow, hasten ST-segment elevation resolution, and enhance myocardial tissue perfusion and reduce MI. The Thrombus Aspiration During Percutaneous Coronary Intervention in Acute Myocardial Infarction (TAPAS) trial showed that patients with STEMI benefit from aspiration thrombectomy. At 1-year follow-up, the study demonstrated a significant correlation between myocardial blush grade and death ($p = 0.001$) and a reduction in mortality ($p = 0.04$). Rheolytic thrombectomy, which employs a more sophisticated mechanism, has greater efficacy toward the removal of large thrombus burden compared to manual aspiration, but in a clinical trial of 480 STEMI patients (including those without visible clot) randomly assigned to PCI alone or PCI with AngioJet catheter thrombectomy, there was a greater infarct size measured by sestamibi imaging at 14 to 28 days with thrombectomy compared to PCI alone (12.5% versus 9.8%).

【 】 EMBOLIZATION PROTECTION DEVICES

Embolization protection devices, including the Percusurge (balloon occluding device) and FilterWire (filter basket device), were designed to enhance myocardial tissue perfusion by reducing distal embolization of atherothrombotic debris. Both the Saphenous Vein Graft Angioplasty Free of Emboli Randomized (SAFER) and FilterWire EX Randomized Evaluation (FIRE) studies demonstrated selective protection in saphenous vein graft interventions only. Several other studies have also failed to illustrate any benefits of these devices in native coronary artery interventions. Although the explanation for such a discrepancy is unclear, smaller thrombus burden in native coronary arteries, embolization due to the crossing a stenotic lesion with the device, delayed reperfusion due to the occlusive nature of the device, and difficulty in protecting vulnerable side branches are thought to be several possibilities.

ADJUNCTIVE ANTICOAGULANT AND ANTIPLATELET AGENTS

Regardless of the reperfusion strategy, the ACC guidelines recommend the inclusion of unfractionated or low-molecular-weight heparin (LMWH) as a class Ia indication. The ExTRACT-TIMI 25 (Enoxaparin and Thrombolysis Reperfusion for Acute Myocardial

TABLE 27-2

Combined Analysis of Randomized Control Trials of Drug-Eluting Stents in Myocardial Infarction

	Death			TLR/TVR			Stent Thrombosis			Restenosis		
	DES	BMS	p	DES	BMS	p	DES	BMS	p	DES	BMS	p
TYPHOON[a] (n = 712)	1.9%	1.4%	0.55	5.6%	13.4%	0.0004	3.3%	3.6%	0.80	7%	20%	NA
PASSION[a] (n = 605)	4%	6.3%	0.20	5.3%	7.6%	0.23	1%	1%	0.99	—	—	
SESAMI[a] (n = 307)	1.8%	4.3%	0.36	5.0%	13.1%	0.015	3.1%	3.7%	0.43	9%	21%	NA
MULTISTRATEGY[b] (n = 745)	3%	4%	0.42	3.2%	10.2%	<0.001	0.8%	1.1%	0.71	—	—	

DES, drug-eluting stent; BMS, bare-metal stent; TLR, target lesion revascularization; TVR, target vessel revascularization.

[a]1 year follow-up.

[b]8 months follow-up.

Modified from Anderson HV, Smalling RW, Henry TD. Drug-eluting stents for acute myocardial infarction. J Am Coll Cardiol. 2007;49:1931–1933.

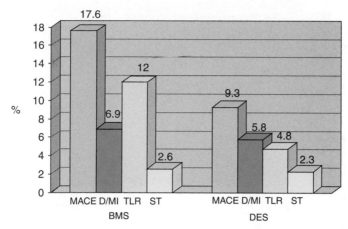

*MACE: major cardiac events; D/MI: death or myocardial infarction; TLR: target vessel revascularization; ST: stent thrombosis; BMS: bare metal stent; DES: drug eluting stent

FIGURE 27-4. Meta-analysis of clinical trials on use of DES for treatment of acute MI.

Infarction Treatment–Thrombolysis in Myocardial Infarction 25) and CLARITY-TIMI 28 (Clopidogrel as Adjunctive Reperfusion Therapy–Thrombolysis in Myocardial Infarction 28) trials demonstrated that LMWH improved clinical outcomes, including a reduction in the rate of composite end point of death and nonfatal reinfarction but associated with modestly increased bleeding when compared with unfractionated heparin (ExTRACT-TIMI 25). The factor Xa inhibitor, fondaparinux, demonstrated improved clinical outcomes in patients who received fibrinolysis or no reperfusion therapy, but not with primary PCI, in contrast to unfractionated heparin or placebo, in the OASIS-6 (Organization for the Assessment of Strategies for Ischemic Syndromes-6) trial, although fondaparinux did not show benefit in STEMI patients undergoing PCI compared to heparin, and was associated with catheter thrombus in 1.6% of patients.

[ ] GLYCOPROTEIN IIB/IIIA INHIBITORS

Abciximab remains the best-studied glycoprotein IIb/IIIa inhibitor in STEMI patients. In the Controlled Abciximab and Device Investigation to Lower Late Angioplasty Complications (CADILLAC) trial, one of the largest studies available, stent implantation resulted in significantly lower rates of death, MI, TVR, or stroke at 30 days and 6 months when compared to balloon angioplasty, regardless of the use of abciximab. Subacute stent thrombosis and recurrent ischemia in index vessels were significantly reduced by the use of abciximab (0% versus 1.0%, $p = 0.03$). The Direct Angioplasty and Stenting in Myocardial Infarction Regarding Acute and Long-Term Follow-up (ADMIRAL) trial evaluated the timing of abciximab administration in STEMI patients, and showed that the greatest benefit of early abciximab administration was improving vessel patency and preserving left ventricular function. While there was no significant different in mortality at 30 days (3.4% versus 6.6%, $p = 0.19$) and 6 months (3.4% versus 7.3%, $p = 0.13$) when compared to placebo, abciximab significantly reduced the combined end point of death, reinfarction, and TVR at 30 days (6.0% versus 14.6%, $p = 0.01$) and 6 months (7.4% versus 15.9%, $p = 0.02$). There was no significant excess in major bleeding with abciximab, but there was an increased rate of minor bleeding (12.1% versus 3.3%, $p = 0.004$).

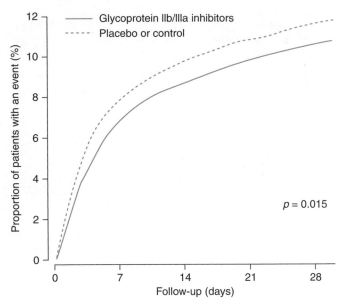

FIGURE 27-5. Kaplan–Meier estimates of cumulative occurrence of death of MI within 30 days with platelet glycoprotein IIB/IIIa. (Reproduced with permission from Boersma E, Harrington RA, Moliterno DJ, et al. Platelet glycoprotein IIb/IIIa inhibitors in acute coronary syndromes: a meta-analysis of all major randomised clinical trials, Lancet. Jan 19; 2002;359(9302):189–98.

A meta-analysis of 6 major randomized clinical trials utilizing glycoprotein IIb/IIIa inhibitors (tirofiban, eptifibatide, lamifiban, and abciximab) in ACS, comprising both STEMI and non-STEMI patients, indicated that the use of glycoprotein IIb/IIIa inhibitors reduce death or MI in patients presenting with ACS (Fig. 27-5).

【 】 DIRECT THROMBIN INHIBITORS

The benefit of bivalirudin in both low- and high-risk patients was elucidated in ACS patients enrolled in the Randomized Evaluation in PCI Linking Angiomax to Reduced Clinical Events (REPLACE-2) and Acute Catheterization and Urgent Intervention Triage Strategy (ACUITY) trials, respectively. Significant protection of bivalirudin against major bleeding without a significant benefit on ischemic outcomes was demonstrated in the ACUITY trial. The Intracoronary Stenting and Antithrombotic Regimen—Rapid Early Action for Coronary Treatment 3 (ISAR-React-3) trial evaluated the efficacy of bivalirudin versus unfractionated heparin in patients pretreated with clopidogrel and, like REPLACE-2, showed less bleeding without any significant overall ischemic end point benefit, when compared to patients treated with unfractionated heparin after preloading with clopidogrel.

【 】 ANTIPLATELET THERAPY

Dual antiplatelet therapy using clopidogrel and aspirin has been shown effective in preventing a composite end point of death, MI, and stroke in patients who have ACS without ST-segment elevation or who have undergone PCI. Recently, two major studies have examined whether aggressive antiplatelet therapy with clopidogrel in combination with aspirin would be beneficial in STEMI patients. The Clopidogrel as Adjunctive Reperfusion Therapy—Thrombolysis in Myocardial Infarction (CLARITY-TIMI 28) trial, conducted in 3,491 patients presenting within 12 hours of onset of STEMI, compared the effects of adding clopidogrel (300 mg loading dose, then 75 mg once daily) or placebo to an aspirin- and heparin-based fibrinolytic regimen. The primary composite end point (occluded infarct-related artery [IRA] upon angiography or recurrent MI/death from any cause before angiography) occurred in 21.7% of placebo-treated patients versus 15% in the clopidogrel group ($p < 0.001$). This 36% improvement was driven largely by a lower incidence of IRA occlusion with clopidogrel than placebo (11.7% versus 18.4%, $p < 0.001$). At 30 days, addition of clopidogrel to aspirin/fibrinolytic therapy produced a 20% relative risk reduction in cardiovascular mortality, recurrent MI, and recurrent ischemia leading requiring urgent revascularization (from 14.1% to 11.6%, $p = 0.03$). The rates of bleeding and other safety outcomes were similar in both treatment groups. A prospectively planned subanalysis of patients who underwent PCI showed that pretreatment with clopidogrel plus aspirin significantly reduced the rate of cardiovascular death, MI, or stroke after PCI to 30 days after randomization (odds ratio 0.54, 95% CI 0.35–0.85, $p = 0.008$).

While the CLARITY trial was not powered to show a survival benefit in STEMI patients, this question was addressed in a separate study, the COMMIT/CCS-2 trial (Clopidogrel and Metoprolol in Myocardial Infarction Trial/Second Chinese Cardiac Study —The Clopidogrel Arm). This randomized, placebo-controlled trial, conducted in 46,000 patients in China, investigated the effects of dual antiplatelet therapy on mortality rates in STEMI patients presenting within 24 hours, who were randomized to ≤ 4 weeks of clopidogrel (75 mg/d) treatment or placebo; all patients received aspirin 162 mg/d for the duration of the study. Clopidogrel treatment produced a 9% reduction in the co-primary composite end point of death, MI, or stroke, compared with placebo (95% CI 3–14, $p = 0.002$). At hospital discharge or day 28 (whichever came first), clopidogrel-treated patients had significantly lower rates of all-cause mortality (7.5% versus 8.1%, $p = 0.03$). Although a loading dose was not used in this trial, the survival curves began to diverge as early as day 1. The benefits appeared to be greatest where clopidogrel was administered early (within 6 hours) after symptom onset. Major bleeding was similar in both groups, but minor bleeding was more common with clopidogrel.

More recently, prasugrel, a new and more powerful P_2Y_{12} inhibitor, has been evaluated in a large ACS trial in which both STEMI and non-STEMI patients were randomized to either prasugrel + aspirin or clopidogrel + aspirin where patients underwent early coronary angiography and either PCI or CABG surgery. Compared to clopidogrel, there was a 20% incremental reduction in the composite of cardiac death, MI, or stroke during long-term follow-up, but with an increase signal of both fatal and major bleeding. This agent is not yet FDA-approved for use in ACS patients.

RESCUE AND FACILITATED ANGIOPLASTY

Rescue angioplasty, the mechanical reopening of an occluded infarct artery after failed thrombolysis, has been used as adjunctive therapy in STEMI patients with failed thrombolysis, but has been associated with inconsistent results. Despite the intuitive benefit of rescue PCI and the well-recognized improvement in procedural results with stenting, the role of rescue PCI for STEMI, based on evidence from multiple randomized trials, remains controversial. However, even in the absence of conclusive clinical benefit, it does appear reasonable to consider acute angiography with rescue angioplasty in patients with anterior or large STEMI who are thought to have failed thrombolysis, as evidenced by persistent chest pain, lack of resolution of ST-segment elevation, or hemodynamic compromise at greater than 90 minutes following treatment.

Similarly, a number of recent studies have evaluated so-called facilitated PCI, where pharmacologic therapy is followed immediately by PCI, but at present the data suggest that it is not beneficial and may be harmful. Worse outcomes were seen with facilitated PCI versus primary PCI in a recent meta-analysis—driven largely by the largest trial to date, the ASSENT-4 PCI (Assessment of the Safety and Efficacy of a New Treatment Strategy with Percutaneous Coronary Intervention) trial, which showed that routine immediate PCI following full-dose fibrinolytic therapy was associated with higher rates of abrupt vessel closure, reinfarction, and death versus primary PCI alone in patients with only modest treatment delays and treated with low-dose heparin. One implication of this trial is that patients receiving full-dose fibrinolytic therapy, together with signs of presumptive reperfusion (e.g., resolution of chest pain and/or ST-segment elevation), should not undergo routine immediate PCI, as there may be an early prothrombotic state following fibrinolytic therapy. Most recently, the Facilitated Intervention with Enhanced Reperfusion Speed to Stop Events (FINESSE) trial results were published, in which STEMI patients were randomized in a 1:1:1 fashion to primary PCI with in-lab abciximab, up-front abciximab-facilitated primary PCI, or half-dose reteplase/abciximab-facilitated PCI. At 90 days, there was no difference among treatment arms for the primary composite end point (all-cause mortality, readmission for heart failure, ventricular fibrillation, or cardiogenic shock). The rates for TIMI non-intracranial major bleeding and minor bleeding were significantly higher for the abciximab/lytic-facilitated PCI strategy as compared with the primary PCI or the abciximab-only group, as were major and minor bleeding combined. Current evidence does not justify the facilitated PCI approach.

In summary, the acute interventional approach to STEMI management has continued to undergo important and profound changes, both in terms of catheter-based treatment approaches and the evolving role of adjunctive pharmacotherapies.

SUGGESTED READING

Ali A, Cox D, Dib N, et al. Rheolytic thrombectomy with percutaneous coronary intervention for infarct size reduction in acute myocardial infarction: 30-day results from multicenter randomized study. *J Am Coll Cardiol.* 2006;48:244–252.

American College of Cardiology. *Clinical Statement and Guidelines.* http://www.acc.org/qualityandscience/clinical/guidelines/stemi. 2005.

Anderson HV, Smalling RW, Henry TD. Drug eluting stents for acute myocardial infarction. *J Am Coll Cardiol.* 2007;49:1931–1933.

Brodie BR, Hansen C, Stuckey TD, et al. Door-to-balloon time with primary percutaneous coronary intervention for acute myocardial infarction impacts late cardiac mortality in high-risk patients and patients presenting early after the onset of symptoms. *J Am Coll Cardiol.* 2006;47:289–295.

Hochman JS, Sleeper LA, Webb JG, et al. Early revascularization in acute myocardial infarction complicated by cardiogenic shock. *N Engl J Med.* 1999;341:625–634.

Kastrati A, Dibra A, Spaulding C, et al. Meta-analysis of randomized trials on drug eluting stents vs. bare-metal stents in patients with acute myocardial infarction. *Eur Heart J.* 2007;28:2706–2713.

O'Neill W, Brodie BR. Mechanical interventions in acute myocardial infarction. In: Fuster V, Alexander RW, O'Rourke RA, et al., eds. *Hurst's The Heart.* 11th ed. New York, NY: McGraw-Hill; 2004:1451–1464.

Smith SC Jr., Feldman TE, Hirshfeld JW Jr., et al. ACC/AHA/SCAI 2005 Guideline Update for Percutaneous Coronary Intervention. A report of the American College of Cardiology/American Heart Association Task Force on Practice Guidelines (ACC/AHA/SCAI Writing Committee to Update the 2001 Guidelines for Percutaneous Coronary Intervention). *J Am Coll Cardiol.* 2006;47:1–121.

Valgimigli M, Campo G, Percoco G, et al. Comparison of angioplasty with infusion of tirofiban or abciximab and with implantation of sirolimus-eluting or uncoated stents for acute myocardial infarction: the MULTISTRATEGY randomized trial. *JAMA.* 2008;299:1788–1799.

Welsh RC, Gordon P, Westerhout CM, et al. A novel enoxaparin regime for ST elevation myocardial infarction patients undergoing primary percutaneous coronary intervention: a West sub-study. *Catheter Cardiovasc Interv.* 2007;70:341–348.

CHAPTER 28

Systemic Hypertension: Pathogenesis and Etiology

Michael E. Hall, John E. Hall, Joey P. Granger, and Daniel W. Jones

A direct positive relationship between blood pressure (BP) and cardiovascular disease (CVD) risk has been observed in men and women of all ages, races, ethnic groups, and countries, regardless of other risk factors for CVD. Observational studies indicate that death from CVD increases linearly as BP rises above 115 mm Hg systolic and 75 mm Hg diastolic pressure. For every 20 mm Hg systolic or 10 mm Hg diastolic increase in BP, there is a doubling of mortality from both ischemic heart disease and stroke in all age groups from 40 to 89 years old. Despite major advances in our understanding of its pathophysiology and the availability of many drugs that can effectively reduce BP in most hypertensive subjects, hypertension continues to be the most important modifiable risk factor for CVD.

BASIC PRINCIPLES OF BLOOD PRESSURE REGULATION

Adequate BP is critical to provide the driving force for tissue blood flow. Consequently, the regulation of BP is a complex physiologic function that depends on the integrated actions of multiple cardiovascular, renal, neural, endocrine, and local tissue control systems.

The multiple local control, hormonal, neural, and renal systems that regulate BP are often discussed in terms of how they influence cardiac pumping or vascular resistance because of the well-known formula: *mean arterial pressure = cardiac output × total peripheral resistance*. This conceptual framework (with the addition of factors that influence vascular capacity and transcapillary exchange) adequately explains short-term BP regulation, but is inadequate when discussing abnormalities of long-term BP regulation, such as hypertension. To explain long-term BP regulation, we must introduce two other concepts: (1) time-dependency of BP control mechanisms and (2) the necessity of maintaining balance between intake and output of water and electrolytes, and the role of BP in maintaining this balance.

【 】 FEEDBACK CONTROL SYSTEMS

Feedback control systems for BP are time dependent. Three important neural control systems begin to function within seconds after a disturbance of BP (Fig. 28-1): (1) the arterial baroreceptors, which detect changes in BP and send appropriate autonomic reflex signals back to the heart and blood vessels to return the BP toward normal; (2) the chemoreceptors, which detect changes in oxygen or carbon dioxide in the blood and initiate autonomic feedback responses that influence BP; and (3) the central nervous system, which responds within a few seconds to ischemia of the vasomotor centers in the

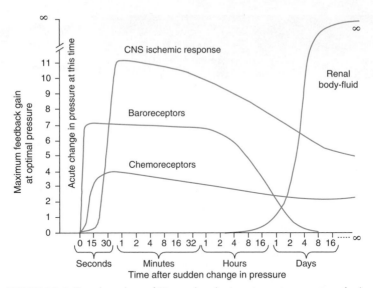

FIGURE 28-1. Time dependency of BP control mechanisms. Approximate maximum feedback gains of various BP control mechanisms at different time intervals after the onset of a disturbance to arterial pressure. (Redrawn with permission from Guyton AC, Hall JE. *Textbook of Medical Physiology.* 11th ed. Philadelphia, PA: Elsevier; 2006:230.)

medulla, especially when BP falls below about 50 mm Hg. Within a few minutes or hours after a BP disturbance, several additional control systems react, including (1) a shift of fluid from the interstitial spaces into the bloodstream in response to decreased BP (or a shift of fluid out of the blood into the interstitial spaces in response to increased BP); (2) the rennin–angiotensin system (RAS), which is activated when BP falls too low and suppressed when BP increases above normal; and (3) multiple vasodilator systems that are suppressed when BP decreases and stimulated when BP rises above normal.

Most of the BP regulators are *proportional* control systems. This means that they will correct a BP abnormality only part of the way back toward the normal level. However, there is one BP control system, the renal–body fluid feedback system, that has *near-infinite feedback gain* if it is given enough time to operate. Thus, the renal–body fluid feedback control mechanism does not stop functioning until the arterial pressure returns all the way back to its original control level, as discussed below.

【 】 RENAL–BODY FLUID FEEDBACK

Renal–body fluid feedback is a dominant mechanism for long-term BP regulation. Figure 28-2 shows the conceptual framework for understanding long-term control of BP by the renal–body fluid feedback mechanism. Extracellular fluid volume is determined by the balance between intake and excretion of salt and water by the kidneys. Under steady-state conditions there must always be a precise balance between intake and output of salt and water; otherwise, there would be continued accumulation or loss of fluid leading to complete circulatory collapse within a few days. In fact, it is more critical to maintain salt and water balance than to maintain a normal level of BP and, as discussed below, increased BP is a means of regulating these balances in the face of impaired kidney function.

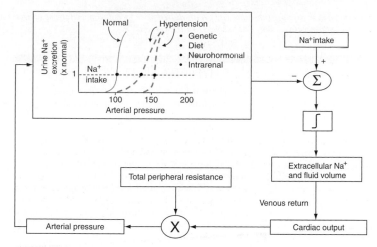

FIGURE 28-2. Block diagram showing the basic elements of the renal–body fluid feedback mechanism for long-term regulation of arterial pressure.

A key mechanism for regulating salt and water balance is pressure natriuresis and diuresis, the effect of increased BP to raise sodium and water excretion. Under most conditions this mechanism stabilizes BP and body fluid volumes. For example, when BP increases above the renal set-point, because of increased TPR or increased cardiac pumping ability, this also increases sodium and water excretion via pressure natriuresis if kidney function is not impaired. As long as fluid excretion exceeds fluid intake, extracellular fluid volume will continue to decrease, reducing venous return and cardiac output, until BP returns to normal and fluid balance is reestablished.

An important feature of pressure natriuresis is that various hormonal and neural control systems can greatly amplify or blunt the basic effects of BP on sodium and water excretion. For example, during chronic increases in sodium intake only small changes in BP are needed to maintain sodium balance in most people. One reason for this insensitivity of BP to changes in salt intake is decreased formation of antinatriuretic hormones, such as angiotensin II (ANG II) and aldosterone, which enhance the effectiveness of pressure natriuresis and allow sodium balance to be maintained with minimal increases in BP. On the other hand, excessive activation of these antinatriuretic systems can reduce the effectiveness of pressure natriuresis, thereby necessitating greater increases in BP to maintain sodium balance.

Another important feature of pressure natriuresis is that it continues to operate until BP returns to the original set-point. In other words, it acts as part of an *infinite gain* feedback control system. As far as we know, it is the only infinite gain feedback system for BP regulation in the body, and it is this property which makes it a dominant long-term controller of BP.

Therefore, in all forms of human or experimental hypertension studied thus far, there is impaired pressure natriuresis that appears to initiate and sustain the hypertension. In some cases, abnormal kidney function is caused by intrarenal disturbances that impair renal hemodynamics or increase tubular reabsorption. In other cases, impaired kidney function is caused by extrarenal disturbances, such as increased SNS activity or excessive formation of antinatriuretic hormones that reduce the kidney's ability to excrete sodium and water and eventually raise BP. *Consequently, effective treatment of hypertension requires interventions that reset pressure natriuresis toward normal levels of BP either by directly increasing renal excretory capability (e.g., with diuretics) or by reducing extrarenal antinatriuretic influences (e.g., with RAS blockers) on the kidneys.*

RENAL MECHANISMS OF HYPERTENSION

An observation that points toward abnormal kidney function as a key factor in hypertension is that almost all forms of experimental hypertension, as well as all monogenic forms of human hypertension thus far discovered, are caused by obvious insults to the kidneys that alter renal hemodynamics or tubular reabsorption. For example, constriction of the renal arteries (e.g., Goldblatt hypertension), compression of the kidneys (e.g., perinephritic hypertension), or administration of sodium-retaining hormones (e.g., mineralocorticoids or ANG II) are all associated with either initial reductions in renal blood flow and glomerular filtration rate (GFR) or increases in tubular reabsorption prior to development of hypertension. Likewise, in all known monogenic forms of human hypertension, the common pathway to hypertension appears to be increased renal tubular sodium reabsorption caused by mutations that directly increase renal electrolyte transport or the synthesis and/or activity of antinatriuretic hormones. As BP rises, the initial renal changes are often obscured by compensations that restore kidney function toward normal. The rise in BP then initiates a cascade of cardiovascular changes, including increased TPR that may be more striking than the initial disturbance of kidney function. The general types of renal abnormalities that can cause chronic hypertension include (1) increased preglomerular resistance, (2) decreased glomerular capillary filtration coefficient, (3) reduced numbers of functional nephrons, and (4) increased tubular reabsorption.

NEUROHUMORAL MECHANISMS OF HYPERTENSION

Although impaired renal pressure natriuresis plays a central role in all forms of experimental and human hypertension studied thus far, not all disorders of pressure natriuresis originate within the kidneys. Inappropriate activation of antinatriuretic hormone systems (e.g., ANG II, aldosterone) that normally regulate sodium excretion or a deficiency of natriuretic influences (e.g., atrial natriuretic peptide, nitric oxide) on the kidneys can impair renal pressure natriuresis and cause chronic hypertension. Likewise, excessive activation of the SNS plays a major role in elevating BP in many hypertensive patients.

【 】 SYMPATHETIC NERVOUS SYSTEM

The SNS is a major short-term and long-term controller of BP. Sympathetic vasoconstrictor fibers are distributed to almost all of regions of the vasculature, as well as to the heart, and activation of the SNS can raise BP within a few seconds by causing vasoconstriction, increased cardiac pumping capability, and increased heart rate. Conversely, sudden inhibition of SNS activity can decrease BP to as low as half normal within less than a minute. Therefore, changes in SNS activity, caused by various reflex mechanisms, central nervous system ischemia, or by activation of higher centers in the brain, provide powerful and rapid, moment-to-moment regulation of BP.

The SNS also is important in long-term regulation of BP and in the pathogenesis of hypertension, in large part by activation of the renal sympathetic nerves. There is extensive innervation of the renal blood vessels, the juxtaglomerular apparatus, and the renal tubules, and excessive activation of these nerves causes sodium retention, increased renin secretion, and impaired renal pressure natriuresis. Evidence for a role of the renal nerves in hypertension comes from multiple studies showing that renal denervation reduces BP in several models of experimental hypertension. Human primary hypertension, especially when associated with obesity, is often associated with increased renal sympathetic activity. Although the mechanisms that cause activation of renal sympathetic nerves in primary hypertension are still unclear, excess weight gain contributes to increased SNS activity in many patients with primary (essential) hypertension, as discussed later.

【 】 RENIN–ANGIOTENSIN SYSTEM

The renin–angiotensin system (RAS) is perhaps the most powerful hormone system for regulating body fluid volumes and BP as evidenced by the effectiveness of various RAS blockers in reducing BP in normotensive and hypertensive subjects. Although the RAS has many components, its most important effects on BP regulation are exerted by angiotensin II (ANG II), which participates in both short-term and long-term control of BP. ANG II is a powerful vasoconstrictor and helps maintain BP in conditions associated with acute volume depletion (e.g., hemorrhage), sodium depletion, or circulatory depression (e.g., heart failure). The long-term effects of ANG II on BP, however, are closely intertwined with volume homeostasis through direct and indirect effects on the kidneys.

Blockade of the RAS, with ANG II receptor blockers (ARBs) or angiotensin-converting enzyme (ACE) inhibitors, increases renal excretory capability so that sodium balance can be maintained at reduced BP. However, blockade of the RAS also reduces the slope of pressure natriuresis and makes BP salt sensitive. Thus, the effectiveness of RAS blockers in lowering BP is greatly diminished by high salt intake and improved by the reduction in sodium intake or addition of a diuretic.

Inappropriately high levels of ANG II impair pressure natriuresis, thereby necessitating increased BP to maintain sodium balance. The mechanisms mediating the potent antinatriuretic effects of ANG II include renal hemodynamic effects (e.g., constriction of efferent arterioles) as well as direct and indirect effects to increase sodium reabsorption in proximal, loop of Henle, and distal tubules.

When renal perfusion pressure is reduced to low levels or when other disturbances such as sodium depletion are superimposed on low BP, the vasoconstrictor effect of ANG II on efferent arterioles is important in preventing excessive decreases in GFR. This effect is especially important in patients with renal artery stenosis and/or sodium depletion or with heart failure who may have substantial decreases in GFR when treated with RAS blockers. On the other hand, RAS blockade may be beneficial when nephrons are hyperfiltering, especially if ANG II is not appropriately suppressed. For example, in diabetes mellitus and in certain forms of hypertension associated with glomerulosclerosis and nephron loss, ANG II blockade, by decreasing efferent arteriolar resistance and arterial pressure, lowers glomerular hydrostatic pressure and attenuates glomerular hyperfiltration and progression of renal injury.

【 】 ALDOSTERONE

Aldosterone is a powerful sodium-retaining hormone and consequently has important effects on renal pressure natriuresis and BP regulation. The primary sites of actions of aldosterone on sodium reabsorption are the principal cells of the distal tubules, cortical collecting tubules, and collecting ducts where aldosterone stimulates sodium reabsorption and potassium secretion. Aldosterone binds to intracellular mineralocorticoid receptors (MRs) and activates transcription by target genes which, in turn, stimulate synthesis or activation of the Na^+-K^+-ATPase pump on the basolateral epithelial membrane and activation of amiloride-sensitive sodium channels on the luminal side of the epithelial membrane. These effects are termed *genomic* because they are mediated by activation of gene transcription and require 60 to 90 minutes to occur after administration of aldosterone. Aldosterone also appears to exert rapid *nongenomic* effects on the cardiovascular and renal systems, although the importance of these actions on renal function and BP regulation is still unclear.

Some investigators suggest that hyperaldosteronism may be more common than previously believed, especially in patients with hypertension that is resistant to treatment with the usual antihypertensive medications. For example, the prevalence of primary aldosteronism is reported to be almost 20% among patients referred to specialty clinics for resistant hypertension. Many of these patients, however, are overweight or obese. Regardless of the prevalence of primary aldosteronism, antagonism of MRs may provide an important therapeutic tool for preventing target-organ injury and reducing BP in patients with resistant hypertension.

【 】 ENDOTHELIN

Endothelin-1 (ET-1), a powerful vasoconstrictor, has receptor binding sites throughout the body, with the greatest numbers in the kidneys and lungs. ET-1 causes vasoconstriction and hypertension by activation of type A (ET_A) receptors but also has antihypertensive effects through activation of type B (ET_B) receptors which cause vasodilation and inhibit sodium reabsorption in the kidneys. Although ET_A receptor activation may play a role in certain forms of hypertension, this effect does not appear to have a major influence on cardiovascular and renal function under normal physiologic conditions.

【 】 NITRIC OXIDE (NO)

Tonic release of NO by the vascular endothelium plays a major role in regulating vascular function and impairment of NO formation causes impaired renal pressure natriuresis and sustained hypertension. The magnitude of the increase in BP during NO inhibition is greater with high sodium intake. Reductions in NO synthesis may decrease renal sodium excretory function by increasing renal vascular resistance directly or by enhancing the renal vascular responsiveness to vasoconstrictors such as ANG II or norepinephrine. Reductions in NO synthesis also increase renal tubular sodium reabsorption via direct effects on renal tubular transport and through changes in intrarenal physical factors, such as renal interstitial hydrostatic pressure and medullary blood flow.

【 】 OXIDATIVE STRESS

Oxidative stress occurs when total oxidant production exceeds antioxidant capacity. Recent studies suggest that reactive oxygen species (ROS) may play a role in the initiation and progression of cardiovascular dysfunction associated with hyperlipidemia, diabetes mellitus, and hypertension. In many forms of hypertension, increased ROS appear to be derived mainly from nicotinamide adenine dinucleotide phosphate oxidases, which could serve as a triggering mechanism for uncoupling endothelial nitric oxide synthase (NOS) by oxidants. ROS produced by migrating inflammatory cells and/or vascular cells have distinct effects on different cell types. These effects include endothelial dysfunction, increased renal tubule sodium transport, cell growth and migration, inflammatory gene expression, and stimulation of extracellular matrix formation. ROS, by affecting vascular and renal tubule function, can also impair renal pressure natriuresis, alter systemic hemodynamics, and raise BP.

【 】 ATRIAL NATRIURETIC PEPTIDE

Atrial natriuretic peptide (ANP) is a peptide synthesized and released from atrial cardiocytes in noresponse to stretch. ANP reduces vascular resistance while enhancing sodium excretion through extrarenal and intrarenal mechanisms. ANP increases GFR but has little effect on renal blood flow. ANP may also inhibit renal tubular sodium reabsorption either directly by inhibiting active tubular transport of sodium or indirectly via alterations in medullary blood flow, physical factors, and intrarenal hormones. ANP reduces renin secretion and reductions in intrarenal ANG II levels likely contribute to ANP-induced natriuresis. ANP also decreases aldosterone release either by direct effects on the adrenal gland or by reducing ANG II secondary to suppression of renin. Long-term physiologic elevations in plasma ANP enhance renal pressure natriuresis and reduce BP.

SECONDARY CAUSES OF HYPERTENSION

In a small percentage of patients, the clinical features, history, and physical examination point to a specific cause of increased BP and the hypertension is therefore said to be *secondary*. Some types of secondary hypertension have a definite genetic basis, whereas others are caused by CVD and target-organ injury associated with various disorders, such as diabetes and kidney disease. In some instances, hypertension can be caused by drugs or treatments that the patient receives. Nearly all forms of secondary hypertension, however, are characterized by impaired renal function or altered activity of the SNS or hormones that, in turn, impair the ability of the kidneys to excrete salt and water.

Table 28-1 lists some of the most frequent causes of secondary hypertension, including those caused by drugs that either themselves raise BP or exacerbate underlying

TABLE 28-1

Some Secondary Causes of Hypertension

A. Renal parenchymal disease
- Acute and chronic glomerulonephritis
- Chronic nephritis (e.g., pyelonephritis, radiation)
- Polycystic disease
- Diabetic nephropathy
- Hydronephrosis
- Neoplasms

B. Renovascular
- Renal artery stenosis/compression
- Intrarenal vasculitis
- Suprarenal aortic coarctation

C. Renoprival (renal failure, loss of kidney tissue)

D. Endocrine disorders
- Renin-producing tumors
- Cushing's syndrome
- Primary aldosteronism
- Pheochromocytoma (adrenal or extraadrenal chromaffin tumors)
- Acromegaly

E. Pregnancy-induced hypertension

F. Sleep apnea

G. Increased intracranial pressure (brain tumors, encephalitis)

H. Exogenous hormones and drugs (partial list)
- Glucocorticoids
- Mineralocorticoids
- Sympathomimetics
- Tyramine-containing foods and monoamine oxidase inhibitors
- Estrogen (e.g., oral contraceptive pills)
- Apparent mineralocorticoid excess (e.g., licorice)
- Nonsteroidal antiinflammatory drugs
- Cyclosporine
- Excess alcohol use
- Drug abuse (e.g., amphetamines, cocaine)

disorders that contribute to hypertension. These drugs include nonsteroidal anti-inflammatory drugs, oral contraceptive agents, glucocorticoids, and sympathomimetics that are used as cold remedies. This chapter discusses only a few of the more common causes of secondary hypertension.

【 】 RENOVASCULAR HYPERTENSION

Renovascular hypertension, although accounting for only 2% to 3% of all hypertension, is one of the most common causes of secondary hypertension. The pathophysiology of renovascular hypertension is related directly to the reduction in renal perfusion that occurs as a result of stenosis of the main renal artery, one of its branches, or stenosis/injury of other smaller preglomerular blood vessels and glomeruli. The majority of renal vascular lesions reflect either fibromuscular dysplasia or atherosclerosis. The predominant lesion found in the main renal artery or its branches in patients greater than 50 years of age is atherosclerotic disease. More subtle functional (constriction) or structural changes in smaller blood vessels (e.g., afferent arterioles, glomeruli), however, are difficult to detect clinically and can also contribute to increased BP. Renal artery stenosis produces a rise in BP that is proportional to the severity of the constriction. Renovascular hypertension can be unilateral, involving only one kidney, or bilateral and can result in a homogeneous or a non-homogeneous ischemia of nephrons. However, there are some important differences in the pathophysiology of homogeneous compared to nonhomogenous impairment of renal perfusion.

【 】 ADRENAL CORTEX HYPERTENSION

Aldosterone normally exerts nearly 90% of the mineralocorticoid activity of adrenocortical secretions. However, cortisol, the major glucocorticoid secreted by the adrenal cortex, can also provide significant mineralocorticoid activity in some conditions. Aldosterone's mineralocorticoid activity is about 3,000 times greater than that of cortisol, but the plasma concentration of cortisol is nearly 2,000 times that of aldosterone. The renal MR is normally protected from activation by cortisol as a result of the effects of 11β–HSD2, which converts active cortisol into inactive cortisone, but when activity of this enzyme is reduced or when cortisol levels are very high, the MR can be activated by cortisol.

Primary aldosteronism (PA) is the syndrome that results from hypersecretion of aldosterone in the absence of a known stimulus. The excess aldosterone secretion almost always comes from the adrenal cortex and is usually associated with a solitary adenoma or bilateral hyperplasia of the adrenal cortex. Secondary aldosteronism refers to increased aldosterone secretion that occurs secondary to a known stimulus, such as activation of the RAS. This is the most common form of aldosteronism and occurs in various conditions associated with increased renin secretion, such as congestive heart failure, sodium depletion, or renal artery stenosis.

Excess aldosterone increases sodium reabsorption and potassium secretion by the principal cells of the renal tubules leading to an expansion of extracellular fluid volume, hypertension, suppression of renin secretion, hypokalemia, and metabolic alkalosis, hallmarks of primary aldosteronism. Most of these effects are highly salt sensitive and low sodium intake can greatly attenuate the hypertension and hypokalemia associated with primary aldosteronism.

Adrenal adenomas and bilateral adrenal hyperplasia account for more than 95% of PA. However, this is a rare form of hypertension, and in most studies of unselected patients, the classic form of PA was found in less than 1% of hypertensive patients. Some adrenal glands in patients with PA may have varying degrees of hyperplasticity, and the term *idiopathic hyperaldosteronism* (IHA) was coined to describe this condition. Clinically, PA and IHA are difficult to distinguish, although patients with PA often have more severe hypertension and hypokalemia compared to those with IHA.

[ ] CUSHING'S SYNDROME (GLUCOCORTICOID EXCESS)

Cushing's syndrome is a serious disorder. Hypertension occurs in approximately 80% of patients with Cushing's syndrome and is difficult to control. Cushing's syndrome can be caused by either administration of excess cortisol (e.g., for treatment of various inflammatory disorders) or by excess endogenous cortisol secretion. The most common cause of endogenous cortisol excess is overproduction of adrenocorticotrophic hormone (ACTH) from a pituitary adenoma, a condition referred to as *Cushing's disease*. The increased ACTH causes adrenal hyperplasia and stimulates cortisol secretion. Cushing's disease can also occur as a result of ectopic secretion of ACTH by tumors outside the pituitary, such as an abdominal carcinoma.

[ ] PHEOCHROMOCYTOMA

This is a rare form of secondary hypertension occurring in approximately 0.05% of hypertensive patients. Although rare, pheochromocytoma can provoke fatal hypertensive crises if unrecognized and untreated. Pheochromocytoma can arise from neuroectodermal chromaffin cells, which are part of the sympathoadrenal system. The chromaffin cells have the capacity to synthesize and store catecholamines and are normally found mainly in the adrenal medulla. The symptoms and severity of hypertension associated with pheochromocytoma are highly variable, depending on the secretory pattern and amount of catecholamines released. Tumors that continuously release large amounts of catecholamines may cause sustained hypertension with few paroxysms, or sudden bursts of very high levels of BP. Tumors that are less active may have cyclical release of catecholamines stores that induce paroxysms of hypertension. The periodic bursts of catecholamine release may cause moderate to severe hypertension and lead to target-organ injury. Consequently, diagnosis and effective treatment of pheochromocytoma is essential.

[ ] PREECLAMPSIA

Preeclampsia in women is characterized by hypertension and proteinuria after 20 weeks gestation and is associated with significantly increased risk for fetal and maternal morbidity and mortality. Although numerous factors—including genetic, immunologic, behavioral, and environmental factors—have been implicated in the pathogenesis of preeclampsia, reduced uteroplacental perfusion as a result of abnormal cytotrophoblast invasion of spiral arterioles appears to play a key role. Placental ischemia is thought to cause widespread activation/dysfunction of the maternal vascular endothelium, which results in enhanced formation of endothelin, thromboxane, and superoxide, increased vascular sensitivity to ANG II, and decreased formation of vasodilators such as nitric oxide and prostacyclin. These endothelial abnormalities, in turn, cause hypertension by impairing renal function and increasing total peripheral vascular resistance.

GENETIC CAUSES OF HYPERTENSION

With the development of superb tools for genetic studies, there has been great enthusiasm for the possibility that genetic causes of primary hypertension can be identified. However, there have been no clear successes in identifying genes that cause human primary hypertension. On the other hand, at least 10 monogenic disorders have been identified that have either high BP or low BP as part of the phenotype (Table 28-2 shows some of these that are associated with high BP). In all monogenic hypertensive disorders thus far, the final common pathway to hypertension is increased sodium reabsorption and volume expansion. Monogenic hypertension, however, is rare, and all of the known forms together account for less than 1% of human hypertension.

TABLE 28-2

Known Genetic Causes of Hypertension

Genetic Disorder	Age of Onset	Pattern of Inheritance	Aldosterone Level	Serum Potassium Level	Treatment[a]
FHI (GRA)[b]	2nd or 3rd decade	Autosomal dominant	High	Decreased in 50% of cases; marked decrease with thiazides	Glucocorticoids
FHII[c]	Middle age	Autosomal dominant	High	Low to normal	Spironolactone, eplerenone
DOC over-secretion due to CAH[c,d]	Childhood	Autosomal recessive	Low	Low to normal	Glucocorticoids
Activating MR mutation exacerbated by pregnancy[e]	2nd or 3rd decade	Unknown	Low	Low to normal	Delivery of fetus
AME2[c,f]	Childhood	Autosomal recessive	Low	Low to normal	Spironolactone, dexamethasone
Liddle's syndrome[g]	3rd decade	Autosomal dominant	Low	Low to normal	Amiloride, triamterene
Gordon's syndrome[h]	2nd or 3rd decade	Autosomal dominant	Low	High	Thiazide diuretic, low-sodium diet

ACTH, adrenocorticotropic hormone; AME, apparent mineralocorticoid excess; CAH, congenital adrenal hyperplasia; DOC, deoxycorticosterone; FHH, familial hyperaldosteronism type I; FHII, familial hyperaldosteronism type II; GRA, glucocorticoid-remediable aldosteronism; MCR, mineralocorticoid receptor.

[a]Treatment for underlying mechanisms; other forms of treatment, including different antihypertensive medications, might be needed to adequately control BP.

[b]Familial hyperaldosteronism.

[c]Excess production of non-aldosterone mineralocorticoids.

[d]Congenital adrenal hyperplasia, DOC-producing tumors.

[e]Because of increased activity of MCRs.

[f]Apparent mineralocorticoid excess caused by either licorice ingestion or ectopic ACTH secretion.

[g]Increased activity of sodium channels.

[h]Increased activity of Na-Cl cotransporter in the distal tubule.

Data adapted from Garovic VD, Hilliard AA, Turner ST. Monogenic forms of low-renin hypertension. Nat Clin Pract Nephrol. 2006;2:624–630.

PATHOPHYSIOLOGY OF PRIMARY (ESSENTIAL) HYPERTENSION

Widespread human primary (essential) hypertension appears to be a relatively modern disorder associated with industrialization and ready availability of food. Studies of industrialized populations have demonstrated that BP, and therefore the prevalence of hypertension, rises with age. Hunter-gatherers living in nonindustrialized societies, however, rarely develop hypertension or progressive increases in BP that occur in the majority of individuals living in industrialized societies. This suggests that environmental factors play a major role in raising BP in many patients with primary hypertension. However, genetic variation almost certainly is responsible for differences in baseline BP that result in normal distribution of BP in a population. When hypertension-producing environmental factors are added to the population baseline BP, the normal distribution is shifted toward higher BP. Experimental, clinical, and population studies suggest some of the key environmental factors that affect BP include excess weight gain, excess sodium intake, and excess alcohol consumption.

【 】 OBESITY

Obesity is a major cause of primary hypertension. Current estimates indicate that more than one *billion* people in the world are overweight or obese. In the United States, 64% of adults are overweight, and almost one-third of the adult population is obese with a body mass index (BMI) greater than 30. Population studies show that excess weight gain is the best predictor we have for the development of hypertension, and the relationship between BMI and BP appears to be nearly linear in diverse populations throughout the world. Clinical studies also indicate that weight loss is effective in reducing BP in most hypertensive subjects and in primary prevention of hypertension.

Mechanisms of Impaired Renal Pressure Natriuresis in Obesity Hypertension

Three mechanisms appear to be especially important in mediating impaired pressure natriuresis in obesity hypertension: (1) increased SNS activity, (2) activation of the RAS, and (3) physical compression of the kidneys by fat accumulation within and around the kidneys.

HYPERLEPTINEMIA AND SNS ACTIVATION Leptin is released from adipocytes and acts on the hypothalamus and brainstem to reduce appetite and increase SNS activity. In rodents, increasing plasma leptin concentration to levels comparable to those found in severe obesity not only increases SNS activity but also raises BP. Moreover, the hypertensive effects of leptin are enhanced when NO synthesis is inhibited, as often occurs in obese subjects with endothelial dysfunction. Leptin's stimulatory effect on SNS activity appears to be mediated by interaction with other hypothalamic factors, especially the proopiomelanocortin pathway. Antagonism of the melanocortin 3/4 receptors (MC3/4-R) completely abolished leptin's chronic BP effects.

RENIN–ANGIOTENSIN–ALDOSTERONE SYSTEM ACTIVATION IN OBESITY Obese individuals, especially those with visceral obesity, often have mild to moderate increases in plasma renin activity, angiotensinogen, ACE activity, ANG II, and aldosterone despite sodium retention, volume expansion, and hypertension, all of which would normally tend to suppress renin secretion and ANG II formation. RAS blockade blunts sodium retention, volume expansion, and increased BP during the development of obesity in experimental studies. Small clinical trials have also shown that ARBs, ACE inhibitors, and MR receptor antagonists are all effective in lowering BP in obese hypertensive patients.

RENAL COMPRESSION CAUSED BY VISCERAL OBESITY   Visceral obesity also leads to physical compression of the kidneys, which impairs renal pressure natriuresis and causes hypertension. Although this cannot account for the initial increase in BP that occurs with rapid weight gain, it may help to explain why abdominal obesity is much more closely associated with hypertension than subcutaneous obesity.

Kidney Injury in Obesity Hypertension

Obese patients often develop proteinuria that is followed by progressive loss of kidney function. The most common types of renal lesions observed in renal biopsies of obese subjects are focal and segmental glomerular sclerosis and glomerulomegaly. The gradual loss of kidney function, as well as the hypertension and diabetes that commonly coexist with obesity, lead to progressive impairment of pressure natriuresis, increasing salt sensitivity, and greater increases in BP. Thus, renal injury in obese subjects makes the hypertension more severe and more difficult to control with antihypertensive drugs.

Effective control of BP is essential in treating patients with obesity and metabolic syndrome, and for preventing CVD. Weight reduction is an essential first step in the effective management of most patients with metabolic syndrome and hypertension, and more emphasis should be placed on lifestyle modifications that help patients to maintain a healthier weight and prevent CVD.

SUGGESTED READING

Chobanian AV, Bakris GL, Black HR, et al. Seventh report of the Joint National Committee on Prevention, Detection, Evaluation, and Treatment of High Blood Pressure. *Hypertension*. 2003;42:1206–1252.

Guyton AC, Hall J E. *Textbook of Medical Physiology*. 11th ed. Philadelphia, PA: Elsevier; 2006.

Hall JE. The kidney, hypertension, and obesity. *Hypertension*. 2003;41:625–633.

Hall JE, Brands MW, Henegar JR. Angiotensin II and long-term arterial pressure regulation: the overriding dominance of the kidney. *Kidney Int*. 1999;10:s258–s265.

Hall JE, Granger JP. Regulation of fluid and electrolyte balance in hypertension: role of hormones and peptides. In: Battegay EJ, Lip GHY, Bakris GL, eds. *Hypertension: Principles and Practice*. Boca Raton, FL: Taylor & Francis; 2005:121–142.

Hall JE, Guyton AC, Brands MW. Pressure-volume regulation in hypertension. *Kidney Int*. 1996;49(suppl 55):S35–S41.

Kaplan NM. *Clinical Hypertension*. 8th ed. Philadelphia, PA: Lippincott William & Wilkins; 2002:89–92.

Lifton RP. Molecular genetics of human blood pressure variation. *Science*. 1996;272:676–680.

CHAPTER (29)

Diagnosis and Treatment of Hypertension

Darrell Rubin, Mahboob Rahman, and
Jackson T. Wright Jr.

EVALUATION OF THE HYPERTENSIVE PATIENT

【 】 BLOOD PRESSURE MEASUREMENT

The Seventh Report of the Joint National Committee on Prevention, Detection, Evaluation, and Treatment of High Blood Pressure (JNC 7) classifies hypertension 1 into four categories (Table 29-1). Accurate measurement of blood pressure requires a trained health care provider using a mercury or *calibrated* alternative sphygmomanometer under standardized conditions. These include the removal of tight clothing, 5 minutes of rest in a chair (not an examination table), back supported with feet on the floor, the arm supported at heart level, and avoidance of talking during the measurement. The bladder of the cuff should encircle at least 80% of the upper arm and be a width that is at least 40% of arm circumference such that the distal margin is at least 3-cm proximal to the antecubital fossa. The cuff should be inflated to a pressure about 30 mm Hg above the point where the palpable pulse disappears, and then deflated at 2 to 3 mm Hg per second. The onset of phase I of the Korotkoff sounds (tapping sounds corresponding to the appearance of a palpable pulse) corresponds to systolic pressure. The disappearance of sounds (phase V) corresponds to diastolic pressure. The fifth phase should be used, except in situations in which the disappearance of sounds cannot reliably be determined because sounds are audible even after complete deflation of the cuff, as in pregnant women. In this case the fourth phase (muffling) may be used to define the diastolic pressure. At least two measurements spaced by 1 to 2 minutes apart should be taken. Blood pressure should be measured in both arms at the first visit to detect possible differences because of peripheral vascular disease; and, if present, the higher value should be used. In those at risk for orthostatic hypotension (e.g., the elderly, diabetics, autonomic instability), blood pressure should be measured after 2 minutes of standing.

【 】 HISTORY, PHYSICAL EXAMINATION, AND LABORATORY EVALUATION

The three main goals of the initial evaluation of the hypertensive patient are to (1) assess the presence of target-organ damage related to hypertension, especially those that might influence choice of therapy; (2) determine the presence of other cardiovascular risk factors and disease; and (3) evaluate for possible underlying secondary causes of hypertension.

TABLE 29-1

Classification of Blood Pressure for Adults

Blood Pressure Classification	Systolic Blood Pressure (mm Hg)	Diastolic Blood Pressure (mm Hg)
Normal	< 120	< 80
Prehypertension	120–139	80–89
Stage 1 hypertension	140–159	90–99
Stage 2 hypertension	≥ 160	≥ 100

Adapted from Chobanian AV, Bakris GL, Black HR, et al. *Seventh Report of the Joint National Committee on Prevention, Detection, Evaluation, and Treatment of High Blood Pressure.* NIH pub. no. 04–5230. Available at: http://www.nhlbi.nih.gov/guidelines/hypertension/jnc7full.htm.

The key issues that need to be addressed in the history include:

- Age of onset, duration, levels of high blood pressure, as well as the impact and adverse effects of previous antihypertensive therapy.
- Symptoms suggestive of secondary causes of hypertension (Table 29-2).
- Lifestyle factors including diet (fat, salt, alcohol), smoking, physical activity, and weight gain since early adult life.
- Symptoms of target-organ damage including neurologic dysfunction, heart failure, coronary heart disease, or peripheral arterial disease.
- Use of medications that influence blood pressure, such as oral contraceptives, licorice, nasal decongestants, cocaine, amphetamines, steroids, nonsteroidal anti-inflammatory drugs, erythropoietin, and cyclosporine.
- Presence of other cardiovascular risk factors.

Routine laboratory investigations before initiation of therapy include urine for protein and blood, serum creatinine (estimated glomerular filtration rate [GFR]) and electrolytes, fasting blood glucose, fasting lipid profile, and electrocardiogram (ECG). Additional workup is guided by the clinical presentation in an individual patient, and the need to evaluate possible causes of secondary hypertension.

【　】 SECONDARY CAUSES OF HYPERTENSION

Secondary hypertension is defined by identifying a specific cause of hypertension, in contrast to the more common essential hypertension, where no direct cause is evident. The most common causes of secondary hypertension are renal artery stenosis, renal parenchymal disease, sleep apnea, primary hyperaldosteronism, Cushing's syndrome, and pheochromocytoma (see Tables 29-2 and 29-3).

【　】 RENAL ARTERY STENOSIS

Renovascular hypertension occurs in 1% to 2% of the overall hypertensive population, but the prevalence may be as high as 10% in patients with resistant hypertension, and even higher in patients with accelerated or malignant hypertension. Renovascular disease may be due to two distinct pathophysiologic processes: fibromuscular dysplasia in younger patients, especially women 15 to 50 years of age, and atherosclerotic renal artery stenosis in older persons often associated with other peripheral vascular disease. Duplex ultrasonography is a useful and noninvasive technique to evaluate for renal artery stenosis. However, the sensitivity and specificity of this measurement are operator dependent. Renal angiography remains the gold standard for diagnosis and provides information

TABLE 29-2

Important Findings in Physical Examination That Might Help to Diagnose Secondary Hypertension or Find End-Organ Damage

	Finding	Significance
Vital sign	Pulse pressure > 60 mm Hg	↑ CVD risk
	Tachycardia	Hyperthyroid, pheochromocytoma, HF
Body habitus	Cushingoid	Cushing syndrome
Skin	Oral-facial tumors	MEN-2A/2B (pheochromocytoma)
	Neurofibromas, café-au-lait spots	Pheochromocytoma
Eyes	AV nicking, hemorrhages, exudates	Hypertensive retinopathy
Neck	Bruits	Carotid disease
	Thyroid	Hypothyroid MEN-2A
Chest wall	Rib bruits	Coarctation of aorta
	Renal bruits heard over the Kidneys	Renal artery stenosis
Lungs	Crackles, wheezes	Heart failure
Cardiac	Gallops, LVH, murmur	Heart failure, valvular disease
Abdomen	Palpable kidneys, bruit, epigastric and post	Polycystic kidneys, renal artery stenosis
Extremities	Diminished pulses, femoral pulse delay	Coarctation of aorta
	Bruits	Vascular damage

AV, atrioventricular; CVD, cardiovascular disease; HF heart failure; LVH, left ventricular hypertrophy; MEN, multiple endocrine neoplasia

Data compiled from 2003 European Society of Hypertension-European Society of Cardiology guidelines for the management of arterial hypertension. *J Hypertens.* 2003;21:1011–1053.

 TABLE 29-3

Clinical and Laboratory Clues for Diagnosis of Secondary Hypertension

Cause	Clues
Renovascular hypertension	Abrupt onset before age 30 years or worsening after age 55 years; renal artery diastolic or lateralizing abominal bruit; resistance to therapy; sustained rise in creatinine after initiation of angiotensin-converting enzyme inhibitor, renal failure of uncertain etiology; retinal hemorrhages, exudates, or papilledema; recurrent "flash" pulmonary edema; coexisting diffuse atherosclerotic vascular disease
Renoparenchymal disease	Abnormal urinalysis (proteinuria, hematuria); elevated serum creatinine; abnormal renal ultrasonography
Sleep apnea	Obesity; gaspy nocturnal breathing with prominent snoring
Primary aldosteronism	Unexplained hypokalemia, metabolic alkalosis
Cushing's syndrome	Truncal obesity, acne, plethora, fat pads, striae, and bruising; hyperglycemia
Pheochromocytoma	Labile blood pressure, paroxysms of, palpitations, pallor, perspiration, headache (pain)

Adapted from Hall WD. Resistant hypertension, secondary hypertension, and hypertensive crises. *Cardiol Clin.* 2002;20:281–289.

about the site and severity of stenoses, thereby suggesting appropriate revascularization strategies. Therapeutic options include renal artery angioplasty with stent placement and surgical revascularization; however, not all patients benefit from renal revascularization. The presence of urinary protein excretion of at least 1 g/d; estimated GFR of < 40 mL/min; age older than 65 years; the presence of coronary artery disease, arterial occlusive disease of the legs, or cerebrovascular disease; and a resistance index > 80 in the segmental arteries of both kidneys; are useful in identifying patients who are less likely to benefit from vascular intervention. Appropriate management of renal artery stenosis requires close collaboration between the internist, interventional radiologist, and vascular surgeon.

【 】 SLEEP APNEA

Obstructive sleep apnea is a common medical condition characterized by abnormal collapse of the pharyngeal airway during sleep causing repetitive arousals from sleep. It may occur in up to 50% of patients with hypertension. The most common clinical presentation of obstructive sleep apnea is loud snoring or breathing pauses observed by the bed partner, nightmares or abrupt awakening from sleep, and excessive daytime sleepiness. There are several questionnaires that can be used in screening for this disorder, although a formal sleep study usually is needed for diagnosis of obstructive sleep apnea and the determination of corrective interventions. Continuous positive airway pressure can reduce nocturnal blood pressure in patients with obstructive sleep apnea.

【 】 PRIMARY HYPERALDOSTERONISM

Screening for hyperaldosteronism should be considered for at least the following patients: hypertensive patients with spontaneous hypokalemia (K^+ less than 3.5 mmol/L); hypertensive patients with marked diuretic-induced hypokalemia (K^+ less than 3.0 mmol/L); patients with hypertension refractory to treatment with three or more drugs; and hypertensive patients found to have an incidental adrenal adenoma. Screening for hyperaldosteronism includes assessment of plasma aldosterone and plasma renin activity measured under standardized conditions, (the collection of morning samples taken from patients in a sitting position after resting at least 15 minutes and after restoration of normokalemia). Antihypertensive drugs, with the exception of aldosterone antagonists, may be continued before initial testing. The screening test is considered positive if the plasma aldosterone/renin activity ratio is greater than 30 pmol/L/ng/mL or 550 SI units. The diagnosis of primary aldosteronism is established by demonstrating inappropriate autonomous hypersecretion of aldosterone after oral or IV saline loading. Imaging with adrenal computed tomography scan or magnetic resonance imaging may help differentiate between adrenal adenoma and bilateral adrenal hyperplasia, although selective adrenal venous sampling may be needed. The treatment of confirmed unilateral aldosterone-producing adenoma is surgical removal of the affected adrenal gland, usually by laparoscopic adrenalectomy. Prior to surgery, patients should be treated medically for 8 to 10 weeks to correct metabolic abnormalities and to control blood pressure. Aldosterone antagonists (spironolactone or eplerenone) should be considered for patients with adrenal hyperplasia, bilateral adenoma, or increased risk of perioperative complications. Amiloride is another alternative for the patient who is intolerant to spironolactone.

【 】 CUSHING'S SYNDROME

Cushing's syndrome is more common in women and results from excessive concentrations of circulating free glucocorticoids, which is corticotropin-dependent in approximately 80% to 85% of cases. The 24-hour urinary free cortisol (> 90 mg/d; sensitivity = 100%; specificity = 98%) is a useful screening test; however, the single-dose (1-mg) overnight dexamethasone suppression test is equally sensitive but less specific. Treatment of Cushing's syndrome is either medical or surgical. Metyrapone, ketoconazole, and mitotane can all be used to lower cortisol by directly inhibiting synthesis and secretion in the adrenal gland.

【 】 PHEOCHROMOCYTOMA

Patients with paroxysmal and/or severe sustained hypertension that is refractory to the usual antihypertensive therapy should be evaluated for pheochromocytoma. Hypertension triggered by beta-blockers, anesthesia induction, monoamine oxidase inhibitors, micturition, or changes in abdominal pressure should increase suspicion for pheochromocytoma. It may also be present with other conditions such as multiple endocrine neoplasias (MEN-2A/2B), von Recklinghausen neurofibromatosis, or von Hippel–Lindau disease. A 24-hour urinary metanephrine is highly sensitive and specific with a cutoff point > 3.70 nmol/d. Plasma metanephrines are easy to obtain, and may represent a good screening test for pheochromocytoma, especially if the patient is symptomatic or blood pressure is elevated. Because they have limited specificity (85%) at cutoffs of metanephrine > 0.66 nmol/L or normetanephrine > 0.30 nmol/L, a positive plasma metanephrine should be confirmed by the 24-hour urinary metanephrine-to-creatinine ratio (cutoff point > 0.354; specificity = 98%) before proceeding to anatomic localization of the tumor. Imaging studies commonly used to localize pheochromocytomas include CT scan and meta-iodobenzylguanidine (MIBG) scintigraphy; the latter is particularly useful when an extraabdominal focus is suspected. Alpha-blockers (prazosin, doxazosin, phenoxybenzamine) should be used as first-line agents in suspected pheochromocytoma, but surgical resection is indicated for confirmed tumors. It is important not to use beta-blockers alone because the unopposed alpha-activity will worsen the vasoconstriction, resulting in a further increase in blood pressure. Thus, beta-blockers should generally be withheld until surgery is performed, unless there are arrhythmias present and adequate alpha-blockade has been achieved. Perioperative care of the patient with pheochromocytoma requires careful monitoring by an experienced anesthesiologist. For patients with inoperable or metastatic malignant pheochromocytoma, blood pressure and adrenergic symptoms may be controlled with alpha-adrenergic blockade plus beta-blockade and/or tyrosine hydroxylase inhibition with metyrosine.

TREATMENT OF ESSENTIAL HYPERTENSION

Hypertension is the most important preventable cause of premature death, and treatment should focus on achieving the recommended blood pressure goal. For most patients, reduction to < 140 mm Hg for the systolic blood pressure and < 90 mm Hg for the diastolic blood pressure are the recommended goals while lower goals (< 130/80 mm Hg) are recommended for those with diabetes and chronic kidney disease.

【 】 LIFESTYLE MODIFICATION

Clear verbal and written guidance on lifestyle measures, such as eating a healthy diet and getting regular exercise, should be provided for all prehypertensive and hypertensive patients (see Table 29-4). Lifestyle interventions reduce the need for drug therapy, enhance the antihypertensive effects of drugs, and favorably influence overall CVD risk. Failure to adopt these measures may attenuate the response to antihypertensive drugs.

【 】 DRUG THERAPY OF HYPERTENSION

The placebo-controlled outcome trials have demonstrated a reduction in cardiovascular disease, renal disease, and stroke with nearly all classes of antihypertensive agents. With few exceptions, the benefit from the various regimens correlated with degree of blood

TABLE 29-4

Lifestyle Modifications to Prevent and Manage Hypertension

Modification	Recommendation	Approximate Systolic Blood Pressure Reduction (Range)
Weight reduction	Maintain normal body weight (body mass index 18.5–24.9 kg/m²)	5–20 mm Hg/10 kg
Adopt DASH (Dietary Approaches to Stop Hypertension) eating plan	Consume a diet rich in fruits, vegetables, and low-fat dairy products with a reduced content of saturated and total fat	8–14 mm Hg
Dietary sodium reduction	Reduce dietary sodium intake to no more than 100 mmol/d (2.4 g sodium or 6 g sodium chloride)	2–8 mm Hg
Physical activity	Engage in regular aerobic physical activity such as brisk walking (at least 30 min/d, most days of the week).	4–9 mm Hg
Moderation of alcohol consumption	Limit consumption to no more than 2 drinks (e.g., 24 oz beer, 10 oz wine, or 3 oz 80-proof whiskey) per day in most men and to no more than one drink per day in women and lighter-weight persons	2–4 mm Hg

Adapted from Chobanian AV, Bakris GL, Black HR, et al. *Seventh Report of the Joint National Committee on Prevention, Detection, Evaluation, and Treatment of High Blood Pressure.* NIH pub. no. 04–5230. Available at: http://www.nhlbi.nih.gov/guidelines/hypertension/jnc7full.htm.

pressure lowering rather than specific drug characteristics. Most patients will require two or more antihypertensives to achieve their blood pressure goal (Table 29-5).

Thiazide-type diuretics, introduced in the early 1950s have been the most studied, most recommended, and most cost-effective of all the antihypertensive drug classes. As initial therapy, they remain unsurpassed by any other antihypertensive class in preventing clinical outcomes and should be included in most multidrug regimens.

Thiazide-Type Diuretics

Thiazide-type diuretics inhibit the Na-Cl cotransporter in the distal tubule to reduce extracellular volume and cardiac output. Diuresis is essential to their antihypertensive action, and their antihypertensive efficacy can be antagonized by high salt intake; however, their mechanism of action is not fully understood and may include reduction in peripheral vascular resistance. Hydrochlorothiazide is the most commonly prescribed agent of this class in the United States. Indapamide, at the recommended doses produces less hypokalemia, although at higher doses it behaves similar to other thiazides. With the exception of metolazone and indapamide, most thiazide diuretics lose their antihypertensive effectiveness when the GFR declines to < 30 to 40 mL/min. Most side effects are related to fluid and electrolyte abnormalities including hypokalemia and hyponatremia; but they can also increase blood glucose and lipids (each approximately 5 mg/dL).

TABLE 29-5

Antihypertensive Drug Classes[a]

Class	Drug (Trade Name)	Usual Dose Range (md/d)	Usual Daily Frequency[a]
Thiazide diuretics			
	Chlorothiazide (Diuril)	125–500	1–2
	Chlorthalidone (generic)	12.5–25	1
	Hydrochlorothiazide (Microzide, HydroDIURIL[b])	12.5–50	1
	Polythiazide (Renese)	2–4	1
	Indapamide (Lozol[b])	1.25–2.5	1
	Metolazone (Mykrox)	0.5–1.0	1
	Bendroflumethiazide	2.5–5	1
	Metolazone (Zaroxolyn)	2.5–10	1–2
Loop diuretics			
	Bumetanide (Bumex[b])	0.5–2	2
	Furosemide (Lasix[b])	20–80	2
	Torsemide (Demadex[b])	2.5–10	1
Potassium-sparing diuretics			
	Amiloride (Midamor[b])	5–10	1–2
	Triamterene (Dyrenium)	50–100	1–2
Aldosterone receptor blockers			
	Eplerenone (Inspra)	50–100	1–2
	Spironolactone (Aldactone[b])	25–50	1
Beta-blockers			
	Atenolol (Tenormin[b])	25–100	1
	Betaxolol (Kerlone[b])	5–20	1
	Bisoprolol (Zebeta[b])	2.5–10	1
	Metoprolol (Lopressor[b])	50–100	1–2
	Metoprolol extended release (Toprol XL)	50–100	1
	Nadolol (Corgard[b])	40–120	1
	Propranolol (Inderal[b])	40–160	2
	Propranolol long-acting (Inderal LA[b])	60–180	1
	Timolol (Blocadren[b])	20–40	2
	Nebivolol (Nebilet[c])	5	1
Beta-blockers with intrinsic sympathomimetic activity			
	Acebutolol (Sectral[b])	200–800	2
	Penbutolol (Levatol)	10–40	1
	Pindolol (generic)	10–40	2

TABLE 29-5

Antihypertensive Drug Classes[a] (Continued)

Class	Drug (Trade Name)	Usual Dose Range (md/d)	Usual Daily Frequency[a]
Combined alpha- and beta-blockers			
	Carvedilol (Coreg[c])	12.5–50	2
	Labetalol (Normodyne, Trandate[b])	200–800	2
ACE inhibitors			
	Benazepril (Lotensin[b])	10–40	1
	Captopril (Capoten[b])	50–200	2
	Enalapril (Vasotec[b])	50–40	1–2
	Fosinopril (Monopril)	10–40	1
	Lisinopril (Prinivil, Zestril[b])	10–40	1
	Moexipril (Univasc)	7.5–30	1
	Perindopril (Aceon)	4–8	1
	Quinapril (Accupril)	10–80	1
	Ramipril (Altace)	2.5–20	1
	Trandolapril (Mavik)	1–4	1
Angiotensin II antagonists			
	Candesartan (Atacand)	8–32	1
	Eprosartan (Teveten)	400–800	1–2
	Irbesartan (Avapro)	150–300	1
	Losartan (Cozaar)	25–100	1–2
	Olmesartan (Benicar)	20–40	1
	Telmisartan (Micardis)	20–80	1
	Valsartan (Diovan)	80–320	1–2
Calcium-channel blockers— nondihydropyridines			
	Diltiazem extended release (Cardizem CD, Dilacor XR, Tiazac[b])	180–420	1
	Diltiazem extended-release (Cardizem LA)	120–540	1
	Verapamil immediate-release (Calan, Isoptin[b])	80–320	2
	Verapamil long acting (Calan SR, Isoptin SR[b])	120–480	1–2
	Verapamil (Covera HS, Verelan PM)	120–360	1
CCBs— dihydropyridines			
	Amlodipine (Norvasc)	2.5–10	1
	Felodipine (Plendil)	2.5–20	1
	Isradipine (Dynacirc CR)	2.5–10	2
	Nicardipine sustained-release (Cardene SR)	6–120	2

TABLE 29-5

Antihypertensive Drug Classes[a] (Continued)

Class	Drug (Trade Name)	Usual Dose Range (md/d)	Usual Daily Frequency[a]
	Nifedipine long-acting (Adalat CC, Procardia XL)	30–60	1
	Nisoldipine (Sular)	10–40	1
Alpha-1 blockers			
	Doxazosin (Cardura)	1–16	1
	Prazosin (Minipress[b])	2–20	2–3
	Terazosin (Hytrin)	1–20	1–2
Central alpha-2 agonists and other centrally acting drugs			
	Clonidine (Catapres[b])	0.1–0.8	2
	Clonidine patch (Catapres-TTS)	0.1–0.3	1 wkly
	Methyldopa (Aldomet[b])	250–1000	2
	Reserpine (generic)	0.1–0.25	1
	Guanfacine (Tenex[b])	0.5–2	1
Direct vasodilators			
	Hydralazine (Apresoline[b])	25–100	2
	Minoxidil (Loniten[b])	2.5–80	1–2
Renin inhibitor			
	Aliskiren	50–600	1

[a]In some patients treated once daily, the antihypertensive effect may diminish toward the end of the dosing interval (trough effect). Blood pressure should be measured just prior to dosing to determine if satisfactory blood pressure control is obtained. Accordingly, an increase in dosage or frequency may need to be considered. These dosages may vary from those listed in the *Physicians' Desk Reference*, 61st ed. (2007).
[b]Available in generic preparations.
[c]License may only exist in some countries.

Adapted from Chobanian AV, Bakris GL, Black HR, et al. *Seventh Report of the Joint National Committee on Prevention, Detection, Evaluation, and Treatment of High Blood Pressure.* NIH pub. no. 04–5230. Available at: http://www.nhlbi.nih.gov/guidelines/hypertension/jnc7full.htm.

Loop Diuretics

Loop diuretics inhibit Na-K-2Cl transport in the thick ascending limb of the loop of Henle and include furosemide, bumetanide, ethacrynic acid, and torsemide. Because of their short half-life, they are less effective than thiazide-type diuretics in lowering blood pressure in patients with normal renal function when prescribed once or twice daily. In those with estimated GFR < 30–40 mL/min/1.73 m^2, their use is essential to achieve blood pressure goals. They are also usually required for volume control in those requiring vasodilators, especially minoxidil. Most adverse reactions are related to electrolyte abnormalities and extracellular volume depletion. NSAIDs and probenecid blunt the effect of loop diuretics, and thiazide diuretics have synergic effects with loop diuretics.

Potassium-Sparing Diuretics

Potassium-sparing diuretics include triamterene and amiloride and inhibit the renal epithelial Na channels and cause small increases in NaCl excretion. They are relatively weak diuretics and rarely used as a single agent in the treatment of hypertension or edema. They are useful in preventing diuretic-induced hypokalemia when prescribed with other diuretics. The most serious side effect of this class of diuretics is hyperkalemia. Use with NSAIDs, angiotensin-converting enzyme (ACE) inhibitors, ARBs, beta-blockers, and in diabetic hypertensives with or without nephropathy increases the risk of this side effect.

Mineralocorticoid receptor antagonists are another class of potassium-sparing diuretics and include spironolactone and eplerenone. Mineralocorticoids bind to the mineralocorticoid receptor to cause salt and water retention and increase the excretion of potassium and H^+. Mineralocorticoid antagonists, often in combination with thiazides or loop diuretics, are effective in treating hypertension, particularly resistant hypertension and hypertension associated with sleep apnea. They are particularly useful in the treatment of primary hyperaldosteronism. The major adverse effects include hyperkalemia, hypertriglyceridemia, and antiandrogen effects like breast pain, gynecomastia, and sexual dysfunction in males. Eplerenone is more selective for the mineralocorticoid receptor than the spironolactone and less likely to produce antiandrogenic effects.

Calcium-Channel Blockers

Calcium-channel blockers (CCBs) inhibit calcium entry into vasculature smooth muscle through the voltage-sensitive L-type Ca^{2+} channels, resulting in vasodilation of coronary and peripheral arteries. Two subclasses of calcium-channel blockers, dihydropyridines (DHPs; e.g., nifedipine, felodipine, amlodipine) and non-dihydropyridines (non-DHPs; e.g., verapamil and diltiazem) are available and have similar antihypertensive efficacy. Non-DHP CCBs substantially reduce contractility and atrioventricular nodal conduction. Thus, they are inappropriate for the patient with significant left ventricular dysfunction or > 1^0 atrioventricular block and should be replaced by DHP-CCBs if used with beta-blockers. Unlike the DHP-CCBs, they are less likely to produce headache, edema, and palpitations. Typical antihypertensive doses of diltiazem range from 180 to 540 mg/d while lower doses are used for their antianginal effect. A common side effect of verapamil is constipation because of its effect on gastrointestinal smooth muscle relaxation.

The DHP-CCBs are potent arteriolar vasodilators and especially effective in the more resistant patient as their antihypertensive action and side-effect profile complements that of beta-blockers when used together. They have little effect on cardiac conduction and contractility. Both felodipine and amlodipine have demonstrated their safety in hypertensives with systolic dysfunction in heart failure trials. The most common side effect of the DHP-CCBs include headache, flushing, and dose-dependent peripheral edema. The edema results from precapillary arteriolar dilatation and transudation of fluid from the vascular compartments into dependent tissues rather than from fluid retention; it does not respond well to treatment with diuretics.

Beta-Blockers

Beta-blockers lower blood pressure predominantly by inhibiting beta1-adrenergic receptors, thereby decreasing cardiac contractility and heart rate and thus reducing cardiac output. Renin release and the generation of angiotensin II are also inhibited by this mechanism. Additionally, beta-blockers are reported to alter baroceptor sensitivity, down-regulate peripheral adrenergic receptors, and increase prostacyclin biosynthesis, thereby facilitating vasodilation. They are particularly beneficial in hypertensive patients with coronary disease and heart failure (Table 29-6). They are less effective in lowering blood pressure in black patients and in the elderly unless accompanied by diuretics or calcium-channel blockers.

TABLE 29-6

Compelling Indications for Individual Drug Classes

Compelling Indication	Recommended Drugs					
	Diuretic	BB	ACEI	ARB	CCB	Aldo ANT
Heart failure	×	×	×	×		×
Postmyocardial infarction		×	×			×
High coronary disease risk	×	×	×		×	
Diabetes	×	×	×	×	×	
Chronic kidney disease			×	×		
Recurrent stroke prevention	×		×			

ACEI, angiotensin-converting enzyme inhibitor; Aldo ANT, aldosterone antagonist; ARB, angiotensin-receptor blocker; BB, beta-blocker; CCB, calcium-channel blocker.

Adapted from Chobanian AV, Bakris GL, Black HR, et al. *Seventh Report of the Joint National Committee on Prevention, Detection, Evaluation, and Treatment of High Blood Pressure*. NIH pub. no. 04–5230. Available at: http://www.nhlbi.nih.gov/guidelines/hypertension/jnc7full.htm.

Inhibitors of the Renin–Angiotensin System

Inhibitors of the renin–angiotensin system (RAS) include the ACE inhibitors, angiotensin-receptor blockers (ARBs), and renin inhibitors. The ACE inhibitors and ARBs (and presumably the renin inhibitors, though outcome data are not yet available) are specifically indicated in hypertensive patients with heart failure and chronic kidney disease and useful in hypertensive patients following myocardial infarction and stroke when combined with thiazide-type diuretics. The incidence of side effects is low; however, angioedema, while rare, can occur at any time during treatment and occurs more frequently in blacks. Cough occurs in up to 25% of all treated patients, but occurs more frequently in blacks. ARBs (and presumably renin inhibitors) are reasonable alternatives for patients with ACE inhibitor-associated cough. Generally, it is recommended to avoid ARBs in patients with a history of ACE inhibitor-related angioedema, although there are case reports of this substitution being done safely.

Alpha-Blockers

Alpha-blockers like prazosin, terazosin, and doxazosin block the activation of the vasoconstricting alpha-1 adrenoreceptors and are indicated as add-on therapy for blood pressure control. They also alleviate some symptoms of benign prostatic hypertrophy. Postural hypotension is an important side effect to keep in mind while using this class of drugs.

Alpha-2 Agonists

Alpha-2 agonists include methyldopa, clonidine, guanabenz, and guanfacine and stimulate central nervous system alpha-2 receptors to reduce central nervous system sympathetic outflow. As monotherapy, their antihypertensive efficacy diminishes with time. Their effect is enhanced with concomitant diuretic, vasodilator, or CCB administration but not with other sympatholytics or RAS inhibitors. The most common side effects include sedation, dry mouth, and fatigue. Liver dysfunction and a Coombs-positive hemolytic anemia can be seen with methyldopa.

Vasodilators

Vasodilators, such as hydralazine and minoxidil have been largely replaced by better-tolerated and more effective drugs such as the CCBs. However, vasodilators can be used to treat resistant hypertension. Their major side effects include fluid retention, including heart failure, and hirsuitism with minoxidil.

The findings of clinical trials to date suggest that for the patient with uncomplicated hypertension, as well as for the patient with diabetes but without nephropathy, initial therapy with "newer therapies" (e.g., ACE inhibitors, CCBs, and ARBs) is effective, but not superior to thiazide-type diuretics at reducing stroke, coronary heart disease morbidity or mortality, or all-cause mortality. Recent studies indicate that beta-blockers may be less effective than ARBs and CCBs in preventing cardiovascular disease outcomes. In addition, compelling indications exist for specific drug classes in those with hypertension and specific target-organ damage (see Table 29–6).

Since most hypertensive patients require multiple agents for blood pressure control, nearly all guideline panels support the initiation of treatment with two or more antihypertensive medications when blood pressure is more than 20/10 mm Hg above goal. Patients with indications for specific agents should obviously have these included in their regimen.

SPECIAL POPULATIONS

【 】 ELDERLY

The prevalence of hypertension is high, 60% to 80%, in populations older than 65 years of age. Systolic blood pressure rises and diastolic blood pressure declines after ages 50 to 55 years in both normotensive and untreated hypertensive subjects. In older hypertensives, measuring standing blood pressure becomes important because of the increased risk of orthostatic hypotension and the greater need for agents that may aggravate this condition. Antihypertensive medications should be initiated at lower doses in the elderly to facilitate a more gradual reduction in blood pressure.

【 】 DIABETES

Diabetes is highly prevalent in hypertensive patients, and increases the risk for complications of both diseases. The goal of appropriate treatment of is to minimize the effects of these disorders on the cardiovascular and renal systems. Multiple studies have demonstrated that blood pressure lowering using either an ACE inhibitor or an ARB slows the progression of both type 1 and 2 diabetic renal disease. Nearly every patient with renal insufficiency will require a diuretic to lower blood pressure, especially to the recommended goal for diabetics (< 130/80 mm Hg). In the ALLHAT, one of the few renal outcome studies able to address this question, there was no loss of protection against renal disease progression when a diuretic-based regimen was compared with one containing an ACE inhibitor, even in participants with diabetes. A CCB-based regimen is less effective in preventing renal outcomes than one containing either an ACE inhibitor or ARB.

【 】 RACE/ETHNICITY

Ethnic and racial differences in hypertension prevalence, severity, and response to therapy have been reported. Hypertension is more common and severe in black populations than in white populations, and has an earlier onset. It is less common and less severe in Mexican Americans and Native Americans, but blood pressure control rates are generally lower when hypertension is present. In general, the treatment of hypertension is similar for all demographic groups. However, African Americans demonstrate somewhat reduced blood pressure lowering in response to monotherapy with beta-blockers, ACE inhibitors, or ARBs, compared to diuretics or CCBs. These differential responses are largely eliminated by drug combinations that include adequate doses of a diuretic or CCB. RAS inhibitors were less effective in preventing many major clinical outcomes (including heart failure, stroke, and coronary events) than diuretics in black participants in several large studies. However, in patients with compelling indications (i.e., heart failure or renal disease), RAS-blocking agents (either ACE inhibitors or ARBs) or beta-blockers should be prescribed regardless of race. Because of the severity of hypertension in black patients, RAS inhibitors will usually be required as part of most multidrug therapy to achieve the blood pressure goal.

【 】 RENAL DISEASE

Hypertension is well-recognized as a risk factor for progression of renal disease. Current Kidney Disease Outcomes Quality Initiative (K/DOQI) Clinical Practice Guidelines on Hypertension and Antihypertensive Agents in Chronic Kidney Disease and the JNC 7 recommend a goal blood pressure of 130/80 mm Hg in patients with chronic kidney disease. Patients with proteinuria > 1 g/d have been shown to benefit from an even lower blood pressure goal (< 125/75 mm Hg). Inhibition of the renin–angiotensin axis is superior to conventional antihypertensive therapy in slowing the decline of renal function in patients with diabetic and nondiabetic nephropathy with proteinuria (total protein/creatinine ratio of 200 mg/g or greater).

【 】 HYPERTENSION DURING PREGNANCY

Hypertension occurring during pregnancy falls into one of four major classifications:

1. Chronic hypertension is the presence of preexisting hypertension or developing within 20 weeks of gestation pregnancy.

2. Gestational hypertension (also called transient hypertension) refers to elevated blood pressure first detected after 20 weeks of gestation without proteinuria.

3. Preeclampsia-eclampsia (also called pregnancy-induced hypertension) is defined by a systolic blood pressure ≥ 140 mm Hg or a diastolic blood pressure ≥ 90 mm Hg after the 20th week of gestation in a previously normotensive woman and which is accompanied by more than 300 mg proteinuria in 24 hours.

4. Preeclampsia superimposed on underlying hypertension.

For management and counseling purposes, chronic hypertension in pregnancy is also categorized as either low risk or high risk. Low-risk pregnant patients have mild essential hypertension without any organ involvement and can expect an outcome similar to that in the general obstetric population. Initiation of therapy is usually considered in women without end-organ damage if systolic blood pressure exceeds 160 mm Hg or diastolic pressure exceeds 110 mm Hg.

In pregnant patients with end-organ damage, it is desirable to keep the blood pressure below 140/90 mm Hg. ACE inhibitors and ARBs are contraindicated, and should be discontinued as soon as pregnancy is detected. If drug therapy is necessary, methyldopa (250 mg twice daily orally, maximum dose 3 g/d) has a long track record of safety and efficacy in pregnant patients, and is often the initial drug of choice. Hydralazine (25 mg twice daily orally; maximum dose 300 mg/d) and beta-blockers, such as labetalol (100 mg twice daily orally, maximum dose 800 mg every 8 hours) can also be used; however, beta-blockers may be associated with reduced intrauterine fetal growth. For severe hypertension, > 160/110 mm Hg, with end-organ damage (encephalopathy, hemorrhage, or eclampsia), IV preparations of labetalol or hydralazine are recommended.

Preeclampsia occurs in approximately 5% of pregnancies. It is associated with significant maternal and fetal risk. The major decisions in the management are obstetrical ones regarding timing of delivery. In preeclamptic hypertension, the reasonable goals for systolic and diastolic blood pressures are 140 to 155 mm Hg and 90 to 105 mm Hg, respectively.

In breastfeeding mothers, the following drugs are considered safe for control of hypertension: captopril, diltiazem, enalapril, hydralazine, HCTZ, labetalol, methyldopa, minoxidil, nadolol, nifedipine, oxprenolol, propranolol, spironolactone, timolol, and verapamil. It should be noted that diuretics may reduce milk production.

【　】 HYPERTENSION ASSOCIATED WITH SOLID-ORGAN TRANSPLANTATIONS

Hypertension is common is patients who undergo solid organ transplantation, and is associated with increased risk for cardiovascular morbidity and graft loss. Preexisting hypertension may be exacerbated by use of calcineurin inhibitors, corticosteroids, and progressive chronic kidney disease. Treatment goals are similar to the goals for the general population, including lower blood pressure goals (< 130/80 mm Hg) in patients with diabetes and chronic kidney disease. Although there are few prospective clinical trials to guide choice of antihypertensive therapy in transplantation patients, dihydropyridine calcium-channel blockers are commonly used in the regimen because of their pharmacologic property to antagonize calcineurin-mediated vasoconstriction. It is important to consider any possible interactions with immunosuppressive therapy when initiating antihypertensive drug therapy in transplantation patients.

【　】 HYPERTENSIVE EMERGENCIES AND URGENCIES

Hypertensive emergency is defined by acute and rapidly evolving end-organ damage, such as aortic dissection, heart failure, symptomatic coronary heart disease, progressive renal disease, stroke, or cerebral dysfunction associated with significant hypertension. Although there is no blood pressure threshold for the diagnosis of hypertensive emergency, most end-organ damage is noted with systolic blood pressures exceeding 220 mm Hg or diastolic blood pressures exceeding 120 mm Hg. In these patients, immediate but monitored reduction, often in a critical care setting, is accomplished with parenteral medications and is essential to prevent long-term organ damage.

Hypertensive urgency is defined by a markedly elevated blood pressure, usually in the same range seen in a hypertension emergency, but without the rapid progression of target-organ damage. If the patient is asymptomatic or clinically stable, the patient can be managed as an outpatient with close follow-up within days. In fact, there is evidence that the rapid reduction of blood pressure in asymptomatic hypertension may also precipitate adverse outcomes.

The initial assessment of hypertensive crisis is straightforward. A history and physical examination will rapidly direct further investigation to the involved organs while appropriate chemistry measurements and ECG will assess their involvement. Urine toxicology for cocaine metabolites is helpful in select populations. Plain chest radiographs are useful for assessing volume status and cardiac size and as a first screen for aortic dissection, but false-positive and false-negative results occur.

In hypertensive emergency, the goal of therapy is to lower the mean arterial pressure by approximately 25% within 2 hours, and to 160/100 mm Hg by 6 hours. Multiple medications are available for the treatment of hypertension crisis (Table 29-7). Sodium nitroprusside produces concomitant venous and arterial dilation, improving forward flow and cardiac output, and is the drug of choice because of its immediate onset of action and short duration of effect (1–2 minutes). Hypertension-induced acute pulmonary edema and acute aortic dissection are best treated with sodium nitroprusside. Prolonged treatment can result in accumulation of thiocyanate, particularly in patients with hepatic or renal insufficiency. Parenteral labetalol is another first-line agent for hypertensive emergency with a fast onset of action. It should be used cautiously in patients who have severe bradycardia, congestive heart failure, or bronchospasm.

TABLE 29-7

Medical Treatment for Management of Hypertension Crises

Agent	Dose	Onset of Action	Precautions
Parenteral Vasodilators			
Sodium nitroprusside	0.25–10 μg/kg/min IV infusion	Immediate	Thiocyanate toxicity with prolonged use
Nitroglycerin	5–100 μg/min IV infusion	2–5 min	
Nicardipine	5–15 mg/h IV infusion	1–5 min	Headache, tachycardia, tolerance Protracted hypotension after pro-longed use
Fenoldopam mesylate	0.1–0.3 μg/kg/min IV infusion	1–5 min	Headache, tachycardia, increased intraocular pressure
Hydralazine	5–10 mg as IV bolus or 10–40 mg IM repeat q4–6h	10 min IV 20 min IM	Unpredictable and excessive falls in pressure; tachycardia; angina exacerbation
Enalaprilat	0.625–1.25 mg q6h IV bolus	15–60 min	Unpredictable and exces-sive falls in pressure; acute renal failure in patients with bilateral renal artery stenosis
Parenteral Adrenergic Inhibitors			
Labetalol	20–80 mg as slow IV injection q10min, or 0.5–2 mg/min IV as infusion	5–10 min	Bronchospasm, heart block, orthostatic hypotension
Metoprolol	5 mg IV q10mi × 3 doses	5–10 min	Bronchospasm, heart block, heart failure, exacerbation of cocaine-induced myocardial ischemia

TABLE 29-7

Medical Treatment for Management of Hypertension Crises (*Continued*)

Agent	Dose	Onset of Action	Precautions
Esmolol	500 µg/kg IV over 3 min then 25–100 mg/kg/min as IV infusion	1–5 min	Bronchospasm, heart block, heart failure
Phentolamine	5–10 mg IV bolus q5–15 min	1–2 min	Tachycardia, orthostatic hypotension

Adapted from Victor R. Arterial hypertension. In: Goldman L, ed. *Cecil Textbook of Medicine.* 22nd ed. Philadelphia, PA: Saunders; 2004:361, with permission from Elsevier Company.

【 】 RESISTANT HYPERTENSION

Resistant hypertension is the failure to reach goal blood pressure in patients who are adhering to full doses of an appropriate three-drug regimen which includes a diuretic. Although white-coat hypertension and substandard measurement techniques, and pseudohypertension (artifactually high blood pressure measured due to a stiffened brachial artery that does not compress with the blood pressure cuff) should be considered, an important etiology of refractory hypertension is poor compliance with therapy. Other causes include dietary indiscretion, volume overload from kidney disease, or inadequate therapy. Some concomitant medications may interfere with blood pressure control, including nonsteroidal antiinflammatory drugs, cyclooxygenase-2 inhibitors, cocaine, amphetamines, other illicit drugs, sympathomimetics (decongestants, anorectics), oral contraceptives, adrenal steroids, cyclosporine and tacrolimus, erythropoietin, licorice (including some chewing tobacco), and selected over-the-counter dietary supplements. After eliminating these contributing factors, secondary causes should be considered as discussed above. A trial of aldosterone antagonists may be effective even in the absence of hyperaldosteronism.

SUGGESTED READING

Chobanian AV, Bakris GL, Black HR, et al. Seventh report of the Joint National Committee on Prevention, Detection, Evaluation, and Treatment of High Blood Pressure. *Hypertension.* 2003;42:1206–1252.

European Society of Hypertension–European Society of Cardiology. 2003 European Society of Hypertension-European Society of Cardiology guidelines for the management of arterial hypertension. *J Hypertens.* 2003;21:1011–1053.

Ezzati M, Lopez AD, Rodgers A, et al. Selected major risk factors and global and regional burden of disease. *Lancet.* 2002;360:1347–1360.

Hemmelgarn BR, Zarnke KB, Campbell NR, et al. The 2004 Canadian Hypertension Education Program recommendations for the management of hypertension: part I—blood pressure measurement, diagnosis and assessment of risk. *Can J Cardiol.* 2004;20:31–40.

Hoffman BB. Therapy of hypertension. In: Brunton LL, Lazo JS, Parker KL, eds. *The Pharmacological Basis of Therapeutics.* New York, NY: McGraw-Hill; 2006:845–868.

K/DOQI clinical practice guidelines for chronic kidney disease: evaluation, classification, and stratification. *Am J Kidney Dis.* 2002;39(suppl 1):S1–S266.

Newell-Price J, Bertagna X, Grossman AB, et al. Cushing's syndrome. *Lancet.* 2006;367:1605–1617.

Pickering TG, Hall JE, Appel LJ, et al. Recommendations for blood pressure measurement in humans and experimental animals: part 1: blood pressure measurement in humans: a statement for professionals from the Subcommittee of Professional and Public Education of the American Heart Association Council on High Blood Pressure Research. *Hypertension.* 2005;45:142–161.

Podymow T, August, P. Update on the use of antihypertensive drugs in pregnancy. *Hypertension.* http://hyper.ahajournal.org. Accessed February 8, 2008.

Report of the National High Blood Pressure Education Program Working Group on High Blood Pressure in Pregnancy. *Am J Obstet Gynecol.* 2000;183:S1–S22.

Wright JT Jr, Dunn JK, Cutler JA, et al. Outcomes in hypertensive black and nonblack patients treated with chlorthalidone, amlodipine, and lisinopril. *JAMA.* 2005;293:1595–1608.

CHAPTER (30)

Pulmonary Hypertension

Lewis J. Rubin

Pulmonary arterial hypertension, a hemodynamic abnormality present in a variety of conditions, is characterized by increased right ventricular afterload and work. The clinical manifestations, natural history, and reversibility of pulmonary hypertension (PH) depend on the nature of the pulmonary vascular lesions and the etiology and severity of the hemodynamic disorder. The degree of pulmonary hypertension that develops is a function of the amount of the pulmonary vascular tree that has been eliminated. PH is usually secondary to cardiac or pulmonary disease. Although idiopathic pulmonary arterial hypertension (IPAH) is uncommon, it is usually considered a distinctive clinical entity in which intrinsic pulmonary vascular disease is free of the complicating features of secondary PH contributed by diseases of the heart and/or lungs. Mild or even moderate PH can exist for a lifetime without becoming evident clinically. When pulmonary hypertension does become manifest clinically, the symptoms tend to be nonspecific.

DEFINITIONS

This chapter deals with *chronic* pulmonary arterial hypertension. Acute pulmonary arterial hypertension is usually a result of either pulmonary embolism or the adult respiratory distress syndrome. Pulmonary *venous* hypertension is usually encountered clinically as a consequence of left ventricular failure or mitral valvular disease. Occasionally it may occur in the course of fibrosing mediastinitis. Only rarely is the entity known as pulmonary venoocclusive disease (PVOD) encountered. The hallmarks of pulmonary venous hypertension are pulmonary congestion and edema. Pulmonary venous hypertension is said to exist when pulmonary venous (or left atrial) pressure rises above 15 mm Hg.

Cor pulmonale signifies the presence of PH in the setting of chronic respiratory disease. The degree of pulmonary hypertension that develops in patients with chronic lung disease tends to be less severe than that in connective tissue diseases, chronic thromboembolic disease, or IPAH. Pulmonary hypertension may be severe, however, in some patients with interstitial lung disease.

HEMODYNAMICS

At *sea level,* a cardiac output of 5 to 6 L/min is associated with a pulmonary arterial pressure of about 20/12 mm Hg, with a mean of about 15 mm Hg. At an altitude of 15,000 ft, the same level of blood flow is associated with somewhat higher pressures. Pulmonary arterial pressures also tend to increase somewhat with age.

A pressure drop of only 5 to 10 mm Hg between the pulmonary artery and left atrium accompanies the cardiac output of 5 to 6 L/min. Determination of pulmonary vascular resistance, calculated as the ratio of the difference in mean pressure at the two ends of the pulmonary vascular bed (pulmonary arterial minus left atrial pressure divided by the cardiac output), is a practical clinical tool for assessing the hemodynamic state of the pulmonary system. In practice, since the left atrium is not readily accessible, pulmonary wedge pressure is generally substituted for left atrial pressure.

PULMONARY HYPERTENSION: GENERAL FEATURES

【 】 CLINICAL MANIFESTATIONS

Pulmonary hypertension is a final common hemodynamic consequence of multiple etiologies and diverse mechanisms. Most cases of PH are secondary. Among the underlying causes of pulmonary hypertension are mechanical compression and distortion of the resistance vessels of the lungs, hypoxic vasoconstriction (e.g., in severe obstructive airways disease or diffuse parenchymal diseases), intravascular obstruction (e.g., thromboemboli or tumor emboli), and combinations of mechanical and vasoconstrictive influences. The significance of PH, however, is that if uncontrolled, it leads to right ventricular failure. Once pulmonary arterial pressures reach systemic levels, right ventricular failure becomes inevitable.

【 】 SPECIAL STUDIES

The "gold standard" for the diagnosis of pulmonary hypertension is right-sided heart catheterization. This technique enables the direct determination of right atrial and ventricular pressures, pulmonary arterial pressure, pulmonary wedge pressure (as an approximation of pulmonary venous pressure), pulmonary blood flow (cardiac output), and the responses of these parameters to interventions (vasodilators, oxygen, exercise). From the measurements and samples obtained during cardiac catheterization, pulmonary vascular resistance can be calculated. In general, noninvasive methods are less reliable and less informative.

CHEST RADIOGRAPHY

The characteristic findings of pulmonary hypertension are enlargement of the pulmonary trunk and hilar vessels in association with attenuation (pruning) of the peripheral pulmonary arterial tree. Right-sided heart enlargement can be best detected radiographically on the lateral view as fullness in the retrosternal air space. In secondary pulmonary hypertension, changes in the lungs (e.g., hyperinflation, fibrosis) and in the position of the heart and diaphragm often mask the radiologic changes of pulmonary hypertension.

THE ELECTROCARDIOGRAM

The electrocardiogram (ECG) can disclose hypertrophy of the right ventricle and is more reliable in respiratory disorders that do not involve the parenchyma of the lungs (e.g., alveolar hypoventilation and sleep apnea) than in obstructive airways disease or parenchymal lung disease. (See also Chapter 2.)

ECHOCARDIOGRAPHY

Echocardiographic techniques have proved useful in providing a measure of right ventricular thickness as an index of right ventricular hypertension. In most clinics, reliable estimates of the level of pulmonary hypertension have been obtained by determining regurgitant flows across the tricuspid and pulmonic valves using continuous-wave Doppler echocardiography.

LUNG SCANS

Ventilation/perfusion scans are of most value in the diagnosis and exclusion of chronic pulmonary thromboembolic disease.

LUNG BIOPSY

The sampling of lung tissue by thoracotomy or thoracoscopy is occasionally helpful in identifying the etiology of the pulmonary hypertension—for example, in the setting of suspected pulmonary vasculitis. However, the procedure carries substantial risk in these hemodynamically compromised individuals.

SECONDARY PULMONARY HYPERTENSION

Cardiac and/or respiratory diseases are the most common causes of secondary pulmonary hypertension. Chronic thromboembolic disease ranks third. Cardiac disease leads to PH by increasing pulmonary blood flow (e.g., with large left-to-right shunts) or by increasing pulmonary venous pressure (e.g., with left ventricular failure). In respiratory disease, the predominant mechanism for the PH is an increase in resistance to pulmonary blood flow arising from perivascular parenchymal changes coupled with pulmonary vasoconstriction due to hypoxia. In chronic thromboembolic disease, clots in various stages of organization and affecting pulmonary vessels of different sizes increase resistance to blood flow.

【 】 ACQUIRED DISORDERS OF THE LEFT SIDE OF THE HEART

Left ventricular failure is the most common cause of pulmonary hypertension. Among the various etiologies, myocardial disorders and lesions of the mitral and aortic valves predominate. Both categories of lesions lead to an increase in pulmonary venous pressure, which in turn evokes an increase in pulmonary arterial pressure. The medical management of myocardial failure is considered elsewhere. The treatment of congenital heart disease and of mitral valvular disease is usually mechanical (e.g., surgical or balloon mitral valvuloplasty). The prospect for relief of the pulmonary venous hypertension, as by mitral valve commissurotomy or replacement, depends on the reversibility of the pulmonary vascular and perivascular lesions.

【 】 CONGENITAL HEART DISEASE

Pulmonary hypertension is part of the natural history of many types of congenital heart disease and is often a major determinant of the clinical course, feasibility of surgical intervention, and outcome. Congenital defects of the heart associated with large left-to-right shunts (e.g., atrial septal defect) or abnormal communication between the great vessels (e.g., patent ductus arteriosus) are commonly associated with pulmonary arterial hypertension. The major cause of PH in congenital heart disease is an increase in blood flow, an increase in resistance to blood flow, or most often, a combination of the two.

Caution is required in administering vasodilator agents to patients with congenital heart disease because of their potential to increase right-to-left shunting by reducing systemic vascular resistance to a greater degree than its pulmonary counterpart. Phlebotomy, with replacement of fluid (e.g., plasma or albumin), is helpful in congenital cyanotic heart disease in which severe hypoxemia has evoked a large increase in red cell mass.

【　】 THROMBOEMBOLIC DISEASE

Thromboembolic disease is a form of occlusive pulmonary vascular disease. It may be acute or chronic. Tumor emboli carried to the lungs from extrapulmonary sites (e.g., the breast) can cause pulmonary hypertension by invading the adjacent minute vessels of the lungs. Intravenous drug use may be associated with talc or cotton fiber embolism to the lungs, which can result in a granulomatous pulmonary arteritis.

CHRONIC PROXIMAL PULMONARY THROMBOEMBOLISM

In some patients who have survived large to massive pulmonary emboli, resolution fails to occur, and the clots become organized and incorporated into the walls of the major pulmonary arteries, leading to pulmonary hypertension. By the time the diagnosis is made, the obstructing lesions in the central pulmonary arteries have become an integral part of the vascular wall through the processes of endothelialization and recanalization.

The importance of recognizing *proximal* pulmonary thromboembolism as a cause of PH lies in the possibility of relieving the pulmonary hypertension by surgical intervention—that is, by pulmonary thromboendarterectomy. Ventilation/perfusion lung scanning is the critical diagnostic test. As a rule, patients with proximal pulmonary thromboembolism show two or more segmental perfusion defects. If the perfusion defects are segmental or larger, selective pulmonary angiography is required to define the location, extent, and number of pulmonary vascular occlusions. Cardiac catheterization for selective pulmonary angiography also enables hemodynamic assessment.

Surgery is advocated for patients with pulmonary hypertension who have persistent clotting in lobar or more proximal pulmonary arteries after at least 6 months of anticoagulation. Thromboendarterectomy is done via a median sternotomy using deep hypothermic cardiopulmonary bypass with intermittent periods of circulatory arrest. Postoperatively, hemodynamic improvement is usually quite dramatic. Reperfusion pulmonary edema can be a severe complication immediately after the obstruction has been relieved. In experienced hands, mortality is of the order of 5%. After the operation, patients are placed on lifelong anticoagulants. A filter is usually placed in the inferior vena cava to further prevent recurrence.

RESPIRATORY DISEASES AND DISORDERS

In addition to intrinsic pulmonary diseases, disturbances in respiratory muscle function or in the control of breathing can also lead to pulmonary hypertension. Among the intrinsic lung diseases are those affecting the airways (e.g., chronic bronchitis) as well as those affecting the parenchyma (i.e., emphysema, pulmonary fibrosis). Among the ventilatory disorders are the syndromes of alveolar hypoventilation due to respiratory muscle weakness and sleep-disordered breathing.

【　】 INTERSTITIAL FIBROSIS

Pulmonary sarcoidosis, asbestosis, idiopathic fibrosis, and radiation-induced fibrosis are common causes of widespread pulmonary fibrosis that culminates in cor pulmonale. Dyspnea and tachypnea generally dominate the clinical picture of interstitial fibrosis; cough is rarely prominent. As a rule, severe PH occurs toward the end of the illness, when hypoxemia and hypercapnia are present at rest. Right ventricular failure is a common sequel.

Systemically administered vasodilators have no proven place in dealing with the pulmonary hypertension associated with interstitial fibrosis and may worsen intra-pulmonary gas exchange. Oxygen therapy, particularly during daily activity or sleep, can be important in attenuating the hypoxic pulmonary pressor response. Glucocorticoids and other potent immunosuppressive agents are the mainstay of therapy and often result in some symptomatic relief. The advent of lung transplantation has greatly widened the therapeutic horizons for dealing with widespread interstitial fibrosis.

【 】 CHRONIC OBSTRUCTIVE AIRWAYS DISEASE

Chronic bronchitis and emphysema (chronic obstructive pulmonary disease [COPD]) are the most common causes of cor pulmonale in patients with intrinsic pulmonary disease. Cystic fibrosis is an example of a mixed airway and parenchymal lung disease in which pulmonary hypertension plays a significant role in outcome.

Cor pulmonale is encountered in two different settings: *acutely* in the setting of decompensation, which is often due to an acute respiratory infection; and *chronically* when progressive lung disease and worsening gas exchange lead to unremitting vascular remodeling.

In the patient with COPD with acute cor pulmonale precipitated by a bout of bronchitis or pneumonia, the goal of therapy is to maintain tolerable levels of arterial oxygenation while waiting for the upper respiratory infection to subside. Supplemental oxygen, such as 28% oxygen delivered by a Venturi mask, generally suffices to relieve arterial hypoxemia and to restore pulmonary arterial pressures toward normal. Considerable improvement may also be accomplished even in the individual who has chronic PH by sustained (> 18 h/d) breathing of oxygen-enriched air.

Arterial blood gas composition is the therapeutic compass for the control of PH in COPD. The degree of hypoxia may be underestimated by blood sampling while the patient is awake and at rest, since hypoxemia is more marked during sleep and with physical activity. Determinations of the oxygen saturation during sleep or with ambulation, using pulse oximetry, are helpful in optimally prescribing supplemental oxygen.

Vasodilators have recently been tried in various types of secondary pulmonary hypertension, including that due to COPD. The agents tried are the same as those outlined for *idiopathic* pulmonary arterial hypertension. They run the risk of aggravating arterial hypoxemia by exaggerating ventilation/perfusion abnormalities. To date, the safest and most effective approach to pulmonary vasodilatation in obstructive lung disease with arterial hypoxemia is the use of supplemental oxygen.

CONNECTIVE TISSUE DISEASES

Pulmonary vascular disease is an important component of certain connective tissue diseases. Among these, the more common are systemic lupus erythematosus (SLE), the scleroderma spectrum of diseases, and dermatomyositis.

In progressive systemic sclerosis (scleroderma) and its variants, such as the CREST syndrome (*c*alcinosis, *R*aynaud's syndrome, *e*sophageal involvement, *s*clerodactyly, and *t*elangiectasis), and in overlap syndromes (e.g., mixed connective tissue disease), the incidence of pulmonary vascular disease is high. In these patients, pulmonary hypertension is the cause of considerable morbidity and mortality. The pulmonary vascular disease may be independent of pulmonary or other visceral disease. As in the case of SLE, the pathology of these lesions is often indistinguishable from that of primary pulmonary hypertension. Vasodilator therapy has not proved to be highly effective; however, continuous intravenous epoprostenol and oral bosentan, an endothelin receptor antagonist, have both been shown to improve hemodynamics and exercise tolerance.

【 】 ALVEOLAR HYPOVENTILATION IN PATIENTS WITH NORMAL LUNGS

In patients who hypoventilate despite normal lungs (alveolar hypoventilation), the primary pathogenetic mechanism is alveolar hypoxia potentiated by respiratory acidosis. These abnormal alveolar and arterial blood gases play the same role in eliciting pulmonary hypertension in patients with alveolar hypoventilation as in those in whom the abnormal alveolar and blood gases are the result of ventilation/perfusion abnormalities. For the patient with alveolar hypoventilation with combined respiratory and cardiac (right ventricular) failure, the highest therapeutic priority is to improve oxygenation. Assisted ventilation, particularly during sleep, may be particularly helpful in improving oxygenation and reducing hypercapnic (e.g., continuous positive airway pressure [CPAP]) breathing.

IDIOPATHIC PULMONARY ARTERIAL HYPERTENSION

【 】 DEFINITION

Idiopathic pulmonary arterial hypertension (IPAH), a disorder intrinsic to the pulmonary vascular bed, is characterized by sustained elevations in pulmonary artery pressure and vascular resistance that generally lead to right ventricular failure and death. The diagnosis of IPAH requires the exclusion on clinical grounds of other conditions that can result in pulmonary artery hypertension. PPH is a rare disease, with an incidence of 1 to 2 per million. Its prevalence is about 0.1% to 0.2% of all patients who come to autopsy.

The clinical diagnosis of IPAH rests on three different types of evidence: (1) clinical, radiographic, and electrocardiographic manifestations of PH; (2) hemodynamic features, consisting of abnormally high pulmonary arterial pressures and pulmonary vascular resistance in association with normal left-sided filling pressures and a normal or low cardiac output; and (3) exclusion of the causes of secondary PH. (see Table 30-1).

【 】 SPECIAL TYPES

Certain associations of IPAH have attracted interest because of their prospects for shedding light on some etiologies. These include so-called anorexigen-induced pulmonary hypertension, familial pulmonary hypertension, human immunodeficiency virus (HIV)-associated pulmonary hypertension, and portal-pulmonary hypertension. In each of these, the clinical findings and the histologic appearance of the lungs at autopsy are identical to those that characterize the sporadic form of IPAH. This diversity in associations underscores the likelihood that so-called IPAH is the final common expression of heterogeneous etiologies.

As a rule, median survival of untreated patients can be predicted on the basis of the New York Heart Association functional classification: 6 months for class IV; 21/2 years for class III; and 6 years for classes I and II. Unless interrupted by sudden death, which occurs in approximately 15% of patients, the usual downhill course terminates in intractable right ventricular failure.

The combination of right-sided heart catheterization and vasodilator testing is particularly useful, not only for defining the hemodynamic state of the patient but also to provide a hemodynamic baseline for future invasive and noninvasive studies, such as serial echocardiograms.

【 】 TREATMENT

A patient with IPAH has several therapeutic options, ranging from oral calcium-channel blockers to continuous infusion of prostacyclin to lung transplantation.

In experienced centers, the trial of nifedipine or diltiazem orally is preceded by testing for acute vasoreactivity using one or more of three agents: (1) inhaled nitric oxide (NO), in concentrations of 10 to 40 ppm for 5 to 10 minutes; (2) prostacyclin (PGI_2; epoprostenol, Flolan), administered intravenously in increasing doses—a starting dose of 1 to 2 ng/kg/min followed by successive increments every 15 minutes of 2 ng/kg/min until a maximal dose of 12 ng/kg/min is reached or side effects preclude further increases; and (3) adenosine, 50 to 200 ng/kg/min. Only patients who manifest significant reductions

TABLE 30-1

Nomenclature and Classification of Pulmonary Hypertension

Diagnostic Classification

1. Pulmonary arterial hypertension
    1.1 Idiopathic familial
    1.2 Related to
        (a) Connective tissue disease
        (b) Congenital systemic to pulmonary shunts
        (c) Portal hypertension
        (d) HIV infection
        (e) Drugs/toxins
            (1) Anorexigens
            (2) Other
        (f) Persistent pulmonary hypertension of the newborn
        (g) Other
2. Pulmonary venous hypertension
    2.1 Left-side atrial or ventricular heart disease
    2.2 Left-side valvular heart disease
    2.3 Extrinsic compression of central pulmonary veins
        (a) Fibrosing mediastinitis
        (b) Adenopathy/tumors
    2.4 Pulmonary venoocclusive disease/pulmonary capillary hemangiomatosis
    2.5 Other
3. Pulmonary hypertension associated with disorders of the respiratory system and/or hypoxemia
    3.1 Chronic obstructive pulmonary disease
    3.2 Interstitial lung disease
    3.3 Sleep-disordered breathing
    3.4 Alveolar hypoventilatory disorders
    3.5 Chronic exposure to high altitude
    3.6 Neonatal lung disease
    3.7 Alveolar-capillary dysplasia
    3.8 Other
4. Pulmonary hypertension caused by chronic thrombotic and/or embolic disease
    4.1 Thromboembolic obstruction of proximal pulmonary arteries
    4.2 Obstruction of distal pulmonary arteries
        (a) Pulmonary embolism (thrombus, tumor, ova and/or parasites, foreign material)
        (b) In situ thrombosis
        (c) Sickle-cell disease
5. Pulmonary hypertension as a consequence of disorders directly affecting the pulmonary vasculature
    5.1 Inflammatory
        (a) Schistosomiasis
        (b) Sarcoidosis
        (c) Other

in pulmonary vascular resistance (usually to a value < 5–6 U), resulting from a fall in pulmonary artery pressure without systemic hypotension and accompanied by an unchanged or increased cardiac output, are considered candidates for chronic therapy with oral calcium-channel blockers.

Intravenous epoprostenol (Flolan, prostacyclin, PGI_2), a metabolite of arachidonic acid, and its analogs continue to be a major focus of attention as treatments for a variety of forms of pulmonary hypertension. Success in long-term management has been reported using aerosolized iloprost and subcutaneous treprostinil, stable prostacyclin analogues. The dual endothelin receptor antagonist bosentan and the selective endothelin-A receptor analogues sitaxsentan and ambrisentan have also been demonstrated to improve exercise tolerance and delay the time to clinical deterioration. Sildenafil, a phosphodiesterase-5 inhibitor used to treat male erectile dysfunction, also improves pulmonary hemodynamics and exercise capacity in pulmonary arterial hypertension.

The use of anticoagulants has been incorporated into the therapeutic regimen in patients with IPAH. The usual goal of anticoagulation is to achieve and maintain an international normalized ratio (INR) of 2 to 2.5.

ATRIAL SEPTOSTOMY

Blade-balloon atrial septostomy has been performed in patients with severe right ventricular pressure and volume overload refractory to maximal medical therapy. The goal of this approach is to decompress the overloaded right heart and improve the systemic output of the underfilled left ventricle. Improvements in exercise function and signs of severe right heart dysfunction, such as syncope and ascites, have been observed. Since the creation of an interatrial communication results in an increased venous admixture, worsening hypoxemia is an expected outcome. The size of the septostomy that is created should be carefully monitored in order to achieve the ideal balance of optimizing systemic oxygen transport and reducing right heart filling pressures without overfilling a noncompliant left ventricle or producing extreme degrees of venous admixture.

LUNG TRANSPLANTATION

Fewer than 20% of patients with IPAH are responsive to long-term oral vasodilator therapy. Of the remainder, approximately 65% to 75% maintain sustained clinical improvement with long-term oral therapies or continuous intravenous prostanoid therapy. When pulmonary hypertensive disease has progressed or threatens to progress to the stage of right ventricular failure, the physician and patient are left with few therapeutic options other than lung transplantation. Lung transplantation is performed at specialized centers and is almost invariably handicapped by shortage of donor lungs, which can lead to long delays. Double-lung transplantation has largely replaced heart-lung transplantation as the procedure of choice for pulmonary arterial hypertension. Rejection phenomena, notably bronchiolitis obliterans, are the major limiting factor to prolonged survival. The median survival after lung transplantation is approximately 3 to 5 years. Recurrence of IPAH after transplantation has not been reported.

SUGGESTED READING

Badesch DB, Abman SH, Simonneau G, et al. Medical therapy for pulmonary arterial hypertension: updated ACCP evidence-based clinical practice guidelines. *Chest.* 2007;131:1917–1928.

Chin K, Rubin LJ. Pulmonary arterial hypertension. *J Am Coll Cardiol.* 2008;51: 1527–1538.

Hoeper M, Meyer E, Simonneau G, et al. Chronic thromboembolic pulmonary hypertension. *Circulation.* 2006;113:2011–2020.

Rubin LJ. Pulmonary hypertension. In: Fuster V, Alexander RW, O'Rourke RA, eds. *Hurst's The Heart.* New York, NY: McGraw-Hill.

Rubin LJ, Badesch DB. Evaluation and management of the patient with pulmonary arterial hypertension. *Ann Intern Med.* 2005;143:282–292.

CHAPTER (31)

Pulmonary Embolism

Gordon L. Yung and Peter F. Fedullo

Despite advances in diagnostic technology, therapeutic approaches, and preventive strategies, pulmonary embolism (PE) remains directly responsible for approximately 100,000 deaths annually in the United States while contributing to an additional 100,000 deaths in patients with concomitant disease. Autopsy studies have repeatedly documented the high frequency with which PE has gone unsuspected and undetected, while clinical studies have established that prophylaxis is underutilized and that death from embolism is unusual once the diagnosis has been confirmed and effective therapy initiated, except in patients who initially present with hemodynamic compromise.

DEEP VENOUS THROMBOSIS: RISK FACTORS AND PATHOGENESIS

Because PE arises from venous thrombosis, the two conditions are considered a continuum of the same condition, venous thromboembolism (VTE). Virchow proposed that the pathogenesis of venous thrombosis was based upon several potential initiating events, including stasis, venous injury, and hypercoagulability. Risk factors for venous thrombosis—which may be acquired or inherited—are based upon these processes (Table 31-1). Frequently more than one risk factor is present. Antecedent pulmonary thromboembolism forecasts an appreciable risk of recurrence in the hospitalized patient. Surgery, trauma, immobility, cancer, anticardiolipin antibodies or a lupus anticoagulant, and pregnancy and the postpartum period are important acquired risks. In addition, several hereditary risk factors have been identified over recent years. These include deficiencies in antithrombin III, protein C, and protein S; the factor V Leiden and the prothrombin gene (G20210A) mutations; hyperhomocysteinemia; and elevated levels of coagulation factors VIII, IX, and XI. The identification of these inherited risk factors has proved useful in providing insight into the etiologic basis for thromboembolism in many patients with idiopathic disease. However, most patients who develop venous thromboembolism do so as the consequence of some clinical predisposition. Even in those with an identified thrombophilic predisposition, interaction with a defined clinical state may be necessary to shift the normal hemostatic balance toward thrombosis.

ACUTE PULMONARY EMBOLISM: PATHOPHYSIOLOGY

The clinical manifestations of pulmonary embolism are related to the size of the emboli and degree of occlusion of the pulmonary vasculature. Secondary neurohumoral responses may also contribute to the pathophysiologic consequences and may explain

TABLE 31-1

Risk Factors for Venous Thromboembolism

Acquired Factors

Age > 40
Prior history of venous thromboembolism
Prior major surgical procedure
Trauma
Hip fracture
Immobilization/paralysis
Venous stasis
Varicose veins
Congestive heart failure
Myocardial infarction
Obesity
Pregnancy/postpartum period
Oral contraceptive therapy
Cerebrovascular accident
Malignancy
Severe thrombocythemia
Paroxysmal nocturnal hemoglobinuria
Antiphospholipid antibody syndrome (including lupus anticoagulant)

Inherited Factors

Antithrombin III deficiency
Factor V Leiden (activated protein C resistance)
Prothrombin gene (G20210A) defect
Protein C deficiency
Protein S deficiency
Dysfibrinogenemia
Disorders of plasminogen

why similar degrees of vascular obstruction may result in different clinical outcomes. The underlying cardiopulmonary status of the patient may have a significant impact on the physiologic response to the event.

【 】 GAS EXCHANGE ABNORMALITIES

Hypoxemia develops in the preponderance of patients with PE and has been attributed to various mechanisms. When no previous cardiopulmonary disease is present, a decrease in the mixed venous oxygen content related to a decrease in cardiac output, redistribution of pulmonary blood flow to lung regions with low ventilation/perfusion ratios, and shunting due to perfusion of atelectatic areas appear to be the predominant mechanisms of hypoxemia.

【 】 HEMODYNAMIC ALTERATIONS

The hemodynamic sequelae of the embolic event depend upon the extent of obstruction of the pulmonary vascular bed, the presence or absence of underlying cardiovascular disease, and the effects of endothelial and platelet-derived mediators on the pulmonary vascular bed. When no underlying cardiopulmonary disease is present, occlusion of 25% to 30% of the vascular bed by emboli is associated with a rise in pulmonary artery pressure. Greater than 40% to 50% obstruction of the pulmonary arterial bed is generally present before there is substantial elevation of the mean pulmonary artery pressure

(PAP), which is associated with a rise in right atrial pressure and a decline in cardiac output. When the extent of embolic occlusion approaches 75%, a previously normal right ventricle becomes incapable of compensating for the increased afterload and subsequently dilates and fails. The maximal *mean* PAP capable of being generated by a previously normal right ventricle is in the range of 40 mm Hg. A mean PAP in excess of 40 mm Hg in the setting of acute embolism strongly suggests an element of chronic cardiopulmonary disease.

DIAGNOSIS OF DEEP VENOUS THROMBOSIS AND PULMONARY EMBOLISM

Most clinically significant pulmonary emboli arise from venous thrombosis of the proximal deep veins (including and proximal to the popliteal veins) of the legs, although upper extremity, abdominal, and pelvic vein thrombi may also result in embolism. Patients with venous thromboembolism may present with symptoms of venous thrombosis, pulmonary embolism, or both.

【 】 HISTORY AND PHYSICAL EXAMINATION

The clinical diagnosis of both venous thrombosis and pulmonary embolism, based upon the history and physical examination, are insensitive and nonspecific. Patients with lower extremity venous thrombosis may be asymptomatic or may have erythema, warmth, pain, swelling, and/or tenderness. These findings, however, while not specific for deep venous thrombosis, suggest the need for further evaluation. The differential diagnosis of venous thrombosis includes cellulitis, edema from other causes, musculoskeletal pain, or trauma (some of these may be concomitant and may or may not be related). The clinical presentation of pulmonary embolism ranges from asymptomatic incidentally discovered events to those that are massive, resulting in cardiogenic shock and death. Dyspnea and pleuritic chest pain are common in embolism, and pulmonary embolism must always be considered when these symptoms are present. Hemoptysis occurs much less frequently. Anxiety, light-headedness, and syncope may also occur but may result from a number of other entities that cause hypoxemia or hypotension. Tachypnea, rales, and tachycardia are the most common signs of PE. Syncope or sudden hypotension should suggest the possibility of massive embolism. With the exception of massive PE, in which the physical examination may disclose findings consistent with right ventricular failure (see Chapter 1), the physical examination findings are nonspecific. The differential diagnosis of embolism includes viral or bacterial pleuritis, pneumonia, pneumothorax, costochondritis, pericarditis, asthma, or an exacerbation of preexisting chronic obstructive pulmonary disease or congestive heart failure. A high clinical suspicion of the possibility of the disease, therefore, must be an integral part of the diagnostic pathway. Diagnostic efforts aimed at possible venous thromboembolism should always be considered if risk factors and the clinical setting are suggestive.

【 】 LABORATORY TESTING FOR ACUTE DEEP VENOUS THROMBOSIS AND PULMONARY EMBOLISM

Routine laboratory testing is not useful in proving the presence of venous thrombosis or pulmonary embolism, but may be helpful in confirming or excluding other diagnoses. Hypoxemia is common in acute PE, although the diagnosis of acute PE *cannot* be excluded based upon a normal PaO_2. Some individuals, particularly young patients without underlying lung disease, may have a normal PaO_2 and even a normal alveolar–arterial O_2 gradient.

Electrocardiography (ECG) cannot be relied upon to confirm or exclude the possibility of embolism, although electrocardiographic evidence of a clear alternative diagnosis, such as myocardial infarction or pericarditis, is useful when PE is among the possible diagnoses. ECG findings in acute PE are generally nonspecific and include T-wave changes, ST-segment abnormalities, and left or right axis deviation. The S1Q3T3 pattern, while commonly considered specific for PE, is seen in only a minority of patients.

The utility of plasma measurements of circulating D-dimer, a specific derivative of cross-linked fibrin, as a diagnostic aid in venous thromboembolism has been extensively evaluated. D-Dimer testing has proven to be highly sensitive but not specific; that is, elevated levels are present in nearly all patients with venous thrombosis and pulmonary embolism but also occur in a wide range of circumstances, including advancing age, pregnancy, trauma, the postoperative period, inflammatory states, and malignancy. The role of D-dimer testing, therefore, is limited to one of thrombotic exclusion. D-Dimer testing has been utilized successfully as part of a number of different diagnostic strategies, and negative results of standardized, highly sensitive enzyme-linked immunosorbent assays (ELISA) have proved to be capable of safely excluding venous thromboembolism in outpatients presenting with a low or intermediate clinical likelihood of disease. It must be emphasized that commercially available D-dimer assays vary in terms of their sensitivity, negative likelihood ratio, and variability, and that the value of D-dimer testing is enhanced when it is incorporated into a comprehensive diagnostic pathway.

【 】 CHEST RADIOGRAPHY IN SUSPECTED PULMONARY EMBOLISM

Most patients with PE have abnormal but nonspecific chest radiographic findings that are incapable of conclusively diagnosing or excluding PE. The main use of the chest radiograph in suspected embolism is to exclude diagnostic possibilities that may simulate the disease. Common radiographic findings include atelectasis, pleural effusion, pulmonary infiltrates, and mild elevation of a hemidiaphragm. Classic findings of pulmonary infarction—such as "Hampton's hump" (pleural-based wedge-shaped density) or decreased vascularity (Westermark's sign)—are suggestive but infrequent. A normal chest radiograph in a patient with otherwise unexplained acute dyspnea or hypoxemia is strongly suggestive of embolism.

【 】 OTHER IMAGING STUDIES FOR SUSPECTED ACUTE PULMONARY EMBOLISM

Until recently, ventilation-perfusion scanning has been the pivotal diagnostic test performed when PE is suspected. Normal and high-probability scans are considered diagnostic. A normal perfusion scan rules out the diagnosis of PE with a high enough degree of certainty that further diagnostic evaluation is unnecessary. Matching areas of decreased ventilation and perfusion in the presence of a normal chest radiograph generally represent a process other than PE. However, scans characterized as low or intermediate-probability (nondiagnostic) scans are commonly found with PE; in such situations, further evaluation depending on the clinical circumstance may be appropriate. In the Prospective Investigation Overview of Pulmonary Embolism Diagnosis (PIOPED) study, for example, embolism was confirmed in 40% of those with low-probability scans when the clinical suspicion of the disease was considered high. The diagnosis of PE should be rigorously pursued even when the lung scan is of low or intermediate probability if the clinical scenario suggests PE. Therefore, while the scan may sometimes be diagnostic of PE or may exclude the possibility with sufficient certainty, it is often nondiagnostic.

Computed tomography has represented a major advance in the diagnosis of PE by providing the capability to directly visualize emboli as well as to detect parenchymal abnormalities that may support the diagnosis of embolism or provide an alternative basis for the patient's complaints. A wide range of sensitivities and specificities for helical CT scanning for embolism diagnosis has been reported. Factors responsible for this wide divergence relate to the proximal extent of vascular obstruction that can be detected and to rapid advances in CT technology that outpace the medical literature. The absence of detectable filling defects reduces the likelihood of embolism, but appears incapable of excluding the possibility with the same degree of certainty as a negative ventilation-perfusion scan.

In the recently published Prospective Investigation of Pulmonary Embolism Diagnosis II (PIOPED II) trial, the sensitivity of CTA alone was 83%. When coupled with simultaneous CT venography, the sensitivity increased to 90%. The positive predictive value of CTA is dependent on the proximal location of the thrombus and the pretest likelihood of the disease. Positive predictive values for CTA in PIOPED II were 97% for emboli in the main or lobar arteries, 68% for segmental vessels, and 25% for subsegmental involvement. In patients with a high or intermediate probability of disease and a positive CTA or CT venogram, the positive predictive value was in excess of 98%. Alternatively, in patients with a low clinical probability of disease and a positive CT angiogram or venogram, the positive predictive value fell to 57%.

Conventional pulmonary angiography remains the accepted "gold standard" for PE diagnosis, although it has a number of limitations as a gold standard. It requires expertise in study performance and interpretation, is invasive, and has associated risks, although published studies would suggest that the use of modern techniques and contrast materials has reduced the reality of those risks well below the lingering perception. Angiography is reserved for the small subset of patients in whom the diagnosis of embolism cannot be established or excluded by less invasive means. Even in this defined set of circumstances, angiography appears to be underutilized.

Echocardiography is not generally useful for proving the presence of PE, although it may offer compelling clues to its presence in certain clinical settings and has been suggested as a potential means by which to determine the need for thrombolytic therapy. Studies of patients with documented PE have revealed that more than 50% have imaging or Doppler abnormalities of right ventricular size or function that may suggest acute PE. Unfortunately, because patients with PE often have underlying cardiopulmonary disease, neither right ventricular dilation nor hypokinesis can be reliably used as even indirect evidence of PE in such settings.

Because the majority of pulmonary emboli arise from the deep veins of the lower extremities, the detection of lower extremity, proximal-vein thrombosis in a patient suspected of embolism, although not confirming that embolism has occurred, is strongly suggestive of that diagnosis and has an equivalent therapeutic implication. Ultrasonography has been reported to be positive in approximately 10% to 20% of patients with suspected embolism and in 50% of patients with proven embolism. A negative ultrasound finding, therefore, cannot exclude the diagnosis.

【 】 IMAGING STUDIES FOR SUSPECTED DEEP VENOUS THROMBOSIS

Doppler ultrasonography is a portable and accurate diagnostic technique for proximal lower extremity venous thrombosis. Its sensitivity and specificity for symptomatic, proximal venous thrombosis have been well above 90% in most recent clinical trials. Limitations include a lack of sensitivity for asymptomatic disease, operator dependence, the inability to accurately distinguish acute from chronic thrombi in symptomatic patients, and a decreased sensitivity for calf vein thrombosis. Compared to other technology, it is portable, noninvasive, and relatively inexpensive, and it has become the most commonly utilized initial diagnostic modality for suspected lower extremity deep venous thrombosis.

CT venography as an adjunct to helical CT scanning has been investigated, and preliminary results suggest that it is capable of detecting femoropopliteal thrombosis with the same accuracy as duplex ultrasonography, while also detecting pelvic and abdominal thrombosis.

While contrast venography remains the diagnostic "gold standard," it has been less commonly performed since the advent of Doppler ultrasonography. Venography should be performed whenever noninvasive testing is nondiagnostic or impossible to perform.

【 】 CLINICAL PREDICTION RULES

A major advance in the diagnostic approach to venous thrombosis and PE has been the derivation and validation of clinical prediction rules that are capable of stratifying patients into probability categories. By combining this derived clinical probability with the results of one or more noninvasive diagnostic techniques, diagnostic accuracy in terms of both the confirmation and the exclusion of venous thromboembolism can be increased well beyond that achieved by the use of either clinical probability or the noninvasive diagnostic techniques alone, and the number of patients who require invasive diagnostic testing can be substantially limited. Standardized prediction rules vary in their complexity and have not been demonstrated to be superior to empiric assessment, but can help avoid variance among practitioners with different levels of experience and training.

【 】 DIAGNOSTIC APPROACH

The recommended diagnostic pathway for outpatients with a low or intermediate probability of pulmonary embolism is to first perform a highly-sensitive D-dimer assay. A negative result is capable of excluding the diagnosis of embolism in these probability categories. Lower extremity evaluation in those with an intermediate probability of disease is recommended and is a prudent and low-cost option. For those with a positive D-dimer result, CTA coupled with either CT venography or a lower extremity ultrasound is recommended. Outcome studies have demonstrated that withholding anticoagulant therapy in patients with a negative CT scan coupled with a negative lower extremity ultrasound study is a safe strategy except in those patients who present with a high clinical likelihood of embolism.

In patients with a high clinical probability of embolism, D-dimer testing is not recommended given that a negative result would not exclude the need for additional evaluation. CTA coupled with either CT venography or a lower extremity ultrasound is recommended. Negative studies will exclude embolism in the large majority of patients. It is prudent to consider additional imaging (conventional pulmonary angiography, ventilation/perfusion scanning) in cases of high clinical suspicion even if CTA is negative, especially when there is coexisting cardiopulmonary disease in which recurrent embolism would be poorly tolerated.

PRINCIPLES OF MANAGEMENT

【 】 PROPHYLAXIS OF DEEP VENOUS THROMBOSIS

A significant reduction in the incidence of deep venous thrombosis (DVT) can be achieved when patients at risk receive appropriate prophylaxis. Such preventive measures appear to be grossly underutilized. Unfractionated heparin (UFH), low-molecular-weight heparin (LMWH), fondaparinux (a synthetic, specific anti-Xa inhibitor), warfarin, and mechanical means of prophylaxis have proven effective in various clinical settings. Surgical and medical patients can be stratified according to their risk of thrombosis, with the intensity of the prophylactic intervention being appropriate to the risk of thrombosis. The American College of Chest Physicians has published guidelines for antithrombotic therapy that offer evidence-based recommendations for the prevention and therapy of venous thromboembolism (VTE). These guidelines offer specific preventive recommendations for general, orthopedic, trauma, stroke, spinal cord injury, and medical patients.

【 】 TREATMENT OF ESTABLISHED VENOUS THROMBOEMBOLISM WITH HEPARIN AND LOW-MOLECULAR-WEIGHT HEPARIN

Anticoagulation has been proven to reduce thromboembolic recurrence and therefore mortality in acute PE. When VTE is diagnosed or strongly suspected, anticoagulation therapy should be instituted promptly unless contraindications exist. Confirmatory testing should always be planned if anticoagulation is to be continued. Heparin and LMWH exert a prompt antithrombotic effect, preventing thrombus growth. While thrombus growth can be prevented, early recurrence can develop even in the setting of therapeutic anticoagulation. With the institution of continuous intravenous heparin, the activated partial thromboplastin time (aPTT) should be followed at 6-hour intervals until it is consistently in the therapeutic range of 1.5 to 2.0 times control values. Standardized dosing regimens should be utilized, thereby decreasing the risk of subtherapeutic anticoagulation. Although supratherapeutic levels are sometimes achieved initially, bleeding complications do not appear to be increased. One such approach utilizes an intravenous bolus of 5000 U followed by a maintenance dose of 30,000 or 40,000 U/24 h by continuous infusion, with the lower dose being administered if the patient is considered at high risk for bleeding. Another commonly employed dosing regimen utilizes an initial intravenous bolus of 80 U/kg of heparin followed by a continuous infusion initiated at 18 U/kg/h; this approach has been demonstrated to reach therapeutic thresholds more quickly than regimens utilizing fixed dosing (Table 31-2). Most recently, a fixed dose regimen of *subcutaneous* heparin administered as an initial dose of 333 U/kg followed by a 250 U/kg every 12 hours was demonstrated to be as effective and safe as LMWH. Warfarin therapy may be initiated as soon as the aPTT is therapeutic, and heparin should be maintained until a therapeutic international normalized ratio (INR) of 2.0 to 3.0 has been overlapped with a therapeutic aPTT for 3 consecutive days.

Although calf-limited thrombi are rarely associated with embolism, approximately 20% may extend proximally. If untreated, calf-limited thrombi should be followed for proximal extension over 10 to 14 days with noninvasive testing.

A number of clinical trials have strongly suggested the efficacy and safety of LMWH for treatment of established acute proximal DVT, using recurrent symptomatic VTE as the primary outcome measure. There are several advantages of these drugs. They have

TABLE 31-2

Weight-Based Nomogram for Heparin Therapy in Acute Venous Thromboembolism

Initial heparin dose = 80-U/kg bolus, then 18 U/kg/h.
Subsequent modifications are shown below.

APTT		Heparin Dose Adjustment
(s)	(Times Control)	
<35	<1.2	80-U/kg bolus, then increase by 4 U/kg/h
35–45	1.2–1.5	40-U/kg bolus, then increase by 2 U/kg/h
46–70	1.5–2.3	No change
71–90	2.3–3	Decrease infusion rate by 2 U/kg/h
>90	>3	Hold infusion 1 h, then decrease rate by 3 U/kg/h

Data adapted from American College of Chest Physicians Guidelines. Hyers TM, Agnelli G, Hull RD, et al. Antithrombotic therapy for venous thromboembolic disease. *Chest.* 1998;114:561S–578S; and Raschke RA, Reilly BM, Guidry JR, et al. The weight-based heparin dosing nomogram compared with a "standard care" nomogram. *Ann Intern Med.* 1993;119:874.

TABLE 31-3

Potential Advantages of Low-Molecular-Weight Heparins Over Unfractionated Heparin

Comparable or superior efficacy
Comparable or superior safety
Superior bioavailability
Once- or twice-daily dosing
No laboratory monitoring
Less phlebotomy
Subcutaneous administration
Earlier ambulation
Home therapy in certain patient subsets

excellent bioavailability and can be administered once or twice daily. No monitoring is required in most patients. Because of the ease of administration of these preparations, home therapy of DVT is becoming frequent. However, many patients may not be candidates for home therapy as a result of hemorrhagic risk, compliance issues, renal insufficiency, significant comorbidity, inadequate cardiopulmonary reserve, or poor likelihood of obtaining adequate outpatient care. Advantages of LMWH preparations are summarized in Table 31-3, and dosing guidelines are outlined in Table 31-4.

TABLE 31-4

Use of FDA-Approved Low-Molecular-Weight Heparins and Pentasaccharides for Treatment of Deep Venous Thrombosis with or without Pulmonary Embolism[a]

Therapeutic Indication	Enoxaparin	Tinzaparin	Fondaparinux
Treatment of acute DVT with or without PE with transition to warfarin	1 mg/kg SC twice daily, or 1.5 mg/kg SC daily	175 U/kg SC daily	<50 kg = 5 mg SC daily 50–100 kg = 7.5 mg SC daily >100 kg = 10 mg SC daily
Outpatient treatment of acute DVT without PE with transition to warfarin	1 mg/kg SC twice daily	X	X
Treatment of acute PE with transition to warfarin	X	X	<50 kg = 5 mg SC daily 50–100 kg = 7.5 mg SC daily >100 kg = 10 mg SC daily

SC, subcutaneously.

[a]There are inadequate data from randomized trials to treat symptomatic pulmonary embolism in the outpatient setting.
[b]Warfarin is initiated within 24 h after the LMWH is started. At least 5 days of therapy with LMWH is appropriate; the international normalized ratio (INR) should be 2.0 or greater for two consecutive mornings prior to discontinuing the LMWH.

【 】 DURATION OF ANTICOAGULATION

Following a first episode of embolism, patients appear to be at lifelong risk for recurrence regardless of whether the event was idiopathic or related to a well-defined predisposing factor. The risk of recurrence appears to be several-fold higher following discontinuation of anticoagulation in those who have experienced an idiopathic event. Among patients with a low risk of recurrence (first episode, provoked PE), 3 to 6 months of anticoagulation is recommended. For those with a high risk of recurrence (recurrent idiopathic events, ongoing predisposition, active malignancy), longer term or indefinite anticoagulation is recommended. The optimal duration of anticoagulation among those with an initial unprovoked event remains undefined. In all circumstances, treatment decisions should be based on the estimated benefits versus the risk of bleeding, the inconvenience of treatment, and the potential hemodynamic consequences of a recurrent event.

【 】 COMPLICATIONS OF ANTICOAGULATION

Complications of heparin include bleeding and heparin-induced thrombocytopenia (HIT). The rates of major bleeding in recent trials using heparin by continuous infusion or high-dose subcutaneous injection are less than 5%. When necessary, the effect of heparin can be reversed with protamine, although this intervention may be associated with hypotension or anaphylaxis. Heparin-induced thrombocytopenia (defined alternatively as a platelet count less than 150,000 mm^3 or a greater than 50% reduction in platelet count) typically develops 5 or more days after the initiation of heparin therapy and occurs in 1% to 5% of patients. Two types of thrombocytopenia are associated with heparin administration: an early-onset (1 to 5 days), non-immune-mediated reduction in platelet count (type I) and a late-onset (greater than 5 days), immune-mediated thrombocytopenia (type II) that may be associated with venous and arterial thrombosis. Development of type II HIT can occur earlier if there has been prior exposure to heparin. The substitution of LMWHs for unfractionated heparin in this circumstance should *not* be considered because of the potential for cross-reactivity. The direct thrombin inhibitors, argatroban, which undergoes hepatic metabolism and excretion, and lepirudin (hirudin), which is renally cleared, are approved for use in heparin-induced thrombocytopenia.

【 】 VENA CAVA INTERRUPTION

If anticoagulation therapy cannot be administered, inferior vena cava (IVC) filter placement can be undertaken. Established indications for filter placement in the therapy of venous thromboembolism include (1) protection against PE in patients with acute venous thromboembolism in whom conventional anticoagulation is contraindicated (recent surgery, hemorrhagic cerebrovascular accident, active bleeding, heparin-associated thrombocytopenia, etc.); (2) protection against PE in patients with acute venous thromboembolism in whom conventional anticoagulation has proven ineffective; and (3) protection of an already compromised pulmonary vascular bed from further thromboembolic risk (massive PE). With the increased ease of percutaneous filter placement and the introduction of retrievable devices, IVC filters have been increasingly utilized for prophylaxis in patients with a high risk of developing venous thrombosis. Prophylactic filter placement has been utilized in patients with traumatic injuries and those undergoing spinal, neurosurgical, and bariatric surgery as an alternative or adjunct to pharmacologic prophylaxis. The evidence that filter placement, whether permanent or temporary, reduces the risk of pulmonary embolism or death in these populations is not conclusive. In general, anticoagulation should be utilized following filter placement if no contraindications exist or as soon as any existing bleeding risk resolves.

【 】 THROMBOLYTIC THERAPY AND ACUTE EMBOLECTOMY

The use of thrombolytic agents in acute PE *remains controversial.* While thrombolytic therapy does appear to accelerate the rate of thrombolysis, there is no convincing evidence to suggest that it decreases mortality, increases the ultimate extent of resolution

TABLE 31-5

Thrombolytic Therapy for Acute Pulmonary Embolism: Approved Regimens

Streptokinase: 250,000 U IV (loading dose over 30 min); then 100,000 U/h
  for 24 h[a]
Urokinase: 4,400 U/kg IV (loading dose over 10 min); then 4400 U/kg/h for 12 h
Tissue-type plasminogen activator: 100 mg IV over 2 h

[a]Streptokinase administered over 24 to 72 h at this loading dose and rate has also been
approved for use in patients with extensive deep venous thrombosis.

when measured at 7 days, reduces thromboembolic recurrence rates, improves symptomatic outcome, or decreases the incidence of thromboembolic pulmonary hypertension. The use of thrombolytic therapy in PE should be limited to those circumstances in which an accelerated rate of thrombolysis may be considered lifesaving—that is, in patients with PE who present with hemodynamic compromise, patients who develop hemodynamic compromise during conventional therapy with heparin, and patients with embolism associated with intracavitary right heart thrombi. Specific thrombolytic regimens are listed in Table 31-5. The role of thrombolytic therapy in patients with anatomically massive embolism or echocardiographic evidence of right ventricular dysfunction in the absence of systemic hypotension is less well defined. Risk stratification approaches using echocardiography and troponin or brain natriuretic peptide (BNP) levels are currently under investigation and may help resolve this area of controversy. At present, urokinase, streptokinase, and recombinant tissue plasminogen activator (rt-PA) are approved for use in the treatment of PE. The method of delivery of thrombolytic agents has also been investigated. Intrapulmonary arterial delivery of thrombolytic agents appears to offer no advantage over the intravenous route. It is reasonable to consider catheter-directed or systemic thrombolytic therapy in patients with proximal occlusive DVT associated with significant swelling and symptoms when there are no absolute or relative contraindications.

The use of systemic thrombolytic agents is associated with a substantially increased risk of bleeding, including intracranial hemorrhage, which has been reported in 1% to 2% of patients undergoing therapy for pulmonary embolism. Hemorrhagic complications due to thrombolytic therapy can be minimized when venous cut-downs, central venous catheters, and unnecessary arterial punctures are avoided. Patients with severe or refractory bleeding should be transfused with blood, cryoprecipitate, and fresh frozen plasma, and heparin can be reversed with protamine.

Pulmonary embolectomy may be performed in the setting of acute massive PE. While many patients die of PE before surgical embolectomy would be feasible, some deteriorate hours after the initial episode and in the setting of maximal medical therapy, suggesting that surgery may occasionally be appropriate. This approach is especially useful when there are contraindications to thrombolytic therapy. Transvenous embolectomy using a suction-catheter device has been utilized by some but has not achieved widespread acceptance. Catheter-directed thrombolytic therapy has been successfully employed in the setting of acute iliofemoral DVT.

[ ] HEMODYNAMIC MANAGEMENT OF MASSIVE PULMONARY EMBOLISM

Once massive PE associated with hypotension and/or severe hypoxemia is suspected, supportive treatment is immediately initiated. Intravenous saline should be infused rapidly but cautiously, since right ventricular function is often markedly compromised, and excessive preload may further distend the right ventricle and increase right ventricular wall tension, resulting in decreased coronary perfusion and right ventricular ischemia. Dopamine or norepinephrine appear to be the favored choice of vasoactive therapy in massive PE and should be administered if the blood pressure is not rapidly restored. Oxygen therapy is administered to minimize hypoxic pulmonary vasoconstriction, and thrombolytic therapy or pulmonary embolectomy should be considered, as described above. Intubation and institution of mechanical ventilation are begun as needed to support respiratory failure.

CHRONIC THROMBOEMBOLISM

See Chapter 30 on pulmonary hypertension.

OTHER FORMS OF EMBOLISM

Because the blood receives all of the blood flow returned from the venous system, the pulmonary vascular bed serves as a "sieve" for all particulates entering the venous blood and is the first vascular bed to be exposed to any toxic substance injected intravenously. As a result of its strategic position, therefore, the pulmonary vascular bed is exposed to a wide variety of potentially obstructing and injurious agents. Other forms of emboli include fat embolism; air embolism; amniotic fluid embolism; tumor embolism; embolism from heroin (talc), bullets, or shotgun shot, cardiac catheters, or indwelling venous catheters; embolism from bone marrow, parasites, and cardiac vegetations; and bile thromboembolism. The acuity and severity of these entities depend upon the specific embolic event and the clinical circumstances.

SUGGESTED READING

Büller HR, Agnelli G, Hull RD, et al. Antithrombotic therapy for venous thromboembolic disease: the seventh ACCP conference on antithrombotic and thrombolytic therapy. *Chest.* 2004;126:401S–429S.

Chagnon I, Bounameaux H, Aujesky D, et al. Comparison of two clinical prediction rules and implicit assessment among patients with suspected pulmonary embolism. *Am J Med.* 2002;113:269–275.

Geerts WH, Pineo GF, Heit JA, et al. Prevention of venous thromboembolism: the seventh ACCP conference on antithrombotic and thrombolytic therapy. *Chest.* 2004;126:338S–400S.

Kearon C, Ginsberg JS, Julian JA, et al. Comparion of fixed-dose weight-adjusted unfractionated heparin and low-molecular weight heparin for acute treatment of venous thromboembolism. *JAMA.* 2006;296:935–942.

Kelly J, Hunt BJ. The utility of pretest probability assessment in patients with clinically suspected venous thromboembolism. *J Thromb Haemost.* 2003;1:1888–1896.

Lutz B, Pieske B, Olschewski M, et al. N-terminal pro-brain natriuretic peptide or troponin testing followed by echocardiography for risk stratification of pulmonary embolism. *Circulation.* 2005;112:1573–1579.

Prandoni P, Noventa F, Ghirarduzzi A, et al. The risk of recurrent venous thromboembolism after discontinuing anticoagulation in patients with acute proximal deep vein thrombosis or pulmonary embolism: a prospective cohort study in 1,626 patients. *Haematologica.* 2007;92:199–205.

Stein PD, Beemath A, Matta F, et al. Clinical characteristics of patients with acute pulmonary embolism: data from PIOPED II. *Am J Med.* 2007;120:871–879.

Stein PD, Fowler SF, Goodman LR, et al. Multidetector computed tomography for acute pulmonary embolism. *N Engl J Med.* 2006;354;2317–2327.

Stein PD, Woodard PK, Weg JG, et al. Diagnostic pathways in acute pulmonary embolism: recommendations of the PIOPED II investigators. *Am J Med.* 2006;119:1048–1055.

Tapson VF. Acute pulmonary embolism. *N Engl J Med.* 2008;358:1037–1052.

Wood KE. Major pulmonary embolism: review of a pathophysiologic approach to the golden hour of hemodynamically significant pulmonary embolism. *Chest.* 2002;121:877–905.

CHAPTER 32

Aortic Valve Disease

Vidya Narayan, Aly Rahimtoola, and
Shahbudin H. Rahimtoola

AORTIC STENOSIS

【 】 DEFINITIONS, ETIOLOGY, AND PATHOLOGY

Aortic stenosis (AS) is obstruction to outflow of blood flow from the left ventricle (LV) to the aorta. The obstruction may be at the valve, above the valve (supravalvular), or below the valve (membranous or subvalvular).

The most common causes of valvular AS are congenital, rheumatic, and calcific ("degenerative"). Calcific AS occurs in patients 35 years of age or older and results from calcification of a congenital or rheumatic valve or of a normal valve. Rare causes of AS include obstructive infective vegetations, homozygous type II hyperlipoproteinemia, Paget's disease of the bone, systemic lupus erythematosus, rheumatoid involvement, ochronosis, and irradiation.

Calcific AS in the older patient is the most common valve lesion requiring valve replacement. Among patients under age 70, a congenital bicuspid valve accounted for one-half of the surgical cases; degenerative changes were the cause in 18%. In contrast, over age 70, degenerative changes accounted for almost one-half of the surgical cases and a congenital bicuspid valve for approximately 25% of the cases.

Supravalvular and membranous subvalvular AS are usually congenital. Congenital bicuspid valves can produce severe obstruction to LV outflow after the first few years of life. The valvular abnormality produces turbulent flow, traumatizes the leaflets, and eventually leads to fibrosis, rigidity, and calcification. In a congenitally abnormal tricuspid aortic valve, the cusps are of unequal size and have some degree of commissural fusion; the third cusp may be diminutive. Eventually, the abnormal structure leads to changes similar to those seen in a bicuspid valve, and significant LV outflow obstruction often results. In calcific AS, early changes show chronic inflammatory cell infiltrate (macrophages and T lymphocytes), lipid within the lesion and in adjacent fibrosa, and thickening of fibrosa with collagen and elastin. These patients also have a higher incidence of risk factors for coronary atherosclerosis.

Rheumatic AS results from adhesions and fusion of the commissures and cusps. The leaflets and the valve ring become vascularized, which leads to retraction, stiffening, and calcification.

Rheumatoid AS is extremely rare and results from nodular thickening of the valve leaflets and the proximal part of the aorta. In severe forms of hypercholesterolemia, lipid deposits may occur in the aortic valve, occasionally producing AS.

The LV is concentrically hypertrophied. The hypertrophied cardiac muscle cells are increased in size. There is an increase of connective tissue and a variable amount of fibrous tissue in the interstitium. Myocardial ultrastructural changes may account for the LV systolic dysfunction that occurs late in the disease.

【 】 PATHOPHYSIOLOGY

The aortic valve must be reduced to one-fourth of its natural size before significant changes occur in the circulation. The normal aortic valve is 3.0 to 4.0 cm²; an area exceeding 0.7 to 1.0 cm² is not usually considered to indicate severe AS. In average-sized individuals, a valve area of greater than 1.0 cm², and in smaller people greater than 0.75 cm², may be adequate.

Based on natural history and hemodynamic studies, AS is graded as mild when the aortic valve area (AVA) is > 1.5 cm² (> 0.9 cm²/m²), moderate when the AVA is > 1.0 to 1.5 cm² (> 0.6 to 0.9 cm²/m²), and severe when the AVA is ≤ 1.0 cm² (≤ 0.6 cm²/m²). The AVA must be reduced by about 50% of normal before a measurable gradient can be demonstrated in humans.

The outflow obstruction imposes a pressure overload on the LV, which compensates by an increase in wall thickness and mass. The concentric left ventricular hypertrophy (LVH) normalizes systolic wall stress and preserves normal systolic function; however, diastolic function may be abnormal. When LVH alone is inadequate to overcome outflow obstruction, the LV uses preload reserve to maintain systolic function. When the preload reserve is no longer adequate, a decrease in systolic function and LV dilatation occurs.

Left atrial contraction is of considerable benefit to these patients. Loss of effective atrial contraction—either due to atrial fibrillation or because of an inappropriately timed atrial contraction—results in elevation of mean left atrial pressure, reduction of cardiac output, or both. This may precipitate clinical heart failure with pulmonary congestion.

In most patients with AS, cardiac output is in the normal range and initially increases normally with exercise. Later, as the severity of AS increases progressively, the cardiac output remains within the normal range at rest. On exercise, however, it either no longer increases in proportion to the amount of exercise undertaken or does not increase at all.

In severe AS, myocardial oxygen needs are increased because of an increased muscle mass, elevations in LV pressures, and prolongation of the systolic ejection time. Patients may have classic angina pectoris even in the absence of coronary artery disease. Associated obstructive CAD further increases the imbalance between myocardial oxygen needs and supply and also of the coronary flow reserve.

【 】 CLINICAL FINDINGS

History

Patients with congenital valvular stenosis may give a history of a murmur since childhood or infancy; those with rheumatic stenosis may have a history of rheumatic fever. Most patients with valvular AS, including some with severe valvular AS, are asymptomatic.

The classic triad of symptoms of AS is *angina pectoris, syncope, and heart failure*. Sudden cardiac death is said to occur in 5% of patients with AS. It occurs only in those with severe AS, however, most of whom have had prior cardiac symptoms.

Angina pectoris may be the initial clinical manifestation. Syncope is the result of reduced cerebral perfusion. Syncope occurring on effort is caused by systemic vasodilatation in the presence of a fixed or inadequate cardiac output, an arrhythmia, or both. Syncope at rest is usually due to a transient tachyarrhythmia from which the patient recovers spontaneously. Other possible causes of syncope include transient atrial fibrillation or transient AV block.

Dyspnea on exertion, orthopnea, paroxysmal nocturnal dyspnea, and pulmonary edema result from varying degrees of pulmonary venous hypertension.

There is an increased incidence of gastrointestinal arteriovenous malformations (often associated with abnormalities of von Willebrand anticoagulation factor). As a result, these patients are susceptible to gastrointestinal hemorrhage and anemia. Calcific systemic embolism may occur.

Physical Findings

There is a spectrum of physical findings in patients with AS, depending on the severity of the stenosis, stroke volume, LV function, and the rigidity and calcification of the valve. The arterial pulse rises slowly, taking longer than normal to reach peak pressure; the peak is reduced (parvus et tardus) (Chapter 1); and the pulse pressure may be narrowed. A systolic thrill may be felt in the carotid arteries. The cardiac impulse is heaving and sustained in character, and there may be a palpable fourth heart sound (S_4). An aortic systolic thrill is often present at the base of the heart. In 80% to 90% of adult patients with severe AS, there is an S_4 gallop sound, a midsystolic ejection murmur that peaks late in systole, and a single second heart sound (S_2) because A_2 and P_2 are superimposed or A_2 is absent or soft. There is often a faint early diastolic murmur of minimal aortic regurgitation. The S_2 may be paradoxically split due to late A_2. In many patients, the midsystolic ejection murmur is atypical and may be heard only at the apex of the heart (Gallaverdin's sign).

In many patients 60 years of age or older, the clinical features may differ from those typical of younger patients. Systemic hypertension is common, being present in over 20% of the patients, half of whom have moderate or severe systolic and diastolic hypertension. Twenty percent first present in congestive heart failure. The male to female ratio is 2:1. Because of thickening of the arterial wall and its associated lack of distensibility, the arterial pulse rises normally or even rapidly, and the pulse pressure is wide.

Chext X-Ray

The characteristic finding is a normal-sized heart. Some patients have poststenotic dilation of the ascending aorta. Calcium in the aortic valve can be seen on the lateral film, but is most easily recognized on two-dimensional echocardiography. Calcium in the aortic valve is the hallmark of AS in adults 40 to 45 years of age. The presence of calcium, however, does not necessarily mean that the valve is stenotic or that the AS is severe. In patients with heart failure, the cardiac size is increased because of dilatation of the LV and left atrium; the lung fields show pulmonary edema and pulmonary venous congestion, and the right ventricle and atrium may be dilated.

Electrocardiogram

The electrocardiogram (ECG) in severe AS shows LV hypertrophy with or without secondary ST-T-wave changes. Conduction abnormalities are common and range from bundle-branch block to first-degree block; higher grades of block occur but are uncommon. The patients are usually in sinus rhythm. Atrial fibrillation indicates the presence of associated mitral valve disease, coronary artery disease (CAD), or heart failure.

【 】 LABORATORY INVESTIGATIONS

Echocardiography/Doppler Ultrasound

Echocardiography/Doppler ultrasound is an extremely important and useful noninvasive test. The aortic valve leaflets normally are barely visible in systole, and the normal range of aortic valve opening is 1.6 to 2.6 cm. In the presence of a bicuspid aortic valve, eccentric valve leaflets may be seen. The aortic valve leaflets may appear to be thickened as a result of calcification and/or fibrosis; however, the older patient without valve stenosis may also have thickened cusps. The aortic valve may have a reduced opening, but this also occurs in other conditions in which the cardiac output is low. The LV hypertrophy often results in thickening of both the interventricular septum and the posterior LV wall. The cavity size is normal. When LV systolic function is impaired, the LV and left atrium are dilated, and the percentage of dimensional shortening is reduced. When properly applied, Doppler echocardiography is extremely useful for estimating the valve gradient and AVA noninvasively. The calculated mean gradient from continuous-waveform Doppler interrogation correlates reasonably closely with that obtained at cardiac catheterization. The AVA can be calculated from the velocity of the jet across the aortic valve and from the velocity and character of the LV outflow tract. Transesophageal echocardiography/Doppler ultrasound is very useful in defining aortic valve abnormality and in assessing its severity when an adequate examination cannot be obtained with the transthoracic technique.

Cardiac Catheterization/Angiography

Cardiac catheterization remains the *standard technique* for assessing the severity of AS "accurately." This is done by measuring simultaneous LV and ascending aortic pressures and the cardiac output by either the Fick principle or the indicator dilution technique. The AVA can be calculated. The state of LV systolic pump function can be quantitated by measuring LV end-diastolic and end-systolic volumes and ejection fraction. *It must be recognized that ejection fraction may underestimate myocardial function in the presence of the increased afterload of severe AS.*

The presence of CAD and its site and severity can be estimated only by selective coronary angiography, which should be performed in all patients 35 years of age or older who are being considered for valve surgery and in those < 35 years if they have LV systolic dysfunction, symptoms or signs suggesting CAD, or two or more risk factors for premature CAD (excluding gender).

Other Laboratory Studies

Gated blood pool radionuclide scans provide information on ventricular function similar to that provided by two-dimensional echocardiography and LV cineangiography.

Exercise testing should be undertaken in patients with severe AS only if there is a specific reason for such studies and there is no associated CAD. Ambulatory ECG recordings may be needed in an occasional patient suspected of having an arrhythmia or painless ischemia.

【　】 NATURAL HISTORY AND PROGNOSIS

Valvular AS is frequently a progressive disease, with the severity increasing over time. The factors that control this progression are unknown. In one study, patients with "mild" stenosis (catheterization-proven AVA > 1.5 cm^2), the rate of progression to severe stenosis was 8% in 10 years and 22% in 20 years. The duration of the asymptomatic period after the development of severe AS is also unknown; some recent data suggest that it may be less than 2 years. In patients aged 63 ± 16 years, the actuarial probability of death or aortic valve surgery was 7 ± 5% at 1 year, 38 ± 8% at 3 years, and 74 ± 10% at 5 years.

Severe disease in adults is lethal, particularly if the patient is symptomatic, with a prognosis that is worse than that for many forms of neoplastic disease. The 3-year mortality is approximately 36% to 52%, the 5-year mortality is about 52% to 80%, and the 10-year mortality is 80% to 90%; the average life expectancy is 2 to 3 years. Almost all patients with heart failure are dead in 1 to 2 years.

【　】 MEDICAL THERAPY

All patients with AS need antibiotic prophylaxis against infective endocarditis (see Chapter 38). Those in whom the valve lesion is of rheumatic origin need additional prophylaxis against recurrence of rheumatic fever. Patients with mild or moderate stenosis rarely have symptoms or complications. In mild stenosis, the patient should be encouraged to lead a normal life. Those with moderate AS should avoid moderate to severe physical exertion and competitive sports. If atrial fibrillation should occur, it should be reverted rapidly to sinus rhythm.

【 】 SURGICAL THERAPY

Operation should be advised for the symptomatic patient who has severe AS. In young patients, if the valve is pliable and mobile, simple commissurotomy or valve repair may be feasible; the operative mortality is < 1%. Such a procedure will relieve outflow obstruction to a major degree. In these patients, catheter balloon valvuloplasty is the procedure of choice in experienced and skilled centers. Both of these are *palliative procedures* that postpone valve replacement. Catheter balloon valvuloplasty is a *temporary palliative procedure* for high-risk elderly patients with advanced symptoms and for emergency situations.

The natural history of symptomatic patients with severe AS is dismal—a 10-year mortality of 80% to 90%—but the outcome after surgery is good, particularly in patients without any comorbid conditions. Given the unknown natural history of the asymptomatic patient with severe AS, which may not be benign, it is reasonable to recommend surgery even to the asymptomatic patient. Some recommend valve replacement in all asymptomatic patients with severe AS, while others would recommend it in those with an AVA ≤ 0.7 cm^2 and in selected patients with an AVA of 0.76 to 1.0 cm^2.

The operative mortality of valve replacement is about 5% or less. In patients without associated CAD, heart failure, or other comorbid factors, it may be 1% to 2% in centers with experienced and skilled staff. Patients with associated CAD should have coronary bypass surgery at the same time as valve surgery because it results in a lower operative and late mortality. Patients with severe AS who need coronary bypass surgery should have aortic valve replacement at the same time. In severe AS, valve replacement results in an improvement in survival, even in those with normal preoperative LV function. Aortic valve replacement is not recommended for asymptomatic patients with severe AS to prevent sudden death (Table 32-1).

For choice(s) of prosthetic valve, see Chapter 36.

AORTIC REGURGITATION

【 】 DEFINITION, ETIOLOGY, AND PATHOLOGY

Aortic regurgitation (AR) is a flow of blood in diastole from the aorta into the LV due to incompetence of the aortic valve. The two most common causes of acute AR are infective endocarditis and prosthetic valve dysfunction. Other common causes include dissection of the aorta, systemic hypertension, and trauma.

In North America, the most common cause of chronic, isolated severe AR is aortic root/annular dilatation that is presumably the result of medial disease. Common causes include a congenital bicuspid valve, previous infective endocarditis, and rheumatic disease. Chronic AR also occurs in association with a variety of other diseases, particularly those that result in dilatation of the aortic root. Between 40% and 60% of the surgically removed valves from patients with isolated severe AR are classified as idiopathic; half show histologic criteria of myxomatous degeneration.

In AR, volume overload of the LV is the basic hemodynamic abnormality. The extent of overload depends on the volume of the regurgitant blood flow, which is determined by the area of the regurgitant orifice, the diastolic pressure gradient between the aorta and the LV, and the duration of diastole.

【 】 PATHOPHYSIOLOGY

The LV diastolic pressure–volume relationship plays a very important role in the pathophysiology of acute AR. The ability of the LV to dilate acutely is limited; as a result, the volume overload of acute AR produces a rapid increase in LV diastolic pressure. If the LV is already stiff or less compliant than normal due to an associated lesion, the LV

TABLE 32-1

Recommendations For Aortic Valve Replacement In Aortic Stenosis[a]

Indication	Class	LOE[b]
1. Symptomatic patients with severe AS	I	B
2. Patients with severe AS undergoing coronary artery bypass surgery	I	B
3. Patients with severe AS undergoing surgery on the aorta or other heart valves	I	B
4. Severe AS and left ventricular systolic dysfunction	I	C
5. Patients with moderate AS undergoing coronary artery bypass surgery or surgery on the aorta or other heart valves	IIa	B
6. Asymptomatic patients with severe AS and abnormal response to exercise (e.g., development of symptoms or hypotension)	IIb	C
7. Adults with severe asymptomatic AS if there is a high likelihood of rapid progression (age, calcification, and CAD) or if surgery might be delayed at the time of symptom onset	IIb	C
8. Patients undergoing CABG who have mild AS when there is evidence, such as moderate-severe valve calcification, that progression may be rapid	IIb	C
9. Asymptomatic patients with extremely severe AS (AVR <0.6 cm², mean gradient >60 mm Hg, and jet velocity >5.0 m/s) when the patient's expected operative mortality is 1.0% or less	IIa	C
10. Prevention of sudden death in asymptomatic patients with none of the findings listed under indication 5	III	C

[a]See also Chapter 39.
[b]LOE, level of evidence.

Reproduced with permission from ACC/AHA 2006 guidelines for the management of patients with valvular heart disease a report of the American College of Cardiology/American Heart Association Task Force on Practice Guidelines (Writing Committee to revise the 1998 guidelines for the management of patients with valvular heart Disease) developed in collaboration with the Society of Cardiovascular Anesthesiologists Endorsed by the Society for Cardiovascular Angiography and Interventions and the Society of Thoracic Surgeons. *J Am Coll Cardiol.* 2006;48(3):e1–e148. Available at: www.acc.org, e24.

diastolic pressure will rise more precipitously as a result of the volume overload of acute AR than if the LV were normal. On the other hand, if the LV is somewhat dilated from a previous lesion—for example, mild AR—the LV pressure will initially rise more gradually with acute AR but may subsequently rise to the same high levels as are seen with a normal or stiff LV. Acute AR that is mild produces little or no hemodynamic abnormality—for example, when associated with systemic hypertension. Increasing severity of AR produces greater degrees of hemodynamic abnormalities, and severe AR often produces the clinical picture of "heart failure."

Acute AR that is severe results in a large volume of regurgitant blood; the increased LV diastolic pressure results in increases in mean left atrial and pulmonary venous pressures and produces varying degrees of pulmonary edema. Two compensatory mechanisms are utilized: an increase in myocardial contractility and tachycardia to maintain an adequate forward cardiac output.

In chronic AR, the AR becomes severe over a period of time; therefore, the LV diastolic pressure–volume relationships are different from those seen in acute AR. If the AR is mild to moderate, the LV end-diastolic volume is increased moderately, the LV diastolic pressure–volume curve is moved to the right of normal, and the LV diastolic pressure is usually normal. In severe AR, the LV diastolic pressure–volume curves are moved further to the right. If the LV systolic pump function is normal, the LV end-diastolic volume can be quite large without significant elevation of LV end-diastolic pressure. If the LV diastolic volume increases further, however, the LV diastolic pressures will be increased. If LV systolic pump dysfunction supervenes, the LV diastolic pressure-volume curve relationships are moved even further to the right, with quite marked LV dilatation and increases in LV diastolic pressure.

In severe chronic AR, the increase in LV end-diastolic volume is a result of the regurgitant volume (and is proportional to the amount of AR) and LV systolic dysfunction. The subsequent large LV stroke volume produces LV systolic hypertension. Both of these increase LV wall stress (afterload), which can result in an impairment of LV function. The heart responds by becoming hypertrophied, and function remains normal. In time, the hemodynamic burden of the volume overload will result in depressed myocardial contractility and decreased LV compliance. Total coronary blood flow is increased, but coronary flow reserve is reduced.

【 】 CLINICAL FEATURES

History

Patients with mild to moderate AR usually do not have symptoms that can be attributed to the heart. Even patients with severe AR may be asymptomatic for many years. The earliest symptom may be an awareness of the increased force of contraction of the dilated heart, which undergoes a large volume change in systole; patients complain of pounding of the heart or palpitations. The main symptoms of severe AR result from elevated pulmonary venous pressures and include dyspnea on exertion, orthopnea, and paroxysmal nocturnal dyspnea. Heart failure and angina occur in 20% of such patients and may be present even in the absence of CAD.

Physical Findings

The arterial pulse is very characteristic and consists of an abrupt distention with a rapid rise and a quick collapse (Corrigan's pulse). The arterial pulse may be bisferiens, a double impulse during systole. The systolic arterial pressure is increased, the diastolic pressure is reduced, and Korotkoff's sounds persist down to 0 mm Hg. The absence of a wide pulse pressure (greater than 50% of peak systolic pressure) or diastolic pressure greater than 70 mm Hg in a patient without heart failure makes severe, chronic aortic regurgitation unlikely. The LV dilatation with severe AR displaces the apical impulse inferiorly and laterally. The AR murmur is a high-pitched, blowing, early diastolic murmur along the left sternal border. A third heart sound (S_3 gallop) and low-pitched diastolic and/or presystolic murmurs (Austin–Flint) may be heard at the apex. The wide pulse pressure, significant LV dilatation, and Austin–Flint murmur are not features of *acute* AR. They occur with *chronic* AR.

Chext X-Ray

The LV is increased in size, and this can be appreciated by an increase in the cardiothoracic ratio. The ascending aorta may be dilated, and there may be calcium in the aortic valve. In the later stages, with increased filling pressures, there might be evidence of an enlarged left atrium and an increased left atrial and pulmonary venous pressure, which are manifest in the pulmonary vascular shadows by a redistribution of blood flow, pulmonary congestion, and pulmonary edema. In the presence of heart failure, enlargement of the right atrium and superior vena cava may be appreciated. Calcification that is limited to the ascending aorta is strongly suggestive of luetic aortitis.

Electrocardiogram

The ECG shows LV hypertrophy with or without associated ST-T-wave changes. In some patients, ECG evidence of LV hypertrophy is absent in spite of severe AR. Conduction abnormalities, such as atrioventricular block or left or right bundle branch block with or without axis deviation, may be present. The PR interval may be prolonged, particularly in patients with ankylosing spondylitis. The presence of atrial fibrillation should make one suspect the presence of associated mitral valve disease or heart failure.

Echocardiography/Doppler

The echocardiogram can provide information about the etiology of AR as well as LV size and function and the severity of AR. Diastolic fluttering of the anterior leaflet of the mitral valve is often present on M-mode and 2-D echocardiography. Echocardiography is of particular value for excluding the presence of associated mitral stenosis in patients with an Austin Flint diastolic murmur. Two-dimensional echocardiography is far superior to the M-mode technique for assessing LV volumes and systolic function. A dilated ascending aorta can be detected on echocardiography, as can an enlarged left atrium. Aortic valve vegetations suggest infective endocarditis. Some other conditions can easily be detected by echocardiography—for example, prolapse of the aortic leaflet into the left ventricle in diastole. Doppler ultrasound is useful for diagnosing and assessing the severity of AR. There is a significant incidence of *false-positive* mild regurgitation. There is also an overlap between the various grades of severity of AR as assessed by Doppler as compared with angiography. Transesophageal echocardiography is a useful technique when transthoracic echocardiography is unsatisfactory; it can be used in certain instances for identifying the anatomy of the valve leaflets and the aortic root/annulus, and it is essential for evaluating whether the valve is suitable for repair. It is also very useful for assessing disease of other valves.

Cardiac Catheterization/Angiography

Cardiac catheterization permits the measurement of intracardiac and intravascular pressures and cardiac output, both at rest and during exercise. In addition, other valvular disease can be excluded. LV angiography demonstrates enlarged LV and allows the calculation of LV volumes and LV ejection fraction. Angiography performed with injection of contrast medium in the ascending aorta demonstrates AR and allows a semiquantitative assessment of the degree of AR. In addition, the angiogram demonstrates the dimensions of the aortic root and the state of the ascending aorta. The indications for selective coronary angiography are the same as for aortic stenosis.

Other Laboratory Tests

Gated blood pool radionuclide scans also allow the measurement of LV volumes and ejection fraction. In addition, with this technique, it is possible to quantify the amount of AR. These scans, however, assess the regurgitation present at both the aortic and mitral valves. This technique also allows measurement of LV ejection fraction on exercise and on serial studies.

A treadmill exercise test provides an objective assessment of the degree of functional impairment and documentation of arrhythmias related to exertion. In some patients, however, the exercise test may remain normal despite deterioration of LV function.

Ambulatory ECG recording may be needed in an occasional patient suspected of having an arrhythmia.

MRI can demonstrate AR but is rarely needed clinically.

【 】 NATURAL HISTORY AND PROGNOSIS

Patients with mild AR that does not progress should have a normal life expectancy. Their major risk is the development of infective endocarditis and further valve destruction. Patients with moderate AR, if their disease did not progress, would be expected to have a life expectancy that is reasonably close to the normal range. The disease does progress, however, and mortality at the end of 10 years appears to be about 15%.

Patients with severe AR are known to have a long asymptomatic period before the condition is discovered. In asymptomatic patients with normal LV function at rest, symptoms and/or LV dysfunction (and/or sudden death) develop at the rate of about 3% to 6% per year. The predictor of development of symptoms is LV systolic dysfunction and/or an increased LV size (LV dimension at end-diastole ≥ 70 mm and at end-systole ≥ 50 mm). Sudden death in asymptomatic patients appears to occur only in those with a massively dilated left ventricle (LV end-diastolic dimension ≥ 80 mm).

【 】 MEDICAL THERAPY

All patients with AR need antibiotic prophylaxis to prevent infective endocarditis. Patients with AR of a rheumatic origin need antibiotic prophylaxis to prevent recurrences of rheumatic carditis. Patients with syphilitic AR need a course of antibiotics to treat syphilis.

Patients with mild AR need no specific therapy. They do not need to restrict their activities and can lead a normal life. Patients with moderate AR also usually need no specific therapy. These patients, however, should avoid heavy physical exertion, competitive sports, and isometric exercise. Asymptomatic patients with severe AR and normal LV systolic function should be treated with a vasodilator (a calcium antagonist such as long-acting nifedipine) unless there is a contraindication to its use. This remains controversial.

【 】 SURGICAL THERAPY

Patients with severe chronic AR need valve surgery. The correct timing of surgical therapy is now better defined, but it is not fully clarified. Valve replacement should be performed before irreversible LV dysfunction occurs (Table 32-2).

Decisions about surgery in AR should be based on the clinical functional class and on the LV ejection fraction. Patients with chronic severe AR who are *symptomatic* (NYHA classes II to IV) need valve replacement. The benefit from valve replacement has been demonstrated even when the LV ejection fraction is 25% or less. Recent data indicate that patients with severe AR, LV end-diastolic dimension on echocardiography ≥ 80 mm, and mild to moderate reduction of LV ejection fraction can obtain benefit from valve replacement. Postoperatively, they are symptomatically improved, LV ejection fraction increases, and LV size is reduced; the 5- and 10-year survival rates are 87% and 71%, respectively.

Patients who are *asymptomatic* and have a reduced ejection fraction at rest should be offered aortic valve replacement. If the ejection fraction is normal at rest, one should consider valve replacement in NYHA functional class I patients if they have severe obstructive CAD and/or if they need surgery for other valve disease. Patients with associated significant CAD should have coronary bypass surgery performed at the time of valvular surgery.

Aortic valve replacement, with or without associated coronary bypass surgery for obstructive CAD, can be performed at many surgical centers with an operative mortality of 5% or less (see Chapter 36). In patients without associated CAD or reduced LV systolic function, the operative mortality may be in the range of 1% to 2%. If aortic valve replacement is successful and uncomplicated, LV volume and hypertrophy regress but do not return to normal. Impaired LV systolic pump function improves postoperatively in

TABLE 32-2

Recommendations For Aortic Valve Replacement In Chronic Severe Aortic Regurgitation[a]

Indication	Class	LOE[b]
1. Symptomatic patients with severe AR irrespective of LV systolic function	I	B
2. Asymptomatic patients with chronic severe AR and LV systolic dysfunction (ejection fraction 0.50 or less) at rest	I	B
3. Patients with chronic severe AR while undergoing CABG or surgery on the aorta or other heart valves	I	C
4. Asymptomatic patients with severe AR with normal LV systolic function (ejection fraction > 0.50) but with severe LV dilatation (end diastolic dimension > 75 mm or end systolic dimension > 55 mm)	IIa	B
5. Patients with moderate AR while undergoing surgery on the ascending aorta	IIb	C
6. Patients with moderate AR while undergoing CABG	IIb	C
7. Asymptomatic patients with severe AR and normal LV systolic function at rest (ejection fraction > 0.50) when the degree of LV dilatation exceeds an end diastolic dimension of 70 mm or end systolic dimension of 50 mm, when there is evidence of progressive LV dilatation, declining exercise tolerance, or abnormal hemodynamic responses to exercise	IIb	C
8. Asymptomatic patients with mild, moderate, severe AR, and normal LV systolic function at rest (ejection fraction > 0.50) when the degree of dilatation is not moderate or severe (end-diastolic dimension < 70 mm, end systolic dimension < 50 mm)	III	B

[a]Lower threshold values should be considered for patients of small stature of either gender. Clinical judgment is required.
[b]LOE, level of evidence.

Reproduced with permission from ACC/AHA 2006 guidelines for the management of patients with valvular heart disease a report of the American College of Cardiology/American Heart Association Task Force on Practice Guidelines (Writing Committee to revise the 1998 guidelines for the management of patients with valvular heart disease) developed in collaboration with the Society of Cardiovascular Anesthesiologists Endorsed by the Society for Cardiovascular Angiography and Interventions and the Society of Thoracic Surgeons. J Am Coll Cardiol. 2006;48(3):e1–e148. Available at: www.acc.org, e24.

50% or more of patients. The 5-year survival of patients with LV ejection fraction $\geq$ 45% is 87%, versus 54% in patients with an ejection fraction < 45%. The recommendations of the American College of Cardiology/American Heart Association (ACC/AHA) Practice Guidelines are shown in Table 32-2. Results of valve repair are encouraging in selected subgroups. It is possible that selected patients may eventually need to have valve repair. New techniques of aortic valve repair are being developed and evaluated.

BICUSPID AORTIC VALVE IN ADULTS

Although a bicuspid aortic valve (BAV) is a congenital lesion, its clinical importance is largely in adults. The incidence of BAV varies from 0.5% to 1.39%, with a male to female ratio of 3:1. The incidence of familial recurrence of BAV is approximately 9%. Inheritance is most likely with an autosomal-dominant inheritance pattern with reduced penetrance. Consequently, screening with echocardiography is recommended for first-degree relatives of patients with BAV.

【 】 PATHOLOGY

Marfan syndrome is known to be a genetic disorder caused by a mutation in the fibrillin gene. Studies have demonstrated histologic and immunohistochemical similarities in the thoracic aorta of patients with BAV and Marfan syndrome. The dimensions of the aortic root are larger in children with BAV than in children with tricuspid AV; and also larger than in young adults. There is a progression of aortic dilation in adults with BAV. The anatomy of the BAV usually includes one large cusp (caused by fusion of two cusps) and a central raphe that is identifiable in most patients with BAV. The raphe does not contain valve tissue. The calcification process that occurs in BAV is similar in its cellular and molecular mechanisms to the processes involved in calcific AS of tricuspid AV, but is accelerated.

【 】 COMPLICATIONS AND ASSOCIATED CONGENITAL CARDIOVASCULAR LESIONS

Complications associated with BAV include infective endocarditis, aortic stenosis, aortic regurgitation, aneurysm of the aortic root or the ascending thoracic aorta, and ascending aortic dissection. Infective endocarditis is a frequent problem partly because patients with BAV are often unaware of their disease and, thus, have not been advised about antibiotic prophylaxis for prevention of infective endocarditis. Congenital cardiovascular lesions associated with BAV include patent ductus arteriosus (PDA), coarctation of the aorta, coronary anatomic variants, and abnormalities involving the mitral and aortic valves.

【 】 PHYSICAL EXAMINATION

A functionally normal BAV may have an ejection sound (systolic ejection click) that may be followed by an early peaking systolic flow murmur. The ejection sound diminishes as the valve cusps become more immobile and stenotic and in the presence of moderate or severe AR. The differential diagnosis of an ejection sound includes a small perimembranous ventricular septal defect with a septal aneurysm, mitral/tricuspid valve prolapse, and mild valvar pulmonary stenosis.

【 】 MANAGEMENT

The serious nature and expected outcomes of patients with BAV should be discussed with the patient and appropriate family members. Echocardiography should be recommended, and its importance emphasized, for first-degree relatives of the patients to detect BAV and/or ascending aorta dilatation. Antibiotic prophylaxis for prevention for infective endocarditis is very important. Considering the similarity of pathologic findings in the ascending aorta in BAV and Marfan's syndrome, it is reasonable to recommend long-term beta-blocker therapy, if there are no contraindications to this use, to patients with a dilated aorta that is not yet in the range of needing surgery. The ACC/AHA Guidelines for management of patients with BAV are given in Table 32-3.

TABLE 32-3

Guidelines For Patients With Bicuspid Aortic Valve (BAV)

Indication	Class	LOE[a]
1. Patients with known BAV should undergo an initial transthoracic echocardiogram to assess diameter of the aortic root and ascending aorta	I	B
2. Cardiac magnetic resonance or cardiac computed tomography is indicated in patients with BAV when morphology of the aortic root or ascending aorta cannot be assessed accurately by echocardiography	I	C
3. Patients with BAV and dilatation of the aortic root or ascending aorta (diameter > 4 cm) should undergo serial evaluation of aortic root/ascending aorta size and morphology by echocardiography, cardiac magnetic resonance, or CT on a yearly basis	I	C
4. Surgery to repair the aortic root or replace the ascending aorta is indicated in patients with BAV if the diameter of the aortic root or ascending aorta is greater than 5.0 cm or if the rate of increase in diameter is 0.5 cm/y or greater	I	C
5. Surgery in patients with bicuspid valves undergoing AVR because of severe AS or AR, repair of the aortic root, or replacement of the ascending aorta is indicated if the diameter of the aortic root or ascending aorta is greater than 4.5 cm	I	C
6. It is reasonable to give beta-adrenergic blocking agents to patients with BAV and dilated aortic roots (diameter > 4.0 cm) who are not candidates for surgical correction and who do not have moderate to severe AR	IIa	C
7. Cardiac magnetic resonance or cardiac computed tomography is indicated in patients with bicuspid aortic valves when aortic root dilatation is detected by echocardiography to further quantify severity of dilatation and involvement of ascending aorta	IIa	B

[a]LOE, level of evidence.

Reproduced with permission from ACC/AHA 2006 guidelines for the management of patients with valvular heart disease a report of the American College of Cardiology/American Heart Association Task Force on Practice Guidelines (Writing Committee to revise the 1998 guidelines for the management of patients with valvular heart disease) developed in collaboration with the Society of Cardiovascular Anesthesiologists Endorsed by the Society for Cardiovascular Angiography and Interventions and the Society of Thoracic Surgeons. *J Am Coll Cardiol.* 2006;48(3):e1–e148. Available at: www.acc.org, e24.

SUGGESTED READING

Bonow RO, Carabello B, Chatterjee K, et al. ACC/AHA Guidelines on the Management of Patients with Valvular Heart Disease: A Report of the ACC/AHA Task Force on Practice Guidelines 2006. Available at: www.acc.org, e24.

Braverman AC, Guven H, Beardslee MA, et al. The bicuspid aortic valve. *Curr Probl Cardiol* 2005; 30:461–522.

Currie PJ, Seward JB, Reeder GS, et al. Continuous-wave Doppler echocardiographic assessment of severity of calcific aortic stenosis: a simultaneous Doppler-catheter correlative study in 100 adult patients. *Circulation.* 1985;71:1162–1169.

Horstkotte D, Loogen F. The natural history of aortic valve stenosis. *Eur Heart J.* 1988;9(suppl E):57–64.

Murphy ES, Lawson RM, Starr A, et al. Severe aortic stenosis in the elderly: state of left ventricular function and result of valve replacement on ten-year survival. *Circulation.* 1981;64(suppl II):184–188.

Otto CM, Knusisto J, Reichenbach D, et al. Characterization of the early lesion of "degenerative" valvular aortic stenosis: historical and immunohistochemical studies. *Circulation.*1994;90:844–853.

Rahimtoola SH. Aortic valve disease. In: Fuster V, O'Rourke RA, Walsh R, et al., eds. *Hurst's The Heart.* 12th ed. New York, NY: McGraw-Hill; 2008:1697–1730.

Rahimtoola SH. Recognition and management of acute aortic regurgitation. *Heart Dis Stroke.* 1993;2:217–221.

Ross J Jr, Braunwald E. Aortic stenosis. *Circulation.*1968;36(suppl IV):61–67.

CHAPTER (33)

Mitral Valve Stenosis

Amardeep K. Singh and Shahbudin H. Rahimtoola

DEFINITION, ETIOLOGY, AND PATHOLOGY

Mitral stenosis (MS), an obstruction to blood flow between the left atrium (LA) and the left ventricle (LV), is caused by abnormal mitral valve function. In virtually all adult patients, the cause of MS is previous rheumatic carditis. About 60% of patients with rheumatic mitral valve disease do not give a history of rheumatic fever or chorea, and about 50% of patients with acute rheumatic carditis do not develop clinical valvular heart disease. Isolated MS occurs in approximately 40% of all patients with rheumatic heart disease. Other infrequent causes of obstruction to LV inflow can be congenital or due to active infective endocarditis, neoplasm, massive annular calcification, systemic lupus erythematosus, carcinoid, methysergide therapy, Hunter-Hurler syndromes, Fabry's disease, Whipple's disease, rheumatoid arthritis, left atrial myxoma, massive left atrial ball thrombus, and cor triatriatum.

Acute rheumatic carditis is a pancarditis involving the pericardium, myocardium, and endocardium. In temperate climates and developed countries, there is usually a long interval (10–20 years) between an episode of rheumatic carditis and the clinical presentation of symptomatic MS. In tropical and subtropical climates and in less developed countries, the latent period is often shorter, and MS may occur during childhood or adolescence.

PATHOPHYSIOLOGY

The histopathologic hallmark of rheumatic carditis is an *Aschoff's* nodule. Rheumatic valvulitis results in scarring and fusion. The combination of commissural fusion, valve leaflet contracture, and fusion of the chordae tendineae results in a narrow, funnel-shaped orifice.

The pathophysiologic features of MS all result from obstruction of the flow of blood between the LA and the LV. With reduction in valve area, energy is lost to friction during the transport of blood from the LA to the LV. Accordingly, a pressure gradient is present across the stenotic valve.

The pressure gradient between the LA and the LV increases markedly with increased heart rate or cardiac output (CO); this is responsible for LA hypertension. The LA gradually enlarges and hypertrophies. Pulmonary venous pressure rises with the increase in LA pressure and is passively associated with an increase in pulmonary arterial (PA) pressure. In up to 20% of patients, the pulmonary vascular resistance is also elevated, which further increases PA pressure. PA hypertension results in right ventricular (RV) hypertrophy and RV enlargement. The changes in RV function eventually result in right atrial (RA) hypertension and enlargement and systemic venous congestion; frequently, tricuspid regurgitation also occurs.

Pulmonary venous hypertension alters the distribution of blood flow in the lung, with a relative increase in flow to the upper lobes and therefore in physiologic dead space. Pulmonary compliance generally decreases with increasing pulmonary capillary pressure, increasing the work of breathing, particularly during exercise. Chronic changes in the pulmonary capillaries and pulmonary arteries include fibrosis and thickening. These changes protect the lungs from the transudation of fluid into the alveoli (alveolar pulmonary edema) yet further add to the abnormalities of ventilation and perfusion.

Long-standing MS with severe PA hypertension and resultant RV dysfunction may be accompanied by chronic systemic venous hypertension. Tricuspid regurgitation is frequently present, even in the absence of intrinsic disease of this valve (see Chapter 35).

CLINICAL MANIFESTATIONS

【 】 HISTORY

An asymptomatic interval is usually present between the initiating event of acute rheumatic fever and the presentation of symptomatic MS. Initially, there is little or no gradient at rest, but with increased cardiac output, LA pressure rises and exertional dyspnea develops. As mitral valve obstruction increases, dyspnea occurs at lower work levels. The progression of disability is so subtle and protracted that patients may adapt by circumscribing their lifestyles. It becomes imperative, therefore, to document what activities the patient can perform without symptoms and at what activity level symptoms begin.

As obstruction progresses, patients note orthopnea and paroxysmal nocturnal dyspnea, apparently resulting from redistribution of blood to the thorax upon assuming the supine position. With severe MS and elevated pulmonary vascular resistance, fatigue rather than dyspnea may be the predominant symptom. Dependent edema, nausea, anorexia, and right-upper-quadrant pain reflect systemic venous congestion resulting from elevated systemic venous pressure and salt and water retention. Symptoms of RV failure (hepatomegaly, edema, and ascites) may predominate in patients with severe pulmonary hypertension.

Palpitations are a frequent complaint in patients with MS and may represent frequent premature atrial contractions or paroxysmal atrial fibrillation/flutter. Fifty percent of patients with severe symptomatic MS have chronic atrial fibrillation.

Systemic embolism, a frequent complication of MS, may result in stroke, occlusion of extremity arterial supply, occlusion of the aortic bifurcation, and visceral or myocardial infarction. Hemoptysis, hoarseness, and exertional chest pain are infrequent manifestations of MS.

Progression of symptoms in MS is generally slow but relentless. Thus, a sudden change in symptoms rarely reflects a change in valve obstruction. Rather, there is usually a noncardiac precipitating event causing tachycardia, which decreases diastolic flow period, or paroxysmal AF in which a loss of atrial transport function occurs.

【 】 PHYSICAL FINDINGS

During the latent, presymptomatic interval, incidental physical findings may be normal or may provide evidence of mild MS. Frequently, the only characteristic finding noted at rest will be a loud S_1 and a presystolic murmur. A short diastolic decrescendo rumble may be heard only with exercise. In patients with symptomatic stenosis, the findings are more obvious, and careful physical examination usually leads to the correct diagnosis (see also Chapter 1).

The jugular venous pressure may be normal or may show evidence of elevated RA pressure. A prominent A wave is a result of RV hypertension/hypertrophy or of associated tricuspid stenosis. A prominent V wave is caused by tricuspid regurgitation. Atrial fibrillation produces an irregular venous pulse with absent A waves. The chest findings may be normal or may reveal signs of pulmonary congestion with rales or pleural fluid.

On palpation, the apical impulse should feel normal or be tapping. An abnormal LV impulse suggests disease other than isolated MS. A diastolic thrill is usually appreciated only when the patient is examined in the left lateral decubitus position. When PA hypertension is present, a sustained RV lift along the left sternal border and pulmonic valve closure may be palpable.

Upon auscultation in the supine position, the only abnormality appreciated may be the accentuated S_1, which is caused by flexible valve leaflets and the wide closing excursion of the valve leaflets. *Failure to examine the patient in the left lateral decubitus position accounts for most of the missed diagnoses of symptomatic MS.* The diastolic rumble is heard best with the bell of the stethoscope applied at the apical impulse. Nevertheless, the murmur may be localized, and so the region around the apical impulse should also be auscultated. The *opening snap* (OS) occurs when the movement of the domed mitral valve into the LV is suddenly stopped. It is heard best with the diaphragm and is often most easily appreciated midway between the apex and the left sternal border. In this intermediate region, the S_1, P_2, and OS can be identified.

The OS occurs after the LV pressure falls below the LA pressure in early diastole. When LA pressure is high, as in severe MS, the snap occurs earlier in diastole. The OS may be absent in patients with stiff, fibrotic, or calcified leaflets. Thus, absence of the OS in severe MS suggests that mitral valve replacement rather than commissurotomy may be necessary.

The low-pitched diastolic rumble follows the OS and is best heard with the bell of the stethoscope. In some patients with low cardiac output or mild MS, brief exercise, such as sit-ups or walking, is adequate to increase flow and bring out the murmur. The murmur is low-pitched, rumbling, and decrescendo. In general, the more severe the MS, the longer the murmur. Presystolic accentuation of the murmur occurs in sinus rhythm and has been reported even in atrial fibrillation.

The two most important auscultatory signs of severe MS are a short A_2–OS interval and a pandiastolic rumble. The diastolic murmur may not be full length in severe MS if the stroke volume is low and there is no tachycardia.

Systolic murmurs also may be heard in association with the murmur of MS. A blowing murmur at the apex suggests associated mitral regurgitation, whereas a systolic blowing murmur heard best at the lower left sternal border that increases with inspiration usually signifies tricuspid regurgitation. The Graham Steell murmur is a high-pitched diastolic decrescendo murmur of pulmonic regurgitation caused by severe PA hypertension. In most patients with MS, such a murmur usually indicates aortic regurgitation.

Chest Roentgenogram

The posteroanterior and lateral chest films are often so typical that experienced clinicians can make the tentative diagnosis from them (see also Chapter 3). The thoracic cage is normal. The lung fields show evidence of elevated pulmonary venous pressure. Blood flow is more evenly redistributed to the upper lobes, resulting in apparent prominence of upper-lobe vascularity. Increased pulmonary venous pressure results in transudation of fluid into the interstitium. Accumulation of fluid in the interlobular septa produces linear streaks in the bases, which extend to the pleura (Kerley B lines). Interstitial fluid may also be seen as perivascular or peribronchial cuffing (Kerley A lines). With transudation of fluid into the alveolar spaces, alveolar pulmonary edema is seen. These changes represent long-standing elevated LA pressure. PA hypertension results in enlargement of the main PA and the right and left main pulmonary arteries.

The cardiac silhouette usually does not show generalized cardiomegaly, but the LA is invariably enlarged. In the posteroanterior chest film, LA enlargement is recognized by a density behind the RA border (double atrial shadow), prominence of the LA appendage on the left heart border between the main PA and LV apex, and elevation of the left main bronchus. The lateral film shows the LA bulging posteriorly. Mitral valve calcification is occasionally seen on the plain chest x-ray.

Electrocardiogram

Patients in sinus rhythm may have a widened P wave caused by interatrial conduction delay and/or prolonged LA depolarization. Classically, the P wave is broad and notched in lead II and biphasic in lead V_1; it measures 0.12 sec or more. AF is common. LV hypertrophy is not present unless there are associated lesions. RV hypertrophy may be present if PA hypertension is marked.

【 】 CLINICAL INDICATIONS OF SEVERE MITRAL STENOSIS

Some clinical features make it virtually certain that MS is severe. These include (1) moderate to severe PA hypertension, as indicated by clinical and ECG evidence of RV hypertrophy, PA hypertension, or both; and/or (2) moderate to severe elevation of LA pressure, as indicated by orthopnea, a short P_2–OS interval, a diastolic rumble that occupies the whole length of a long diastolic interval in patients with AF, and pulmonary edema on the chest x-ray. In both of these clinical circumstances, one must be certain that there is no other cause for elevated LA pressure and that LA hypertension is not caused mainly by a correctable transient elevation of LV diastolic pressure.

LABORATORY TESTS

【 】 ECHOCARDIOGRAPHY/DOPPLER ULTRASOUND

Echocardiography/Doppler ultrasound has proved to be both sensitive and specific for MS when adequate studies are done. The characteristic M-mode echocardiographic features are a decreased EF slope of the anterior mitral leaflet. Two-dimensional (2D) echocardiography will demonstrate the valve orifice and allow calculation of mitral valve area. Doppler echocardiography will provide estimates of the gradient across the valve and of pulmonary artery pressure.

Transesophageal echocardiography (TEE) is a useful technique to assess LA thrombus, the anatomy of the mitral valve and subvalvular apparatus, and the suitability of the patient for catheter balloon commissurotomy or surgical valve repair.

Echocardiography/Doppler ultrasound is a useful test in MS and should be performed in all patients. It is essential for determining the suitability of the valve for commissurotomy and/or repair and for determining the likely result.

【 】 CARDIAC CATHETERIZATION/ANGIOGRAPHY

In most patients with disabling symptoms from presumed MS, right and left heart catheterization should be performed as part of a preoperative assessment. Simultaneous measurement of cardiac output and the gradient between the LA and the LV and calculation of valve area remain the "gold standard" for assessing the severity of MS. LV angiography assesses the competence of the mitral valve, an important determinant of operability for mitral commissurotomy. Quantification of LV function provides a useful prognostic indicator of operative and late survival and of the expected functional result. Aortic valve function should be evaluated in all patients. Selective supraventricular aortography should be performed in all patients unless there is a contraindication. Tricuspid valve function can be assessed when there is a question of coexisting lesions. In certain circumstances, dynamic exercise in the catheterization laboratory with measurement of mitral valve gradient, CO, and LA and PA pressures can be extremely useful. Selective coronary arteriography establishes the site, severity, and extent of coronary artery disease and should be performed in patients with angina, LV dysfunction, and/or risk factors for coronary artery disease and in those 35 years of age or older.

[   ] OTHER LABORATORY STUDIES

Occasionally, a treadmill exercise test to evaluate functional capacity may be very useful clinically—for example, when a patient denies symptoms in spite of severe hemodynamic abnormalities.

NATURAL HISTORY AND PROGNOSIS

The population presenting with MS is changing because of the sharp decline in the incidence of acute rheumatic fever in the past 40 years. Native-born American citizens with symptomatic MS are presenting at an older age. Young adults in the third and fourth decades with symptomatic MS are more likely to come from low socioeconomic backgrounds and from the inner city or to be immigrants, particularly from Latin America, the Middle East, Africa, or Asia. The mechanism for the progression from no symptoms to mild to severe symptoms is progressive stenosis of the mitral valve. Approximately 50% of patients develop symptoms gradually. Sudden deterioration is usually the result of AF, systemic embolization, or other conditions that result in tachycardia and/or increased cardiac output.

The 10-year survival rate of patients with MS who are asymptomatic is approximately 84%, and that of those who are mildly symptomatic is 34% to 42%. Patients in NYHA functional class IV have very poor survival without treatment: 42% at 1 year and 10% or less at 5 years. All are dead within 10 years.

MEDICAL TREATMENT

All streptococcal infections should be diagnosed rapidly and correctly treated. All patients with known previous acute rheumatic fever/rheumatic carditis with or without obvious valve disease should receive appropriate antibiotic prophylaxis against recurrent streptococcal infection (see Chapter 38). Secondary prevention against infective endocarditis is a lifelong requirement. If AF is present, digitalis plays a critical role in controlling ventricular rate. In selected patients, beta-adrenergic blocking agents, diltiazem, or amiodarone may be added if digoxin alone is not satisfactory in controlling ventricular rate at rest or exercise. Diuretics reduce pulmonary congestion and peripheral edema, and allow most patients freedom from severe salt restriction. For the patient with mild symptoms, maintenance of sinus rhythm is desirable. Cardioversion of AF and maintenance of sinus rhythm using antiarrhythmic therapy with either digitalis and quinidine or digitalis and amiodarone should be offered to these patients. In patients who need interventional therapy, cardioversion is usually performed after completion of the procedure. Anticoagulation with warfarin is usually begun about 3 weeks in advance of cardioversion and continued for 4 weeks after the procedure. Alternatively, if left atrial thrombus is excluded by TEE, 2 to 3 days of intravenous heparin should be instituted, the patient cardioverted to sinus rhythm, and warfarin therapy continued for at least 4 weeks. Patients with chronic AF and those with a previous history of embolism should receive anticoagulation with warfarin (International Normalized Ratio [INR] of 2 to 3) unless there is a specific contraindication. Systemic embolization necessitates permanent anticoagulation. A single systemic embolic episode is not an *absolute* indication for mitral valve surgery, as emboli can and do occur in patients with mild mitral stenosis (see Algorithms 33-1 to 33-3).

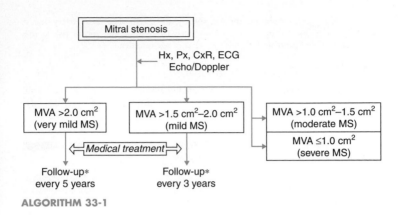

ALGORITHM 33-1

INTERVENTIONAL THERAPY

Unless there is a contraindication, surgery or catheter balloon commissurotomy (CBC) should be recommended to an MS patient with functional class III or IV symptoms. For younger patients with a pliable, noncalcified valve and without important mitral regurgitation, this means valve repair or CBC. The hemodynamic results of surgical commissurotomy or CBC are excellent. Because of the low morbidity and mortality of CBC/valve repair, surgery is also offered to patients when functional class II symptoms are present (Table 33-1). The results of successful commissurotomy are excellent; in

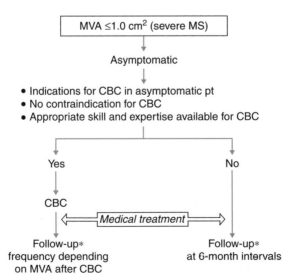

ALGORITHM 33-2

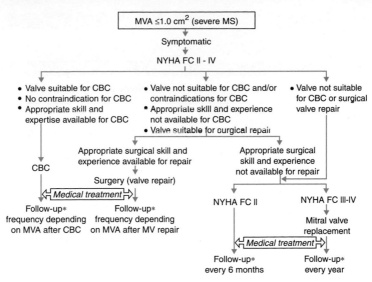

ALGORITHM 33-3

TABLE 33-1

Indications for Percutaneous Mitral Balloon Valvotomy

Indication	Class
1. Symptomatic patients (NYHA functional class II, III, or IV), moderate or severe MS and valve morphology favorable for percutaneous balloon valvotomy in the absence of left atrial thrombus or moderate to severe MR	I
2. Asymptomatic patients with moderate or severe MS and valve morphology favorable for percutaneous balloon valvotomy who have pulmonary hypertension (pulmonary artery systolic pressure >50 mm Hg at rest or >60 mm Hg with exercise) in the absence of left atrial thrombus or moderate to severe MR	I
3. Patients with NYHA functional class III to IV symptoms, moderate or severe MS, and a nonpliable calcified valve who are either not candidates for surgery or at high risk for surgery in the absence of left atrial thrombus or moderate to severe MR	IIa
4. Asymptomatic patients, moderate or severe MS, and valve morphology favorable for percutaneous balloon valvotomy who have new onset of atrial fibrillation in the absence of left atrial thrombus or moderate to severe MR	IIb
5. Symptomatic patients (NYHA functional class II, III, or IV) with MV area ≥ 1.5 cm^2 if there is evidence of hemodynamically significant MS based on pulmonary artery systolic pressure greater than 60 mm Hg, pulmonary artery wedge pressure ≥ 25, or mean MV gradient >15 mm Hg during exercise	IIb
6. Patients in NYHA functional class III to IV with moderate or severe MS and a nonpliable calcified valve as an alternate to surgery	IIb

TABLE 33-1

Indications for Percutaneous Mitral Balloon Valvotomy (*Continued*)

Indication	Class
7. Percutaneous mitral balloon valvotomy is not indicated in patients with mild MS	III
8. Percutaneous mitral balloon valvotomy should not be performed in patients with moderate to severe MR or left atrial thrombus	III

Reproduced with permission from ACC/AHA 2006 guidelines for the management of patients with valvular heart disease a report of the American College of Cardiology/American Heart Association Task Force on Practice Guidelines (Writing Committee to revise the 1998 guidelines for the management of patients with valvular heart disease) developed in collaboration with the Society of Cardiovascular Anesthesiologists Endorsed by the Society for Cardiovascular Angiography and Interventions and the Society of Thoracic Surgeons. *J Am Coll Cardiol.* 2006; 48:e1–e148.

    TABLE 33-2

Indications for Surgery for Mitral Stenosis

Indication	Class
1. Mitral valve surgery (repair if possible) is indicated in patients with symptomatic (NYHA functional class III to IV), moderate to severe MS and valve morphology favorable for repair if (1) percutaneous mitral balloon valvotomy is not available, (2) percutaneous mitral balloon valvotomy is contraindicated because of left atrial thrombus despite anticoagulation or concomitant moderate to severe MR is present, or (3) the valve morphology is not favorable for percutaneous mitral balloon valvotomy in a patient with acceptable operative risk	I
2. Symptomatic patients with moderate to severe MS who also have moderate to severe MR should receive MV replacement, unless valve repair is possible at the time of surgery	I
3. MV replacement is reasonable for patients with severe MS and severe pulmonary hypertension (pulmonary artery systolic pressure > 60 to 80 mm Hg) with NYHA functional class I to II symptoms who are not considered candidates for percutaneous mitral balloon valvotomy or surgical MV repair	IIa
	IIb
4. Asymptomatic patients with moderate or severe MS and valve morphology favorable for repair who have had recurrent episodes of embolic events on adequate anticoagulation	
5. MV repair for MS is not indicated for patients with mild MS	III
6. Closed commissurotomy should not be performed on patients undergoing MV repair; open commissurotomy is the preferred approach	III

Reproduced with permission from ACC/AHA 2006 guidelines for the management of patients with valvular heart disease a report of the American College of Cardiology/American Heart Association Task Force on Practice Guidelines (Writing Committee to revise the 1998 guidelines for the management of patients with valvular heart disease) developed in collaboration with the Society of Cardiovascular Anesthesiologists Endorsed by the Society for Cardiovascular Angiography and Interventions and the Society of Thoracic Surgeons. *J Am Coll Cardiol.* 2006; 48:e1–e148.

experienced and skilled centers, surgical mortality is less than 1%. Late mortality at 10 years is less than 5%, the thromboembolism rate is 2% per year or less, and the reoperation rate ranges from 0.5% to 4.5% per year.

For the older patient with a stiff or calcified valve, or when moderate mitral regurgitation is present, mitral valve replacement is usually performed. Valve replacement carries a higher operative mortality than does commissurotomy (up to 5%) and the morbidity associated with prostheses. Hemodynamic results of mitral valve replacement are often not ideal (see also Chapter 36). Survival at 10 years after mitral valve replacement for functional class III and IV patients is better than 60% (Table 33-2).

Use of the double-balloon technique or the Inoue balloon produces immediate and 3-month hemodynamic and clinical results comparable to those obtained by surgical commissurotomy. The mitral valve area increases from a mean of 1.0 to 2.0 cm^2. There are reductions of LA and PA pressures at rest and on exercise and an increase of exercise capacity. The immediate results of CBC are greatly influenced by the characteristics of the valve and its supporting apparatus, which are best determined by 2D echocardiography (transthoracic and/or transesophageal) (Table 33-1). Echocardiographic scores ≤ 8 (MGH) or of 0 to 1 (USC) determined by the two different methods provide a clue to the best immediate results. Repeat CBC or mitral valve replacement is needed in 20% of patients within 5 to 7 years. Late survival is poorer in those in whom functional class IV, higher echocardiographic score, higher LV enddiastolic pressure, or higher PA systolic pressure is present prior to the CBC.

SUGGESTED READING

Bonow RO, Carabello B, Chatterjee K, et al. ACC/AHA guidelines for the management of patients with valvular heart disease: a report of the ACC/AHA taskforce on practice guidelines. *J Am Coll Cardiol*. 2006;48:1–148.

Committee on Rheumatic Fever, Endocarditis, and Kawasaki Disease of the Council on Cardiovascular Disease in the Young of the American Heart Association. Treatment of streptococcal pharyngitis and prevention of rheumatic fever: a statement for health professionals. *Pediatrics*.1995;96:758–764.

Currie PJ, Seward JB, Chan KL, et al. Continuous wave Doppler determination of right ventricular pressure: a simultaneous Doppler-catheterization study in 127 patients. *J Am Coll Cardiol*. 1985;6:750–756.

Hatle L, Angelsen B, Tromsdal A. Noninvasive assessment of atrioventricular pressure half-time by Doppler ultrasound. *Circulation*. 1979;60:1096–1104.

Manning WJ, Silverman DI, Keighley CS, et al. Transesophageal echocardiographically facilitated early cardioversion from atrial fibrillation using short-term anticoagulation: final results of a prospective 4.5 year study. *J Am Coll Cardiol*. 1995; 256:1354–1361.

Nishimura RA, Rihal CS, Tajik AJ, et al. Accurate measurement of the transmitral gradient in patients with mitral stenosis: a simultaneous catheterization and Doppler echocardiographic study. *J Am Coll Cardiol*. 1994;2:52–158.

Rahimtoola SH. Mitral valve stenosis. In: Fuster V, O'Rourke RA, Walsh RA, et al., eds. *Hurst's The Heart*. 12th ed. New York, NY: McGraw-Hill; 2008:1757–1769.

Reid CL, McKay CR, Chandraratna PA, et al. Mechanisms of increase in mitral valve area and influence of anatomic features in double-balloon, catheter balloon valvuloplasty in adults with rheumatic mitral stenosis: a Doppler and two-dimensional echocardiographic study. *Circulation*. 1987;76:628 636.

Tuzcu EM, Block PC, Griffin DF, et al. Immediate and long-term outcome of percutaneous mitral valvotomy in patients 65 years and older. *Circulation*. 1992;85:963–971.

CHAPTER (34)

Mitral Regurgitation (Including Mitral Valve Prolapse)

Robert A. O'Rourke

MITRAL REGURGITATION

【 】 DEFINITION, ETIOLOGY, AND PATHOLOGY

Mitral regurgitation (MR) is characterized by an abnormal reversed blood flow from the left ventricle (LV) to the left atrium (LA) due to abnormalities in the mitral apparatus.

Prolapse of the mitral valve leaflets into the left atrium during systole is now the most common cause of MR, followed by coronary artery disease. MR due to rheumatic valvulitis remains an important cause. Additional causes include infective endocarditis, mitral annular calcification, hypertrophic cardiomyopathy, trauma, connective tissue disorders, and congenital deformities. The competence of the mitral valve depends on the normal structure and function of every part of the mitral apparatus—that is, the leaflets, chordae tendineae, annulus, left atrium, papillary muscles, and LV myocardium surrounding the papillary muscles. There are reports of MR and AR associated with the use of anorectic drugs that are no longer manufactured. In many cases, the prolapsing mitral valve on echocardiography is associated with other features of what has been termed the "mitral valve prolapse syndrome," as discussed later.

【 】 PATHOPHYSIOLOGY

In MR, the abnormal coaptation of the mitral leaflets creates a *regurgitant orifice* during systole. The systolic pressure gradient between the LV and the LA is the driving force for the regurgitant flow, which results in a *regurgitant volume.* This regurgitant volume represents a percentage of the total ejection of the LV and may be expressed as the *regurgitant fraction.* The regurgitant volume creates a volume overload by entering the LA in systole and the LV in diastole, modifying LV loading and function; it is additive to the systolic output of the right ventricle.

In *acute MR*, the hemodynamic burden is different. The sudden burden of the MR does not allow compensatory dilatation of the LA and LV. Consequently, marked elevations of the LA and pulmonary venous pressures are produced, leading to acute pulmonary edema.

LV dysfunction is a frequent complication of MR; its exact mechanism is unknown. The changes in myofiber contractility parallel changes in global LV function and are associated with reduced myofiber content. During diastole, LV relaxation is frequently abnormal, but chamber stiffness is usually reduced. Age and decreased systolic function are associated with increased chamber stiffness.

【 】 CLINICAL MANIFESTATIONS

History

Patients with MR often are asymptomatic. Even severe MR may be associated with no or minimal symptoms. Fatigue and mild dyspnea on exertion are most common symptoms and are rapidly improved by rest; these progress to orthopnea, paroxysmal nocturnal dyspnea, and peripheral edema. Often, the history provides clues to the etiology—for example, a history of angina/myocardial infarction, rheumatic carditis, infective endocarditis, chronic heart failure (HF) with a markedly dilated heart, or sudden onset of severe symptoms with a normal-sized heart.

With severe MR of *acute onset,* symptoms are usually more dramatic—pulmonary edema or congestive heart failure—but may progressively subside with administration of diuretic and increased LA compliance.

【 】 PHYSICAL FINDINGS

Blood pressure is usually normal. The arterial upstroke is brisk, especially when ejection time is reduced in MR (see also Chapter 1).

On palpation, the cardiac impulse (enlarged LV) is often laterally displaced, diffuse, and brief. An apical thrill is characteristic of very severe MR. A left sternal border lift is observed with right ventricular dilatation and may be difficult to distinguish from the LA lift in *later systole* due to the dilated, expansive LA, which is more substernal and lower (see Chapter 1).

The first heart sound is often included in the murmur but may be increased in rheumatic disease. The second heart sound is usually normal but may be paradoxically split if the LV ejection time is markedly shortened. The presence of a third heart sound (S_3) is directly related to the volume of the regurgitation. MR is often associated with an early diastolic rumble due to the increased mitral flow in diastole even without mitral stenosis. The S_3 and diastolic rumble are low-pitched sounds that may be difficult to detect except in the left lateral decubitus position. An atrial gallop (S_4) is heard mainly in MR of recent onset and in ischemic and/or functional MR in sinus rhythm. Midsystolic clicks are markers of mitral valve prolapse and are due to sudden tension of the chordae (discussed later).

The hallmark of MR is the systolic murmur, most often holosystolic, including first and second heart sounds. If an opening snap or S_3 is mistakenly interpreted as S_2, the murmur may appear midsystolic. The murmur is of a high-pitched and blowing type but may be harsh, especially in mitral valve prolapse syndrome. The maximum intensity is usually at the apex, but it may radiate to the axilla when the anterior leaflet results in greater regurgitation and to the left sternal border when the posterior leaflet results in greater regurgitation. When the posterior leaflet prolapses, the jet is usually superiorly and medially directed, and the murmur radiates toward the base of the heart. When the anterior leaflet prolapses, the murmur may be heard in the back, in the neck, and sometimes on the skull. In those cases where the murmur radiates to the base, it may be difficult to distinguish from the murmur of aortic stenosis or obstructive cardiomyopathy. The murmur decreases with reduction of afterload or LV size and increases with increase of afterload or LV size. Murmur intensity does not increase with postextrasystolic beats because the degree of MR is not increased (see Chapter 1).

Murmurs of shorter duration usually correspond to mild MR; they may be mid- or late systolic in mitral valve prolapse or early systolic in functional MR.

Electrocardiogram

Chronic MR produces LA or LV enlargement, typically manifest by increased amplitude of the P waves and QRS complex. If atrial fibrillation is present, the LA enlargement is associated with coarse fibrillatory waves. RV hypertrophy is uncommon. The electrocardiogram, especially in acute MR, may be entirely normal. When papillary muscle ischemia or infarction is the cause of MR, evidence of inferior or posterior infarction (old or new) may be present.

Chest Roentgenogram

In chronic severe MR, the chest x-ray shows LA and LV enlargement. In rheumatic disease, the valve leaflets may be calcified; with degenerative disease, a calcified mitral annulus is often present. Acute severe MR is usually associated with normal cardiac size and pulmonary edema.

【 】 LABORATORY TESTS

Echocardiography/Doppler

The echocardiogram is used for defining the etiology of the MR (e.g., flail leaflets, severe prolapse, mitral annulus calcification, systolic anterior motion of the anterior leaflet, and endocarditis vegetation) and determining its consequences. The echocardiography/Doppler technique provides an estimate of the severity of the regurgitation by assessing the velocity, width, and length of the regurgitant jet. Color-flow imaging demonstrates the origin and direction of the jet. Accordingly, the jet length, the ratio of the jet area to the left atrial (LA) area, or more simply the size of the jet area have been suggested as good indices of the severity of MR. Small jets, such as those seen in normal subjects, consistently correspond to mild regurgitations. Color-flow imaging for defining regurgitant lesions has significant limitations. The extent of a jet is determined by its momentum and thus is determined as much by regurgitant velocity as by regurgitant flow. Also, jets are constrained by the LA and expand more in large atria. The eccentric jets of valvular prolapse depend on the left atrial wall and tend to underestimate regurgitation. In contrast, the central jets of ischemic and functional MR expand markedly in a large atrium and tend to overestimate regurgitation. Transesophageal echocardiography usually shows larger jets, but does not eliminate these limitations of color-flow imaging. The pulmonary venous velocity profile is useful to assess the degree of regurgitation. Systolic reversal of flow in the pulmonary veins is a strong argument for severe MR. The reliability of several techniques for the quantitative assessment of MR remains to be demonstrated.

Cardiac Catheterization and Angiography

Cardiac catheterization is utilized to assess hemodynamic status, the severity of MR, LV function, and coronary artery anatomy. It confirms the diagnosis of MR as well. A large V wave in the pulmonary capillary wedge pressure tracings suggests MR, but its absence does not exclude MR. A balloon flotation catheter, inserted at the bedside to determine oxygen saturation in the right heart chambers and the presence or absence of the V wave in the pulmonary capillary pressures, is helpful in establishing the cause of a new systolic murmur that develops in a patient after acute myocardial infarction. The assessment of the degree of regurgitation can be obtained by LV contrast angiography and can be qualitatively graded in three or four grades on the basis of the degree and persistence of opacification of the LA. The assessment of LV function can be performed using quantitative angiography.

LV volumes are determined by the regurgitant volume, duration of regurgitation, etiology of regurgitation, and LV function. The most frequently utilized indices of LV function are the end-systolic volume and the LV ventricular ejection fraction. Both have been shown to be useful prognostically. The hemodynamic response to exercise (e.g., cardiac output, pulmonary artery pressure) often helps to determine the need for valve replacement in borderline circumstances.

Regional wall-motion abnormalities have been observed in patients with MR even in the absence of coronary lesions. Selected coronary angiography is at present the only technique for defining the coronary artery anatomy. It is usually performed in patients above 35 years of age or in those with angina or multiple risk factors for coronary artery disease.

Other Laboratory Studies

Radionuclide angiography can be used to estimate the LV end-diastolic and end-systolic volumes as well as the RV and LV ejection fractions. The detection of exercise-induced LV dysfunction is frequent; however, the significance of such measurements for the long-term prognosis has not been analyzed in large series of patients. Comparison of the counts measured over the RV and LV allows the calculation of the mitral valve regurgitant fraction. Exercise testing is often useful for determining the patient's exercise capacity, particularly in those who appear relatively asymptomatic despite severe MR.

【 】 NATURAL HISTORY AND PROGNOSIS

Because of the qualitative and imprecise assessment of the degree of regurgitation, the natural history of MR is poorly defined. Patients with mild rheumatic MR appear to have a good prognosis. The prognosis of patients with echocardiographic mitral valve prolapse and no or mild regurgitation is usually excellent. Some deaths may occur in patients with murmurs of MR, more often when LV function is markedly decreased.

The predictors of poor outcome in patients with MR who are treated medically include severe symptoms (functional classes III to IV), even if the symptoms are transient; pulmonary hypertension; markedly increased LV end-diastolic volume; decreased cardiac output; and reduced LV ejection fraction. A comparison of the outcome of medically and surgically treated patients shows a trend in favor of surgical treatment, especially early surgery, with a definite improvement of outcome with surgery in patients who have decreased systolic LV function.

【 】 MEDICAL TREATMENT

Prevention of infective endocarditis with use of antibiotics is necessary in patients with MR. Young patients with rheumatic MR should receive rheumatic fever prophylaxis. In patients with AF, rate control is achieved using digoxin and/or beta-blockers, diltiazem, and amiodarone. Long-term maintenance of sinus rhythm after cardioversion in patients with severe MR or enlarged LA who are treated medically is usually not possible. Oral anticoagulation should be used in patients with atrial fibrillation (international normalized ratio [INR] 2.0–3.0).

Afterload reduction decreases the amount of regurgitation, not only by reducing the LV systolic pressure but also by decreasing the effective regurgitant orifice area. The acute utilization of sodium nitroprusside in unstable patients with severe MR, especially in the context of myocardial infarction, may be lifesaving in patients being prepared for mitral valve surgery. Chronic afterload reduction is usually not indicated for chronic MR. Diuretic treatment is extremely useful for the control of heart failure and for the chronic control of symptoms, especially dyspnea.

【 】 SURGICAL TREATMENT

Mitral valve reconstruction for MR is often possible. The frequency with which valve repair can be used in patients with MR varies with the experience of the operating team (up to 90% success rate) and the spectrum of underlying valve disease; repair is more often feasible in patients with degenerative valve disease than in those with regurgitation caused by rheumatic valvulitis or endocarditis. LV systolic function and late survival in general are better with mitral valve repair than with mitral valve replacement because of the lesser decline in or maintenance of normal LV function when the chordae are preserved at the time of surgery. In patients whose mitral valves cannot be repaired, mitral valve replacement with chordal preservation is less likely to depress LV function than mitral valve replacement without preservation of the chordae tendineae. Patients with severe symptoms due to MR should be treated surgically even if their symptoms are markedly improved by medical treatment (see Table 34-1 and Chapter 59). Patients who are functional class I or II but have signs of overt LV dysfunction (LV ejection fraction < 60%, end-systolic diameter > 45 mm) should be treated surgically, particularly if they are candidates for valve repair or valve replacement with chordal preservation. In patients with *severe* MR who have no or minimal symptoms and no signs of LV dysfunction,

TABLE 34-1

Recommendations for Mitral Valve Surgery in Nonischemic Severe Mitral Regurgitation

Indication	Class
1. Acute symptomatic MR in which repair is likely	I
2. Patients with NYHA functional class II, III, or IV symptoms with normal LV function defined as ejection fraction > 0.60 and end-systolic dimension < 45 mm	I
3. Symptomatic or asymptomatic patients with mild LV dysfunction, ejection fraction 0.50 to 0.60, and end-systolic dimension 45 to 50 mm	I
4. Symptomatic or asymptomatic patients with moderate LV dysfunction, ejection fraction 0.30 to 0.50, and/or end-systolic dimension 50 to 55 mm	I
5. Asymptomatic patients with preserved LV function and atrial fibrillation	IIa
6. Asymptomatic patients with preserved LV function and pulmonary hypertension (pulmonary artery systolic pressure > 50 mm Hg at rest or > 60 mm Hg with exercise)	IIa
7. Asymptomatic patients with ejection fraction 0.50 to 0.60 and end-systolic dimension < 45 mm and asymptomatic patients with ejection fraction > 0.60 and end-systolic dimension 45 to 55 mm	IIa
8. Patients with severe LV dysfunction (ejection fraction < 0.30 and/or end-systolic dimension > 55 mm) in whom chordal preservation is highly likely	IIa
9. Asymptomatic patients with chronic MR with preserved LV function in whom mitral valve repair is highly likely	IIb
10. Patients with MVP and preserved LV function who have recurrent ventricular arrhythmias despite medical therapy	IIb
11. Asymptomatic patients with preserved LV function in whom significant doubt about the feasibility of repair exists	III

*a*The committee recognizes that there may be variability in the measurement of mitral valve area and that the mean transmitral gradient, pulmonary artery wedge pressure, and pulmonary artery pressure at rest or during exercise should also be taken into consideration.

Reproduced with permission from Bonow RO, Carabello BA, Chatterjee K, et al. ACC/AHA 2006 guidelines for the management of patients with valvular heart disease a report of the American College of Cardiology/American Heart Association Task Force on Practice Guidelines (Writing Committee to revise the 1998 guidelines for the management of patients with valvular heart disease) developed in collaboration with the Society of Cardiovascular Anesthesiologists Endorsed by the Society for Cardiovascular Angiography and Interventions and the Society of Thoracic Surgeons. *J Am Coll Cardiol.* 2006;48(3):e1–e148. Erratum in: *J Am Coll Cardiol.* 2007;49(9):1014.

surgery is a reasonable option when it is likely that the mitral valve can be repaired with chordal preservation. This pertains to patients with a low operative risk (1%–2%) and valvular lesions that can be repaired as indicated by echocardiography. Intraoperative transesophageal echocardiography (TEE) should be performed by physicians prior to operation and to monitor the repair procedure and help with decisions warranted by an imperfect result.

Patients who have *no symptoms* due to *severe* MR and normal LV systolic function who are candidates for mitral valve repair and have severe pulmonary hypertension at rest or with exercise, atrial fibrillation, or recurrent thromboemboli despite anticoagulation therapy are commonly recommended for early surgery if mitral valve repair with preservation of the chordae is the likely procedure.

MITRAL VALVE PROLAPSE

Mitral valve prolapse (MVP) is defined echocardiographically as the systolic billowing of one or both mitral leaflets into the left atrium, with or without mitral regurgitation. The *MVP syndrome* often occurs as a clinical entity with no or only mild mitral regurgitation, and it is frequently associated with unique clinical characteristics when compared with the other causes of mitral regurgitation. Nevertheless, MVP is the most common cause of significant MR and the most frequent substrate for mitral valve endocarditis in the United States. The mitral valve apparatus is a complex structure composed of the mitral annulus, valve leaflets, chordae tendineae, papillary muscles, and supporting left ventricular, left atrial, and aortic walls. Disease processes involving any one or more of these components may result in dysfunction of the valvular apparatus and prolapse of the mitral leaflets toward the left atrium during systole, when LV pressure exceeds left atrial pressure.

In primary MVP (Table 34-2), there is interchordal hooding due to leaflet redundancy involving both the rough and the clear zones of the involved leaflets. The basic microscopic feature of primary MVP is marked proliferation of the spongiosa, the delicate myxomatous connective tissue between the atrialis (a thick layer of collagen and elastic tissue forming the atrial aspect of the leaflet) and the fibrosa or ventricularis, which is composed of dense layers of collagen and forms the basic support of the leaflet. In primary MVP, myxomatous proliferation of the mucopolysaccharide-containing spongiosa tissue causes focal interruption of the fibrosa. Secondary effects of the primary MVP syndrome include

TABLE 34-2

Classification of Mitral Valve Prolapse

Primary mitral valve prolapse
    Familial
    Nonfamilial
    Marfan's syndrome
    Other connective tissue diseases
    Cardiomyopathies
    "Flail" mitral valve leaflet(s)
Secondary mitral valve prolapse
    Coronary artery disease
    Rheumatic heart disease
Normal variant
    Inaccurate auscultation
    "Echocardiographic" heart disease

fibrosis of the surface of the mitral valve leaflets, thinning and/or elongation of the chordae tendineae, and ventricular friction lesions. Fibrin deposits often form at the mitral valve–left atrial angle. The primary form of MVP may occur in families, where it appears to be inherited as an autosomal dominant trait with varying penetrance. The primary MVP syndrome has also been found with increasing frequency in patients with Marfan's syndrome and in other heritable connective tissue diseases.

In secondary forms of MVP, echocardiographic myxomatous proliferation of the spongiosa portion of the mitral valve leaflet is absent. Echocardiographic evidence of MVP, often with MR, can be produced in closed-chest dogs undergoing transient coronary artery occlusion. Serial studies in patients with known ischemic heart disease have occasionally documented unequivocal MVP following an acute coronary syndrome that was previously absent; however, in most patients with coronary artery disease (CAD) and MVP, the two entities are coincident but unrelated.

Recently, several studies have indicated that valvular regurgitation due to prolapsing mitral valve leaflets may result from postinflammatory changes, including those following rheumatic fever. Mitral valve prolapse has also been observed in patients with hypertrophic cardiomyopathy, in whom posterior MVP may result from a disproportionally small left ventricular cavity, altered papillary muscle alignment, or a combination of factors. Patients with the primary MVP syndrome and those with secondary MVP must be distinguished from those with normal variations on cardiac auscultation or echocardiograms that are misinterpreted as showing MVP.

【 】 PATHOPHYSIOLOGY OF MVP SYNDROME

In patients with MVP, there is frequently LA and LV enlargement, depending upon the presence and severity of mitral regurgitation. In patients with connective tissue syndromes, the mitral annulus is usually dilated and sometimes calcified; it does not decrease its circumference by the usual 30% during left ventricular systole. The hemodynamic effects of mild to moderate MR are similar to those from other causes of MR.

【 】 CLINICAL MANIFESTATIONS OF MVP SYNDROME

Symptoms

The diagnosis of MVP is most commonly made by cardiac auscultation in asymptomatic patients or by echocardiography performed for some other purpose. The patient may be evaluated because of a family history of cardiac disease or occasionally may be referred because of an abnormal resting electrocardiogram. The most common presenting complaint is palpitations, which are usually due to premature ventricular beats. Supraventricular arrhythmias are also frequent; the most common sustained tachycardia is paroxysmal reentry supraventricular tachycardia.

Chest pain is a frequent complaint in patients with the MVP syndrome. It is atypical in most patients without coexistent ischemic heart disease and rarely resembles classic angina pectoris. Dyspnea and fatigue are also frequent symptoms in patients with MVP, including many without severe MR. Objective exercise testing often fails to show an impairment in exercise tolerance, and some patients exhibit distinct episodes of hyperventilation. Neuropsychiatric complaints are not uncommon in patients with MVP: some have panic attacks and others frank manic-depressive syndromes. Transient cerebral ischemic episodes occur with increased incidence in patients with MVP, and some develop stroke syndromes. Reports of amaurosis fugax, homonymous field loss, and retinal artery occlusion have been described; occasionally the visual loss persists. These signs likely are due to embolization of platelets and fibrin deposits occurring on the atrial side of the mitral valve leaflets. It is important to note that both MVP and panic attacks occur relatively frequently. Accordingly, the occurrence of both syndromes in the same individual would be expected to occur frequently by chance.

TABLE 34-3

Response of the Murmur of Mitral Valve Prolapse to Interventions

Intervention	Timing	Intensity
Standing upright	←	↑
Recumbent	→	↓ or 0
Squatting	→	↓ or 0
Hand grip	←	±
Valsalva	←	±
Amyl nitrite	±	↑

↑, increase; ↓, decrease; 0, no change; ±, variable; ← , earlier; → , later.

Physical Examination

The presence of thoracic skeletal abnormalities—the most common being scoliosis, pectus excavatum, straightened thoracic spine, and narrowed anteroposterior diameter of the chest—may suggest the diagnosis of the MVP syndrome. The principal cardiac auscultatory feature of this syndrome is the midsystolic click, a high-pitched sound of short duration. The click may vary considerably in intensity and location in systole according to LV loading conditions and contractility. It results from the sudden tension of the mitral valve apparatus as the leaflets prolapse into the left atrium during systole. Multiple systolic clicks may be generated as different portions of the mitral leaflets prolapse at various times during systole. The major feature differentiating the midsystolic click of MVP from that due to other causes is that its timing during systole may be altered by maneuvers that change hemodynamic conditions.

Dynamic auscultation is often useful for establishing the clinical diagnosis of the MVP syndrome (Table 34-3). Changes in the LV end-diastolic volume lead to changes in the timing of the midsystolic click and murmur. When end-diastolic volume is decreased, the critical volume is achieved earlier in systole, and the click-murmur complex occurs shortly after the first heart sound. In general, any maneuver that decreases the end-diastolic LV volume, increases the rate of ventricular contraction, or decreases the resistance to LV ejection of blood causes the MVP to occur early in systole and the systolic click and murmur to move toward the first heart sound. This occurs when the patient suddenly stands from the supine position, does submaximal hand-grip exercise, or performs the Valsalva maneuver (see Table 34-3).

【 】 DIAGNOSTIC STUDIES

Electrocardiogram

The electrocardiogram (ECG) is usually normal in patients with the MVP syndrome. The most common abnormality in the MVP syndrome is the presence of ST-T-wave depression or T-wave inversion in the inferior leads. MVP is associated with an increased incidence of false-positive exercise ECG results in patients with normal coronary arteries, especially females. Myocardial perfusion imaging with thallium or technetium sestamibi has been useful for differentiating false from true abnormal exercise ECG findings in patients with MVP.

Although arrhythmias may be observed on the resting ECG or during treadmill or bicycle exercise, they are detected more frequently by continuous ambulatory ECG recordings. The reported incidence of documented arrhythmias is higher in patients with MVP; however, most are not life-threatening, and they often do not correlate with the patient's symptoms.

Chest Roentgenogram

Posteroanterior and lateral chest x-ray films usually show normal cardiopulmonary findings. The skeletal abnormalities described above can be seen. When severe MR is present, enlargement of both the LA and LV often results. Various degrees of pulmonary venous congestion are evident when left heart failure results. Acute chordal rupture with a sudden increase in the amount of mitral regurgitation may present as pulmonary edema without obvious LV or LA dilatation. Calcification of the mitral annulus may be seen, particularly in adults with Marfan's syndrome.

Echocardiography

As indicated earlier, echocardiography is the most useful noninvasive test for defining MVP. The M-mode echocardiographic definition of MVP includes ≥ 2-mm posterior displacement of one or both leaflets or holosystolic posterior "hammocking" > 3 mm. On two-dimensional (2D) echocardiography, systolic displacement of one or both mitral leaflets, particularly when they coapt on the left atrial side of the annular plane in the parasternal long-axis view, indicates a high likelihood of MVP. There is disagreement concerning the reliability of an echocardiographic diagnosis of MVP when these signs are observed only in the apical four-chamber view. The diagnosis of MVP is even more certain when the leaflet thickness is > 5 mm during ventricular diastole. Leaflet redundancy is often associated with an elongated mitral annulus and elongated chordae tendineae. On Doppler velocity recordings, the presence or absence of MR is an important consideration, and MVP is more likely when the MR is detected as a high-velocity jet in late systole, midway, or more posterior in the left atrium.

There is no consensus on 2D echocardiographic criteria for MVP. Since echocardiography is a tomographic cross-sectional technique, no single view should be considered diagnostic. The parasternal long-axis view permits visualization of the medial aspect of the anterior mitral leaflet and the middle scallop of the posterior leaflet. If the findings of prolapse are localized to the lateral scallop in the posterior leaflet, they would be best visualized by the apical four-chamber view. All available echocardiographic views should be utilized, with the provision that anterior leaflet billowing in the four-chamber apical view is not in itself evidence of prolapse; however, a displacement of the posterior leaflet or the coaptation point in any view, including the apical views, suggests the diagnosis of prolapse. The echocardiographic criteria for MVP should include structural changes, such as leaflet thickening, redundancy, annular dilatation, and chordal elongation.

Patients with echocardiographic criteria for the MVP syndrome but without evidence of thickened/redundant leaflets or definite MR are more difficult to classify. If such patients have auscultatory findings typical of MVP, the echocardiogram usually confirms the diagnosis. Two-dimensional/Doppler echocardiography is also useful for defining LA size as well as LV size and function and for the detection and semiquantitation of MR. Recommendations for echocardiography in MVP are listed in Table 34-4 (see also Chapter 59).

Cardiac Catheterization

Cardiac catheterization is rarely used as a diagnostic technique for MVP. Also, contrast ventriculography is unnecessary for determining LV function, since it can usually be quantitated by 2D echocardiography or radionuclide ventriculography. While contrast cineventriculography is often useful for assessing the severity of mitral regurgitation, cardiac catheterization and angiography are most commonly used in patients with MVP to exclude the possibility of CAD.

TABLE 34-4

Recommendations for Echocardiography in Mitral Valve Prolapse

Indication	Class
1. Diagnosis, assessment of hemodynamic severity of MR, leaflet morphology, ventricular compensation in patients with physical signs of MVP	I
2. To exclude MVP in patients who have been given the diagnosis where there is no clinical evidence to support the diagnosis	
3. To exclude MVP in patients with first-degree relatives with known myxomatous valve disease	IIa
4. Risk stratification in patients with physical signs of MVP with no or mild regurgitation	IIa
5. To exclude MVP in patients in the absence of physical findings suggestive of MVP positive family history	III
6. Routine repetition of echocardiography in patients with MVP with no or mild regurgitation and no changes in clinical signs or symptoms	III

Class   I: Conditions for which there is evidence and/or general agreement that a given procedure or treatment is useful and effective

Class II: Conditions for which there is conflicting evidence and/or a divergence of opinion about the usefulness/efficacy of a procedure or treatment

Class IIa: Weight of evidence/opinion is in favor of usefulness/efficacy

Class IIb: Usefulness/efficacy is less well established by evidence/opinion

Class III: Conditions for which there is evidence and/or general agreement that the procedure/treatment is not useful/effective and in some cases may be harmful

MR, mitral regurgitation; MVP, mitral valve prolapse (See also Chapter 59).

Reproduced with permission from ACC/AHA 2006 guidelines for the management of patients with valvular heart disease a report of the American College of Cardiology/American Heart Association Task Force on Practice Guidelines (Writing Committee to revise the 1998 guidelines for the management of patients with valvular heart disease) developed in collaboration with the Society of Cardiovascular Anesthesiologists Endorsed by the Society for Cardiovascular Angiography and Interventions and the Society of Thoracic Surgeons. *J Am Coll Cardiol.* 2006;48(3):e1–e148. Erratum in: *J Am Coll Cardiol.* 2007;49(9):1014.

Intracardiac pressures and cardiac output are usually normal in uncomplicated MVP; however, these measurements become progressively more abnormal as MR becomes more severe. LV angiography usually confirms the presence of MVP. LV wall motion is usually normal in patients with the primary MVP syndrome, but some patients show abnormal contraction patterns in the absence of CAD.

Other Diagnostic Tests

Exercise myocardial perfusion imaging with thallium or technetium sestamibi has been recommended as an adjunct to exercise ECG for determining the presence or absence of coexistent myocardial ischemia in patients with MVP. Most MVP patients with clinical evidence of CAD have an abnormal exercise scintigram. The indications for electrophysiologic testing in a patient with MVP are similar to those in general practice. The upright tilt test with monitoring of blood pressure and rhythm may be valuable in patients with light-headedness or syncope and in diagnosing autonomic dysfunction.

TABLE 34-5

Recommendations For Antibiotic Endocarditis Prophylaxis For Patients With Mitral Valve Prolapse Undergoing Procedures Associated With Bacteremia

Indication	Class
1. Patients with characteristic systolic click-murmur complex	I
2. Patients with isolated systolic click and echo evidence of MVP and MR	I
3. Patients with isolated systolic click and echo evidence of high-risk MVP	IIa
4. Patients with isolated systolic click and no or equivocal evidence of MVP	III

MR, mitral regurgitation; MVP, mitral valve prolapse.

Data compiled from ACC/AHA guidelines for the clinical application of echocardiography. *Circulation.* 1997;95:1686–1744.

【 】 NATURAL HISTORY, PROGNOSIS, AND COMPLICATIONS

In most patient studies, the MVP syndrome is associated with a benign prognosis. The age-adjusted survival rate for both males and females with MVP is similar to that for patients without this common clinical entity. The gradual progression of mitral regurgitation in patients with mitral prolapse, however, may result in progressive dilatation of the LA and LV. LA dilatation often results in atrial fibrillation, and moderate to severe MR eventually results in left ventricular dysfunction and the development of congestive heart failure in certain patients. Several long-term prognostic studies suggest that complications occur most commonly in patients with a mitral systolic murmur, thickened redundant mitral valve leaflets, or increased LV or LA size. Sudden death is uncommon but is obviously the most severe complication of mitral valve prolapse. Although sudden death is infrequent, its highest incidence has been reported in the familial form of MVP. Infective endocarditis is a serious complication of MVP, and MVP is the leading predisposing cardiovascular lesion in most series of patients reported with endocarditis. Recommendations for antibiotic endocarditis prophylaxis for patients with MVP undergoing procedures associated with bacteremia are listed in Table 34-5.

In some patients, fibrin emboli are responsible for visual problems consistent with involvement of the ophthalmic or posterior cerebral circulation. Therefore, it has been recommended that antiplatelet drugs such as aspirin be administered to patients who have MVP syndrome and suspected cerebral emboli. Warfarin therapy is usually reserved for patients with MVP who have atrial fibrillation or poststroke patients with prolapse, particularly when symptoms occur on aspirin therapy. However, neither antiplatelet drugs nor anticoagulants should be prescribed routinely for patients with MVP, since the incidence of embolic phenomena is very low.

【 】 TREATMENT

The majority of patients with the MVP syndrome are asymptomatic and lack the high-risk profile described earlier. These patients—those with mild or no symptoms and findings of milder forms of prolapse—should be assured of a benign prognosis. A normal lifestyle and regular exercise are encouraged. Patients with MVP and palpitations associated with sinus tachycardia or mild tachyarrhythmias and those with chest pain, anxiety, or fatigue often respond to therapy with beta-blockers. Symptoms of orthostatic hypotension are best treated with volume expansion, preferably by liberalizing fluid and salt intake. In survivors of sudden cardiac death and patients with symptomatic complex arrhythmias, specific antiarrhythmic therapy should be guided by monitoring techniques, including electrophysiologic testing when indicated. Restriction from competitive sports is recommended when moderate LV enlargement, LV dysfunction, uncontrolled tachyarrhythmias, long QT interval, unexplained syncope, prior sudden death, or aortic root enlargement is present, individually or in combination. Asymptomatic patients with MVP and no significant MR can be evaluated clinically every 2 to 3 years. Patients with MVP who have high-risk characteristics, including those with moderate to severe regurgitation, should be followed more frequently, even if no symptoms are present.

Surgical Considerations

Certain patients with MVP may require valve surgery, particularly those who develop a flail mitral leaflet due to rupture of the chordae tendineae or their marked elongation. Most such valves can be repaired successfully by surgeons experienced in mitral valve repair, especially when the posterior leaflet valve is predominantly affected. Symptoms of heart failure, the severity of MR, the presence or absence of atrial fibrillation, LV systolic function, LV end-diastolic and end-systolic volumes, and pulmonary artery pressure (rest and exercise) all influence the decision to recommend mitral valve surgery. Recommendations for surgery in patients with MVP and MR are the same as for those with other forms of nonischemic severe MR and include class III to IV symptoms, LV ejection fraction ≤ 60%, and/or marked increases in LV end-diastolic and end-systolic volumes. Repair is being recommended with increased frequency for functional class II symptoms and suitable anatomy.

SUGGESTED READING

Bonow RO, Carabello B, Chatterjee K, et al. ACC/AHA guidelines for the management of patients with valvular heart disease. *J Am Coll Cardiol.* 2006; 48:e1–e148. Erratum appears in *J Am Coll Cardiol.* 2007;49:1014.

Crawford MH, Souchek J, Oprian CA, et al. Determinants of survival and left ventricular performance after mitral valve replacement. Department of Veterans Affairs cooperative study on valvular heart disease. *Circulation.* 1990;81:1173–1181.

Gilon D, Buonanno FS, Jaffee MM, et al. Lack of evidence of an association between mitral valve prolapse and stroke in young patients. *N Engl J Med.* 1999;341:8–13.

Ling LH, Enriquez-Sarano M, Seward JB, et al. Clinical outcome of mitral regurgitation due to flail leaflet. *N Engl J Med.* 1996;335:1417.

Nishimura R, McGoon MD. Perspectives on mitral valve prolapse. *N Engl J Med.* 1999;341:48–58.

O'Rourke RA. The syndrome of mitral valve prolapse. In: Albert JA, ed. *Valvular Heart Disease.* New York, NY: Lippincott-Raven; 1999:157–182.

O'Rourke RA, Dell'Italia LJ. Mitral valve regurgitation including the mitral valve prolapse syndrome. In: Fuster V, O'Rourke RA, Walsh RA, et al., eds. *Hurst's The Heart.* 12th ed. New York, NY: McGraw-Hill; 2008:1731–1756.

CHAPTER 35

Tricuspid Valve and Pulmonic Valve Disease

John T. Schindler and James A. Shaver

Right-sided cardiac valve disease is encountered less frequently when compared to left-sided valve disease. Despite the lower incidence of right-sided disease, there have been significant advances in the noninvasive imaging leading to increased recognition and improved understanding of the natural history of the disease process. In addition, improved therapy for the treatment of congenital heart disease (CHD), which can involve the right-sided valves, has resulted in a higher percentage of patients surviving into adulthood with simple or complex CHD. Despite these advances in diagnostic modalities, treatment options, and the formation of clinical practice guidelines, many of the indications for intervention remain uncertain or controversial. In general, the treatment of right-sided valve disease requires collaboration between the cardiologist, interventional cardiologist, and cardiothoracic surgeon.

TRICUSPID VALVE DISEASE

【 】 NORMAL ANATOMY

The normal anatomy of the tricuspid valve consists of five components. The three leaflets (anterior, posterior, and septal), annulus, and commisures form the valvular apparatus. The chordae tendinae and papillary muscles form the tensor apparatus. The saddle-shaped tricuspid annulus is part of the fibrous skeleton of the heart where the leaflets attach to the junction of the right atrium and right ventricle. There is intermittent loose connective tissue making the tricuspid annulus much more prone to dilation when the ventricular cavity enlarges as compared to the mitral valve annulus.

The commisures represent the site along the annulus where the leaflets meet. They always have an underlying papillary muscle and a fanlike array of tendinous cords to anchor and support the leaflets. The papillary muscles can be single or multi-headed and receive tendinous cords from two adjacent leaflets. This dual insertion facilitates closure of the valve in right ventricular systole due to pulling of the leaflets toward each other.

The orifice of the tricuspid valve is triangular in shape and is the largest orifice of the four cardiac valves. This results in lower early and late diastolic inflow velocities into the RV when compared to mitral inflow velocities into the LV. The anterior leaflet is the largest and most mobile of the three leaflets and attaches to the anterior and medial papillary muscles. The posterior leaflet is smaller and appears to be of lesser importance to normal valve function. The septal leaflet attaches directly to the membranous and muscular portions of the ventricular septum leading to its relatively immobile state.

【 】 TRICUSPID VALVE REGURGITATION

Etiology

Up to 70% to 90% of patients with *structurally normal valves have some degree of tricuspid regurgitation* (TR) in large part due to incomplete coaptation of the leaflets. The vast majority of these patients are asymptomatic and the valve finding is considered a normal variant. Pathologic TR can be due to primary (intrinsic) valve disease or the more common secondary or functional TR (Table 35-1). With increasing TR severity, there is an associated worsening prognosis that is independent of ventricular systolic function and pulmonary pressures.

The most common form of primary TR is due to infective endocarditis associated with intravenous drug use. The most common causative organism is *Staphylococcus aureus* followed by coagulase negative staphylococci and beta-hemolytic streptococci. These patients can be extremely difficult to manage due to high recurrence rates associated with medical noncompliance. Another less common condition is valvulopathy related to prescription drug use. The first medications implicated were the anorectics fenfluramine (Pondimin) and dexfenfluramine (Redux). Transthoracic echocardiography (TTE) revealed leaflet retraction and thickening in a subset of patients who subsequently developed murmurs after exposure to the drugs. In a subset of patients who then required valve replacement, histologic evidence displayed a plaque-like process extending across the leaflet surfaces and encasing the chordae tendinae. These findings are similar to the valve changes noted in patients with serotonin-secreting carcinoid tumors and patients taking certain antimigraine drugs (methysergide and ergotamine). In March 2007, the FDA voluntarily withdrew pergolide (Permax), an anti-parkinsonian dopamine agonist with potent serotonin activity, due to similar valulopathic findings suggesting a causal association. Subsequent research has suggested specific affinity with the 5-HT$_{2B}$ receptor to be a key step in the development of drug-induced valvular disease.

The most common cause of TR is not intrinsic disease of the valve as noted above, but rather due to dilation of the right ventricle and of the annulus in the setting of RV hypertension. This pathophysiology results in secondary or functional TR. With

---

TABLE 35-1

Etiology of Tricuspid Valve Disease

Primary (Intrinsic) Valve Disease	Secondary (Functional) Valve Disease
Infective endocarditis (IV drug use)	Primary RV disease/dilation
Rheumatic heart disease (never isolated)	Right ventricular infarction
Carcinoid	Dilated cardiomyopathy
Myxomatous disease (prolapse)	Elevated right ventricular systolic pressure
Endomyocardial fibrosis	Left-sided heart failure
Ebstein anomaly	Aortic, mitral, or pulomonic valve disease
Medication use (anorectics and ergot derivatives)	Primary pulmonary disease including pulmonary arterial HTN of any cause
Thoracic trauma	Left-to-right shunt
Iatrogenic (pacemaker lead and repeated endomyocardial biopsies)	
Congenital (non-Ebstein)	
Radiation inury	

continued pressure and volume overload of the RV, TR begets TR. Therefore, it is critically important to determine the underlying cause of the dilated annulus since specific therapy aimed at the primary disorder will improve the severity of the TR.

Diagnosis

The symptoms associated with severe functional TR are those of the associated diagnoses leading to the secondary TR. With time as the RV begins to fail, dyspnea, fatigue, and exercise intolerance are common due to impaired forward cardiac output. Some patients will also complain of chest pain and abdominal pain due to hepatosplenomegaly. On physical exam (PE), distended and pulsatile jugular veins with prominent V waves are appreciated (Fig. 35-1). Other findings include an accentuated precordial impulse of the RV, a holosystolic murmur at either sternal border that increases with inspiration, an accentuated or attenuated P2 (in the setting of pulmonary hypertension [HTN] or RV outflow obstruction), a pulsatile liver, ascites, peripheral cyanosis, and lower extremity edema. Rivero–Carvallo's sign is an accentuation of the TR murmur with inspiration and possibly lengthening of the murmur if it is not completely holosystolic due to increased venous return to the right side of the heart with negative intrathoracic pressure.

In primary (intrinsic) TR, the physical findings are entirely isolated to the right-sided cardiac exam. The precordial impulse, the pulsitile jugular venous pulse (JVP), distended liver, and peripheral edema are similar to functional TR. However, in the absence of RV hypertension, even with severe TR, the murmur maybe very soft or absent due to the small pressure gradient between the RA and RV (Fig. 35-2).

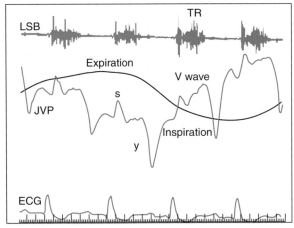

FIGURE 35-1. Physical findings of severe tricuspid regurgitation in the setting of right ventricular systolic pressure overload due to pulmonary hypertension. The jugular venous pulse shows a very prominent S (systolic wave) and V wave. With inspiration, there is a significant increase in the height of the S-V wave and the rate of Y descent. There is also a simultaneous increase in the intensity of the pansystolic regurgitant tricuspid murmur. With diuresis, the degree of tricuspid regurgitation and the intensity of the pansystolic regurgitant murmur may decrease or disappear. (Reproduced with permission from Salemi R, et al. Noninvasive graphic evaluation: phonocardiography and echocardiography. In: Frankl WS, Brest AN, eds. *Cardiovascular Clinics: Valvular Heart Disease: Comprehensive Evaluation and Management.* Philadelphia, PA: Davis; 1986;16(2):173-210.)

Hemodynamics of
Severe Organic Tricuspid Regurgitation

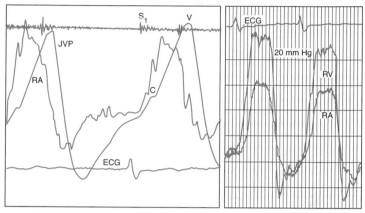

FIGURE 35-2. In the left panel, a phonocardiogram has been recorded simultaneously with the jugular venous pulse and the right atrial pressure. Only minimal early systolic vibrations are recorded on the phonocardiogram, and a huge C-V wave is present on the jugular venous pulse and right atrial tracing. In the right panel, simultaneous right ventricular and right atrial pressures are recorded, demonstrating ventricularization of the right atrial pressure. There is only a minimal pressure gradient across the tricuspid valve during systole resulting in a low-velocity retrograde flow and absence of a significant murmur. (Reproduced with permission from Hurst JW, Schlant RC, Rackley CE, et al., eds. *The Heart.* 7th ed., vol. 1. New York, NY: McGraw-Hill; 1990:224.)

The electrocardiogram (ECG) frequently shows nonspecific findings compatible with the underlying diagnosis causing the functional TR. Atrial fibrillation is often present, but if sinus rhythm (SR) prevails, right atrial enlargement is often seen with tall and narrow P waves in the inferior leads. In rheumatic disease, there is often biatrial enlargement due to concomitant involvement of the mitral valve. The chest x-ray (CXR) often shows cardiomegaly and obliteration of the retrosternal clear space on the lateral view due to RV enlargement. Prominence of the superior vena cava, distension of the azygous vein, and pleural effusions are often present. The diaphragms may be displaced superiorly due to ascites.

Echocardiography is the reference standard for diagnosis and evaluation of TR. Often identification of other cardiac abnormalities that might influence tricuspid valve function can be determined from the full interrogation using two-dimensional images, pulsed- and continuous-wave Doppler, and color flow Doppler. This allows for assessment of the valvular apparatus, determination of RV function, and an estimation of the pulmonary pressures using the modified Bernoulli equation. Color flow Doppler is widely used to determine the severity of the regurgitation allowing for visualization of the width of the jet (vena contracta), the spatial orientation of the regurgitant jet area in the receiving chamber (jet area), and flow convergence into the regurgitant orifice (proximal isovelocity surface area [PISA]). The major criteria for diagnosing severe TR are a vena contracta width greater than 0.7 cm; a PISA radius greater than 0.9 cm; and evidence of systolic flow reversal in the hepatic veins, although this finding is inaccurate in the presence of atrial fibrillation.

In functional TR, dilation of the RA, RV, and tricuspid annulus are by definition present. In addition, there can be findings of paradoxical septal movement reflecting the increased volume within the right ventricle. Specific findings of an apically displaced tricuspid valve and atrialization of the ventricular tissue is seen in Ebstein's anomaly. In patients with endocarditis, vegetations may be seen on the atrial side of the tricuspid valve and/or an associated flail leaflet. Prolapse of the valve may be readily apparent with TTE. Thickened and retracted leaflets are the hallmark of carcinoid valvular disease, which is similar to the findings seen in drug-induced valvular disease due to elevated serotonin levels.

Transesophageal echocardiography (TEE) is rarely needed for TR assessment due to the excellent assessment provided by TTE. Only in those patients with poor acoustic windows should TEE be utilized. Occasionally, in the intraoperative setting, TEE is used to measure the tricuspid annulus diameter and may contribute to surgical decisions regarding TV annuloplasty.

Cardiac catheterization has no role in the diagnosis of TR due to distortion of the TV with placement of catheters into the RV and leading to false assessments with respect to the severity of the TR. However, right heart catheterization is strongly advised in the clinical setting of right ventricular hypertension in order to properly document the right ventricular, pulmonary artery, pulmonary capillary wedge pressure, and measurement of cardiac output. These values allow calculation of the transpulmonary gradient and the pulmonary vascular resistance, which aids in the management of the patient. A systolic PA pressure greater than 55 mm Hg is likely to cause TR with an anatomically normal tricuspid valve, whereas TR occurring with a systolic PA pressure less than 40 mm Hg is likely to reflect a structural abnormality of the valve apparatus (Fig. 35-2).

Treatment

TR in the absence of right ventricular hypertension is generally well tolerated, as exemplified in patients who have undergone tricuspid valvectomy due to endocarditis where dilation of the RV occurs months or years later. The majority of these patients can be managed with efforts directed to control systemic venous congestion with diuretics, although some patients may go on to develop atrial arrhythmias that will require additional therapy. Certain patients with severe TR may benefit from surgical intervention, especially if there is concomitant mitral valve disease requiring operative treatment and if there is a class I indication (Level of Evidence: B) according to the most recently published ACC/AHA guidelines (Chapter 59). As a whole, though, the timing of surgical intervention for TR remains controversial, as do the surgical techniques. Differing annuloplasty procedures with and without a supporting ring have been utilized with varying degrees of success. These include plication of the posterior leaflet annulus (bicuspidization), partial purse string reduction in the anterior and posterior leaflet annulus (DeVega annuloplasty), placement of a semirigid ring (Carpentier–Edwards), and placement of a flexible band (Cosgrove annuloplasty system). More recently, there have been clinical evaluations utilizing a three-dimensional annuloplasty system (MC3 ring) in an attempt to preserve atrioventricular dynamics. All of these techniques tend to reduce but do not eliminate TR and every effort should be made to reduce the RV pressure with medications.

Tricuspid valve replacement (TVR) is performed only when annuloplasty is not feasible due to diseased or abnormal valve leaflets and receives a class IIa (Level of Evidence: C) indication for those patients with severe primary TR. When possible, a bioprosthesis is preferred due to high rates of thromboembolic complications in patients with a mechanical prosthesis in the tricuspid position. In patients with conduction system disease, insertion of a permanent epicardial pacing wire at the time of valve surgery can obviate the need for a subsequent transvenous lead across the prosthetic valve.

In contrast to the recommendation for correction of severe symptomatic TR, the guidelines conclude that the weight of evidence is less well established for TV annuloplasty in patients with less than severe TR, who are to undergo MV surgery with a dilated tricuspid annulus in the presence of RV hypertension. Often with correction of the mitral valve disease, the lowering of the left atrial and right ventricular pressures result in significant improvement of the TR; therefore clinical judgment is essential.

Currently, there are no acceptable approved percutaneous techniques available. However, with continued experience and refinement, edge-to-edge valve repair may be an option in the future for those symptomatic patients who are not considered to be optimal surgical candidates.

TRICUSPID STENOSIS

【 】 ETIOLOGY

Tricuspid stenosis (TS) is a rare clinical entity with RHD accounting for greater than 90% of the cases. In patients with rheumatic mitral valve disease, only 5% to 15% have concurrent TS. There are several conditions that mimic TS by causing obstruction to tricuspid inflow. These include tricuspid atresia, right atrial myxomas (or other tumors), carcinoid syndrome (more likely to cause regurgitation), right atrial thrombus, and bacterial endocarditis.

【 】 DIAGNOSIS

Due to the pressure gradient across the tricuspid valve, the patient with TS notices signs and symptoms related to the elevated RA pressure. The obstruction to forward flow leads to decreased cardiac output and fatigue. Due to the low cardiac output, the lung fields may be clear and the patient may be comfortable while lying supine despite the profound ascites and occasional anasarca. Cardiac findings may be masked by the concomitant mitral stenosis, requiring a high index of suspicion that TS is present.

The cardiac examination may reveal an opening snap at the left lower sternal border. The murmur is usually softer, higher pitched, and shorter in duration than the murmur of MS and increases in intensity with maneuvers which increase tricuspid flow. The presystolic component has a scratchy quality and is the result of atrial contraction when sinus rhythm is present (Fig. 35-3). In the presence of sinus rhythm, jugular venous pulsations reveal a prominent A wave and a diminished rate of Y descent. In atrial fibrillation, it is extremely difficult to diagnose due to the loss of the A wave and the reduction in the intensity of the murmur.

The ECG in sinus rhythm reveals right atrial enlargement and commonly biatrial enlargement due to the concomitant MS. Atrial fibrillation is present in the majority of patients. The CXR is notable for cardiomegaly and enlargement of the right heart border without dilation of the pulmonary artery.

Echocardiographic findings included restricted and thickened leaflets with diastolic doming. There is less calcification and thickening of the tricuspid valves when compared to the mitral valve in patients with combined RHD. A diastolic pressure gradient of 3 to 5 mm Hg is enough to lead to elevated systemic vascular congestion and it rarely exceeds 10 mm Hg. It is extremely important to accurately define the degree of TR as this can impact the decision to proceed with balloon valvotomy.

Right heart catheterization can be performed with simultaneous pressure measurements of the RA and RV (Fig. 35-4). Because a clinically significant obstruction may be present with a minimal gradient (2–4 mm Hg), it is imperative that the transducers be calibrated equisensitive. However, catheterization is not usually necessary, because accurate measurements may be obtained by noninvasive means.

【 】 TREATMENT

Initially, diuretics and sodium restriction may improve the symptoms due to fluid retention. Definitive therapy includes balloon valvotomy; however, reported experience in the literature is limited. Severe TR is a known consequence of this procedure, thus limiting its long-term success when it develops. In patients with severe concomitant MS, TS should not be corrected alone, as this can exacerbate the symptoms of the mitral valve

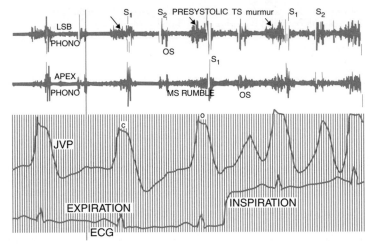

FIGURE 35-3. A phonocardiogram at the left sternal border and apex are recorded together with the jugular venous pulse in a patient with combined mitral stenosis and tricuspid stenosis. At the apex, a loud opening snap introduces a long diastolic rumble that terminates with a loud S_1. At the left sternal border, a crescendo-decrescendo presystolic murmur increases in intensity with inspiration and occurs simultaneously with a prominent A wave of the jugular venous pulse (JVP). There is no respiratory variation in the intensity of the apical mitral rumble. The gradual Y descent of the JVP is typical of tricuspid stenosis. (Reproduced with permission from Shaver JA. Current uses of phonocardiography in clinical practice. In: Rapaport E, ed. *Cardiology Update: Reviews for Physicians.* New York, NY: Elsevier; 1981:366.)

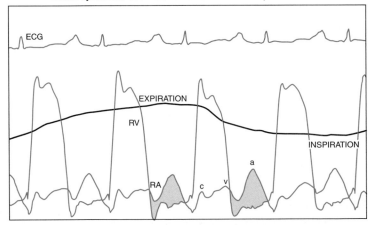

FIGURE 35-4. Reproduced with permission from Shaver JA. Hemodynamics in valvular heart disease. In: Lewis RP, O'Gara PT, Hirsch G. *ACCSAP Version 6 (Core Cardiology. Adult Clinical Cardiology Self-Assessment Program).* Bethesda, MD: American College of Cardiology Foundation; 2005.

disease due to increased forward cardiac output across the left-sided valve. Therefore, surgical treatment of the TS should be carried out at the same time as the MS.

PULMONARY VALVE DISEASE

【 】 NORMAL ANATOMY

The pulmonic valve consists of the annulus, leaflets, and commisures. There are no chordal attachments, thus making the opening and closing a passive process. It lies closest to the chest wall of all cardiac valves with its orifice is directed toward the left shoulder.

【 】 PULMONARY REGURGITATION

Etiology

The most common etiology of pulmonary regurgitation (PR) is due to dilation of the annulus as a result of pulmonary HTN. Dilation of the pulmonary artery itself may occur in the absence of pulmonary HTN, such as in Marfan's syndrome and idiopathic dilatation of the pulmonary artery. PR may also be caused by infective endocarditis or as a late manifestation of previously treated CHD. The two most commonly encountered congenital disorders associated with PR include prior treatment of congenital PS and repair of tetralogy of Fallot (TOF). PR can also develop as a result of primary lesions affecting the valve such as absent or malformed leaflets, which usually occur with other congenital abnormalities.

Diagnosis

In the setting of severe pulmonary hypertension (PH), the symptoms of the patient are primarily related to the cause of the PH (idiopathic pulmonary arterial hypertension, severe mitral stenosis, Eisenmenger syndrome, etc.). *The functional murmur (Graham Steell's murmur) is identical to the murmur of aortic regurgitation because the hemodynamics responsible for their production are identical. The differential diagnosis is made by the "company the murmur keeps," and the ancillary findings of both diseases establish the diagnosis.*

The symptoms of organic pulmonary regurgitation may be well tolerated for many years. However, in some patients, the chronic RV overload may cause clinical right ventricular failure. The murmur of organic regurgitation is quite different than the Graham Steell's murmur (PR) associated with pulmonary arterial hypertension (PAH). This organic PR murmur is frequently delayed from the pulmonic closure sound, and then builds up quickly to a crescendo followed by a decrescendo, which ends well before S_1 (Chapter 1). Since organic pulmonic regurgitation is usually in the setting of a normal pulmonary artery pressure, the diastolic gradient between the pulmonary artery and right ventricle is very small, resulting in a low-velocity retrograde flow and a lower-pitched murmur. Frequently, there is an associated systolic ejection murmur due to the large stroke volume of the right ventricle.

In the absence of PAH, the ECG may only manifest incomplete right bundle-branch block (RBBB) due to diastolic volume overload. However, when associated with PAH, the ECG traditionally shows RVH. The CXR shows nonspecific signs of prominence of the main pulmonary artery and RV enlargement and the associated findings related to the cause of the PR.

TTE will allow for a complete noninvasive evaluation of the morphology and physiology of the PV as well as the size and function of the RV. Abnormal flattening of the interventricular septum may be noted in diastole due to the increased volume in the RV displacing the septum toward the LV cavity. The degree of septal flattening has been shown to correlate with the severity of the PAH. Abnormal Doppler signals in the right ventricular outflow tract (RVOT) with velocity sustained throughout diastole are generally observed in patients with a dilated annulus. In contrast, when the velocity falls during diastole, the PA pressure is usually normal and the PR is due to a primary abnormality of the valve itself.

Due to limitations in imaging of the pulmonic valve secondary to adjacent lung tissue and near-field artifact, cardiac magnetic resonance imaging (CMR) is a useful and complimentary tool in the assessment of the severity of PR. In particular, CMR may play a role in the assessment of post-TOF repair patients and assist with decisions regarding the timing of surgical intervention.

Treatment

PR alone is rarely severe enough to require specific treatment. Treatment of the primary condition responsible for the PR will often dramatically improve the degree of PR. However, in the rare CHD patient with severe PR secondary to remote successful repair of TOF and New York Heart Association (NYHA) class II or III symptoms (Chapter 59), surgical consideration may be indicated for those with RV dilation and RV dysfunction. There are no current published guidelines to assist with decision-making in this group of patients, although intuitively PVR would seem to make sense in highly symptomatic patients with evidence of increased RV end-systolic or end-diastolic volumes. Under such circumstances, low-risk PVR has been performed with insertion of a homograft or xenograft. Pulmonary percutaneous valve implantation has been performed in the pediatric population with reported success.

PULMONIC STENOSIS

【 】 ETIOLOGY

Because the pulmonary valve is the least likely valve to be affected by acquired heart disease, virtually all cases of pulmonic stenosis (PS) are congenital. Less common noncongenital causes include the carcinoid syndrome, rheumatic fever, and stenosis of a bioprosthetic valve. Infundibular stenosis is rare as an isolated condition but often accompanies valvular PS due to hypertrophy of the RVOT and typically regresses after correction of the valvular PS.

In congenital PS, the valve is either dome shaped due to fusion of the valve leaflets, or thickened and dysplastic resulting in inability of leaflet separation during ventricular systole.

【 】 DIAGNOSIS

Mild and moderate degrees of PS are generally well tolerated. When symptoms from PS develop, they mainly consist of dyspnea on exertion and fatigue due mainly to the limitation of augmentation of right ventricular cardiac output. Severe PS may lead to RV failure and cyanosis in the presence of a concomitant interatrial communication.

The PE reveals a basal systolic murmur heard best in the second left interspace and similar to aortic stenosis in intensity, configuration, and pitch. With increasing degrees of obstruction, both the duration of the murmur and the width of the splitting increase. The pulmonic component of the second heart sound may be widely split or difficult to hear. When an ejection click is present, it suggests a valvular lesion as opposed to a supravalvular or infravalvular stenosis, although it may be absent with severe stenosis as it occurs earlier in systole and can be superimposed with the first heart sounds. A parasternal impulse and a prominent A wave in the JVP are present with significant RV hypertrophy.

The ECG is often normal in mild to moderate PS; however, as the stenosis becomes severe, RA abnormalities, RVH, and RAD are present. In addition RBBB is common, except in Noonan's syndrome, where left bundle-branch block may be seen.

Echocardiography is the gold standard to assess the severity of the PS as well as to determine the size and function of the RV. It is a class I recommendation in the ACC/AHA Guidelines (Chapter 59) for the initial evaluation and serial 5- to 10-year follow-up examinations. The guidelines define the severity of the lesion based on the following findings using Doppler techniques:

1. Peak velocity across the PV greater than 4 m/s (peak gradient >60 mm Hg)—severe.

2. Peak velocity across the PV greater than 3 m/s and less than 4 m/s (peak gradient 36–60 mm Hg)—moderate.

3. Peak velocity across the PV less than 3 m/s (peak gradient <36 mm Hg)—mild.

Cardiac catheterization is rarely recommended unless a therapeutic intervention is being considered. Diagnostic cardiac catheterization actually receives a class III indication from the most recent ACC/AHA guidelines as an initial diagnostic strategy (Chapter 59).

【 】 TREATMENT

The clinical course of children and young adults with PS has been well described. Mild congenital PS is a benign disease that rarely progresses. Those with moderate or severe disease can be improved with either surgery or endovascular techniques. The exception is the presence of Noonan's syndrome, which generally requires PVR due to the severely dysplastic valve. Otherwise, either procedure can be performed with low risk to the patient by experienced operators. Both treatment modalities afford excellent long-term outcomes as manifested by a low rate of recurrent PS.

SUGGESTED READING

Baddour LM, Wilson WR, Bayer AS, et al. Infective endocarditis: diagnosis, antimicrobial therapy, and management of complications. *Circulation.* 2005;112: 3167–3184.

Bonow RO, Carabello BA, Chatterjee K, et al. ACC/AHA 2006 practice guidelines for the management of patients with valvular heart disease. *J Am Coll Cardiol.* 2006;48:598–675.

Edwards WD. Cardiac anatomy and examination of cardiac specimens. In: Allen HD, Driscoll DJ, Shaddy RE, et al., eds. *Moss & Adams Heart Disease in Infants, Children & Adolescents.* Baltimore, MD: Lippincott Williams & Wilkins; 2007:2–34.

Khambadkone S, Coats. L, Taylor A, et al. Percutaneous pulmonary valve implantation in humans. *Circulation.* 2005;112:1189–1197.

McCarthy PM, Bhudia SK, Rajeswaran J, et al. Tricuspid valve repair: durability and risk factors for failure. *J Thorac Cardiovasc Surg.* 2004;127:674–685.

Nath J, Foster E, Heidenreich PA. Impact of TR on long-term survival. *J Am Coll Cardiol.* 2004;43:405–409.

Rizzoli G, Vendramin I, Nesseris G, et al. Biologic or mechanical prostheses in the tricuspid position? A meta analysis of intra-institutional results. *Ann Thorac Surg.* 2004;77:1607–1614.

Roth BL. Drugs and valvular heart disease. *N Engl J Med.* 2007;356:6–9.

Sorrell VL, Altbach MI, Kudithpudi V, et al. Cardiac MRI is an important complementary tool to Doppler echocardiography in the management of patients with pulmonary regurgitation. *Echocardiography.* 2007;24:316–328.

Zoghbi WA, Enriquez-Sarano M, Foster E, et al. Recommendations for evaluation of the severity of native valvular regurgitation with two dimensional and Doppler echocardiography. *J Am Soc Echocardiogr.* 2003;16:777–802.

CHAPTER (36)

Prosthetic Heart Valves: Choice of Valve and Management of the Patient

YingXing Wu, Gary L. Grunkemeier, Albert Starr,
and Shahbudin H. Rahimtoola

A heart valve prosthesis consists of an orifice through which blood flows and an occluding mechanism that closes and opens the orifice. There are two classes of prosthetic heart valves (PHVs): *mechanical prostheses*, with rigid, manufactured occluders; and *biological* or *tissue valves*, with flexible leaflet occluders of animal or human origin. Among the mechanical valves, there are three basic types, depending on whether the occluding mechanism is a reciprocating ball, a tilting disk, or two semicircular hinged leaflets. The biological valves include those whose origin is from the patient, from another human, or from another species.

PROSTHETIC HEART VALVES

〖 〗 MECHANICAL VALVES

The first successful PHV, which led to long-term survivors, used a ball-in-cage design and was introduced in 1960. Then came the low-profile disk valves in the early 1970s, followed by bileaflet valves since the early 1980s. Currently, most mechanical valves being implanted are bileaflet valves. Nevertheless, the "current" Starr-Edwards ball valves (models A1200/A1260 and M6120) that were introduced in 1965 have endured until today.

〖 〗 BIOLOGICAL VALVES

Bioprosthesis (heterograft or xenograft) is a term that was introduced by Carpentier for nonviable valves of biological origin, such as the porcine and bovine pericardial valves. Bioprostheses are mounted on rigid or flexible stents (stented) to which the leaflets and the sewing ring are attached. Nonstented versions are also available (stentless). Pericardial valves are tailored and sewn into a valvular configuration using bovine pericardium as a fabric, resulting in a valve that opens more completely than a porcine valve and thus provides better hemodynamics. Other biological valves are homografts (or allograft) and autografts. A homograft valve is transplanted from another human; the homograft is obtained at autopsy.

GUIDELINES FOR CLINICAL REPORTING

The reporting of clinical results of heart valves has evolved since the first successful implants in 1960. In 1994, the Food and Drug Administration (FDA) issued a guidance

432

document for submission of premarket approval (PMA) applications for heart valves that emphasize confidence interval estimation and comparison to objective performance criteria (OPC). OPC are complication rates for critical complications, representing averages that were achieved by the best currently used valves at that time.

Standards that specified which complications should be collected and how they should be defined were proposed by a joint committee of the American Association for Thoracic Surgery and the Society of Thoracic Surgeons (AATS/STS) and were revised. Complications that were determined to be of critical importance by these guidelines include *structural valvular deteriorations* and *nonstructural dysfunction* (including *prosthesis–patient mismatch*), *valve thrombosis, embolism, bleeding event,* and *operated valvular endocarditis.* The *consequences* of these morbid events include reoperation, valve-related mortality, sudden unexpected unexplained death, cardiac death, total deaths, and permanent valve-related impairment.

CHOICE OF PROSTHETIC HEART VALVE

When considering a PHV for an individual patient one has to account for known patient outcomes (survival and complications) with use of a particular PHV. The known patient outcomes are influenced by factors related to publications and to patients. Factors related to publications include reporting center, data analysis, selection bias, and publication. Table 36-1 lists patient factors influencing operative and late mortality. Table 36-2 lists the factors that need to be considered when choosing a PHV.

The most frequent issue is whether to choose a mechanical or bioprosthetic PHV. The choice is based on balancing the advantages and disadvantages of these two types of PHV. Mechanical valves are durable but have the problem of thrombogenicity, and thus require lifetime anticoagulation therapy. Biological valves have low thrombogenicity but have the problem of structural valve deterioration (SVD), and thus the risk of reoperation. Figure 36-1 shows the recommendations based on age (and therefore rate of SVD) and ability to take warfarin anticoagulant therapy. Figure 36-2 shows the factors to be considered in the choice of PHV for young women with valvular heart disease. Table 36-3 lists the American College of Cardiologists/American Heart Association (ACC/AHA)

TABLE 36-1

Factors Influencing Operative and Late Mortality After PHV[a]

- Decade of age
- Other valve disease
- Complications of PHV
- Comorbid conditions
- Cardiac
  LV dysfunction, heart failure, NYHA functional class III and IV, CAD, myocardial infarction, CABG, arrhythmias (e.g., atrial fibrillation), pulmonary hypertension
- Noncardiac
  Impaired renal function (creatinine clearance), renal dialysis, diabetes, hypertension, dyslipidemia, metabolic syndrome, smoking, liver disease, lung disease (e.g., COPD)

CABG, coronary artery bypass graft; CAD, coronary artery disease; COPD, chronic obstructive pulmonary disease; LV, left ventricle; NYHA, New York Heart Association; PHV, prosthetic heart valve.

[a]For operative (30-day mortality) additional factors include emergency surgery > urgent > elective; previous cardiac surgery; perioperative myocardial infarction; and duration of the operation and of aortic cross-clamp time.

Copyright by S. H. Rahimtoola.

TABLE 36-2

Deciding Which Prosthetic Heart Valve to Choose

Factors to be considered
Age of the patient
Comorbid conditions
    Cardiac
    Noncardiac
Expected life span of patient
Long-term known outcomes with prosthetic heart valve
Skill and experience with procedure(s) and prosthetic heart valve at the Medical
    Center and of Physicians
Patient's "wishes"
Other extenuating circumstances

Copyright by S. H. Rahimtoola.

 TABLE 36-3

Major Criteria for Aortic Valve Selection[a]

Class I

1. A mechanical prosthesis is recommended for aortic valve replacement (AVR) in patients with a mechanical valve in the mitral or tricuspid position. *(Level of Evidence: C)*
2. A bioprostheses is recommended for AVR in patients of any age who will not take warfarin or who have major medical contraindications to warfarin therapy. *(Level of Evidence: C)*

Class IIa

1. Patient preference is a reasonable consideration in the selection of aortic valve operation and valve prosthesis. A mechanical prosthesis is reasonable for AVR in patients less than 65 years of age who do not have a contraindication for anticoagulation. A bioprosthesis is reasonable for AVR in patients under 65 years of age who elect to receive this valve for lifestyle considerations after detailed discussions of the risk of anticoagulation versus the likelihood that a second AVR may be necessary in the future. *(Level of Evidence: C)*
2. A bioprosthesis is reasonable for AVR in patients age 65 years or older without risk factors for thromboembolism. *(Level of Evidence: C)*
3. Aortic valve re-replacement with a homograft is reasonable for patients with active prosthetic valve endocarditis. *(Level of Evidence: C)*

Class IIb

1. A bioprosthesis might be considered for AVR in a woman of childbearing age. *(Level of Evidence: C)*

[a]See also Chapter 59.

Reproduced with permission from American College of Cardiology/American Heart Association Task Force on Practice Guidelines; Society of Cardiovascular Anesthesiologists; Society for Cardiovascular Angiography and Interventions; Society of Thoracic Surgeons, Bonow RO, Carabello BA, Kanu C, et al. ACC/AHA 2006 guidelines for the management of patients with valvular heart disease: a report of the American College of Cardiology/American Heart Association Task Force on Practice Guidelines (Writing Committee to revise the 1998 guidelines for the management of patients with valvular heart disease): developed in collaboration with the Society of Cardiovascular Anesthesiologists: endorsed by the Society for Cardiovascular Angiography and Interventions and the Society of Thoracic Surgeons. *Circulation.* 2006;114(5):e84–e231.

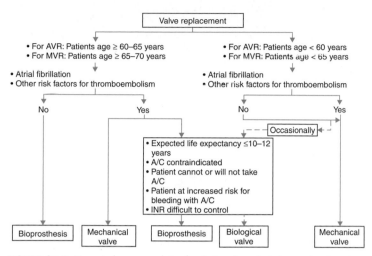

FIGURE 36-1. Suggested recommendation for choice of prosthetic heart valves based on age of the patient and the presence of risk factors. (A/C, anticoagulation with warfarin; AVR, aortic valve replacement; INR, international normalized ratio; MVR, mitral valve replacement.) (Rahimtoola SH. Choice of prosthetic heart valve in adult patients. *J Am Coll Cardiol.* 2003;41:893–904.)

recommendations for aortic valve selection. It must be emphasized that all such recommendations cannot apply to each and every patient because there are exceptions, and several factors that must be considered are shown in Table 36-2.

VALVE REPAIR

When practicable, mitral valve repair is preferable to replacement. Mitral valve repair also provides good results for treating infective endocarditis and for valve problems in elderly patients. It has been suggested that it improves survival and has lower complication rates. However, the weakness of valve repair is its durability which increases the risk of future reoperation.

Aortic valve repair is performed less often and is more technically difficult than mitral valve repair. Patients considered for aortic valve repair are generally young (who wish to avoid anticoagulation) with aortic regurgitation without a component of stenosis.

MANAGEMENT

Patients who have undergone valve replacement are not cured; they still have serious heart disease. They have exchanged native valvular disease for prosthetic valvular disease, and must be followed with great care. Table 36-4 lists major complications of valve replacement. Besides the complications specified in the AATS/STS guidelines, valve prosthesis–patient mismatch (VP–PM) is another type of complication that has been studied in the past three decades. No PHV currently used has an effective orifice as large as that of the native valve; consequently, VP–PM occurs. This is most important in a large patient in whom a prosthesis that is considered "small" in relation to body size must be placed for technical reasons. The resulting VP–PM (Table 36-5) contributes to

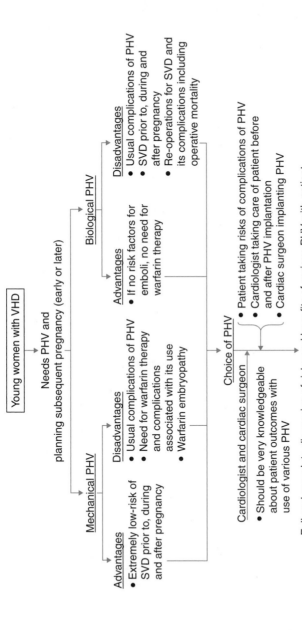

FIGURE 36-2. Factors to be considered in the choice of prosthetic heart valve (PHV) for young women with valvular heart disease (VHD). (SVD, structural valve deterioration.) (Hung L, Rahimtoola SH. Prosthetic heart valve and pregnancy. *Circulation.* 2003;107:1240–1246.)

TABLE 36-4

Major Complications of Valve Replacement

1. Operative mortality
2. Perioperative myocardial infarction
3. Prosthetic endocarditis
4. Prosthetic dehiscence
5. Prosthetic dysfunction
    a. Obstruction: usually thrombotic, occasionally caused by item 3, 4, or 8
    b. Regurgitation
    c. Hemolysis
    d. Structural failure
6. Thromboemboli
7. Hemorrhage with anticoagulant therapy
8. Valve prosthesis–patient mismatch
9. Prosthetic replacement often caused by items 3,4, or 5; occasionally caused by items 6,7, or 8
10. Late mortality, including sudden, unexplained death

From Rahimtoola SH. Valvular. Heart disease: a perspective. *J Am Coll Cardiol.* 1983;3:199–215. Reproduced with permission of the publisher and author.

 TABLE 36-5

Valve Prosthesis–Patient Mismatch

Aortic Valve		
Severity of Stenosis and of VP–PM after AVR	Valve Area (cm^2/m^2)	Clinical Status
Mild	> 0.9	Asymptomatic
Moderate	> 0.6–0.9	Asymptomatic (symptoms with associated conditions)
Severe	≤ 0.6	Asymptomatic or symptomatic[a]
Mitral Valve		
Severity of Mitral Valve Stenosis and VP–PM after MVR	Valve Area (cm^2)	Clinical Status
Very mild	> 2.0 cm^2	Asymptomatic
Mild	>1.5–2.0	Asymptomatic
Moderate	1.1–1.5	Usually asymptomatic, some symptomatic
Severe	≤ 1.0 cm^2	Asymptomatic or symptomatic[b]

AVR, aortic valve replacement; MVR, mitral valve replacement; VP–PM, valve prosthesis–patient mismatch.

[a]Symptoms: angina, syncope, dyspnea, heart failure, sudden death.
[b]Symptoms associated with left atrial and pulmonary arterial hypertension and low/reduced cardiac output and their consequences.

From Rahimtoola SH. Choice of prosthetic heart valve in adult patients. *J Am Coll Cardiol.* 2003;41:893–904. Reproduced with permission of the publisher and author.

incomplete relief of symptoms. Patients with VP–PM have been reported to have worse short-term and long-term outcomes.

All patients with prosthetic valves need appropriate antibiotics for prophylaxis against infective endocarditis (Chapter 38). Patients with rheumatic heart disease continue to need antibiotics as prophylaxis against the recurrence of rheumatic carditis. Adequate antithrombotic therapy is needed for appropriate patients (Chapter 38).

During the 4 to 6 weeks after surgery, the physician and surgeon jointly manage the patient, directing their attention toward relieving postoperative discomfort, readjusting cardiac medications, and instituting anticoagulation if not contraindicated. A graduated plan of activity is started that enables the patient to return to full activity in 4 to 6 weeks.

Several syndromes are peculiar to the postoperative period. The postperfusion syndrome usually appears in the third or fourth postoperative week. It is characterized by fever, splenomegaly, and atypical lymphocytes; it is benign and self-limited. The postpericardiotomy syndrome is characterized by fever and pleuropericarditis. It usually develops in the second or third postoperative week, but can appear as late as 1 year after surgery and sometimes recurs. Although this syndrome is usually self-limited, most patients benefit from taking anti-inflammatory drugs, such as aspirin or indomethacin; a short course of glucocorticoids is also occasionally required. Even though the pericardium is left open at the end of surgery, cardiac tamponade may occur during the first 6 weeks and needs to be relieved. Usually, anticoagulants have been given and the fluid is hemorrhagic.

The 4- to 6-week postoperative visit is critical, because by this time the patient's physical capabilities and expected improvement in functional capacity can usually be assessed. The recommendations for follow-up strategy are shown in Table 36-6.

Multiple noninvasive tests have emerged for assessing valvular and ventricular function. Echocardiography/Doppler is the most useful noninvasive test. Other noninvasive tests include fluoroscopy and radionuclide angiography.

TABLE 36-6

Suggestions for Follow-Up Strategy of Patient with Prosthetic Heart Valve

History, physical examination, ECG, chest radiograph, echocardiogram/Doppler, complete blood count, serum chemistries, and INR (if indicated) at first postoperative outpatient evaluation.[a]

Radionuclide angiography/CMR to assess LV function if result of echocardiography/Doppler is unsatisfactory.

CMR to assess native and PHV function if results of echocardiography/Doppler are unsatisfactory.

Routine follow-up visits at yearly intervals with earlier reevaluations for change in clinical status.

Routine serial echocardiograms at time of annual follow-up visit at 5 years after bioprosthetic MVR and at 8 years after bioprosthetic AVR even in the absence of change in clinical status.

Other tests, if indicated.

AVR, aortic valve replacement; CMR, cardiovascular magnetic resonance; INR, international normalized ratio; LV, left ventricle; MVR, mitral valve replacement; PHV, prosthetic heart valve.

[a]This evaluation should be performed 4 to 6 weeks after hospital discharge. In some settings, the outpatient echocardiogram may be difficult to obtain; if so, an inpatient echocardiogram may be obtained before hospital discharge. An echocardiogram/Doppler study at 6 to 12 months is essential for proper assessment of severity of valve prosthesis–patient mismatch.

Copyright by S. H. Rahimtoola.

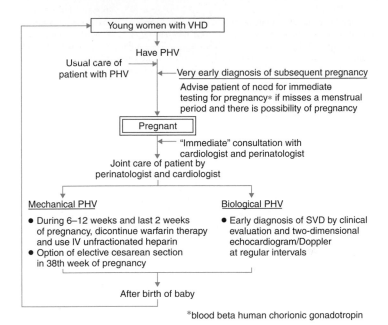

FIGURE 36-3. Management of the patient with prosthetic heart valve who becomes pregnant. (PHV, prosthetic heart valve; SVD, structural valve deterioration; VHD, valvular heart disease.) (Hung L, Rahimtoola SH. Prosthetic heart valve and pregnancy. *Circulation.* 2003;107;1240–1246.)

Figure 36-3 describes management of the patient with PHV who becomes pregnant.

"Heart failure" after valve replacement may be the result of (1) preoperative left ventricular dysfunction that improved partially or not at all, (2) perioperative myocardial damage, (3) progression of other valve disease, (4) complications of PHV, or (5) associated heart disease such as CAD and systemic arterial hypertension.

Any patient with a PHV who does not improve after the surgery or who later shows deterioration of functional capacity should undergo appropriate testing to determine the cause. For the patient with catastrophic dysfunction, surgery is clearly indicated and urgent.

ANTITHROMBOTIC THERAPY

All patients with mechanical valves require anticoagulant therapy. With the use of warfarin, the risk of thromboemboli in these patients is reduced but is still 1% to 2% per year; the risks are higher in the mitral than in the aortic position. Therefore, the international normalized ratio (INR) of the patient with an aortic mechanical valve should be about 2.5 (range, 2–3), and the INR of the patient with a mitral mechanical valve should be about 3.0 (range, 2.5–3.5). Many authorities recommend the addition of low-dose aspirin (81 mg) to warfarin unless there is a contraindication to its use. Importantly, the risk of thromboemboli is increased early after the insertion of a prosthetic valve (mechanical or biological); this is a reason to start heparin within 24 to 48 hours of surgery, as soon as it is safe to do so with maintenance of the activated partial thromboplastin time (aPPT) between 60 and 80 seconds until the recommended

INR level is achieved. Patients with biological valves can have the warfarin discontinued after 2 to 3 months. However, *even patients with biological valves* need continued warfarin therapy (INR 2.5; range, 2–3) if they have atrial fibrillation, severe left ventricular dysfunction, previous thromboembolism, and/or a hypercoagulable condition. The management of antithrombotic therapy is discussed in Chapter 37.

SUGGESTED READING

Bonow RO, Carabello B, Chatterjee K, et al. ACC/AHA 2006 guidelines for the management of patients with valvular heart disease: a report of the American College of Cardiology/American Heart Association Task Force on Practice Guidelines (writing committee to revise the 1998 Guidelines for the Management of Patients with Valvular Heart Disease). Developed in collaboration with the Society of Cardiovascular Anesthesiologists. Endorsed by the Society for Cardiovascular Angiography and Interventions and the Society of Thoracic Surgeons. *Circulation.* 2006;114:e84–e231. Erratum appears in *Circulation.* 2007;115:e409.

Edmunds LH Jr., Clark RE, Cohn LH, et al. Guidelines for reporting morbidity and mortality after cardiac valvular operations. *J Thorac Cardiovasc Surg.* 1996;112: 708–711.

Hammermeister K, Sethi GK, Henderson WG, et al. Outcomes 15 years after valve replacement with a mechanical vs bioprosthetic valve: final report of the VA randomized trial. *J Am Coll Cardiol.* 2000;36:1152–1158.

Hung L, Rahimtoola SH. Prosthetic heart valve and pregnancy. *Circulation.* 2003;107;1240–1246.

McAnulty JH, Rahimtoola SH. Antithrombotic therapy for valvular heart disease. In: Fuster V, Alexander RW, O'Rourke RA, et al., eds. *Hurst's The Heart.* 12th ed. New York, NY: McGraw-Hill; 2008:1800–1807.

Rahimtoola SH. Choice of prosthetic heart valve in adult patients. *J Am Coll Cardiol.* 2003;41:893–904.

Rahimtoola SH, YingXing Wu, Grunkemeier GL, et al. Prosthetic heart valves: choice of valve and management of the patient. In: Fuster V, O'Rourke RA, Walsh R, et al., eds. *Hurst's The Heart.* 12th ed. New York, NY: McGraw-Hill; 2008:1783–1799.

Turpie AG, Gent M, Laupacis A, et al. A double blind randomized trial of acetylsalicylic acid (100 mg) versus placebo in patients treated with oral anticoagulants following heart valve replacement. *N Engl J Med.* 1991;329:1365–1369.

CHAPTER 37

Antithrombotic Therapy for Valvular Heart Disease

Eric C. Stecker, John H. McAnulty, and
Shahbudin H. Rahimtoola

Although bleeding is a risk with all antithrombotic agents, the frequency and consequences of a stroke outweigh the bleeding risks associated with drug therapy in many patients with valve disease. This is particularly true in patients with prosthetic heart valves (PHV), but is also true in patients with native valve disease accompanied by comorbid conditions associated with thromboemboli (Table 37-1).

Antithrombotic therapy includes antiplatelet agents and anticoagulants. Warfarin, aspirin, unfractionated heparin, and thrombolytic agents are the only antithrombotic agents currently recommended for preventing or treating thromboemboli related to valve disease, although low-molecular-weight heparin is also widely used. *There are no randomized trials and few comparative data to guide therapy in preventing thromboemboli in valve-disease patients.*

NATIVE VALVE DISEASE

Patients with native valve disease require antithrombotic therapy only in the presence of an associated stroke *risk factor*. The two most common associated risk factors are atrial fibrillation and left ventricular (LV) systolic dysfunction.

【 】 RISK OF THROMBOEMBOLI WITH NATIVE VALVE DISEASE

Atrial Fibrillation

In six large, prospective, randomized trials assessing the value of antithrombotic therapy for primary stroke prevention in patients with nonvalvular, constant or paroxysmal, atrial fibrillation, the embolic rate (essentially a stroke) was 3% to 8% per year in the placebo or untreated patients. Some patients in the studies had valve disease, although patients with severe valvular disease (including all with mitral stenosis or PHV) were excluded. When an individual with native valve disease has associated intermittent or continuous atrial fibrillation, *antithrombotic treatment should be selected* based on the existing clinical trial evidence. Warfarin (with a target international normalized ratio [INR] of 2–3) is recommended in the setting of prior systemic embolus or if a patient has two or more of the following: diabetes mellitus, a history of hypertension, congestive heart failure, and age older than age 75 years. Those with none or only one of the risk factors can reasonably be given aspirin 325 mg/d as an alternative.

Left Ventricular Dysfunction

Systemic or pulmonary thromboemboli occur at a rate of over 5% per year in patients with LV systolic dysfunction. While antithrombotic therapy is of unproven value, the

TABLE 37-1

Valve Disease and Antithrombotic Therapy

1. Prevention of thromboemboli should be addressed each time a patient with valve disease is seen.
2. Lifelong antithrombotic therapy is required in patients with atrial fibrillation (paroxysmal or persistent), severe left ventricular dysfunction, or prior thromboembolism.
3. Warfarin therapy is required in all patients with a mechanical prosthesis (see Table 37-2).
4. Antithrombotic therapy should be started early after valve surgery.
5. Warfarin should be avoided in the first trimester of pregnancy.
6. Antithrombotic therapy should be individualized during noncardiac surgery and cardiovascular procedures.

risk of an embolic event is sufficient that, with or without valve disease, consideration should be given to treatment. Warfarin (INR 2–3) may be used if the LV ejection fraction (EF) is ≤ 0.30, or aspirin (325 mg daily) may be used if warfarin use is judged to be associated with excessive risk

Previous Thromboemboli

A thromboembolic event defines patients who are at high risk for having a recurrent event in clinical situations unrelated to native valve disease (e.g., in patients with atrial fibrillation or with a PHV). It is unclear whether this is true in patients with native valve disease, but lifelong warfarin therapy should be considered if there are no contraindications to its use.

Hypercoagulable Conditions

The presence of protein C, protein S, or antithrombin III deficiencies; the anticardiolipin antibody syndrome; resistance to activated protein C; or an associated malignancy increase risk of venous thrombosis. Concomitant native valve disease should be factored into the decision regarding anticoagulation, although there are no direct data to guide therapy.

【 】 OTHER POTENTIAL THROMBOEMBOLI RISK FACTORS

Beyond an assessment of LV systolic function, the use of transthoracic and transesophageal echocardiography to determine which patients are at risk of thromboemboli is not yet well defined. Left atrial enlargement or thrombi, a patent foramen ovale, an atrial septal aneurysm, or spontaneous echo contrast are findings of concern. The value of treatment based on these findings is unproven.

PROSTHETIC HEART VALVES

All patients with mechanical valves require warfarin therapy. Even with the use of warfarin, the risk of thromboemboli in these patients is 1% to 2% per year. The risk of an embolus in patients with biological valves in sinus rhythm is approximately 0.6% to 0.7% per year without antithrombotic therapy.

【 】 ANTITHROMBOTIC TREATMENT FOR PROSTHETIC VALVES

Table 37-2 gives an overview of antithrombotic treatment for prosthetic valves.

TABLE 37-2

Antithrombotic Therapy—Prosthetic Heart Valves[a]

	Mechanical Prosthetic Valves				Biological Prosthetic Valves		
	Warfarin INR 2–3	Warfarin INR 2.5–3.5	Aspirin 50–100 mg	Warfarin INR 2–3	Warfarin INR 2.5–3.5	Aspirin 50–100 mg
First 3 months after valve replacement		+	±		+	±
After first 3 months						
Aortic valve	+					
Aortic valve	+		±			+
Aortic valve + risk factor[b]		+	+	+		+
Aortic valve + embolus[c]		+	±	+		+
Mitral valve		+	+			+
Mitral valve + risk factor		+	±		+	±
Mitral valve + embolism[c]		+	+		+	+

+, Positive for prevention of thrombosis on prosthetic valves; ±, may prevent prosthetic clots; clinical judgment very important for addition of aspirin therapy; INR, international normalized ratio.

[a]Depending on the clinical status of patient, antithrombotic therapy must be individualized (see special situations in text).
[b]Risk factors: atrial fibrillation, left ventricle dysfunction, and hypercoagulable state.
[c]Embolus = previous thromboembolism.

NOTE: In an individual patient, there is a need for clinical judgment ± if aspirin is added to warfarin therapy.

Mechanical Valves

All patients with mechanical valves require anticoagulation, usually with warfarin. In patients with an aortic prosthesis without risk factors for emboli, the INR should be between 2.0 and 3.0; in those with risk factors and those with a mitral prosthesis, the INR should be between 2.5 and 3.5. The addition of low-dose aspirin (70–100 mg/d) to warfarin therapy further decreases the risk of thromboembolism and is recommended unless there is a contraindication.

Biological (Tissue) Valves

Because of an increased risk of thromboemboli during the *first 3 months* after implantation of a biological prosthetic valve, anticoagulation with warfarin is indicated. After that time, the tissue valve can be treated in the same way as native valve disease, and warfarin can be discontinued in approximately two-thirds of patients with biological valves. *Associated atrial fibrillation or an LV ejection fraction $\leq$ 30% are reasons for lifelong warfarin therapy.*

SPECIAL CLINICAL SITUATIONS

【 】 ALTERED NATIVE VALVES

Valve disease is treated increasingly by interventional catheter techniques. The recommendations given for treatment of native valve disease would seem most applicable in such patients; that is, antithrombotic treatment depends on associated stroke risk factors.

【 】 SURGERY AND DENTAL CARE

Although antithrombotic therapy must be individualized, some generalizations apply. For procedures in which bleeding is unlikely or would be inconsequential if it occurred, antithrombotic therapy should not be stopped. This can apply to surgery on the skin, dental prophylaxis, or simple treatment for dental caries.

When bleeding is likely or its potential consequences are severe, antithrombotic treatment should be altered. If a patient is on aspirin, it should be discontinued 1 week before the procedure and restarted as soon as it is considered safe by the surgeon or dentist.

For most patients taking warfarin, the drug should be stopped 72 hours before the procedure to achieve an INR $\leq$ 1.5. Unless postoperative hemorrhage occurs, warfarin can be restarted within 24 hours after the procedure. Admission to the hospital or a delay in discharge to give heparin is usually unnecessary. Deciding who is at very high risk of thrombosis and thus should require "bridging" with heparin until warfarin can be reinstated may be difficult; clinical judgment is required. Heparin can usually be reserved for patients who have had a prior thromboembolism, patients with demonstrated thrombotic problems when previously off therapy, and patients with two or more risk factors. When used, heparin should be started 24 hours after warfarin is stopped (i.e., 48 hours before surgery) and stopped 6 to 12 hours before the procedure. Heparin should be restarted as early after surgery as bleeding stability allows and the partial thromboplastin time (aPTT) maintained at a "therapeutic level" until warfarin is restarted and the desired INR can be achieved. Home administration and management of heparin (and warfarin) can be arranged to minimize hospitalization.

【 】 CARDIAC CATHETERIZATION AND ANGIOGRAPHY

Neither antiplatelet therapy nor heparin need be stopped for these procedures. Cardiac catheterization can be performed with a patient taking warfarin, but preferably, the drug should be stopped 72 hours before the procedure and restarted after the procedure on the same day. If a patient is at very high risk of thromboembolism, heparin should be started 48 hours before the procedure and continued until warfarin is restarted and the desired INR is achieved. If the catheterization procedure is to include a transseptal puncture (especially in a patient who has not had previous opening of the pericardium), patients should be off all antithrombotic therapy and the INR should be < 1.2.

【 】 CORONARY ARTERY STENTS

Many patients with valve disease require a stent as treatment for coronary artery disease. A thienopyridine agent, usually clopidogrel, is used for at least 1 month (and up to 12 months or more for drug-eluting stents) to prevent in-stent thrombosis. Clopidogrel has no proven efficacy in preventing thromboemboli in patients with a PHV, so continuation of warfarin is recommended in patients with mechanical prostheses. If these patients are also on aspirin (along with warfarin), it would seem prudent that it be stopped given concerns of bleeding, but this is unproved. Patients with tissue valves taking aspirin should continue that drug after stent insertion.

【 】 PREGNANCY

Indications for antithrombotic therapy are not altered by pregnancy but treatment regimens have to be adjusted. This is because of risks to fetal development but also because of concerns about fetal and maternal bleeding. The incidence of warfarin-caused embryopathy is 3% to 25% when the drug is taken in the first 3 months (particularly weeks 6 to 12). It can essentially be eliminated by avoiding warfarin during this time and possibly be using doses of less than 5 mg/d. Heparin does not cross the placenta, but like warfarin, can be ineffective or cause maternal bleeding. Given these concerns, in the pregnant women requiring anticoagulant for her valve, it is recommended that she use heparin for the first 3 months and then switch to warfarin. At 1 to 3 weeks before labor and delivery, when it can be predicted, she should switch back to heparin. The return to heparin is with the hope of better control of maternal bleeding with labor and delivery, should it occur, and to prevent fetal hemorrhage as the baby will be anticoagulated if the mother is taking warfarin. If the mother has a PHV, use of low-molecular-weight heparin should be individualized for the reasons outlined in the previous discussion of "bridging."

【 】 THERAPY AT THE TIME OF A THROMBOEMBOLIC EVENT

Acute Management

Data and opinions about optimal timing for initiating or continuing anticoagulants in patients in whom an embolus is the presumed cause of a stroke are conflicting. Antithrombotic therapy should be withheld or stopped for 72 hours because of excessive rates of conversion from nonhemorrhagic to hemorrhagic stroke. If a computed tomography (CT) scan at 3 days reveals little or no hemorrhage, heparin should be administered to maintain an aPTT at the lower end of the therapeutic level until warfarin, started at the same time, results in the desired INR. If the CT scan demonstrates significant hemorrhage, antithrombotic therapy should be withheld until the bleed has been treated or has stabilized (7–14 days). Anticoagulation can then be started as just described.

Long-Term Management

If the embolic event occurs when a patient is *off* antithrombotic therapy, long-term warfarin therapy is required. If the embolic event occurs while the patient is *on* adequate antithrombotic treatment, therapy should be altered as follows:

- If on warfarin, with an INR of 2 to 3: increase dose to achieve an INR of 2.5 to 3.5.
- If on warfarin, with an INR of 2.5 to 3.5: add aspirin 50 to 100 mg/d.
- If on warfarin, with an INR of 2.5 to 3.5, plus aspirin 80 to 100 mg/d: aspirin dose may also need to be increased to 325 mg/d.
- If on aspirin 325 mg/d: switch to warfarin to achieve an INR of 2 to 3.

Embolism occurring after this medical approach should lead to consideration of possible valve surgery if the valve is the likely source of the thrombus.

【　】 EXCESSIVE ANTICOAGULATION

In most patients with INR above the therapeutic range, excessive anticoagulation can be managed by withholding warfarin. Patients with PHVs with an INR of 5 to 10 who are not bleeding can be managed by withholding warfarin and administering oral vitamin K, often as an inpatient to monitor for bleeding. In emergency situations, the use of fresh-frozen plasma is preferable to high-dose vitamin K_1, especially *parenteral vitamin K_1*, because use of the latter increases the *risks of overcorrection to a hypercoagulable state and of anaphylaxis.* Human recombinant factor (rFVIIa), dose 15 to 19 µg/kg body weight, has been used to reverse critically prolonged INR and bleeding complications safely and rapidly.

【　】 THERAPY AT THE TIME OF A BLEED

With significant bleeding, antithrombotic therapy should be stopped and, if the patient is at risk, drug effects should be reversed. If possible, the cause of bleeding should be corrected and antithrombotic therapy restarted as soon as possible. If this is not possible, treatment decisions are difficult. In patients with a mechanical prosthesis or multiple risk factors for thromboemboli, acceptance of intermittent bleeding with acute management of bleeding may be necessary. In valve patients who are at lower risk of emboli or in whom the role of antithrombotic treatment is less clear (e.g., LV dysfunction), it may be optimal to withhold chronic therapy or, if a patient is on warfarin, to switch to aspirin. With mechanical PHVs, consideration should be given to replacing the mechanical valve with a biologic valve in some patients (e.g., in those who have had multiple, large, life- or organ-threatening bleeds).

【　】 THROMBOSIS OF PROSTHETIC HEART VALVES

PHV obstruction is caused by thrombus in approximately 50%, pannus in 10%, and pannus plus thrombus in 40% of cases. Diagnosis can be difficult and requires knowledge of the clinical presentation and results of Doppler echocardiography (transthoracic and/or transesophageal). Pannus is tissue in-growth; therefore, thrombolytic therapy is ineffective and if obstruction is severe, valve replacement is indicated. If a patient has a thrombotic obstruction of a right-sided PHV, thrombolytics are the first choice of therapy as they are successful in 80% to 100% of treated patients.

Left-sided PHV thrombosis (aortic and mitral) is more serious. With use of thrombolytics, studies show a mortality of 2% to 16% depending on New York Heart Association (NYHA) functional status, thromboembolism in 12% to 15%, major bleeding in 5%, and nondisabling bleeding in 14%. Best results were obtained in patients who are in NYHA functional classes I and II and who have a "small" thrombus. Surgical replacement of the thrombosed PHV is associated with a mortality of 10% to 60%.

【　】 INFECTIVE ENDOCARDITIS

If a patient with valve disease develops endocarditis, antithrombotic therapy should be continued. If the patient presents with or develops an embolic event involving the central nervous system, therapy should be as described above for acute embolic events.

Additionally, the issue of whether or not the embolus is caused by thrombus or infected vegetation should be addressed. If thrombus is likely, the chronic anticoagulation program will also require alteration.

SUGGESTED READING

Bates SM, Greer IA, Hirsh J, et al. Use of antithrombotic agents during pregnancy. The seventh ACCP conference on antithrombotic and thrombolytic therapy. *Chest.* 2004;126 (suppl):627S–644S.

Bonow RO, Carabello B, Chatterjee K, et al. ACC/AHA 2006 guidelines for the management of patients with valvular heart disease: a report of the American College of Cardiology/American Heart Association Task Force on Practice Guidelines (Writing Committee to Revise the 1998 Guidelines for the Management of Patients with Valvular Heart Disease). Developed in collaboration with the Society of Cardiovascular Anesthesiologists. Endorsed by the Society for Cardiovascular Angiography and Interventions and the Society of Thoracic Surgeons. *Circulation.* 2006;114:e84–e231.

Hammermeister K, Sethi GK, Henderson WG, et al. Outcomes 15 years after valve replacement with a mechanical versus a bioprosthetic valve: final report of the veterans affairs randomized trial. *J Am Coll Cardiol.* 2000;36:1152–1158.

McAnulty JH, Rahimtoola SH. Antithrombotic therapy for valvular heart disease. In: Fuster V, O'Rourke RA, Walsh RA, et al., eds. *Hurst's The Heart.* 12th ed. New York, NY: McGraw-Hill; 2008:1800–1807.

Rahimtoola SH. Choice of prosthetic heart valve for adult patients. *J Am Coll Cardiol.* 2003;41:893–904.

Salem DN, Stein PD, Al Ahmad A, et al. Antithrombotic therapy in valvular heart disease—native and prosthetic. *Chest.* 2004;126 (suppl):457S–482S.

CHAPTER (38)

Infective Endocarditis

Christian T. Ruff, Saptarsi Haldar, and Patrick T. O'Gara

Infective endocarditis (IE) is a disease caused by microbial infection of the endothelial lining of intracardiac structures and is invariably fatal if untreated. Infection most commonly resides on one or more heart valve leaflets, but may involve mural endocardium, chordal structures, myocardium, and pericardium. The presence of an intracardiac or endovascular device provides a nidus for infection, as well as a barrier to eradication. Despite the diagnosis and treatment of IE, the 6-month mortality rates still approach 25%. Changes in both patient demographics and microbial biology have challenged conventional wisdom.

EPIDEMIOLOGY

In the first half of the 20th century, IE was predominantly a complication of rheumatic heart disease and poor dentition. In developing countries, rheumatic heart disease remains the most frequent predisposing cardiac condition. However, the epidemiologic features in developed countries have changed considerably. With the aging of the population increases in the prevalence of degenerative heart valve disease and in the use of implanted heart valve substitutes and intracardiac devices are now common. The numbers of patients with chronic, predisposing medical comorbidities, such as diabetes, HIV infection, and end-stage renal disease, have also increased, as has the commensurate risk of exposure to nosocomial bacteremia, often with antibiotic resistance. These changing demographics are reflected in two observations. First, the median age of patients with IE gradually increased from 30 to 40 years in the pre-antibiotic era, to 47 to 69 years in the first decade of 21st century. Second, the incidence of IE in developed countries has remained unchanged, despite the reduction in rheumatic heart disease over the last half-century.

PATHOGENESIS

The hallmark of IE is persistent endocardial or endovascular infection causing continuous bacteremia. Importantly, IE is a relatively uncommon consequence of transient bacteremia and not all organisms can effectively colonize or invade the endovascular space. It is apparent that complex series of host–pathogen interactions conspire in the development of IE lesions, including the integrity of the vascular endothelium, the host immune system, hemostatic mechanisms, cardiac anatomic characteristics, microbial properties, and the peripheral events that cause the bacteremia. Experimental data suggest that host endothelial damage is the key predisposing insult, supported by the observation that vegetations are most likely to form in areas where blood-flow injury is likely to occur—on the ventricular side of semilunar valves and the atrial side of AV valves.

MICROBIOLOGY

A wide range of microorganisms can cause IE, but only a few species account for the vast majority of cases. Streptococci and staphylococci are the cause of over 80% of IE cases in which a responsible organism is identified. Streptococcal species were historically the most common group of pathogens, but more recent data identify *Staphylococcus aureus* as the most frequently isolated agent worldwide. Moreover, the rate of antibiotic resistance among causative organisms is increasing.

【 】 NATIVE VALVE ENDOCARDITIS

Streptococci

Viridans group streptococci, or alpha-hemolytic streptococci, are a frequent cause of community-acquired native valve endocarditis (NVE) and are responsible for 30% to 65% of cases of NVE in older children and adults. They are normal residents of the oropharynx and easily gain access to the circulation following dental or gingival trauma. The viridans streptococci comprise several species, of which *S. sanguis*, *S. bovis*, *S. mutans*, and *S. mitior* are most commonly isolated in cases of IE. *S. bovis*, a normal inhabitant of the human gastrointestinal (GI) tract, is noteworthy as IE caused by this organism is strongly suggestive of GI malignancy, polyp formation, or diverticular disease. Colonoscopy should be performed when this organism is detected in the blood.

The *Enterococcus* spp., formerly classified as group D streptococci, are now defined as a distinct genus. The incidence of enterococcal endocarditis appears to be rising, responsible for 5% to 18% of cases of NVE, the vast majority of which are due to *E. faecalis* (80%) or *E. faecium* (10%) These organisms are normal inhabitants of the GI and genitourinary tracts and may enter the bloodstream after manipulation of the colon, urethra, or bladder (e.g., Foley catheterization, colonoscopy).

Group A *Streptococcus* rarely cause IE in the contemporary era. Before 1945, however, *S. pneumoniae* caused approximately 10% of IE cases, often resulting in an acute, fulminant illness associated with severe valve damage, perivalvular extension, embolic complications, pericarditis, meningitis, and high mortality (25%–50%).

Group B streptococci (e.g., *S. agalactiae*) are chiefly responsible for infections in the neonate and parturient, although the organism can also be isolated from diabetic foot ulcers. Risk factors for group B streptococcal bacteremia in adults include obstetric complications, diabetes, carcinoma, liver failure, alcoholism, and injection drug use (IDU).

Staphylococci

Staphylococcus aureus causes 80% to 90% of staphylococcal IE and is the most common cause of "acute" IE. Emerging data from the International Consortium on Endocarditis (ICE) suggest that *S. aureus* has become the leading cause of IE worldwide. The mucous membranes of the anterior nasopharynx are the most common sites of colonization, and approximately 30% of normal persons carry *S. aureus*. High-risk individuals include patients on dialysis, type I diabetics, burn victims, persons with HIV, injection drug users, patients with certain chronic dermatologic conditions, and patients with recent surgical incisions. *S. aureus* IE is frequently fulminant when it involves left-sided cardiac valves and often results in major complications such as heart failure, perivalvular extension with conduction disturbances, embolization and metastatic infection. Not surprisingly, *S. aureus* as a causative organism is an independent predictor of poor prognosis in IE and is associated with a 25% to 30% mortality rate. As many as 50% of patients with left-sided native valve IE (NVE) due to *S. aureus* will require surgery. Right-sided (tricuspid valve) IE with *S. aureus*, by contrast, is most frequently a complication of IDU, is associated with a high incidence of septic pulmonary embolization, but carries only a 2% to 4% case fatality rate.

The coagulase negative staphylococci (CoNS) are constituents of normal human skin flora and are much less likely to infect normal endocardial surfaces. *S. epidermidis* is an important causative agent in prosthetic valve and device-related endocarditis. NVE caused by CoNS occurs mainly in patients with preexisting valvular heart disease.

Gram-Negative Bacilli

IE due to gram-negative bacilli (GNB) is uncommon and tends to occur in IDUs, immunocompromised patients, patients with advanced liver disease, and prosthetic heart valve recipients. The fastidious gram-negative rods of the HACEK group reside normally in the oropharynx and are responsible for a very small (~1%) proportion of cases of NVE, usually involving abnormal valve tissue. Because of their growth requirements (CO_2), they may take 3 to 4 weeks to grow in culture and have gained notoriety for their implicated role in certain cases of culture-negative IE.

The ricksettial organism, *Coxiella burnetii,* is the causative agent of Q fever and is a relevant cause of IE in areas where cattle, sheep, and goat farming are common. Cases of IE caused by *C burnetii* are well documented in the developed world. As the organism is extremely difficult to culture, the diagnosis is best made serologically using antibody titers. *Bartonella* species, the etiologic agent in cat scratch disease, have been recently described as an important cause of IE among both homeless men and HIV-infected patients. The diagnosis can be confirmed with special culture or polymerase chain reaction (PCR) techniques.

Fungal IE

Fungal endocarditis is a relatively new syndrome associated with exceedingly high mortality (survival rates < 20%). Patients who develop fungal IE often have multiple predisposing conditions that include an immunocompromised state, the use of endovascular devices, and previous reconstructive cardiac surgery. *Candida* and *Aspergillus* species are the most common causes of fungal IE and are associated with large, bulky vegetations that can obstruct valve orifices and embolize to large vessels. Blood cultures are usually positive in cases of *Candida* IE, whereas they are rarely positive with *Aspergillus*. Fungal endocarditis is an indication for surgical replacement of an infected valve. Cure usually requires combination fungicidal (amphotericin) and surgical treatment, followed by long-term suppressive therapy with an oral antifungal agent.

Culture-Negative IE

Blood cultures are negative in up to 20% of patients with IE diagnosed by strict criteria. Failure to isolate a microorganism may be the result of inadequate culture technique, a highly fastidious organism or a nonbacterial pathogen as the causative agent, or previous administration of antimicrobial therapy prior to blood culture acquisition. The latter is an extremely important consideration as the administration of antibiotics prior to drawing blood cultures can reduce the recovery rate of bacterial pathogens by nearly one-third. There are numerous noninfectious causes of endocarditis that may behave like culture negative IE, including those that are related to neoplasia (nonbacterial thrombotic endocarditis, NBTE), autoimmune diseases (antiphospholipid antibody syndrome, SLE), or the post-cardiac surgical state (thrombi, stitches).

【 】 PROSTHETIC VALVE ENDOCARDITIS (PVE)

Prosthetic valve endocarditis represents approximately 10% to 30% of all IE cases. Although many of the general principles applicable to native valve IE are relevant, there are important considerations specific to PVE (see also Chapter 36). After valve replacement, the incidence of PVE is approximately 1% to 3% at 1 year and 3% to 6% at 5 years. Although the current evidence is not definitive, PVE can be broadly divided into two groups based on the time of onset after valve surgery—early PVE and late PVE. Early PVE is defined as endocarditis that develops within the first 2 months to 1 year after valve surgery. During this period, the vast majority of causative organisms are nosocomially acquired with a predominance of staphylococci, notably coagulase-negative species (*S epidermidis*). In contrast to early PVE, the spectrum of causative organisms in late PVE resembles that of NVE. Complication rates with PVE are high and surgery is often required even in the absence of documented perivalvular extension.

APPROACH TO THE PATIENT WITH SUSPECTED INFECTIVE ENDOCARDITIS

The history should focus on predisposing factors such as IDU, a prior history of IE, recent exposures, the presence of an intracardiac device or indwelling central venous catheter, congenital or acquired valvular heart disease, and other congenital heart disease. The patient may report fever, fatigue, anorexia, weight loss, night sweats, joint pain, or back pain. Features on clinical examination that raise suspicion for IE include fever, a new heart murmur, signs of heart failure, and vascular and immunologic phenomena. Examples of classic IE-related findings include major arterial emboli with pulse deficits, septic pulmonary emboli (with right-sided IE), mycotic brain aneurysms with intracranial hemorrhage, mucosal or conjunctival petechiae, splinter hemorrhages of the nailbeds, palpable purpuric skin rashes, Janeway's lesions (small, flat, irregular erythematous spots on the palms and soles), Osler's nodes (tender, erythematous nodules occurring in the pulp of the fingers), Roth spots (cytoid bodies and associated hemorrhage caused by microinfarction of retinal vessels), and urinary red cell casts suggestive of glomerulonephritis.

The diagnosis of IE rests on the ability to demonstrate endocardial involvement of infection and persistent bacteremia. The proper acquisition of blood cultures prior to initiation of antimicrobial therapy is essential. Echocardiography should be used to assess for the presence of endocardial involvement (vegetations, abscess formation, and new valvular regurgitation). These clinical, microbiologic, and echocardiographic features are the foundation for the Modified Duke Criteria, a set of integrated findings, which has become the standard for diagnosis of IE (Tables 38-1 and 38-2).

Once the diagnosis is made and appropriate therapy initiated, patients should be closely monitored for complications and repeat blood cultures should be obtained to ensure sterilization. Persistent fever beyond 1 week of appropriate therapy should raise suspicion for intracardiac extension or satellite abscess formation. In the absence of complications, the first several days of intravenous antibiotics are administered in the hospital and the remaining course provided via a central venous catheter (PICC line) as an outpatient with careful follow-up. Patients should be maintained on telemetry while in hospital; the need for surveillance electrocardiograms (ECGs) during outpatient therapy is dictated by the location of the infection and the predicted likelihood of conduction disturbances. Patients should also be monitored for antimicrobial toxicity, particularly with aminoglycoside use. Routine surveillance echocardiography during therapy is not necessary unless complications develop or cardiac surgery is considered. At the completion of therapy, transthoracic echocardiography (TTE) may be performed to establish a new "post-IE baseline." After successful therapy, patients with IE should be followed longitudinally for progressive valvular and ventricular dysfunction. Patients with successfully treated IE are at high risk for the development of future episodes of IE and should receive antibiotic prophylaxis for procedures, as recommended by current guidelines.

[ ] DIAGNOSIS OF INFECTIVE ENDOCARDITIS

IE is defined as an infection on any structure within the heart, including on normal or damaged endothelial surfaces (e.g., myocardium and valvular structures), prosthetic

TABLE 38-1

Definition of Terms Used in the Proposed Modified Duke Criteria for the Diagnosis of Infective Endocarditis[a]

Major Criteria
Blood culture positive for IE
    Typical microorganisms consistent with IE from two separate blood cultures:
        Viridans streptococci, *Streptococcus bovis*, HACEK group, *Staphylococcus aureus;*
        or community-acquired enterococci in the absence of a primary focus; or
    Microorganisms consistent with IE from persistently positive blood cultures, defined
    as follows:
        At least two positive cultures of blood samples drawn more than 12 h apart; or
        All of three or a majority of greater than four separate cultures of blood (with first
        and last sample drawn at least 1 h apart)
    Single positive blood culture for *Coxiella burnetti* or anti-phase 1 IgG
    antibody titer greater than 1:800
Evidence of endocardial involvement
Echocardiogram positive for IE (TEE recommended in patients with prosthetic valves,
    rated at least "possible IE" by clinical criteria, or complicated IE [paravalvular
    abscess]; TTE as first test in other patients), defined as follows:
    Oscillating intracardiac mass on valve or supporting structures, in the path of
        regurgitant jets, or on implanted material in the
    Absence of an alternative anatomic explanation; or
    Abscess; or
    New partial dehiscence of prosthetic valve
New valvular regurgitation (worsening or changing of preexisting murmur not sufficient)

Minor Criteria
Predisposition, predisposing heart condition, or injection drug use
Fever, temperature greater than 38°C
Vascular phenomena, major arterial emboli, septic pulmonary infarcts, mycotic
aneurysm, intracranial hemorrhage, conjunctival
Hemorrhages, and Janeway's lesions
Immunologic phenomena; glomerulonephritis, Osler's nodes, Roth's spots, and
rheumatoid factor
Microbiological evidence: positive blood culture but does not meet a major criterion,[b]
or serologic evidence of active infection
With organism consistent with IE
Echocardiographic minor criteria eliminated

IE, infective endocarditis; TEE, transesophageal echocardiography; TTE, transthoracic echocardiography.

[a]Modifications are shown in bold type.
[b]Excludes single positive cultures for coagulase-negative staphylococci and organisms that do not cause endocarditis.
Reprinted with permission from Li JS, Sexton DJ, Mick N, et al. Proposed modifications to the Duke criteria for diagnosis of infective endocarditis. *Clin Infect Dis.* 2000;30:8.

heart valves, and implanted devices (e.g., pacemakers, ICDs, ventricular assist devices, and surgical shunts). The diagnosis of IE relies chiefly on the following factors: (1) an initial clinical suspicion, especially in a patient with identifiable risk factors; (2) microbiologic data (blood cultures demonstrating continuous bacteremia or cultures of vegetative lesions removed surgically); and (3) the results of echocardiographic imaging. Diagnosis is straightforward in only a minority of patients who present with a defined

TABLE 38-2

Definition of Infective Endocarditis According to the Proposed Modified Duke Criteria[a]

Definite infective endocarditis
   Pathologic criteria
     (1) Microorganisms demonstrated by culture or histological examination of a vegetation, a vegetation that has embolized; or Intracardiac abscess specimen; or
     (2) Pathologic lesions; vegetation, or intracardiac abscess confirmed by histological examination showing active endocarditis
   Clinical criteria
     (1) Two major criteria; or
     (2) One major criterion and three minor criteria; or
     (3) Five minor criteria
   Possible infective endocarditis
     (1) **One major criterion and one minor criterion;** or
     (2) **Three minor criteria**
   Rejected
     (1) Firm alternate diagnosis explaining evidence of infective endocarditis; or
     (2) Resolution of infective endocarditis syndrome with antibiotic therapy for less than 4 days; or
     (3) No pathologic evidence of infective endocarditis at surgery or autopsy, with antibiotic therapy for less than 4 days; or
     (4) Does not meet criteria for possible infective endocarditis, as noted above

[a]Modifications are shown in bold type.

Reprinted with permission from Li JS, Sexton DJ, Mick N, et al. Proposed modifications to the Duke criteria for the diagnosis of infective endocarditis. *Clin Infect Dis.* 2000;30:633–638.

predisposing condition and the classic manifestations of fever, evidence of active valvulitis, peripheral emboli, immunologic or vascular phenomena, and bacteremia. In the majority of patients, however, IE has an extremely variable clinical presentation.

【 】 CLINICAL CRITERIA

The modified Duke criteria (Tables 38-1 and 38-2) have become the current standard for diagnosis and clinical research and have been validated in numerous subsequent studies. A diagnosis of "definite IE" is established clinically by evidence of two major criteria, one major plus three minor criteria, or five minor criteria. Patients identified with "possible IE" (one major plus one minor criterion or three minor criteria) should be treated for IE until the diagnosis is satisfactorily excluded.

The importance of obtaining blood cultures by appropriate methods, prior to the institution of antibiotics, cannot be overemphasized. Three separate sets of blood cultures obtained from different venipuncture sites over 24 hours are recommended.

【 】 ECHOCARDIOGRAPHY IN INFECTIVE ENDOCARDITIS

All patients with suspected IE should undergo prompt echocardiographic assessment. There are several TTE findings suggestive of endocarditis, including vegetations, evidence of periannular tissue destruction, aneurysms or fistula formation, leaflet perforation, or prosthetic valve dehiscence.

Although there remains some debate regarding the optimal initial approach, the vast majority of patients undergo transthoracic (TTE) imaging first because of its immediate availability. A low threshold to pursue transesophageal (TEE) imaging is appropriate, as

TABLE 38-3

Aggregate Performance Characteristics of TTE and TEE in the Diagnosis of IE

	Sensitivity (%)	Specificity (%)
TTE	60–65	98
TEE	85–95	85–98

dictated by the clinical circumstances, the adequacy of the TTE images, and the potential need for early surgical planning and intervention. The performance characteristics of TTE and TEE are summarized in Table 38-3. TEE should be performed expeditiously in patients with high-risk clinical features at presentation (e.g., suspected *S. aureus* infection of the aortic valve and root), known congenital heart disease, or suboptimal TTE images. For patients undergoing cardiac surgery for IE, intraoperative TEE is routine. TEE should also be considered for patients with catheter-associated *S. aureus* bacteremia to predict the indicated duration of antibiotic therapy (i.e., 2 weeks versus 4 weeks). In uncomplicated cases of IE, a single echocardiographic study is usually sufficient. However, with complex IE, serial echocardiographic examinations may help determine prognosis and guide surgical intervention.

ACUTE COMPLICATIONS

Complication rates with IE have remained relatively unchanged despite advances in diagnosis and antimicrobial therapy. Complications can generally be related to local extension of infection (e.g., valve ring abscess, fistulae, conduction block), destruction of or interference with intracardiac structures (e.g., leaflet perforation or valvular obstruction), embolization (e.g., stroke, septic pulmonary emboli), bacteremia /sepsis (e.g., multisystem organ failure), and immune complex disease (e.g., glomerulonephritis).

【 】 HEART FAILURE

Heart failure is the most frequent major complication of IE; its development portends an adverse outcome with medical therapy alone and is usually an indication for surgical intervention. Reduced LV systolic function is the most powerful predictor of an adverse outcome following surgery. Heart failure in IE is most often related to acute, severe valvular dysfunction owing either to leaflet destruction or interference with normal coaptation. It may also occur from rupture of infected mitral chordae, obstruction due to bulky vegetations, the development of intracardiac shunts, or prosthetic valve dehiscence. Heart failure may also develop more gradually as a function of continued valve incompetence and worsening ventricular function, following otherwise successful antibiotic treatment. Heart failure is most commonly associated with aortic valve IE, followed by mitral valve, and then tricuspid valve involvement. Inappropriate bradycardia, which can develop if the infection extends into the conduction system leading to atrioventricular block or if the patient receives a beta-blocker, can be catastrophic.

【 】 EMBOLIZATION

Embolization is a dreaded complication of IE. Central nervous system (CNS) involvement is most common; stroke comprises up to 65% of embolic events and may be the presenting sign of IE in up to 14% of cases. CNS embolization can present with subtle neurologic abnormalities, as seen with microembolization, or with sudden hemiplegia and obtundation, as seen with a ruptured mycotic aneurysm and intracranial hemorrhage (ICH) (Fig. 38-1A) or with a large embolic stroke. Up to 90% of CNS emboli

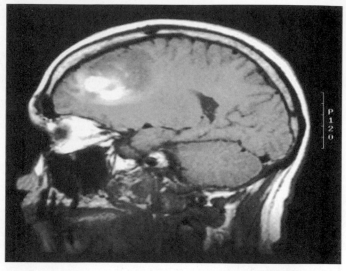

A

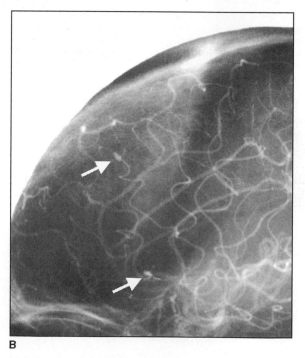

B

FIGURE 38-1 A. Large right frontal hemorrhage in a patient with *S. aureus* mitral valve endocarditis. **B.** Mycotic aneurysms (*arrows*) along the course of the branches of the middle cerebral artery. (Adapted with permission from Mauri L, de Lemos JA, O'Gara PT. Infective endocarditis. *Curr Probl Cardiol.* 2001;26:562–610.)

lodge in the distribution of the middle cerebral artery, and carry a high mortality rate. Any patient with suspected or definite IE who develops neurologic symptoms should promptly undergo neurologic imaging and be considered to have CNS embolization until proved otherwise.

Emboli may also involve other organ systems including the liver, spleen, kidneys, and lungs. Metastatic sites of infection may appear in the spine or para-spinous space, and may be the cause of prolonged fever or bacteremia despite appropriate antimicrobial therapy. Septic pulmonary emboli are present in the majority of cases of right-sided IE related to IDU.

[ ] MYCOTIC ANEURYSMS

Mycotic aneurysms (MA) represent a small but dangerous subset of embolic complications. They occur most frequently in the intracranial arteries and have a particular predilection for the middle cerebral artery and its branches (Fig. 38-1B). The overall mortality rate among IE patients with intracranial MAs is 60%, and approaches 80% if rupture occurs. Screening patients with definite IE for the presence of intracranial MAs is not currently recommended and neurovascular imaging is reserved for symptomatic patients or for selected patients undergoing surgery for IE.

[ ] PERIANNULAR EXTENSION OF INFECTION

Extension or spread of infection beyond the valve annulus is a very concerning development that usually presages the need for surgical therapy. Findings such as persistent fever and bacteremia despite antibiotic therapy, heart failure, or new conduction block should raise suspicion for this complication. Periannular extension may occur in 10% to 40% of all native valve IE and > 50% of prosthetic valve IE and complicates aortic valve IE more commonly than either mitral or tricuspid valve IE.

[ ] RENAL DYSFUNCTION

Renal dysfunction is a common complication of IE and is often multifactorial in nature given the high incidence of preexisting renal disease, immune complex disease, drug-induced nephrotoxicity, and hemodynamic perturbations.

ANTIMICROBIAL THERAPY

[ ] GENERAL PRINCIPLES

Rapid institution of appropriate parenteral antibiotic therapy is the single most important initial intervention in the treatment of suspected or proven IE. Given the rising rate of antimicrobial resistance among causative organisms, therapy is predicated on the identification of the causative isolate and delineation of its antibiotic sensitivities. An infectious disease specialist should supervise the dose, duration, and method of delivery (IV or IM) of antimicrobial therapy with longitudinal follow-up. Serum antibiotic levels should be monitored where appropriate and renal and hepatic function assayed when indicated. A recent American Heart Association Scientific Statement addresses antimicrobial therapy for IE in detail (Tables 38-4 to 38-10).

[ ] CHOICE OF ANTIBIOTICS

The lesions of IE are extremely difficult to eradicate, as the infection exists in a sequestered area of impaired host defense. Thus, IE requires weeks of parenteral antibiotic therapy, preferably with a drug with bactericidal activity against the offending organism.

TABLE 38-4

Therapy of Native Valve Endocarditis Caused by Highly Penicillin-Susceptible Viridans-Group Streptococci and *Streptococcus bovis*

Regimen	Dosage^a and Route	Duration (wk)	Comments
Aqueous crystalline penicillin G sodium	12–18 million U per 24 h IV either continuously or in 4–6 equally divided doses	4	Preferred in most patients greater than 65 y of age or patients with impairment of 8th cranial nerve function or renal function
Or Ceftriaxone sodium	2 g per 24 h IV/IM in 1 dose Pediatric dose ^b: penicillin 200,000 U/kg per 24 h IV in 4–6 equally divided doses; ceftriaxone 100 mg per 24 h IV/IM in 1 dose	4	
Aqueous crystalline penicillin G sodium	12–18 million U per 24 h IV either continuously or in 6 equally divided doses	2	2 wk regimen not intended for patients with known cardiac or extracardiac abscess or for those with creatinine clearance of less than 20 mL/min, impaired 8th cranial nerve function, or *Abiotrophia, Granulicatella,* or *Gemella* spp. infection. Gentamicin dosage should be adjusted to achieve peak serum concentration of 3–4 μg/mL and trough serum concentration of less than 1 μg/mL when 3 divided doses are used; nomogram used for single daily dosing
Or Ceftriaxone sodium	2 g per 24 h IV/IM in 1 dose	2	

457

Therapy of Native Valve Endocarditis Caused by Highly Penicillin-Susceptible Viridans-Group Streptococci and *Streptococcus bovis* (*Continued*)

Regimen	Dosage[a] and Route	Duration (wk)	Comments
Plus			
Gentamicin sulfate[c]	3 mg/kg per 24 h IV/IM in 1 dose Pediatric dose: penicillin 200,000 U/kg per 24 h IV in 4–6 equally divided doses; ceftriaxone 100 mg/kg per 24 h IV/IM in 1 dose; gentamicin 3 mg/kg per 24 h IV/IM in 1 dose or 3 equally divided doses[d]	2	
Vancomycin hydrochloride[e]	30 mg/kg per 24 h IV in 2 equally divided doses not to exceed 2 g per 24 h unless concentrations in serum are inappropriately low Pediatric dose: 40 mg/kg per 24 h IV in 2 or 3 equally divided doses	2	Vancomycin therapy recommended only for patients unable to tolerate penicillin or ceftriaxone; vancomycin dosage should be adjusted to obtain peak (1 h after infusion completed) serum concentration of 30–45 μg/mL and a trough concentration range of 10–15 μg/mL

Minimum inhibitory concentration less than or equal to 0.12 μg/mL.

[a]Dosages recommended are for patients with normal renal function.
[b]Pediatric dose should not exceed that of a normal adult.
[c]Other potentially nephrotoxic drugs (e.g., nonsteroidal anti-inflammatory drugs) should be used with caution in patients receiving gentamicin therapy.
[d]Data for once-daily dosing of aminoglycosides for children exist, but no data for treatment of infective endocarditis exists.
[e]Vancomycin dosages should be infused during course of at least 1 h to reduce risk of histamine-release "red man" syndrome.

Modified from Baddour LM, Wilson WR, Bayer AS, et al. Infective endocarditis: diagnosis, antimicrobial therapy, and management of complications. A statement for healthcare professionals from the Committee on Rheumatic Fever, Endocarditis, and Kawasaki Disease, Council on Cardiovascular Disease in the Young, and the Councils on Clinical Cardiology, Stroke, and Cardiovascular Surgery and Anesthesia, American Heart Association. *Circulation*. 2005;111:e394-e434.

TABLE 38-5

Therapy of Native Valve Endocarditis Caused by Strains of Viridans Group Streptococci and *Streptococcus bovis* Relatively Resistant to Penicillin

Regimen	Dosage[a] and Route	Duration (wk)	Comments
Aqueous crystalline penicillin G sodium	24 million U per 24 h IV either continuously or in 4–6 equally divided doses	4	Patients with endocarditis caused by penicillin-resistant (MIC greater than 0.5 μg/mL) strains should be treated with regimen recommended for enterococcal endocarditis
Or			
Ceftriaxone sodium	2 g per 24 h IV/IM in 1 dose	4	Recommended for enterococcal endocarditis (see Table 38-6)
Plus			
Gentamicin sulfate[b]	3 mg/kg per 24 h IV/IM in 1 dose Pediatric dose[c]: penicillin 300 000 U per 24 h IV in 4–6 equally divided doses; ceftriaxone 100 mg/kg per 24 IV/IM in 1 dose, gentamicin 3 mg/kg per 24 h IV/IM in 1 dose or 3 equally divided doses	2	

TABLE 38-5

Therapy of Native Valve Endocarditis Caused by Strains of Viridans Group Streptococci and *Streptococcus bovis* Relatively Resistant to Penicillin (*Continued*)

Regimen	Dosage[a] and Route	Duration (wk)	Comments
Vancomycin hydrochloride	30 mg/kg per 24 h IV in 2 equally divided doses not to exceed 2 g per 24 h, unless serum concentration are inappropriately low Pediatric dose: 40 mg/kg per 24 h in 2 or 3 equally divided doses	4	Vancomycin[d] therapy is recommended only for patients unable to tolerate penicillin or ceftriaxone therapy

IM, intramuscular; IV, intravenous; MIC, minimum inhibitory concentration.

Minimum inhibitory concentration (MIC) greater than 0.12 μg/mL to less than or equal to 0.5 μg/mL.

[a] Dosages recommended are for patients with normal renal function.

[b] See Table 38-7 for appropriate dosages of gentamicin.

[c] Pediatric dose should not exceed that of a normal adult.

[d] See Table 38-7 for appropriate dosages of vancomycin.

Modified from Baddour LM, Wilson WR, Bayer AS, et al. Infective endocarditis: diagnosis, antimicrobial therapy, and management of complications. A statement for healthcare professionals from the Committee on Rheumatic Fever, Endocarditis, and Kawasaki Disease, Council on Cardiovascular Disease in the Young, and the Councils on Clinical Cardiology, Stroke, and Cardiovascular Surgery and Anesthesia, American Heart Association. *Circulation.* 2005;111:e394–e434.

TABLE 38-6

Therapy for Native Valve or Prosthetic Valve Enterococcal Endocarditis Caused by Strains Susceptible to Penicillin, Gentamicin, and Vancomycin

Regimen	Dosage^a and Route	Duration (wk)	Comments
Ampicillin sodium	12 g per 24 h IV in 6 equally divided doses	4–6	Native valve: 4-wk therapy recommended for patients with symptoms of illness less than or equal to 3 mo; 6-wk therapy recommended for patients with symptoms greater than 3 mo
Or			
Aqueous crystalline penicillin G sodium	18–30 million U per 24 h IV either continuously or in 6 equally divided doses	4–6	Prosthetic valve or other prosthetic cardiac material: minimum of 6-wk therapy recommended
Plus			
Gentamicin sulfate ^{b}	3 mg/kg per 24 h IV/IM in 3 equally divided doses Pediatric dose^c: ampicillin 300 mg/kg per 24 h IV in 4–6 equally divided doses; penicillin 300,000 U/kg per 24 h IV in 4–6 equally divided doses; gentamicin 3 mg/kg per 24 h IV/IM in 3 equally divided doses	4–6	

TABLE 38-6

Therapy for Native Valve or Prosthetic Valve Enterococcal Endocarditis Caused by Strains Susceptible to Penicillin, Gentamicin, and Vancomycin (*Continued*)

Regimen	Dosage[a] and Route	Duration (wk)	Comments
Vancomycin hydrochloride[d]	30 mg/kg per 24 h IV in 2 equally divided doses	6	Vancomycin therapy is recommended only for patients unable to tolerate penicillin or ampicillin
Plus Gentamicin sulfate	3 mg/kg per 24 h IV/IM in 3 equally divided doses Pediatric dose: vancomycin 40 mg/kg per 24 h IV in 2 or 3 equally divided doses; gentamicin 3 mg/kg per 24 h IV/IM in 3 equally divided doses	6	6 wk of vancomycin therapy recommended because of decreased activity against enterococci

IM, intramuscular; IV, intravenous.

[a]Dosages recommended are for patients with normal renal function.

[b]Dosage of gentamicin should be adjusted to achieve peak serum concentration of 3–4 µg/mL and a trough concentration of less than 1 µg/mL. Patients with a creatinine clearance of less than 50 mL/min should be treated in consultation with an infectious diseases specialist.

[c] Pediatric dose should not exceed that of a normal adult.

[d]See Table 38-7 for appropriate dosing of vancomycin.

Modified from Baddour LM, Wilson WR, Bayer AS, et al. Infective endocarditis: diagnosis, antimicrobial therapy, and management of complications. A statement for healthcare professionals from the Committee on Rheumatic Fever, Endocarditis, and Kawasaki Disease, Council on Cardiovascular Disease in the Young, and the Councils on Clinical Cardiology, Stroke, and Cardiovascular Surgery and Anesthesia, American Heart Association. *Circulation.* 2005;111:e394–e434. See full document for treatment regimens of resistant organisms.

TABLE 38-7

Therapy for Endocarditis Caused by Staphylococci in the Absence of Prosthetic Materials

Regimen	Dosage[a] and Route	Duration	Comments
Oxacillin-susceptible strains			
Nafcillin or oxacillin [b]	12 g per 24 h IV in 4–6 equally divided doses	6 wk	For complicated right-sided IE and for left-sided IE; for uncomplicated right-sided IE, 2 wk
With			
Optional addition of gentamicin sulfate [c]	3 mg/kg per 24 h IV/IM in 2 or 3 equally divided doses Pediatric dose[d]: nafcillin or oxacillin 200 mg/kg per 24 h IV in 4–6 equally divided doses; gentamicin 3 mg/kg per 24 h IV/IM in 3 equally divided doses	3–5 d	Clinical benefit of aminoglycosides has not been established
For penicillin-allergic (nonanaphylactoid type) patients			
Cefazolin	6 g per 24 h IV in 3 equally divided doses	6 wk	Consider skin testing for oxacillin-susceptible staphylococci and questionable history of immediate-type hypersensitivity to penicillin Cephalosporins should be avoided in patients with anaphylactoid-type hypersensitivity to beta-lactams; vancomycin should be used in these cases [d]

TABLE 38-7

Therapy for Endocarditis Caused by Staphylococci in the Absence of Prosthetic Materials (*Continued*)

Regimen	Dosage[a] and Route	Duration	Comments
With Optional addition of gentamicin sulfate	3 mg/kg per 24 h IV/IM in 2 or 3 equally divided doses Pediatric dose: cefazolin 100 mg/kg per 24 h IV in 3 equally divided doses; gentamicin 3 mg/kg per 24 h IV/IM in 3 equally divided doses	3–5 d	Clinical benefit of aminoglycosides has not been established
Oxacillin-resistant strains vancomycin[e]	30 mg/kg per 24 h IV in 2 equally divided doses Pediatric dose: 40 mg/kg per 24 h IV in 2 or 3 equally divided doses	6 wk	Adjust vancomycin dosage to achieve 1-h serum concentration of 30–45 μg/mL and trough concentration of 10–15 μg/mL

IE, infective endocarditis; IM, intramuscular; IV, intravenous.

[a]Dosages recommended are for patients with normal renal function.
[b] Penicillin G 24 million U per 24 h IV in four to six equally divided doses may be used in place of nafcillin or oxacillin if strain is penicillin susceptible (minimum inhibitory concentration less than or equal to 0.1 μg/mL) and dose does not produce beta-lactamase.
[c] Gentamicin should be administered in close temporal proximity to vancomycin, nafcillin, or oxacillin dosing.
[d]Pediatric cose should not exceed that of a normal adult.
[e]For specific dosing adjustment and issues concerning vancomycin, see Table 38-7 footnotes.

Modified from Baddour LM, Wilson WR, Bayer AS, et al. Infective endocarditis: diagnosis, antimicrobial therapy, and management of complications. A statement for healthcare professionals from the Committee on Rheumatic Fever, Endocarditis, and Kawasaki Disease, Council on Cardiovascular Disease in the Young, and the Councils on Clinical Cardiology, Stroke, and Cardiovascular Surgery and Anesthesia, American Heart Association. *Circulation*. 2005;111:e394–e434.

TABLE 38-8

Therapy for Prosthetic Valve Endocarditis Caused by Staphylococci

Regimen	Dosage[a] and Route	Duration (wk)	Comments
Oxacillin-susceptible strains			
Nafcillin or oxacillin	12 g per 24 h IV in 6 equally divided doses	At least 6	Penicillin G 24 million U per 24 h IV in four to six equally divided doses may be used in place of nafcillin or oxacillin if strain is penicillin susceptible (minimum inhibitory concentration less than or equal to 0.1 μg/mL) and does not produce beta-lactamase; vancomycin should be used in patients with immediate-type-hypersensitivity reactions to beta-lactam antibiotics (see Table 38-3 for dosing guidelines); cefazolin may be substituted for nafcilin or oxacillin in patients with nonimmediate-type hypersensitivity reactions to penicillins
Plus Rifampin	900 mg per 24 h IV/PO in 3 equally divided doses	At least 6	
Plus Gentamicin[b]	3 mg/kg per 24 h IV/IM in 2 or 3 equally divided doses Pediatric dose[c]: nafcillin or oxacillin 200 mg/kg per h IV in 4–6 equally divided doses; rifampin 20 mg/kg per 24 h IV/PO in 3 equally divided doses; gentamicin 3 mg/kg per 24 h IV/IM in 3 equally divided doses	2	

465

TABLE 38-8

Therapy for Prosthetic Valve Endocarditis Caused by Staphylococci (*Continued*)

Regimen	Dosage[a] and Route	Duration (wk)	Comments
Oxacillin-resistant strains			
Vancomycin	30 mg/kg per 24 h in 2 equally divided doses	At least 6	Adjust vancomycin to achieve 1-h serum concentration of 30–45 μg/mL and trough concentration of 10–15 μg/mL
Plus Rifampin	900 mg/kg per 24 h IV/PO in 3 equally divided doses	At least 6	
Plus Gentamicin	3 mg/kg per 24 h IV/IM in 2 or 3 equally divided doses Pediatric dose: vancomycin 40 mg/kg per 24 h IV in 2 or 3 equally divided doses; rifampin 20 mg/kg per 24 h IV/PO in 3 equally divided doses (up to adult dose); gentamicin 3 mg/kg per 24 h IV or IM in 3 equally divided doses	2	

IM, intramuscular; IV, intravenous; PO, by mouth.

[a]Dosages recommended are for patients with normal renal function.

[b]Gentamicin should be administered in close proximity to vancomycin, nafcillin, or oxacillin dosing.

[c]Pediatric cose should not exceed that of a normal adult.

Modified from Baddour LM, Wilson WR, Bayer AS, et al. Infective endocarditis: diagnosis, antimicrobial therapy, and management of complications. A statement for healthcare professionals from the Committee on Rheumatic Fever, Endocarditis, and Kawasaki Disease, Council on Cardiovascular Disease in the Young, and the Councils on Clinical Cardiology, Stroke, and Cardiovascular Surgery and Anesthesia, American Heart Association. *Circulation*. 2005;1:e394-e434.

TABLE 38-9

Therapy for Both Native and Prosthetic Valve Endocarditis Caused by HACEK[a] Microorganisms

Regimen	Dosage and Route	Duration (wk)	Comments
Ceftriaxone sodium	2 g per 24 h IV/IM in 1 dose[b]	4	Cefotaxime or another third- or fourth-generation cephalosporin may be substituted
Or			
Ampicillin-sulbactam[c]	12 g per 24 h IV in 4 equally divided doses	4	
Or			
Ciprofloxacin[c,d]	1000 mg per 24 h PO or 800 mg per 24 h IV in two equally divided doses Pediatric dose[e]: ceftriaxone 100 mg/kg per 24 h IV/IM once daily; ampicillin-sulbactam 300 mg/kg per 24 h IV divided into 4 or 6 equally divided doses; ciprofloxacin 20–30 mg/kg per 24 h IV/PO in 2 equally divided doses	4	Fluoroquinolone therapy recommended only for patients unable to tolerate cephalosporin and ampicillin therapy; levofloxacin, gatifloxacin, or moxifloxacin may be substituted; fluoroquinolones generally not recommended for patients less than 18 y old. Prosthetic valve: patients with endocarditis involving prosthetic cardiac valve or other prosthetic cardiac material should be treated for 6 wk

IM, intramuscular; IV, intravenous; PO, by mouth.

[a]*Haemophilus parainfluenzae, Haemophilus aphrophilus, Actinobacillus actinomycetemcomitans, Cardiobacterium hominis, Eikenella corrodens,* and *Kingella kingae.*
[b]Patients should be informed that intramuscular injection of ceftriaxone is painful.
[c]Dosage recommended for patients with normal renal function.
[d]Fluoroquinolones are highly active in vitro against HACEK microorganisms. Published data on use of fluoroquinolone therapy for endocarditis caused by HACED are minimal.
[e]Pediatric dose should not exceed that of a normal adult.

Modified from Baddour LM, Wilson WR, Bayer AS, et al. Infective endocarditis: diagnosis, antimicrobial therapy, and management of complications. A statement for healthcare professionals from the Committee on Rheumatic Fever, Endocarditis, and Kawasaki Disease, Council on Cardiovascular Disease in the Young, and the Councils on Clinical Cardiology, Stroke, and Cardiovascular Surgery and Anesthesia, American Heart Association. *Circulation.* 2005;111:e394–e434.

TABLE 38-10

Therapy for Culture-Negative Endocarditis Including *Bartonella* Endocarditis

Regimen	Dosage[a] and Route	Duration (wk)	Comments
Native Valve			
Ampicillin-sulbactam	12 g per 24 h IV in 4 equally divided doses	4–6	Patients with culture-negative endocarditis should be treated with consultation with an infectious diseases specialist
Plus			
Gentamicin sulfate[b]	3 mg/kg per 24 h IV/IM in 2 equally divided doses	4–6	
Vancomycin[c]	30 mg/kg per 24 h IV in 2 equally divided doses	4–6	Vancomycin recommended only for patients unable to tolerate penicillins
Plus			
Gentamicin sulfate	3 mg/kg per 24 h IV/IM in 3 equally divided doses	4–6	
Plus			
Ciprofloxacin	1000 mg per 24 h PO or 800 mg per 24 h IV in 2 equally divided doses Pediatric dose[d]: ampicillin-sulbactam 300 mg/kg per 24 h IV in 4–6 equally divided doses; gentamicin 3 mg/kg per 24 h IV/IM in 3 equally divided doses; vancomycin 40 mg/kg per 24 h in 2 or 3 equally divided doses; ciprofloxacin 20–30 mg/kg per 24 h IV/PO in 2 equally divided doses	4–6	

Prosthetic valve (early— less than or equal to 1 y)		
Vancomycin	30 mg/kg per 24 h IV in 2 equally divided doses	6
Plus		
Gentamicin sulfate	3 mg/kg per 24 h IV/IM in 3 equally divided doses	2
Plus		
Cefepime	6 g per 24 h IV in 3 equally divided doses	6
Plus		
Rifampin	900 mg per 24 h PO/IV in 3 equally divided doses Pediatric dose: vancomycin 40 mg/kg per 24 h IV in 2 or 3 equally divided doses; gentamicin 3 mg per kg per 24 h IV/IM in 3 equally divided doses; cefepime 150 mg/kg per 24 h IV in 3 equally divided doses; rifampin 20 mg/kg per 24 h PO/IV in 3 equally divided doses	6
Prosthetic valve (late— greater than 1 y)		Same regimens as listed above for native valve endocarditis	6
Suspected *Bartonella*, culture negative		
Ceftriaxone sodium	2 g per 24 h IV/IM in 1 dose	6 Patients with *Bartonella* endocarditis should be treated in consultation with an infectious diseases specialist
Plus		
Gentamicin sulfate	3 mg/kg per 24 h IV/IM in 3 equally divided doses	2
with/without		
Doxycycline	200 mg/kg per 24 h IV/PO in 2 equally divided doses	

469

TABLE 38-10

Therapy for Culture-Negative Endocarditis Including *Bartonella* Endocarditis (*Continued*)

Regimen	Dosage[a] and Route	Duration (wk)	Comments
Documented *Bartonella* culture positive			
Doxycycline	200 mg per 24 h IV or PO in 2 equally divided doses	6	If gentamicin cannot be given, then replace with rifampin, 600 mg per 24 h PO/IV in 2 equally divided doses
Plus			
Gentamicin sulfate	3 mg/kg per 24 h IV/IM in 3 equally divided doses Pediatric dose: ceftriaxone 100 mg/kg per 24 h IV/IM once daily; gentamicin 3 mg/kg per 24 h IV/IM in 3 equally divided doses; doxycycline 2–4 mg/kg per 24 h IV/PO in 2 equally divided doses; rifampin 20 mg/kg per 24 h PO/IV in 2 equally divided doses	2	

IM, intramuscular; IV, intravenous; PO, by mouth.

[a]Dosages recommended are for patients with normal renal function.
[b]See Table 38-7 for appropriate dosing of gentamicin.
[c]See Table 38-7 for appropriate dosing of vancomycin.
[d]Pediatric dose should not exceed that of a normal adult.

Modified from Baddour IM, Wilson WR, Bayer AS, et al. Infective endocarditis: diagnosis, antimicrobial therapy, and management of complications. A statement for healthcare professionals from the Committee on Rheumatic Fever, Endocarditis, and Kawasaki Disease, Council on Cardiovascular Disease in the Young, and the Councils on Clinical Cardiology, Stroke, and Cardiovascular Surgery and Anesthesia, American Heart Association. *Circulation.* 2005;111:e394–e434.

Combination antimicrobial therapy may provide more rapid bactericidal effect and in certain circumstances acts synergistically. All patients should have surveillance blood cultures obtained 2 to 3 days after the initiation of antibiotic therapy to ensure efficacy. Most patients will require long-term venous access via a PICC or Hickman line for a 4- to 6-week course of antibiotics. Patients should remain in an inpatient setting during the initial phase of treatment when complications are most likely, after which selected low-risk patients can be considered for outpatient parenteral antibiotic therapy (OPAT).

【　】 EMPIRIC ANTIBIOTIC THERAPY

Initial empiric antibiotic therapy (i.e., before blood culture results are available) should cover *S aureus*, the many species of streptococci that can cause IE, and *E faecalis*. Thus, a combination of a beta-lactamase-resistant penicillin (nafcilllin), or vancomycin for penicillin allergic patients, and gentamicin, is often used.

ANTIPLATELET AND ANTITHROMBIN THERAPY

Despite their theoretical benefit, there are no human studies that support the use of either antiplatelet or antithrombin therapy to prevent embolic complications or to hasten antibiotic cure. Moreover, small uncontrolled studies suggest that antithrombin therapy actually increases the risk of intracranial hemorrhage following CNS embolization. For patients who generally require anticoagulation (e.g., patients with chronic atrial fibrillation or a mechanical heart valve), warfarin should be immediately discontinued on admission and IV unfractionated heparin cautiously substituted at the time when bleeding risk is deemed acceptably low.

SURGICAL THERAPY

The decision to undertake cardiac surgery for the treatment of IE can be extremely challenging, and there are no randomized clinical trials to guide practice. The most recent ACC/AHA guidelines for surgery in IE are summarized in Tables 38-11 and 38-12.

For NVE, the primary indication for surgery in the active phase of infection is the development of heart failure from either valve stenosis or regurgitation. Valve surgery is indicated for treatment of fungal or other highly resistant organisms, and for treatment of intracardiac abscess, perforation, fistulous tracts, and false aneurysms. Surgery is reasonable for patients with recurrent emboli and persistent vegetations and for patients with persistent bacteremia despite several days (5–7) of appropriate antibiotic therapy in the absence of a metastatic focus of infection. Surgery to prevent embolization can be considered for treatment of large valve repair. Indications for surgery in patients with PVE are similar, although early surgery may be considered for selected patients with PVE despite demonstration of perivalular extension or heart failure.

The timing of surgery following CNS embolization in either native or prosthetic valve endocarditis is problematic, due to the risk of hemorrhagic transformation. It is generally advisable to wait at least 5 to 7 days after bland CNS infarction, and as long as 4 weeks after primary CNS hemorrhage (e.g., from a ruptured mycotic aneurysm) before undertaking cardiac surgery.

> ## TABLE 38-11

Indications for Surgery for Native Valve Endocarditis

Class I

1. Surgery of the native valve is indicated in patients with acute infective endocarditis who present with valve stenosis or regurgitation resulting in heart failure. *(Level of Evidence: B)*
2. Surgery of the native valve is indicated in patients with acute infective endocarditis who present with AR or MR with hemodynamic evidence of elevated LV end-diastolic or left atrial pressures (e.g., premature closure of MV with AR, rapid decelerating MR signal by continuous-wave Doppler (V-wave cutoff sign), or moderate to severe pulmonary hypertension). *(Level of Evidence: B)*
3. Surgery of the native valve is indicated in patients with infective endocarditis caused by fungal or other highly resistant organisms. *(Level of Evidence: B)*
4. Surgery of the native valve is indicated in patients with infective endocarditis complicated by heart block, annular or aortic abscess, or destructive penetrating lesions (e.g., sinus of Valsalva to right atrium, right ventricle, or left atrium fistula; mitral leaflet perforation with aortic valve endocarditis; or infection in annulus fibrosa). *(Level of Evidence: B)*

Class IIa

Surgery of the native valve is reasonable in patients with infective endocarditis who present with recurrent emboli and persistent vegetations despite appropriate antibiotic therapy. *(Level of Evidence: C)*

Class IIb

Surgery of the native valve may be considered in patients with infective endocarditis who present with mobile vegetations in excess of 10 mm with or without emboli. *(Level of Evidence: C)*

Reproduced with permission from American College of Cardiology; American Heart Association Task Force on Practice Guidelines (Writing Committee to revise the 1998 guidelines for the management of patients with valvular heart disease); Society of Cardiovascular Anesthesiologists, Bonow RO, Carabello BA, Chatterjee K, et al. ACC/AHA 2006 guidelines for the management of patients with valvular heart disease: a report of the American College of Cardiology/American Heart Association Task Force on Practice Guidelines (Writing Committee to revise the 1998 guidelines for the management of patients with valvular heart disease) developed in collaboration with the Society of Cardiovascular Anesthesiologists endorsed by the Society for Cardiovascular Angiography and Interventions and the Society of Thoracic Surgeons. *J Am Coll Cardiol.* 2006;48(3):e1–e148.

PROGNOSIS

Patients with IE are an extremely heterogeneous group with varying comorbidities, causative organisms, and complications. Overall mortality can approach 20% to 25%. Accurate prognostic classification may help inform individual treatment decisions. Retrospective studies have identified high-risk features that include advanced age, diabetes mellitus, female gender, heart failure, renal dysfunction, *S aureus*, an embolic event, and vegetation length > 1.5 cm. Although the decision to undertake early surgery for the treatment of IE must be made on an individual basis, these data provide a useful means to target aggressive medical and surgical interventions to high-risk patient groups.

TABLE 38-12

Indications for Surgery for Prosthetic Valve Endocarditis

Class I

1. Consultation with a cardiac surgeon is indicated for patients with infective endo-carditis of a prosthetic valve. *(Level of Evidence: C)*
2. Surgery is indicated for patients with infective endocarditis of a prosthetic valve who present with heart failure. *(Level of Evidence: B)*
3. Surgery is indicated for patients with infective endocarditis of a prosthetic valve who present with dehiscence evidence by cine fluoroscopy or echocardiogra-phy. *(Level of Evidence: B)*
4. Surgery is indicated for patients with infective endocarditis of a prosthetic valve who present with evidence of increasing obstruction or worsening regurgitation. *(Level of Evidence: C)*
5. Surgery is indicated for patients with infective endocarditis of a prosthetic valve who present with complications, for example, abscess formation. *(Level of Evidence: C)*

Class IIa

Surgery is reasonable for patients with infective endocarditis of a prosthetic valve who present with evidence of persistent bacteremia or recurrent emboli despite appropriate antibiotic treatment. *(Level of Evidence: C)*
Surgery is reasonable for patients with infective endocarditis of a prosthetic valve who present with relapsing infection. *(Level of Evidence: C)*

Class III

Routine surgery is not indicated for patients with uncomplicated infective endocardi-tis of a prosthetic valve caused by first infection with a sensitive organism. *(Level of Evidence: C)*

Reproduced with permission from American College of Cardiology; American Heart Association Task Force on Practice Guidelines (Writing Committee to revise the 1998 guide-lines for the management of patients with valvular heart disease); Society of Cardiovascular Anesthesiologists, Bonow RO, Carabello BA, Chatterjee K, et al. ACC/AHA 2006 guide-lines for the management of patients with valvular heart disease: a report of the American College of Cardiology/American Heart Association Task Force on Practice Guidelines (Writing Committee to revise the 1998 guidelines for the management of patients with valvular heart disease) developed in collaboration with the Society of Cardiovascular Anesthesiologists endorsed by the Society for Cardiovascular Angiography and Interventions and the Society of Thoracic Surgeons. *J Am Coll Cardiol.* 2006;48(3):e1–e148.

PREVENTION

Antibiotic prophylaxis for IE remains challenging, as there is little evidence from well-designed human trials regarding its efficacy. The prophylaxis guidelines have recently been revised resulting in substantially fewer patients being recommended for IE prophy-laxis. The changes reflect consensus that IE is much more likely to result from frequent exposure to random bacteremias associated with daily activities than from bacteria caused by a dental, GI tract, or GU tract manipulation. In addition, the population-wide risk of antibiotic-associated adverse events is thought to exceed the benefits from widespread prophylactic antibiotic therapy.

Antibiotic prophylaxis is now only recommended for cardiac conditions associated with the highest risk of adverse outcome (Table 38-13). Patients at highest risk should

TABLE 38-13

Cardiac Conditions Associated with Highest Risk of Adverse Outcome from Endocarditis for Which Prophylaxis is Dental and Respiratory Procedures is Reasonable

Prosthetic cardiac or prosthetic material used for cardiac valve repair
Previous IE
Congenital heart disease (CHD)[a]
    Unrepaired cyanotic CHD, including palliative shunts and conduits
    Completely repaired congenital heart defect with prosthetic material or device, whether placed by surgery or by catheter intervention, during the first 6 months after the procedure[b]
    Repaired CHD with residual defects at the site or adjacent to the site of a prosthetic patch or prosthetic device (which inhibit endothelialization)
Cardiac transplantation recipients who develop cardiac valvulopathy

[a]Except for the conditions listed above, antibiotic prophylaxis is no longer recommended for any other forms of CHD.
[b]Prophylaxis is reasonable because endothelialization of prosthetic material occurs within 6 months after the procedure.

Aadapted with permission from Wilson T, Taubert KA, Gewitz M, et al. Prevention of infective endocarditis: guidelines from the American Heart Association. A guideline from the American Heart Association Rheumatic Fever, Endocarditis, and Kawasaki Disease Committee, Council on Cardiovascular Disease in the Young, and the Council on Clinical Cardiology, Council on Cardiovascular Surgery and Anesthesia, and the Quality of Care and Outcomes Research Interdisciplinary Working Group. *Circulation.* 2007;116:1745.

TABLE 38-14

Antibiotic Regimens for IE Prophylaxis

Situation	Agent	Single Dose 30–60 min Before Procedure	
		Adults	Children
Oral	Amoxicillin	2 g	50 mg/kg
Unable to take oral medication	Ampicillin OR	2 g IM or IV	50 mg/kg IM or IV
	cefazolin or ceftriaxone	1 g IM or IV	50 mg/kg IM or IV
Allergic to penicillins or ampicillins—oral	Cephalexin [a,b] OR	2g	50 mg/kg
	clindamycin OR	600 mg	20 mg/kg
	azithromycin or clarithromycin	500 mg	15 mg/kg
Allergic to penicillins or ampicillin and	Cefazolin or ceftriazone [b] OR	1 g IM or IV	50 mg/kg IM or IV
unable to take oral medication	clindamycin	600 mg IM or IV	20 mg/kg IM or IV

IM, intramuscular; IV, intravenous.

[a]Or other first- or second-generation oral cephalosporin in equivalent adult or pediatric dosage.
[b]Cephalosporins should not be used in an individual with a history of anaphylaxis, angioedema, or urticaria with penicillins or ampicillin.

Adapted with permission from Wilson T, Taubert KA, Gewitz M, et al. Prevention of infective endocarditis: guidelines from the American Heart Association. A guideline from the American Heart Association Rheumatic Fever, Endocarditis, and Kawasaki Disease Committee, Council on Cardiovascular Disease in the Young, and the Council on Clinical Cardiology, Council on Cardiovascular Surgery and Anesthesia, and the Quality of Care and Outcomes Research Interdisciplinary Working Group. *Circulation.* 2007;116:1747.

receive prophylaxis when undergoing dental procedures that involve the manipulation of gingival tissue, periapical region of the teeth, or perforation of the oral mucosa. Prophylaxis is also reasonable for invasive procedures of the respiratory tract that involve incision or biopsy of respiratory mucosa. Importantly, antibiotic prophylaxis is no longer recommended for GU or GI tract procedures. Recommendations for procedure-specific antibiotic prophylaxis regimens are provided in Table 38-14.

SUGGESTED READING

Baddour LM, Wilson WR, Bayer AS, et al. Infective endocarditis: diagnosis, antimicrobial therapy, and management of complications. A statement for healthcare professionals from the Committee on Rheumatic Fever, Endocarditis, and Kawasaki Disease, Council on Cardiovascular Disease in the Young, and the Councils on Clinical Cardiology, Stroke, and Cardiovascular Surgery and Anesthesia, American Heart Association. Endorsed by the Infectious Diseases Society of America. *Circulation*. 2005;111:e394–e434.

Bonow RO, Carabello BA, Kanu C, et al. ACC/AHA 2006 guidelines for the management of patients with valvular heart disease: a report of the American College of Cardiology/American Heart Association Task Force on Practice Guidelines (writing committee to revise the 1998 Guidelines for the Management of Patients with Valvular Heart Disease). Developed in collaboration with the Society of Cardiovascular Anesthesiologists. Endorsed by the Society for Cardiovascular Angiography and Interventions and the Society of Thoracic Surgeons. *Circulation*. 2006;114:e84–e231.

Cheitlin MD, Armstrong WF, Aurigemma GP, et al. ACC/AHA/ASE 2003 guideline update for the clinical application of echocardiography: summary article. A report of the American College of Cardiology/American Heart Association Task Force on Practice Guidelines (ACC/AHA/ASE Committee to Update the 1997 Guidelines for the Clinical Application of Echocardiography). *J Am Soc Echocardiogr*. 2003;16:1091–1110.

Haldar SM, O'Gara PT. Infective endocarditis. In: Fuster V, O'Rourke RA, Walsh RA, et al., eds. *Hurst's The Heart*. 12th ed. New York, NY: McGraw-Hill; 2008:1975–2004.

Levy DM. Centenary of William Osler's 1885 Gulstonian lectures and their place in the history of bacterial endocarditis. *J R Soc Med*. 1985:78:1039–1046.

Li JS, Sexton DJ, Mick N, et al. Proposed modifications to the Duke criteria for the diagnosis of infective endocarditis. *Clin Infect Dis*. 2000;30:633–638.

Mylonakis E, Calderwood SB. Infective endocarditis in adults. *N Engl J Med*. 2001; 345:1318–1330.

Netzer RO, Altwegg SC, Zollinger E, et al. Infective endocarditis: determinants of long term outcome. *Heart*. 2002;88:61–66.

Vikram HR, Buenconsejo J, Hasbun R, et al. Impact of valve surgery on 6-month mortality in adults with complicated, left-sided native valve endocarditis: a propensity analysis. *JAMA*. 2003; 290:3250–3521.

Wilson, T, Taubert, KA, Gewitz, M, et al. Prevention of infective endocarditis: a guideline from the American Heart Association Rheumatic Fever, Endocarditis, and Kawasaki Disease Committee, Council on Cardiovascular Disease in the Young, and the Council on Clinical Cardiology, Council on Cardiovascular Surgery and Anesthesia, and the Quality of Care and Outcomes Research Interdisciplinary Working Group. *Circulation*. 2007;116:1736–1754.

CHAPTER (39)

Dilated Cardiomyopathies

Luisa Mestroni, Edward M. Gilbert,
Brian D. Lowes, and Michael R. Bristow

BACKGROUND AND HISTORICAL PERSPECTIVE

The primary and secondary dilated cardiomyopathies are the most common causes of chronic heart failure. The clinical syndrome of heart failure is a complex process where the primary pathophysiology is quickly obscured by a variety of superimposed secondary adaptive, maladaptive, and counterregulatory processes. Despite improvements in the treatment of heart failure introduced in the last 10 years, including the general availability of cardiac transplantation and better medical treatment, clinical outcome following the onset of symptoms has not changed substantially. The mortality remains high (median survival of 1.7 years for men and 3.2 years for women), the natural history is progressive, the cost excessive, and disability and morbidity among the highest of any disease or disease syndrome.

THE CLASSIFICATION OF CARDIOMYOPATHIES

The 1995 World Health Organization/International Society and Federation of Cardiology (WHO/ISFC) classification of cardiomyopathies was recently revised to accommodate several rapidly emerging realities, in particular the identification of new disease entities, advances in diagnosis, and knowledge of etiology of previously unknown types of heart muscle disease.

The classifications of cardiomyopathies are shown in Table 39-1. The WHO/ISFC classification of cardiomyopathy was mainly based on the global anatomic description of chamber dimensions in systole and diastole. Thus, the dilated and restrictive categories had definitions based on left ventricular (LV) dimensions or volume, which also define function via calculated ejection fraction. The novel AHA Scientific Statement emphasizes the genetic determinants of cardiomyopathies. Thus, dilated and restrictive cardiomyopathies are defined as *mixed* cardiomyopathies (predominantly nongenetic); however, hypertrophic cardiomyopathy (HCM), caused by mutations in contractile proteins, and other rare forms of cardiomyopathy including arrhythmogenic right ventricular cardiomyopathy/arrhythmogenic right ventricular dysplasia (ARVC/ARVD) and left ventricular noncompaction (LVNC), which also turned out to be completely genetic in basis, are defined as *genetic* cardiomyopathies. The third category concerns *acquired* cardiomyopathies, such as peripartum- and tachycardia-induced cardiomyopathies. Conversely, genetic cardiomyopathies without unique phenotypes and involvement of a generalized multiorgan disorder, such as the dilated cardiomyopathy of Becker–Duchenne, are defined as *secondary* cardiomyopathies. This distinction is arbitrary and may inevitably cause significant overlap between primary and secondary cardiomyopathies.

TABLE 39-1

Classification of the Cardiomyopathies

Category	Definition
Genetic	
I. Hypertrophic (HCM)	↑↑ septal and ↑ posterior wall thickness, myofibrillar disarray
	Mutation in sarcomeric protein, autosomal dominant inheritance
II. Arrhythmogenic RV (ARVC/ARVD)	Fibrofatty replacement of RV myocardium
III. LV noncompaction	Spongy LV cavity (apex)
IV. Glycogen storage diseases	Danon disease, PRKAG2
V. Ion channelopathies	Conduction defects, LQTS, Brugada syndrome, SQTS, CPVT, Asian SUNDS
Mixed	
I. Dilated (DCM)	↑ EDV ↑ ESV; low EF
II. Restrictive (RCM)	↑ EDV, ↔ ESV; ↑ FP, ↔ EF
Acquired	
I. Myocarditis	Inflammatory process
II. Stress provoked (tako-tsubo)	Reversible LV dysfunction
III. Peripartum	Third trimester or 5 months after pregnancy
IV. Tachycardia induced	Following prolonged periods of SVT or VT
V. Infants of insulin-dependent diabetic mothers	

ARVC, arrhythmogenic right ventricular cardiomyopathy; ARVD, arrhythmogenic right ventricular dysplasia; CM, cardiomyopathy; CPVT, catecholaminergic polymorphic ventricular tachycardia; EDV, end-diastolic volume; ESV, end-systolic volume; EF, LV ejection fraction; FP, LV filling pressure; HCM, hypertrophic cardiomyopathy; LQTS, long QT syndrome; LV, left ventricular; RV, right ventricular; SQTS, short QT syndrome; SVT, supraventricular tachycardia; SUNDS, sudden unexplained death syndrome; VT, ventricular tachycardia.

Finally, the novel classification suggests abandoning the term *specific* cardiomyopathies and excludes valvular, hypertensive, and ischemic cardiomyopathy from the classification; but many mechanisms responsible for the natural history of myocardial dysfunction are qualitatively similar in primary versus these specific dilated cardiomyopathies, which accurately predicted a qualitatively similar response to treatment targeted at these mechanisms. In particular this is the case of *ischemic dilated cardiomyopathy* related to previous myocardial infarction (MI) and the subsequent remodeling process, or *hypertensive dilated* (or *restrictive* depending on the chamber dimensions) *cardiomyopathy*, definitions that are still widely used in the clinical practice in the literature.

MOLECULAR MECHANISMS IN CARDIOMYOPATHIES AND MYOCARDIAL FAILURE: DISEASE PHENOTYPE PRODUCED BY ALTERATIONS IN GENE EXPRESSION

There are three general categories of mechanisms whereby altered gene expression can lead to a phenotypic change in cardiac myocytes:

1. A single gene defect, such as lamin A/C gene mutations or alpha-myosin heavy chain

2. Polymorphic variation in modifier genes, such as is present in many components of the renin–angiotensin, adrenergic, and endothelin systems

3. Maladaptive regulated expression of completely normal genes, such as for the mechanisms responsible for progressive myocardial dysfunction and remodeling in secondary dilated cardiomyopathies.

【 】 GENETIC CAUSES OF DILATED CARDIOMYOPATHIES IN HUMANS AND ANIMAL MODELS

Multiple gene defects have been identified that can produce a dilated cardiomyopathy in humans, as discussed in more detail in the section on familial forms of dilated cardiomyopathy. As listed in Table 39-2, these include mutations in genes encoding proteins of the cytoskeleton, such as dystrophin; nuclear envelope, such as lamin A/C; sarcomere, such as cardiac beta-myosin heavy chain (beta-MHC) and alpha-myosin heavy chain (alpha-MHC); ion channels, like SCN5A; desmosome; and signaling pathways, such transcriptional and Ca^{2+}-cycling regulators.

【 】 POLYMORPHIC VARIATION IN MODIFIER GENES

Genes exhibit polymorphic variation; for example, normal variants of genes exist in the population that are of slightly different size or sequence. Some gene polymorphisms are associated with differences in function of the expressed protein gene product, and some differences in function likely account for the *biological variation* routinely encountered in population studies of disease susceptibility or clinical response to treatment.

Examples of modifier genes that may have an impact on the natural history of a dilated cardiomyopathy include the angiotensin-converting enzyme (ACE) *DD* genotype, where individuals are homozygous for the *deletion* variant, which is associated with increased circulating and cardiac tissue ACE activity. The *DD* genotype appears to be a risk factor for early remodeling after MI and for the development of end-stage ischemic and idiopathic dilated cardiomyopathy. Other potentially important polymorphic variants that may influence the natural history of a cardiomyopathy involve the angiotensin AT_1 receptor, beta-2-adrenergic receptors, the alpha-2C-adrenergic receptor with or without a beta-1-receptor polymorphism, and the endothelin receptor type A.

Finally, recent pharmacogenomic studies have shown that polymorphic variations can influence the response to medications. Patients with the *DD* genotype, who were found to have a worse prognosis, at the same time appeared to respond significantly better to beta-blocker therapy compared to the other genotypes (*II* and *ID*). Similarly, a polymorphism within a conserved region of the beta-1-adrenergic receptor ([389]arginine) increases the response to isotropic therapy (isoproterenol) and is associated with a reduction of mortality in patients treated with the beta-blocker bucindolol.

【 】 ALTERED, MALADAPTIVE EXPRESSION OF A COMPLETELY NORMAL GENE

The third way for altered gene expression to contribute to the development of a cardiomyopathy is altered, maladaptive expression of a completely normal *wild-type* gene. This occurs most commonly in the context of progression of heart muscle disease and myocardial failure, which is the natural history of virtually all cardiomyopathies once they are established. Examples in this category (see Table 39-2) include down-regulation of beta-1-adrenergic receptors, alpha-MHC, and the *SERCA2* (sarcoplasmic reticulum [SR] Ca^{2+} adenosine triphosphatase [ATPase]) genes and upregulation in the atrial natriuretic peptide (*ANP*), beta-*MHC, ACE,* tumor necrosis factor alpha (*TNF*-alpha), endothelin, and beta-adrenergic receptor kinase (*BARK*) genes. Recent data have shown that in patients who respond to treatment by increasing LV ejection fraction, beta-blocker therapy may

TABLE 39-2

Known Familial DCM Genes, Loci, and their OMIM Identifiers

Phenotype	Estimated Frequency (%)	Chromosomal Location	Locus Identifier	OMIM Symbol	Gene	Gene
Autosomal dominant familial DCM	56	1q32	CMD1D	191045	TNNT2	Cardiac troponin T
		3p21.1		191040	TNNC1	Cardiac troponin C
		2q31	CMD1G	188840	TTN	Titin
		2q35	CMD1I	125660	DES	Desmin
		6q12–q16	CMD1K	172405	PLN	Phospholamban
		9	CMD1B			
		10q21–q23	CMD1C	193065	VCL	Metavinculin
		11p11		600958	MYBPC3	Myosin-binding protein C
		11p15.1	CMD1M	600824	CSRP3	Cysteine-glycine–rich protein 3
		12q22	CMD1T	188380	LAP2	Thymopoietin
		14q12	CMD1A	160760	MYH7	Cardiac beta-myosin heavy chain
		14q12		160710	MYH6	Cardiac alpha-myosin heavy chain
		15q14	CMD1A	102540	ACTC	Cardiac actin alpha
		15q22.1		191010	TPM1	Tropomyosin
		17q12	CMD1N	604488	TCAP	Titin-cap (teletonin)
		10q23.2		605906	LDB3	Cypher/ZASP
		12p12.1		601439	ABCC9	Regulatory SUR2A subunit of cardiac K_{ATP} channel

479

TABLE 39-2

Known Familial DCM Genes, Loci, and their OMIM Identifiers (*Continued*)

Phenotype	Estimated Frequency (%)	Chromosomal Location	Locus Identifier	OMIM Symbol	Gene	Gene
Autosomal recessive familial DCM	16	19q13.42		191044	TNNI3	Cardiac troponin I
X-linked DCM	10	unknown Xp21 Xq24	XLCM	212110 300377 300257	 DMD LAMP2	 Dystrophin Lysosome-associated membrane protein-2
Autosomal dominant familial DCM with skeletal muscle disease	7.7	1q11–q23	LGMD1B	150330	LMNA	Lamin A/C
		5q33–34 4q11 6q23	LGMD2F LGMD2E CMD1F	601411 602900 602067	SGCD SGCB	Delta-sarcoglycan B sarcoglycan
Autosomal dominant familial DCM with conduction defects	2.6	1q1–q1	CMD1A	150330	LMNA	Lamin A/C
		2q14–q22 3p22.2	CMD1H CMD1E	604288 600163	 SCN5A	 Na channel, voltage- gated, type V, alpha polypeptide

480

Rare familial DCM	7.7					
Left ventricular noncompaction		Xq28		300069	*TAZ*	G4.5 (tafazzin)
		18q12.1–q12.2		601239	*DTNA*	Alpha-dystrobrevin
		10q23.2		605906	*LDB3*	Cypher/ZASP
		6q23-q24	CMD1J	605362	*EYA4*	Transcriptional coactivator EYA4
Autosomal recessive with retinitis pigmentosa and deafness		6p24		125647	*DSP*	Desmoplakin
Mitochondrial DCM		mtDNA		510000		

DCM, dilated cardiomyopathy; mtDNA, mitochondrial DNA; OMIM, Online Mendelian Inheritance in Man.

Modified from Taylor MRG, Carniel E, Mestroni L. Cardiomyopathy, familial dilated. *Orphanet J Rare Dis*. 2006;1:27.

restore some aspects of altered gene expression, increasing the expression of sarcoplasmic-reticulum calcium ATPase and of alpha-MHC, and decreasing beta-MHC.

【 】 PATHOPHYSIOLOGIC PROCESSES INVOLVED IN MYOCARDIAL DYSFUNCTION/REMODELING AND THEIR PROGRESSION

Tissue preparations and myocytes isolated from failing human hearts exhibit evidence of decreased contractile function. Assuming that loading conditions and ischemia are not adversely affecting cardiac myocyte function, in the setting of chronic systolic dysfunction from a dilated cardiomyopathy, progressive myocardial failure is most likely caused by myocardial cell loss or changes in the gene expression of proteins that regulate or produce muscle contraction. Figures 39-1 and 39-2 summarize these general points and emphasize the central roles of the renin–angiotensin system (RAS) and adrenergic nervous system (ANS) in promoting cell loss, growth and remodeling, and altered gene expression.

SELECTED COMMON TYPES OF DILATED CARDIOMYOPATHIES

【 】 ISCHEMIC CARDIOMYOPATHY

Ischemic cardiomyopathy is commonly defined as a dilated cardiomyopathy in a subject with a history of MI or evidence of clinically significant (i.e., ≥ 70% narrowing of a major epicardial artery) coronary artery disease, in whom the degree of myocardial dysfunction and ventricular dilatation is not explained solely by the extent of previous

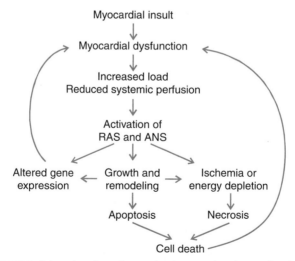

FIGURE 39-1. Relationship of neurohormonal activation and production of cardiac myocyte loss due to apoptosis and necrosis and altered gene expression. Cell loss and altered gene expression result in more myocardial dysfunction, and a vicious cycle is established. (RAS, renin–angiotensin system; ANS, autonomic nervous system.)

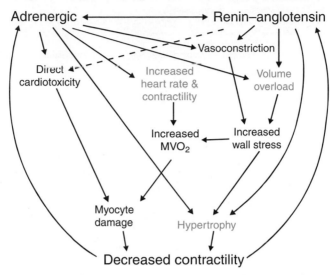

FIGURE 39-2. Heart failure compensatory mechanisms activated to support the failing heart. Lighter-colored type areas indicate physiologic mechanisms that stabilize pump function.

infarction or the degree of ongoing ischemia (see Table 39-3). Dilatation of the LV and a decrease in ejection fraction occurs in 15% to 40% of subjects within 12 to 24 months following an anterior MI and in a smaller percentage of subjects following an inferior MI. The gross pathology of ischemic cardiomyopathy includes transmural or subendocardial scarring, representing old MIs, that may comprise up to 50% of the LV chamber. The histopathology of the noninfarcted regions is similar to changes that occur in DCM, as discussed below. Several studies conclude that patients with ischemic cardiomyopathy have a worse prognosis than subjects with a *nonischemic* dilated cardiomyopathy, probably because the risk of ischemic events is added to the risk of having a dilated cardiomyopathy.

The treatment of ischemic dilated cardiomyopathy consists of the use of (1) ACE inhibitors in asymptomatic or symptomatic patients, (2) beta-blockers in symptomatic patients, (3) diuretics in volume-overloaded subjects, (4) spironolactone in advanced patients, and (5) digoxin in symptomatic patients. Recent data have demonstrated the effectiveness of devices in treating ischemic dilated cardiomyopathies, including implantable cardioverters/defibrillators (ICDs) for patients without intraventricular conduction defects (IVCDs), and biventricular pacing plus ICD for patients with IVCDs. Additionally, adjunctive therapy includes anticoagulation in subjects with lower LV ejection fraction to prevent thromboembolic complications, amiodarone to treat symptomatic arrhythmias, maintenance of potassium levels in the high normal (4.3–5.0 meq/L) range to prevent sudden death, keeping digoxin levels ≤ 1.0 ng/mL, frequent clinic visits to adjust medications, and an aggressive approach to treating ischemia, including revascularization.

【 】 HYPERTENSIVE CARDIOMYOPATHY

A *hypertensive dilated cardiomyopathy* is diagnosed when myocardial systolic function is depressed out of proportion to the increase in wall stress. In other words, a subject presenting in heart failure with a hypertensive crisis would not carry this diagnosis unless

TABLE 39-3

Types of Dilated Cardiomyopathies

Ischemic insult (*ischemic cardiomyopathy*)
Valvular disease (mitral regurgitation, aortic stenosis); (*valvular cardiomyopathy*)
Chronic hypertension (*hypertensive cardiomyopathy*)
Tachyarrhythmias (supraventricular, ventricular, atrial flutter)
Familial (autosomal dominant, autosomal recessive, X-linked, matrilinear)
Idiopathic
Toxins
    Ethanol
    Chemotherapeutic agents (anthracyclines such as doxorubicin and daunorubicin)
    Cobalt
    Antiretroviral agents (zidovudine, didanosine, zalcitabine)
    Phenothiazines
    Carbon monoxide
    Lithium
    Lead
    Cocaine
    Mercury
Metabolic abnormalities
    Nutritional deficiencies (thiamine, selenium, carnitine, protein)
    Endocrinologic disorders (hypothyroidism, acromegaly, thyrotoxicosis, Cushing's
    disease, pheochromocytoma, catecholamines, diabetes mellitus)
    Electrolyte disturbances (hypocalcemia, hypophosphatemia)
Infectious
    Viral (coxsackievirus, cytomegalovirus, HIV, adenovirus, HSV)
    Rickettsial
    Bacterial
    Mycobacterial
    Spirochetal
    Fungal
    Parasitic (toxoplasmosis, trichinosis, Chagas' disease)
Autoimmune/collagen disorders
    Systemic lupus erythematosus
Juvenile rheumatoid arthritis
    Polyarteritis nodosa
    Kawasaki disease
    Collagen vascular disorders (scleroderma, lupus erythematosus, dermatomyosits)
Infiltrative disorders
    Hemochromatosis
Amyloidosis
    Sarcoidosis
Endomyocardial disorders
    Hypereosinophilic syndrome (Löffler endocarditis)
    Endomyocardial fibrosis
Hypersensitivity myocarditis
Peripartum/postpartum dysfunction
    Arrhythmogenic right ventricular dysplasia or cardiomyopathy
Infantile histiocytoid
Neuromuscular dystrophies
    Becker or Duchenne muscular dystrophy, X-linked cardioskeletal myopathy
Facioscapulohumeral muscular dystrophy
    Erb limb-girdle dystrophy
    Myotonic dystrophy
Friedreich ataxia
    Emery–Dreifuss muscular dystrophy
Inborn errors of metabolism
Mitochondrial cardiomyopathies
Keshan cardiomyopathy

ventricular dilatation and depressed systolic function remained after correction of the hypertension. In addition to producing a *pure* form of hypertensive cardiomyopathy, hypertension is a major risk factor for heart failure from any cause. Within the 1995 WHO/ISFC classification, *hypertensive heart disease* may present in the *dilated, restrictive,* or *unclassified* categories. However, the 2006 AHA Scientific Statement has not included the hypertensive myocardial disease in the formal classification of cardiomyopathies. The phenotypic expression is variable and can include dilation and systolic dysfunction without increased wall thickness, concentric hypertrophy with or without systolic dysfunction, and systolic dysfunction without concentric hypertrophy. The prognosis depends on the presence of other comorbid conditions such as diabetes mellitus and coronary artery disease as well as the extent of control of afterload. Compared to other forms of cardiomyopathy, in the absence of comorbid conditions, the prognosis of hypertensive cardiomyopathy in subjects whose afterload is controlled is probably better than for most other types of dilated cardiomyopathy.

The treatment is as for ischemic dilated cardiomyopathy except that afterload must be vigorously controlled. This consists of the addition of pure antihypertensive vasodilators such as amlodipine, hydralazine, nitrates, or even alpha-blocking agents to standard heart failure therapy.

【　】 VALVULAR CARDIOMYOPATHY

A *valvular cardiomyopathy* occurs when a valvular abnormality is present and myocardial systolic function is depressed out of proportion to the increase in wall stress. This most commonly occurs with left-sided regurgitant lesions (mitral regurgitation and aortic regurgitation), less commonly with aortic stenosis, and never as a consequence of pure mitral stenosis. A disturbing and fairly commonly observed phenomenon is the development of a dilated cardiomyopathy after surgical correction of mitral and sometimes aortic valve disease in subjects who preoperatively had only mild LV dysfunction. These cases are likely caused by the superimposition of myocardial damage resulting from open heart surgery and/or underlying dysfunction that was likely greater than may have been appreciated preoperatively. The prognosis is variable and depends on the number of associated conditions. In general, *severely depressed myocardial function will not improve much with surgical repair of aortic regurgitation or mitral regurgitation, but the prognosis is likely to be improved because of elimination of some of the hemodynamic insult.* Replacement of the mitral valve should not be attempted in most subjects with severe mitral regurgitation and LV ejection fraction < 25% because of prohibitively high operative/perioperative mortality rates. Conversely, there is no impairment of LV systolic function severe enough to preclude valve replacement of severe aortic stenosis, because function invariably improves on relief of the hemodynamic insult and the prognosis is relatively good.

The treatment of a valvular dilated cardiomyopathy is surgical valve replacement or repair as soon as the cardiomyopathy is detected. Catheter valvuloplasty may be an option for patients with severe aortic stenosis who are not good surgical candidates for reasons other than heart failure. Medical treatment may be the only option in subjects with aortic insufficiency or mitral regurgitation whose LV function is severely impaired. The medical treatment of either disorder should be as above for ischemic cardiomyopathy plus aggressive afterload reduction, usually hydralazine/nitrates on top of ACE inhibitors. The calcium-channel blocker amlodipine is another option for afterload reduction, particularly for aortic insufficiency, where calcium-blocker therapy has been shown to improve survival.

【　】 IDIOPATHIC DILATED CARDIOMYOPATHY, INCLUDING FAMILIAL FORMS

DCM is diagnosed by excluding significant coronary artery disease, valvular abnormalities, and other causes. DCM is a relatively common cause of heart failure, with an estimated prevalence rate of 0.04%; incidence rates vary from 0.005% to 0.006%. The incidence of DCM increases with age and males are affected at a higher rate than females. Although the diagnosis is not difficult, problems arise when an apparent DCM presents in someone with a history of hypertension or excessive alcohol intake. In such cases it is best to reassign the etiology to alcohol only when the intake has exceeded 80 g/d for males and 40 g/d for females for > 5 years and to hypertensive heart disease when blood pressure has been uncontrolled and high (> 160/100 mm Hg), as well as sustained (for years). All subjects with an unexplained dilated cardiomyopathy need a thyroid-stimulating hormone level done to exclude hypo- or hyperthyroidism, and subjects with diastolic dysfunction may need to have an infiltrative process excluded by endomyocardial biopsy.

Histologic features are nonspecific and consist of myocardial cell hypertrophy and varying amounts of increased interstitial fibrosis. DCM may be familial in as many as 35% to 50% of the cases when first-degree relatives are carefully screened. The analysis of the phenotype identifies a wide range of clinical and pathologic forms indicating genetic heterogeneity. Accordingly, several chromosomal assignments for gene location have been made, and recently (Table 39-2) several genes have been identified. Most familial patients present with autosomal dominant inheritance and a phenotype characterized by low and age-related penetrance (which is the proportion of carriers who manifest the disease). It is estimated that only 20% of gene carriers younger than the age of 20 display the disease phenotype.

Familial dilated cardiomyopathy can be caused by mutations of a large number of genes involved in various myocardial functions including the *sarcomere,* the *cytoskeleton/sarcolemma/nuclear envelope, ion channels,* the *desmosome,* and *signaling pathways.* Specific characteristics of the phenotype can help in the identification of the disease gene. The detection of an altered creatine kinase (CK) level can indicate the existence of a subclinical skeletal muscle disease. In these patients an X-linked inheritance suggests mutations in the dystrophin gene that maps on the X chromosome. Skeletal muscle and endomyocardial biopsy shows abnormalities of dystrophin protein expression by immunocytochemistry. An autosomal dominant transmission and the presence of conduction defects, arrhythmia, and increased CK levels suggest mutations in the lamin A/C gene. In *laminopathies* the phenotype of the affected relatives can be very variable, from a pure DCM to a mild Emery-Dreifuss–like or limb-girdle–like muscle dystrophy. An autosomal recessive transmission of dilated cardiomyopathy may occur in mutations of sarcoglycan genes, which encode for dystrophin complex–associated proteins. Other structural proteins, such as *desmosomal* proteins, can cause a DCM phenotype. This is the case of the *desmoplakin* gene that causes Carvajal syndrome (DCM, woolly hair, and keratoderma).

Although still incomplete, new knowledge on the genetics of DCM has important clinical implications. The frequency of familial forms indicates the need for family screening in DCM, which can allow genetic counseling, an early detection of the disease, and early therapeutic interventions in affected relatives. The complexity of the phenotype requires an accurate skeletal muscle investigation, which can direct the diagnosis toward a specific type of familial myopathy. Family investigations require more sensitive diagnostic criteria that are able to detect minor cardiac abnormalities as initial signs of the disease. These include initial dilatation without marked systolic dysfunction, arrhythmia, segmental wall hypokinesis, and abnormal activity. Finally, the systematic screening of genes causing DCM can identify those genes or mutations that are more prevalent and predictive of a worse outcome, so that carriers of such genes can be clinically tested. This is the case of lamin A/C gene, which is frequently mutated in patients with conduction delays and associated with high mortality and morbidity.

Several immune regulatory abnormalities have been identified in DCM, including humoral and cellular autoimmune reactivity against myocytes, decreased natural killer cell activity, and abnormal suppressor cell activity. A clinical and pathologic syndrome that is similar to DCM may develop after resolution of viral myocarditis in animal models and biopsy-proven myocarditis in human subjects. This has led to speculation that DCM may develop in some individuals as a result of subclinical viral myocarditis.

Analysis of human viruses other than enteroviruses suggests that adenoviruses, herpes, and cytomegalovirus can also cause myocarditis and potentially DCM, particularly in children and young subjects. Endomyocardial biopsy may be a valuable diagnostic adjunct for diagnosing specific myocardial processes that can produce a dilated phenotype, such as myocarditis and infiltrative cardiomyopathies: endomyocardial biopsy should be performed in specialized cardiomyopathy/ heart failure centers.

The prognosis of primary DCM is generally better than for ischemic cardiomyopathy; prior to the routine use of ACE inhibitors, the survival was approximately 50% in 5 years. The prognosis has been substantially improved since then, inasmuch as ACE inhibition, beta-adrenergic blockade, cardiac resynchronization with biventricular pacing, implantable cardioverter-defibrillator, and cardiac transplantation (in the high-risk group) are all effective treatments in this condition. Approximately 10% of DCM subjects treated with beta-adrenergic blockade normalize their myocardial function, and this form of treatment should be offered to all DCM subjects who do not have a contraindication before cardiac transplantation is considered. The risk of thromboembolic complications may be higher than in ischemic cardiomyopathy, resulting in a lower threshold for anticoagulation. Among genetic causes of DCM, *laminopathies* (caused by mutations in the lamin A/C gene) have been associated with poorer prognosis, high mortality for congestive heart failure or sudden death, and need of transplant, making molecular genetic testing an important tool in the clinical management of these patients.

SELECTED SECONDARY DILATED CARDIOMYOPATHIES WITH UNIQUE MANAGEMENT ISSUES

【 】 ANTHRACYCLINE CARDIOMYOPATHY

The commonly used and highly efficacious anthracycline antibiotic anticancer agents doxorubicin and daunorubicin produce a cardiomyopathy that depends on the total cumulative dose. For doxorubicin (Adriamycin), the incidence of heart failure due to cardiomyopathy dramatically increases above total cumulative doses of 450 mg/m^2 in subjects without underlying cardiac problems or other risk factors. Mediastinal radiation involving the heart, regardless of timing, is a powerful risk factor for anthracycline cardiomyopathy. In subjects with risk factors, anthracycline cardiomyopathy can present at cumulative doses lower than 450 mg/m^2.

Although the diagnosis of anthracycline cardiomyopathy can be made clinically, the definitive diagnosis depends on the demonstration of a substantial number of cardiac myocytes exhibiting the characteristic anthracycline effect. Tissue sampling is best done by endomyocardial biopsy, which allows for "thin-section" electron microscopic processing of the sample and more definitive resolution of the anthracyline effect with light microscopy. With increasing exposure to anthracyclines, there is cell vacuolization progressing to cell dropout. Myocardial dysfunction results when 16% to 25% of the total number of sampled cells exhibit this morphology.

【 】 POSTPARTUM CARDIOMYOPATHY

Post- or peripartum cardiomyopathy is defined as the presentation of systolic dysfunction and clinical heart failure during the last trimester of pregnancy or within 6 months of delivery. Postpartum cardiomyopathy is likely a heterogeneous group of disorders, consisting of the addition of the hemodynamic load of pregnancy to a variety of underlying myocardial processes including hypertensive heart disease, familial or idiopathic dilated cardiomyopathy, and myocarditis. Approximately half of subjects who develop postpartum cardiomyopathy will completely recover, and most of the rest will improve. Subjects who have developed a postpartum cardiomyopathy should never become pregnant again, even if myocardial function has fully recovered.

【 】 ALCOHOL CARDIOMYOPATHY

An *alcohol cardiomyopathy* is said to be present when other causes of a dilated cardiomyopathy have been excluded and there is a history of heavy, sustained alcohol intake. The requirement in terms of alcohol amount is 80 g of alcohol per day for males and 40 g for females, typically over several years. However, in susceptible individuals it is likely that lower amounts of intake can produce a cardiomyopathy. The histologic features of alcohol cardiomyopathy are nonspecific and do not differ from DCM. Other than history the only potentially distinguishing feature between DCM and alcohol cardiomyopathy is that the latter may present with a relatively high cardiac output. The pathophysiology of alcohol cardiomyopathy is thought to be related to the toxic effects of alcohol, plus, in some subjects, nutritional components such as thiamine deficiency. Genetic factors may predispose to alcoholic cardiomyopathy, like the ACE *DD* polymorphism. The prognosis depends on the degree of impairment of myocardial function and the extent of abstinence from alcohol and, in an extremely compromised patient, the administration of thiamine. There is evidence that the prognosis is somewhat better for alcohol cardiomyopathy than for DCM.

The treatment of alcohol cardiomyopathy does not differ from that of DCM except for the need for total abstinence from alcohol. Obviously, these subjects are not good candidates for cardiac transplantation because of their high relapse rate to alcoholism.

【 】 CHAGAS' CARDIOMYOPATHY

Chagas' disease is a cause of myocarditis and is the most common cause of nonischemic cardiomyopathy in South and Central America, afflicting over 10 million people. It is caused by a parasite, the leishmanial or tissue form of the protozoan *Trypanosoma cruzi*. Chagas' disease may be transmitted by blood transfusions; as a result, it could become relatively more important in the United States. The natural history consists of an initial myocarditis—most commonly presenting in childhood—associated with acute myocardial infection, followed by recovery and in some individuals the development of a dilated cardiomyopathy 10 to 30 years later. The diagnosis of Chagas' cardiomyopathy is based on clinical criteria and a positive serologic test for *T. cruzi*. The histologic lesion of chronic Chagas' consists of mononuclear infiltrates, fibrosis, and foci of the leishmanial form of *T. cruzi* in myocardial fibers. The basis for the Chagas' cardiomyopathy is unknown but may be immunologic, whereby antibodies generated against *T. Cruzi* cross-react with cardiac myocyte antigens, including myosin.

There is no definitive treatment for Chagas' cardiomyopathy. Nonspecific treatment includes pacemaker implantation for heart block and heart failure treatment, as for idiopathic dilated cardiomyopathy. The one exception may be the more frequent use of amiodarone, which appears to be particularly effective in treating arrhythmias associated with Chagas' cardiomyopathy. The role of cardiac transplantation is still somewhat uncertain, but transplantation can be done at acceptable risk, especially when coupled with trypanocidal agent.

SUGGESTED READING

Armstrong SC. Anti-oxidants and apoptosis: attenuation of doxorubicin induced cardiomyopathy by carvedilol. *J Mol Cell Cardiol*. 2004;37:817–821.

Bristow MR. β-Adrenergic receptor blockade in chronic heart failure. *Circulation*. 2000;101:558–569.

Bristow MR, Saxon LA, Boehmer J, et al. Cardiac-resynchronization therapy with or without an implantable defibrillator in advanced chronic heart failure. *N Engl J Med*. 2004;350:2140–2150.

Fett JD, Christie LG, Carraway RD, et al. Five-year prospective study of the incidence and prognosis of peripartum cardiomyopathy at a single institution. *Mayo Clin Proc.* 2005;80:1602–1606.

Mann DL, Bristow MR. Mechanisms and models in heart failure: the biomedical model and beyond. *Circulation.* 2005;111:2837–2849.

Maron BJ, Towbin JA, Thiene G, et al. Contemporary definitions and classification of the cardiomyopathies. *Circulation.* 2006;113:1807–1816.

McKusick VA. Online Mendelian Inheritance in Man (OMIM). In: McKusick-Nathans Institute for Genetic Medicine, Johns Hopkins University (Baltimore, MD) and National Center for Biotechnology Information, National Library of Medicine (Bethesda, MD); 2000. Available at www.ncbi.nim.nih.gov/Omim/

Mestroni L, Maisch B, McKenna WJ, et al. Guidelines for the study of familial dilated cardiomyopathies. *Eur Heart J.* 1999;20:93–102.

Taylor MRG, Carniel E, Mestroni L. Cardiomyopathy, familial dilated. *Orphanet J Rare Dis.* 2006;1:27.

Taylor MRG, Fain P, Sinagra G, et al. Natural history of dilated cardiomyopathy due to lamin A/C gene mutations. *J Am Coll Cardiol.* 2003;41:771–780.

CHAPTER 40

Hypertrophic Cardiomyopathy

Lian R. Shaw and Robert A. O'Rourke

Hypertrophic cardiomyopathy (HCM) was first introduced by Jeare in 1958, when he published the pathologic findings of young patients who had died suddenly. Described as idiopathic hypertrophic subaortic stenosis, muscular subaortic stenosis, and hypertrophic obstructive cardiomyopathy, *HCM* is now the preferred term by the World Health Organization for the massive hypertrophy of the ventricular septum and small ventricular cavity characteristic of this entity. HCM is perhaps the most common genetic cardiovascular disease caused by a missense mutation in one of at least ten genes encoding proteins of the sarcomere and contractile apparatus. Two-hundred different mutations have now been identified; these lead to myofibrillar disarray and fibrosis. HCM is an autosomal dominant trait with a prevalence of approximately 1 per 500 people, and it is a common cause of sudden death in young people, particularly in trained athletes below 30 years of age. The characteristic features of HCM include an increase in left ventricular (LV) wall thickness without ventricular chamber dilatation and normal or hypercontractile LV function. LV outflow tract obstruction (LVOT) is present in < 30% of cases. The most common sites of ventricular involvement include the septum, apex, and midventricle. The pathophysiologic abnormalities in patients with HCM consist of interrelated processes including dynamic LVOT obstruction, diastolic dysfunction, mitral regurgitation (MR), myocardial ischemia, and cardiac arrhythmias.

PATHOLOGY

Pathologic examination of the heart in HCM often reveals asymmetrical septal hypertrophy (ASH) with a small- or normal-sized LV cavity and left atrial (LA) enlargement. Many variants of HCM exist, including asymmetrical posterior hypertrophy, asymmetrical basal free wall hypertrophy, asymmetrical apical hypertrophy, asymmetrical midventricular septal hypertrophy, and HCM with myocardial disarray without hypertrophy. The mitral valve is usually normal but may be thickened, enlarged, and elongated. Endocardial thickening in the LVOT may be present. There may be anomalous papillary muscle insertion into the anterior mitral leaflet.

Histologic examination reveals myocardial disarray consisting of short runs of hypertrophied, nonparallel myofibers distributed in a disorganized fashion and interrupted by connective tissue, resulting in the characteristic "whirling" pattern of HCM. These areas of disorganization and fibrosis are thought to be the source for the ventricular arrhythmias commonly found in HCM.

The intramural coronary arteries may be small secondary to intimal hyperplasia, which results in thickened walls and narrowed lumina. These abnormal intramural coronary arteries may contribute to myocardial ischemia occurring in the presence of epicardial coronaries found to be free of atherosclerotic disease.

CLINICAL MANIFESTATIONS

Dyspnea, angina pectoris, presyncope/syncope, and sudden death are symptoms found in patients with HCM. Although the majority of such patients are asymptomatic, dyspnea is the most common complaint, occurring in 90% of symptomatic patients. Dyspnea occurs as a result of a stiff, noncompliant ventricle, resulting in an elevated LV end-diastolic pressure (LVEDP) and abnormal ventricular relaxation. Concomitant dynamic LVOT obstruction and MR may be present. Angina pectoris occurs in approximately 80% of symptomatic patients. Angina occurring in the absence of atherothrombotic coronary heart disease may result from small abnormal intramural coronary arteries, intramural arterial compression from myocardial hypertrophy, diastolic dysfunction, and supply/demand mismatch. Patients frequently experience impaired consciousness (syncope, near-syncope, or dizziness), palpitations, and occasionally orthopnea or paroxysmal nocturnal dyspnea when more advanced stages of heart failure evolve. Syncope occurs in approximately 20% of patients with HCM, resulting from either a hemodynamic abnormality or a rhythm disturbance. Some 20% of older patients with HCM may experience atrial fibrillation, which can lead to clinical deterioration and increase the risk of systemic embolization.

【 】 PHYSICAL EXAMINATION

The classic physical findings of HCM usually occur only in the presence of an LVOT pressure gradient. Examination of the neck veins reveals a prominent A wave due to a stiff, noncompliant ventricle, elevated pulmonary pressures, or right ventricular outflow obstruction. The carotid pulse is typically bifid with a brisk upstroke, declining in midsystole (secondary to a sudden deceleration of the blood due to midsystolic obstruction) and then having a secondary rise (the subsequent tidal wave), which reflects the classic "spike and dome" configuration. Palpation of the precordium may reveal an apical impulse that is usually sustained and frequently bifid; it may have the classic "triple ripple" (a presystolic and a double systolic movement of the apical impulse). On auscultation, S_1 may be normal or loud; S_2 may be physiologic or paradoxically split if there is severe LVH, left bundle-branch block, or severe LVOT obstruction. An S_4 is usually present. The murmur of HCM is a harsh crescendo-decrescendo systolic murmur heard best along the left lower sternal border and at the apex. The murmur decreases with maneuvers that increase LV volume, such as squatting, leg lifting, or handgrip. Conversely, maneuvers that decrease LV volume—such as standing, the Valsalva maneuver, or amyl nitrite inhalation—tend to increase LVOT obstruction and cause the murmur to increase in intensity. The most useful maneuver is squatting. The murmur may radiate to the base, apex, or axilla but seldom to the neck. Concomitant MR is often present and may be distinguished from the murmur of HCM by location (apical) and character; MR is more holosystolic and does not increase in intensity in the post-premature ventricular contraction (PVC), as does HCM.

DIAGNOSTIC TESTS

【 】 ELECTROCARDIOGRAM

The 12-lead electrocardiogram (ECG) is very useful in screening for HCM, as a normal ECG virtually eliminates the diagnosis. Thus, the ECG is typically abnormal in patients with HCM. Common ECG findings include LV hypertrophy (found in 80% of patients), left atrial enlargement, left anterior hemiblock, left bundle-branch block, PVCs, left axis deviation, abnormal Q waves, or poor R-wave progression across the precordium (representing pseudoinfarction). Prominent T-wave inversion across the precordium may be found in patients with the apical variety of HCM. Findings of preexcitation (delta wave) may be present. Atrial fibrillation is not uncommonly found. There is no pattern that is unique to HCM.

【 】 HOLTER MONITORING

Holter monitoring is frequently utilized to identify patients with high-risk features of sudden cardiac death (SCD). Although the rhythm is typically normal sinus, monitoring may reveal atrial fibrillation, PVCs, and episodes of supraventricular and ventricular arrhythmias.

【 】 CHEST X-RAY

The chest x-ray may be completely normal in the asymptomatic patient. Left atrial enlargement, pulmonary artery engorgement, and edema may be present when LV filling pressures are elevated. The cardiac silhouette is often enlarged, and the left cardiac border may be prominent secondary to LVH. Mitral annular calcification may be seen. The absence of aortic root dilation and aortic valve calcium help to differentiate these patients from those with aortic valve stenosis.

DIAGNOSTIC EVALUATION

【 】 ECHOCARDIOGRAPHY

M-mode, two-dimensional (2D), pulse-wave (PW), continuous-wave (CW) and color-flow Doppler echocardiography have been widely used to screen, diagnose, and follow patients with HCM. Two-dimensional echocardiography is considered the "gold standard" for diagnosing HCM. Echocardiographic features of HCM include LVH (typically asymmetrical) in a nondilated left ventricle with normal systolic function and impaired diastolic function. Although asymmetrical septal hypertrophy is the most common morphologic type of HCM, there is considerable variability in the pattern of hypertrophy found in HCM, including involvement of the free wall, the LV apex, the posterior-basal walls, and frequently only localized thickening of small portions of the LV wall. There is often abnormal anterior displacement of the mitral valve as a result of posterior bulging of the septum. Systolic anterior motion (SAM) of the mitral valve with ventricular septal contact is responsible for dynamic obstruction to LV outflow. Doppler echocardiography can accurately assess the magnitude and dynamic characteristics of the outflow pressure gradient, the severity of dynamic outflow obstruction (with color-flow Doppler), and the diastolic filling and relaxation abnormalities commonly present in HCM. All first-degree family members should undergo echocardiography: every year for the adolescent child aged 12 to 18 and then every 5 years until the sixth to seventh decades of life (Table 40-1).

【 】 RADIONUCLIDE IMAGING/EXERCISE STRESS TESTING

Gated radionuclide ventriculography permits evaluation of cavity size, septal motion, and LV ejection fraction. Myocardial perfusion imaging with thallium 201 or technetium 99m may demonstrate fixed or reversible perfusion defects suggesting areas of myocardial scar or ischemia even in the absence of atherothrombotic coronary heart disease and is therefore of limited utility.

Exercise stress testing is useful for the objective measurement of exercise tolerance and may help in prognostic evaluation. PVCs, arrhythmias such as atrial fibrillation,

TABLE 40-1

Echocardiographic Features of Obstructive Hypertrophic Cardiomyopathy

Decreased LV systolic dimensions
Asymmetrical septal hypertrophy with a ratio of septum to posterior wall 1.5:1 or greater
Systolic anterior motion of the mitral valve
Delayed closure of the mitral valve
Midsystolic closure of the aortic valve
Left atrial enlargement
Mitral regurgitation
Dagger-shaped late peaking continuous-wave Doppler with resting gradient > 30 mm Hg

ventricular tachycardia, and nonsustained ventricular tachycardia may be provoked during exercise. An abnormal blood pressure response to exercise may occur (Table 40-2).

【 】 MAGNETIC RESONANCE IMAGING/ULTRAFAST CT

Magnetic resonances imaging (MRI) and ultrafast computed tomography (CT) have both been used in the evaluation of patients with HCM. MRI is useful in defining the diverse myocardial abnormalities, demonstrating anterior mitral displacement during systole, the narrowing of the LVOT, and left atrial enlargement. MRI can also be utilized to determine the pressure gradients across the LVOT, which are comparable to gradients measured at the time of cardiac catheterization.

【 】 HEMODYNAMICS

Cardiac catheterization and angiography should be performed only when mechanical intervention is contemplated or there is overwhelming evidence of myocardial ischemia.

 TABLE 40-2

Risk Factors for Sudden Cardiac Death in Patients with Hypertrophic Cardiomyopathy

Cardiac arrest (ventricular fibrillation)
Spontaneous sustained ventricular tachycardia
Family history of sudden HCM related death (two or more first-degree relatives < 40 years of age)
Syncope (two or more episodes in 1 year)
Nonsustained ventricular tachycardia on Holter ECG monitoring or exercise testing (three or more consecutive PVCs)
Abnormal blood pressure response with exertion (drop in BP > 10 mm Hg or failure to rise > 25 mm Hg)
Massive LV hypertrophy (LV thickness > 30 mm by echocardiography) LV outflow tract obstruction
Presence of microvascular obstruction detected on MRI or nuclear imaging
High-risk genetic defect within the beta-myosin heavy-chain Arg403Gln, Arg453Cys, and Arg719Trp

When cardiac catheterization is performed, both left and right heart catheterization should be done—in addition to standard coronary angiography—to evaluate for pulmonary hypertension. Left ventriculography should be performed with the RAO projection at 30 degrees and the LAO projection at 60 degrees, with cranial angulation so as to better visualize the septum. Ideally, simultaneous aortic and LV pressures should be measured as the pigtail catheter is pulled back to the LVOT obstruction. Aortic pressure tracings may demonstrate the "spike and dome" configuration (Fig. 40-1). The Brockenbrough, Braunwald, and Morrow phenomena may occur in the beat following a PVC, which leads to an increase in the LV volume and contractility, resulting in an increase of the LVOT gradient and a decrease in the aortic pulse pressure. Patients who have minimal resting gradients during catheterization should undergo provocation with Valsalva, post-PVC, or exercise. Provocation with dobutamine is generally not recommended, as this can elicit a significant gradient in a hyperdynamic LV without true HCM. A significant gradient can occur without provocation in elderly patients with hypertension and hypovolemia and in the hypovolemic postoperative patient receiving inotropic support (Fig. 40-1).

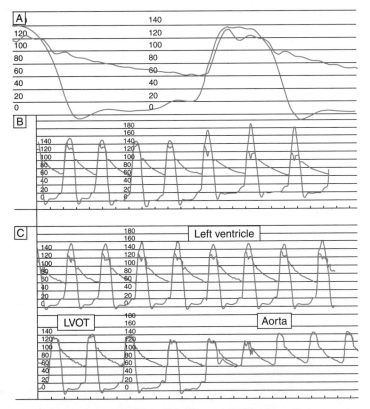

FIGURE 40-1. Left ventricular (LV) and LV outflow tract (LVOT) tracings. **A.** Aortic tracing demonstrating spike and dome. **B.** LV and aortic pressure tracing demonstrating increase in peak-to-peak gradient with Valsalva maneuver. **C.** Simultaneous LV and aortic pressure tracings during pull-back from LV to LVOT to aorta.

NATURAL HISTORY

The natural history of HCM is widely variable. Published studies from tertiary referral centers indicate that the annualized mortality from HCM is between 2% and 6%. However, these centers tend to evaluate a higher proportion of symptomatic and functionally limited patients. Mortality from unselected regional populations is reported at an annual rate of about 1%. The majority of patients are asymptomatic and experience little or no disability, many achieving normal life expectancy. Children between 1 and 15 years of age have an annual mortality of about 6%. Patients with and without LVOT obstruction are equally at risk for sudden death. Premature SCD may occur in the asymptomatic or symptomatic patient. HCM is the most common cause of sudden death in young competitive athletes, frequently occurring during or immediately following physical activity. The primary mechanism of sudden death usually is ventricular tachycardia or fibrillation; however, it is not uncommon for patients to succumb to complete atrioventricular (AV) block, asystole, electromechanical dissociation, or atrial fibrillation with rapid ventricular response. Several risk factors are associated with a higher probability of sudden death (Table 40-2). Progressive symptoms of heart failure may occur and can be exacerbated by atrial fibrillation.

Although many patients live their entire lives without functional limitation, some may begin to experience heart failure after having no symptoms for many decades. A small group of patients will have progressive symptoms of heart failure and will eventually develop the "end stage" or "burned out" stage of HCM, when LV systolic function becomes significantly impaired. This occurs as a result of dilation of the LV cavity due to continued wall stress/tension, causing LV wall thinning and eventual loss of the dynamic outflow tract gradient. In addition to heart failure, other complications of HCM include atrial fibrillation, systemic embolization, and infective endocarditis. Pregnancy is usually well tolerated as long as the patient is kept well hydrated (Table 40-2).

TREATMENT

All patients with HCM should be evaluated on an annual basis and risk-stratified for the occurrence of SCD. Reevaluation should take place whenever there is a perceived change in clinical status. Patients should be advised against isometric exercise such as weight lifting, which can increase myocardial thickness. The implantable cardioverter/defibrillator (ICD) can be offered to the high-risk patient to prevent SCD (Table 40-2). Symptomatic patients can be started on pharmacologic therapy, usually a beta-blocker or a calcium-channel blocker, but their regimen can also include disopyramide. The therapeutic dose of either beta-blocker or verapamil should be titrated for symptomatic relief or a resting heart rate of 50 to 60 beats per minute. Alternatives to medical therapy in obstructive HCM include surgical septal myectomy, alcohol ablation, and dual-chamber pacing or afterload reduction and heart transplantation in the nonobstructive end stage of HCM (Fig. 40-2).

Beta-blockers are negative inotropic agents, which act by decreasing the heart rate and allowing prolonged diastolic filling, ventricular relaxation, and reduction of myocardial oxygen consumption. Beta-blockers are the preferred drug strategy for symptomatic patients with outflow tract gradients provoked by exertion and should be initiated when symptoms of exertional dyspnea appear. Standard doses are often sufficient to relieve disabling symptoms and decrease the outflow tract gradient. Massive doses of propranolol have been advocated when standard doses are insufficient to ameliorate symptoms.

The calcium-channel blocker verapamil has been shown to decrease myocardial oxygen consumption and LVOT obstruction; it is also known to increase LV volume and improve LV isovolumic relaxation. However, in patients with elevated LV filling pressures and a high resting LVOT gradient, verapamil has been associated with provoking

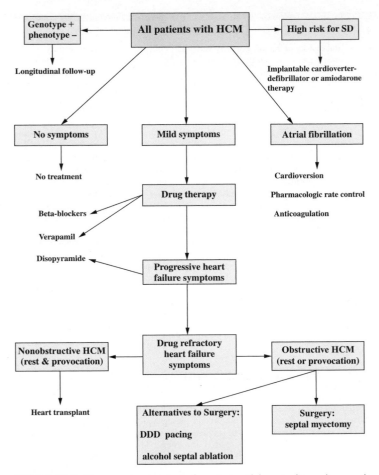

FIGURE 40-2. Primary treatment strategies for patients with hypertrophic cardiomyopathy.

pulmonary edema and SCD. It should therefore be used cautiously or only in patients who are not responsive to beta-blocker therapy or who have severe asthma.

Dysopyramide is a type IA antiarrhythmic agent with negative inotropic properties. In patients with a resting gradient and severe symptoms, dysopyramide has been shown to reduce the LVOT gradient and myocardial contractility and to improve LV diastolic filling. A dosage of 300 to 600 mg/d has been shown to provide relief of symptoms. The combination of dysopyramide and a beta-blocker should be considered in instances when patients remain symptomatic despite maximization of beta-blocker therapy.

The use of afterload-reducing agents is usually *contraindicated* in patients with HCM; however, a small percentage of patients develop systolic heart failure during the "burnt out" stage of HCM. Appropriate medical therapy can include afterload reduction with agents such as angiotensin-converting enzyme (ACE) inhibitors or angiotensin II receptor blockers, digitalis, or even diuretics. Cardiac transplantation is a consideration in this small subgroup of patients.

Despite maximal medical therapy, a small subgroup of patients with HCM will continue to have severe, debilitating symptoms. Patients who have symptoms of New York Heart Association (NYHA) class III or IV, are on maximal medical therapy, and have a resting or provocable LVOT gradient ≥ 50 mm Hg, may be candidates for *surgical septal myectomy*. *Alcohol septal ablation* and *dual-chamber pacing* are less invasive alternative methods to septal myectomy.

Surgical septal myectomy has been performed for well over 40 years; The Morrow procedure is considered the gold standard for ameliorating LVOT obstruction and symptoms in both adults and in children. Although septal myectomy is successful in relieving symptoms, the occurrence of SCD is not diminished. Occasionally, amelioration of the LVOT gradient may not correct the MR that can accompany HCM with LVOT obstruction; concomitant mitral valve repair/replacement should then be performed during septal myectomy. Although the operative risk of septal myectomy is acceptably low, between 1% and 2%, possible complications of septal myectomy include left bundle-branch block, complete heart block, aortic regurgitation, and iatrogenic ventricular septal defects.

A relatively new alternative to surgical myectomy is *alcohol septal ablation*. Septal ablation is an intervention based on the use of a percutaneous catheter, which involves the introduction of alcohol into a septal perforator, which causes a "controlled" myocardial infarction of the proximal ventricular septum. This procedure was first performed in 1995; it produces akinesis or hypokinesis of the proximal septum, thus reducing LVOT obstruction and decreasing SAM of the mitral valve and MR. Results are comparable to those of septal myectomy. Mortality and morbidity associated with septal ablation in *experienced* centers are similar to those of septal myectomy. Complications include right bundle-branch block, AV block, coronary artery dissection, and large anteroseptal myocardial infarction. Septal ablation creates an arrhythmogenic substrate that can lead to an increased risk of lethal arrhythmias. Although long-term follow-up (> 10 years) is lacking, septal ablation has been performed 15 to 20 times more often than myectomy, resulting in over 3,000 septal ablations performed worldwide since its inception.

Dual-chamber pacing was initially reported to provide a substantial reduction in LVOT gradients and amelioration of symptoms in many patients. Results from subsequent randomized, crossover studies have been greeted with little enthusiasm, with an average decrease in the LVOT gradient amounting to only 25% to 40% of that previously reported, and one study showing no change from the preoperative state. Subjective evidence of improvement did not correlate with objective measurements of exercise capacity and oxygen consumption. Compared to surgical myectomy, dual-chamber pacing proved to be inferior to surgical myectomy both in improving hemodynamics and relieving symptoms.

Infective endocarditis occurs in 4% to 5% of patients with HCM, usually on the anterior mitral leaflet and on the area of the outflow tract apposed to the anterior mitral leaflet during SAM. Prophylaxis of *infective endocarditis* is therefore indicated in patients who have evidence of LVOT obstruction (Fig. 40-2).

SUGGESTED READING

Maron BJ. Hypertrophic cardiomyopathy: a systemic review. *JAMA*. 2002:1308–1320.

Maron BJ, McKenna WJ, Danielson GK, et al. ACC/ESC clinical expert consensus document on hypertrophic cardiomyopathy: a report of the American College of Cardiology Task Force on Clinical Expert Consensus Documents and the European Society of Cardiology Committee for Practice Guidelines (Committee to Develop an Expert Consensus Document on Hypertrophic Cardiomyopathy). *J Am Coll Cardiol*. 2003;42:1678–1713.

Maron BJ, Nishimura RA, McKenna WJ, et al. Assessment of permanent dual-chamber pacing as a treatment for drug-refractory symptomatic patients with obstructive hypertrophic cardiomyopathy: a randomized, double-blind, crossover study (M-PATHY). *Circulation*.1999;99:2927–2933.

Maron BJ, Shen W-K, Link MS, et al. Efficacy of implantable cardioverter-defibrillators for the prevention of sudden death in patients with hypertrophic cardiomyopathy. *N Engl J Med*. 2000;342:365–373.

Nishimura RA, Holmes DR Jr. Hypertrophic obstructive cardiomyopathy. *N Engl J Med*. 2004;350:1320–1327.

Nishimura RA, Ommen SR, Tajik AJ. Hypertrophic cardiomyopathy. In: Fuster V, O'Rourke RA, Walsh RA, et al., eds. *Hurst's The Heart*. 12th ed. New York, NY: McGraw-Hill; 2008.

Spirito P, Bellone P, Harris KM, et al. Magnitude of left ventricular hypertrophy predicts the risk of sudden death in hypertrophic cardiomyopathy. *N Engl J Med*. 2000;342: 1778–1785.

CHAPTER (41)

Restrictive, Obliterative, and Infiltrative Cardiomyopathies

Christopher D. McCoy and Brian D. Hoit

RESTRICTIVE CARDIOMYOPATHY

According to a recent consensus document from the American Heart Association, the preferred classification of cardiomyopathies should be either primary (i.e., predominantly confined to the heart) or secondary (i.e., as part of a generalized systemic disorder). *Restrictive cardiomyopathy* refers to an idiopathic or systemic myocardial disorder characterized by restrictive filling, normal or reduced ventricular volumes, and normal or nearly normal systolic ventricular function (Table 41-1). Striking elevation of the jugular venous pulse and prominent X and especially Y descents are characteristic. A diastolic arterial pulse due to a reduced stroke volume and tachycardia may be seen in severe cases. The apical impulse is nondisplaced and systolic murmurs of atrioventricular regurgitation and filling sounds marking the abrupt cessation of rapid early diastolic filling may be present.

Electrocardiographic abnormalities, such as abnormal voltage, atrial and ventricular arrhythmias, and conduction disturbances are frequent. Atrial enlargement and pericardial effusion may produce an enlarged cardiac silhouette on the chest radiogram, and pleural effusions and signs of pulmonary congestion may also be present. Echocardiographic findings are nonspecific.

Several clinical, imaging, and hemodynamic features are helpful in distinguishing restrictive cardiomyopathy from constrictive pericarditis (Table 41-2). Although Doppler techniques have assumed an important role in characterizing the nature of transvalvular filling and helping to make this clinically crucial distinction, rigorous studies of the sensitivity and specificity of these Doppler findings are lacking. Thus, the diagnostic certainty is related to the number of "pathognomonic" findings in concert with clinical information and additional imaging studies. Magnetic resonance imaging (MRI) and computed tomography (CT) are useful in that pericardial thickness can be accurately assessed. B-type natriuretic peptide (BNP) levels are markedly elevated in patients with restrictive cardiomyopathy compared to constrictive pericarditis.

Right- and left-sided heart catheterization is performed to document the diagnosis, assess severity, and sometimes establish the etiology by means of endomyocardial biopsy. The venous pressure is elevated and the deep decline of the right atrial Y descent is striking. The right ventricular (RV) systolic pressure is often elevated, and the early portion of diastole is characterized by a deep, sharp dip followed by a plateau (square root sign), during which no further increase in right ventricular pressure occurs. These hemodynamic features are similar to those of *constrictive pericarditis* and may create further diagnostic confusion. Although it is not uncommon for the pulmonary wedge and the right atrial pressures to be identical, a higher left than RV filling pressure strongly favors the diagnosis of restrictive cardiomyopathy.

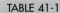
TABLE 41-1

Classification of the Restrictive Cardiomyopathies

Myocardial

1. Noninfiltrative cardiomyopathies
   Idiopathic
   Familial
   Pseudoxanthoma elasticum
   Scleroderma
2. Infiltrative cardiomyopathies
   Amyloidosis
   Sarcoidosis
   Gaucher's disease
3. Storage disease
   Hemochromatosis
   Fabry's disease
   Glycogen storage diseases

Endomyocardial

1. Obliterative
   Endomyocardial fibrosis
   Hypereosinophilic syndrome
2. Nonobliterative
   Carcinoid
   Malignant infiltration
   Iatrogenic (radiation, drugs)

Treatment of restrictive cardiomyopathy is empiric and directed toward the treatment of diastolic heart failure. Judicious use of diuretics is warranted in view of the steep pressure–volume relation of the ventricles and the need to maintain a relatively high filling pressure. Vasodilators may also jeopardize ventricular filling and should be used cautiously.

【 】 NONFILTRATIVE RESTRICTIVE CARDIOMYOPATHIES

Idiopathic restrictive cardiomyopathy may involve myocardium, conduction tissue, and skeletal muscle, with resultant restrictive ventricular filling and heart failure, atrioventricular (AV) block, and distal skeletal myopathy, respectively. Although not generally considered familial, several small families with both autosomal dominant and recessive patterns of inheritance have been reported, and missense mutations in human cardiac troponin I (genetic causes of hypertrophic cardiomyopathy) have been reported to cause restrictive cardiomyopathy. In addition, a heterogeneous group of autosomal dominant disorders are characterized by skeletal myopathy and cardiac conduction abnormalities and are causally related to the desmin gene (which may also cause a dilated cardiomyopathy). Myocyte hypertrophy and fibrosis on endomyocardial biopsy are characteristic. Echocardiography reveals normal or reduced ventricular dimensions, variable systolic function, and increased atrial dimensions. A dominant early diastolic mitral "E" velocity (increased E/A ratio), an increased pulmonary venous atrial systolic "A" reversal velocity and duration, as well as shortened mitral deceleration time are typical features on Doppler. Although idiopathic restrictive cardiomyopathy initially may have a protracted course, the prognosis is poor in older patients (particularly males) with increasing signs

TABLE 41-2

Clinical and Hemodynamic Features that Help to Distinguish Restrictive Cardiomyopathy from Constrictive Pericarditis

	Restrictive Cardiomyopathy	Constrictive Pericarditis
History	Systemic disease that involves the myocardium, multiple myeloma, amyloidosis, cardiac transplant	Acute pericarditis, cardiac surgery, radiation therapy, chest trauma, systemic disease involving the pericardium
Chest radiogram	Absence of calcification	Helpful when calcification persists
	Massive atrial enlargement	Moderate atrial enlargement
Electrocardiogram	Bundle branch blocks, AV block	Abnormal repolarization
CT/MRI	Normal pericardium	Helpful if thickened (> 4 mm) pericardium
Hemodynamics	Helpful if unequal diastolic pressures	Diastolic equilibration
	Concordant effect of respiration on diastolic pressures	Dip and plateau
Biopsy	Fibrosis, hypertrophy, infiltration	Normal

AV, atrioventricular; CT, computed tomography; MRI, magnetic resonance imaging.

of systemic and pulmonary venous congestion, atrial fibrillation, and marked left atrial enlargement (> 60 mm); in that group, the Kaplan–Meier 5-year survival rate is 64%, compared with the expected 85% survival rate.

Pseudoxanthoma elasticum is a rare disorder, characterized by fragmentation and calcification of elastic fibers that uncommonly causes restrictive cardiomyopathy.

Myocardial fibrosis is found in the majority of patients with scleroderma at autopsy, but heart failure due to either restrictive or dilated cardiomyopathy is rare. Pericardial involvement and electrocardiographic abnormalities (heart block, supraventricular and ventricular tachycardia, and pseudoinfarction patterns) are common. Pulmonary hypertension is a leading cause of morbidity and mortality in patients with scleroderma.

【 】 INFILTRATIVE RESTRICTIVE CARDIOMYOPATHIES

Amyloidosis

Amyloidosis is a systemic disorder characterized by interstitial deposition of amyloid protein fibrils in multiple organs. Cardiac involvement is most common in immunoglobulin amyloidosis (AL type), which is caused by several conditions including primary amyloidosis, multiple myeloma, and other plasma cell dyscrasias. Cardiac deposition of amyloid protein (protein A) may also occur in secondary amyloidosis due to chronic inflammation or autoimmune disease. The familial form is characterized by mutations of the protein transthyretin, which produce peripheral and autonomic neuropathy in addition to cardiac disease. Senile amyloidosis, which typically involves the atria, can affect one-quarter of patients over the age of 80 years. Although it carries the most favorable prognosis, the condition is not always benign, resulting in atrial fibrillation, conduction disturbances, heart failure, and cardiac death. Cardiac involvement is uncommon in hemodialysis-associated (beta-2) amyloidosis.

Amyloid deposits may be interstitial and widespread, resulting in restrictive cardiomyopathy or localized to (1) conduction tissue, resulting in heart block and ventricular arrhythmias (especially in familial amyloidosis); (2) the cardiac valves, resulting in valvular regurgitation; (3) the pericardium, resulting in constriction; (4) the coronary arteries, resulting in ischemia; and (5) the pulmonary vasculature, causing pulmonary hypertension and cor pulmonale. In some cases, the clinical picture is dominated by autonomic neuropathy and nephropathy and cardiac involvement is unrecognized. Cardiac manifestations often progress from being asymptomatic to biventricular failure. The cardiac silhouette on the chest radiogram may be normal or moderately enlarged. Electrocardiographic changes may be manifest as decreased voltage, pseudoinfarction, and left axis deviation. Arrhythmias and conduction disturbances may dominate the clinical course. The echocardiogram may reveal symmetrical wall thickness involving the right and left ventricles (LV wall thickness is an important prognostic variable), a small or normal LV cavity with variably depressed systolic function, atrial and vena caval dilatation, thickening of the interatrial septum and valves, and a small pericardial effusion. Highly reflective echoes producing a "granular or sparkling appearance" and occurring in a patchy distribution are characteristic echocardiographic findings but are neither sensitive nor specific.

The earliest sign of amyloid cardiomyopathy is impaired LV relaxation, manifest by a mitral Doppler E/A ratio < 1 and increased isovolumic relaxation and transmitral diastolic deceleration times. The restrictive pattern of LV filling—a transmitral E/A ratio ≥ 2 without respiratory variation, transmitral diastolic deceleration time < 150 ms, and an isovolumic relaxation time ≤ 70 ms—is a strong predictor of cardiac death. The infiltrative pathology associated with amyloidosis may be detected by tissue characterization using MRI

The variable clinical, diagnostic, and prognostic features reflect the location, nature, and extent of amyloid deposition and the temporal course of the disease. Serum and urine protein electrophoresis is diagnostic in most cases of primary amyloidosis, but monoclonal protein may not be secreted. Endomyocardial biopsy of the right ventricle, which is most helpful if an abdominal fat aspirate is negative, provides the diagnosis and quantifies myocardial damage.

The treatment of amyloidosis is fraught with hazard. Patients are sensitive to digoxin and calcium-channel blockers, and hypotension with vasodilators and diuretics is a threat due to the steep LV pressure–volume relation. Angiotensin-converting enzyme inhibitors have been used with varying response rates. Amiodarone and ibutalide are effective drugs for patients with atrial fibrillation. For patients with symptomatic bradycardia or high-grade conduction system disease, a pacemaker should be implanted. Immunosuppressive therapy with melphalan and prednisone is established conventional therapy for primary amyloidosis. Autologous stem cell infusion reduces the monoclonal gammopathy, but has little effect on existing infiltrative amyloid. Orthotopic cardiac transplantation is generally not recommended, but liver transplantation may be lifesaving in patients with familial amyloidosis.

Other Infiltrative Cardiomyopathies

Noncaseating granulomas involve the heart in *sarcoidosis* in as many as 25% of patients but are frequently subclinical. The combination of extracardiac manifestations and cardiac abnormalities favors a presumptive diagnosis of sarcoidosis without biopsy. Interstitial granulomatous inflammation initially produces diastolic dysfunction and later may produce systolic abnormalities. Localized thinning and dilatation of the basilar left ventricle, resembling ischemic heart disease, are characteristic. Restrictive cardiomyopathy is uncommon; more often, sarcoid pulmonary involvement produces pulmonary hypertension and right heart failure. High-grade AV block and ventricular arrhythmias are principal manifestations and may result in syncope and sudden cardiac death. The electrocardiogram (ECG) most commonly demonstrates T-wave and conduction abnormalities and with extensive myocardial involvement, pseudoinfarct patterns may appear. Thallium 201 and gallium 67 have been used to indicate areas of myocardial involvement and are used to predict the response to corticosteroids. MRI may detect sarcoid granulomata or scar. Endomyocardial biopsy is useful but, because of sampling error, may be falsely negative. Treatment with prednisone for symptomatic patients is warranted in highly suspicious or proven cases because the cardiac granuloma may be sensitive. High-grade AV nodal block usually requires a permanent pacemaker, and in patients at high risk for sudden cardiac death, an implantable cardioverter defibrillator is appropriate. Calcium-channel blockers may ameliorate diastolic dysfunction in patients with restrictive cardiomyopathy; patients with dilated cardiomyopathy are treated for congestive heart failure. Cardiac transplantation is an appropriate consideration for intractable heart failure or arrhythmia.

Gaucher's disease is due to an inherited deficiency of beta-glucocerebroside, which results in the accumulation of cerebroside in the reticuloendothelial system, brain, and heart. Diffuse interstitial infiltration of the left ventricle occurs, leading to reduced LV compliance and decreased cardiac output, but is often subclinical. Ventricular and valvular thickening and pericardial effusions are seen on echocardiography. Enzyme replacement therapy with alglucerase (the placental derivative) and imiglucerase (the recombinant form) has revolutionized the treatment of Gaucher's disease but its high cost still limits its availability in many countries.

STORAGE DISEASES

Myocardial iron deposition in *hemochromatosis* (the primary variety owing to an autosomal dominant or recessive mutation in one of five genes involved in iron metabolism) *usually produces dilated cardiomyopathy*, but it may cause restrictive cardiomyopathy; congestive heart failure, arrhythmia, and conduction disturbances are common. The clinical features of hemochromatosis are due to accumulation of iron in the heart, pancreas, skin, liver, anterior pituitary, and gonads. Interstitial fibrosis is variable and unrelated to the extent of iron deposition, which occurs within the myocyte; secondarily, myocardial fibrosis may develop. Findings consistent with either dilated or restrictive cardiomyopathy may be seen. Granular sparkling and atrial enlargement may be observed but are nonspecific signs. CT and MRI may demonstrate subclinical cardiac involvement, and tissue characterization may be possible with MRI. Endomyocardial biopsy is confirmatory. Repeated phlebotomy is recommended for primary hemochromatosis, and the chelating agent desferroxamine is often beneficial in secondary hemochromatosis. Cardiac transplantation (with or without liver transplantation) may be considered in selected cases.

Fabry's disease is characterized by glycolipid accumulation in the myocardium as well as the vascular and valvular endothelium and may present with a restrictive, hypertrophic, or dilated cardiomyopathy, mitral regurgitation, ischemic heart disease, or aortic degeneration. Echocardiographic findings in restrictive cardiomyopathy mimic those seen in amyloid, and LV mass correlates with the severity of disease. Definitive diagnosis may require endomyocardial biopsy. Enzyme replacement therapy has proven effective but is limited by cost and the availability of the enzyme

Pompe's disease is due to an autosomal recessive deficiency of acid maltase that causes glycogen deposition in the heart and skeletal muscles. The echocardiographic manifestations may be indistinguishable from those of hypertrophic obstructive cardiomyopathy. Adults with *glycogen storage type III disease* (debranching enzyme deficiency) may have marked LVH on echocardiography.

Two new disorders belonging to the subgroup that includes Pompe's and Fabry's disease have clinical manifestations predominantly limited to the heart. The nonsarcomeric protein mutations in two genes involved in cardiac metabolism (the gama-2-regulatory subunit of the AMP-activated protein kinase and lysosome-associated membrane protein-2) are reported to be responsible for primary cardiac glycogen storage diseases in older children and adults; the clinical presentation resembles hypertrophic cardiomyopathy.

ENDOMYOCARDIAL OBLITERATIVE DISEASES

Endomyocardial diseases that cause obliterative cardiomyopathy include *endomyocardial fibrosis* (EMF) and *hypereosinophilic (Loeffler's)* syndrome (Table 41-3). Endomyocardial disease is characterized by endocardial fibrosis of the apex and subvalvular regions of one or both ventricles, resulting in restriction to inflow to the affected ventricle. Although the clinical presentations of the endomyocardial diseases differ, their pathology and therefore the cardiac imaging studies are generally similar. Echocardiography reveals apical obliteration of the ventricles, apical thrombus, echodensities in the endocardium, and small ventricular and large atrial cavities. Involvement of the posterior mitral and tricuspid valve leaflets results in mitral and tricuspid regurgitation; less commonly, restricted motion may produce stenosis. Sparing of the outflow tracts is characteristic. Typical patterns of restriction, mitral and tricuspid regurgitation, and less often, stenosis are seen on Doppler. Not surprisingly, the location, extent, and severity of involvement determine the clinical picture.

Medical therapy of Loeffler's is often ineffective and frustrating. Treatment consists of symptomatic relief, anticoagulants, corticosteroids, and hydroxyurea, and most recently, interferon alpha, as well as palliative surgery in the late, fibrotic stage. Surgical excision of fibrotic endocardium and valve replacement may offer symptomatic improvement, but at the expense of high operative mortality. The prognosis of advanced disease is grave (50% 2-year mortality) but is considerably better in those with milder disease.

TABLE 41-3

Endomyocardial Obliterative Disease—Endomyocardial Fibrosis (EMF) versus Hypereosinophilic (Loeffler's) Syndrome

	EMF	Loeffler's Syndrome
Distribution	Worldwide; 10%–20% of cardiac-related deaths in equatorial Africa	Temperate climates
Gender predilection	None; affects children and young adults	Primarily affects males
Etiology	Endemic form associated with high levels of cerium and low levels of magnesium	Parasitic infections, leukemia, and immunologic reactions
Onset	Insidious	Rapid
Course	Indolent	Aggressive and rapidly progressive; 50% 2-year mortality in advanced cases
Cardiac involvement	Biventricular in only 50% of cases; atrial fibrillation common	Biventricular in majority of cases; Thromboembolic phenomena; > 1,500 eosinophils/mL

NONOBLITERATIVE ENDOMYOCARDIAL DISEASES

Carcinoid syndrome results from metastatic carcinoid tumors and consists of cutaneous flushing, diarrhea, and bronchoconstriction; involvement of the heart occurs as a late complication of carcinoid syndrome in approximately 50% of patients. Although tricuspid and pulmonic stenosis and regurgitation dominate the clinical picture, restrictive cardiomyopathy may occur.

Infiltrating tumors of the heart are generally metastatic and rarely produce restriction to ventricular filling unless the pericardium is involved. Infiltration on echocardiography is suggested by a localized increase in wall thickness, often associated with abnormal wall motion and pericardial effusion.

Pericardial disease frequently complicates radiation therapy to the chest (see Chapter 43) and may produce constrictive pericarditis. Anthracyclines and methysergide can cause EMF. A restrictive pattern of LV filling is common soon after orthotopic cardiac transplantation and may persist for at least a year.

SUGGESTED READING

Asher CR, Klein AL. Diastolic heart failure: restrictive cardiomyopathy, constrictive pericarditis, and cardiac tamponade. Clinical and echocardiographic evaluation. *Cardiol Rev.* 2002;10:218–229.

Fatkin D, Graham RM. Molecular mechanisms of inherited cardiomyopathies. *Physiol Rev.* 2002:945–980.

Hoit BD, Gupta S. Restrictive, obliterative, and infiltrative cardiomyopathies. In: Fuster V, O'Rourke RA, Walsh RA, et al., eds. *Hurst's The Heart.* 12th ed. New York, NY: McGraw-Hill; 2008:851–862.

Maron BJ, Towbin JA, Thiene G, et al. American Heart Association; Council on Clinical Cardiology, Heart Failure and Transplantation Committee; Quality of Care and Outcomes Research and Functional Genomics and Translational Biology Interdisciplinary Working Groups; Council on Epidemiology and Prevention. Contemporary definitions and classification of the cardiomyopathies: an American Heart Association Scientific Statement from the Council on Clinical Cardiology, Heart Failure and Transplantation Committee; Quality of Care and Outcomes Research and Functional Genomics and Translational Biology Interdisciplinary Working Groups; and Council on Epidemiology and Prevention. *Circulation.* 2006;113:1807–1816.

CHAPTER 42

Myocarditis and Specific Cardiomyopathies

Sean P. Pinney, Ajith P. Nair, and
Donna M. Mancini

Cardiomyopathies encompasses a wide spectrum of diseases with widely divergent pathogenic mechanisms that have as their final common pathway the syndrome of congestive heart failure (CHF). These heart muscle diseases may be primary or secondary—that is, resulting from specific cardiac or systemic disorders. Etiologies associated with the development of cardiomyopathy are presented in Table 42-1. Hypertrophic cardiomyopathy, HIV-associated cardiomyopathy, and cardiomyopathies due to coronary artery or valvular disease are discussed elsewhere. Although endomyocardial biopsy is generally of low-yield, in this group of diseases it can be diagnostic (Table 42-2).

MYOCARDITIS

Myocarditis means inflammation of the myocardium. Myocardial dysfunction from viral myocarditis can be caused by two distinct phases of myocardial cell damage—the first caused by direct viral infection and the second caused by the host's immune response or apoptotic death. Multiple infectious etiologies (Table 42-1) have been implicated as the cause of myocarditis, the most common being viral, specifically, the enterovirus coxsackie virus B. The discovery of myocarditis in 1% to 9% of routine postmortem examinations suggests that myocarditis is a major cause of sudden, unexpected death.

The clinical manifestations of myocarditis are variable, ranging from an asymptomatic or self-limited disease to profound cardiogenic shock. Cardiac involvement typically occurs 7 to 10 days following an antecedent viral syndrome or systemic illness, which occurs in 60% of patients. Chest pain can occur in up to 35% of patients and may be associated with pericarditis or result from myocardial ischemia. Syncope and sudden cardiac death can be the initial presentations of myocarditis in some patients, presumably due to complete heart block or ventricular tachycardia.

Physical examination findings include fever, tachycardia, and signs of CHF. The first heart sound may be soft and a summation gallop may be present. An apical systolic murmur of mitral regurgitation may be auscultated. A pericardial friction rub may be present. Laboratory findings are generally nondiagnostic and demonstrate leukocytosis, eosinophilia, elevated ESR, and occasionally elevated titers to cardiotropic viruses. A fourfold rise in IgG or IgM antibody titers documents only the response to a recent viral infection and does not indicate active myocarditis. An increase in the myocardial band (MB) of creatine phosphokinase (CPK) is observed in approximately 10% of patients, although troponin assays are proving to be more sensitive. The classic clinical triad of preceding viral illness, pericarditis, and associated laboratory abnormalities used to diagnose coxsackie virus B–induced myocarditis is present in fewer than 10% of histologically proven cases.

TABLE 42-1

Causes of Myocarditis

Disease	Etiologies	Comment
Infectious myocarditis Viral	Viruses Coxsackievirus, echovirus, HIV, Epstein–Barr virus, influenza, cytomegalovirus, adenovirus, hepatitis (A and B), mumps, poliovirus, rabies, respiratory synctyial virus, rubella, vaccinia, varicella zoster, arbovirus	The most common etiology of infectious myocarditis in North America is viral infection by coxsackie- or echoviruses. Most episodes are self-limited and asymptomatic. In patients with symptoms of congestive heart failure (CHF), acute and chronic viral titers are needed along with endomyocardial biopsy to confirm the diagnosis.
Bacteria[1]	Bacteria Corynebacterium diphtheriae, Streptococcus pyogenes, Staphylococcus aureus, Haemophilus pneumoniae, Salmonella spp., Neisseria gonorrhoeae, leptospirosis, Lyme disease, syphilis, brucellosis, tuberculosis actinomycosis, Chlamydia spp., Coxiella burnetii, Mycoplasma pneumoniae, Rickettsia spp.	In South America, the most common cause of myocarditis is Chagas' disease, caused by the bite of the reduviid bug carrying the parasite Trypanosoma cruzi.
Fungal	Fungi Candida spp., Aspergillus spp., histoplasmosis, blastomycosis, cryptococcosis, coccidioidomycosis	
Parasitic	Parasites Toxoplasmosis, schistosomiasis, trichinosis	
Dilated cardiomyopathy	Unknown	May represent prior undiagnosed episode of myocarditis, untreated hypertension, or occult alcohol use.
Infiltrative	Amyloid Sarcoid Hemochromatosis	Myocardial inflammation may be present on biopsy. Routine and special stains are extremely valuable in confirming these diagnoses.

TABLE 42-1

Causes of Myocarditis (*Continued*)

Disease	Etiologies	Comment
Hypersensitivity/ eosinophilic	Carcinoid syndrome Hypereosinophilic (Loeffler's) heart disease Glycogen storage disease *Antibiotics* Sulfonamides, penicillins, cefaclor, chloramphenicol, amphotericin B, tetracycline, streptomycin *Antituberculous drugs* Isoniazid, para-aminosalicylic acid *Anticonvulsants* Phenindione, phenytoin, carbamazepine, phenobarbital *Antidepressants* Amitriptyline, desipramine *Anti-inflammatories* Indomethicin, phenylbutazone, oxyphenylbutazone *Diuretics* Acetazolamide, chlorthalidone, hydrochlorothiazide, spironolactone *Others* Methyldopa, sulfonylureas, interleukin-2, interleukin-4, tetanus toxoid	Treatment is discontinuation of the offending agent with or without steroids. Potentially reversible.

Toxins	Cocaine, cyclophosphamide, emetine, lithium, methysergide, phenothiazines, interferon alpha, interleukin-2, doxorubicin, cobalt, lead, chloroquine, hydrocarbons, carbon monoxide, anabolic steroids	Potentially reversible for some toxins.
Radiation	Past history of lymphoma	
Giant-cell myocarditis	Unknown	Generally a fulminant disease with a high mortality. May recur after transplant.
Postpartum cardiomyopathy	Unknown	CHF onset in last trimester or first 5 months after delivery in patient with no structural heart disease or known cause of CHF.
Genetic	Fabry's disease, Kearns–Sayre syndrome, right ventricular dysplasia	Patients with right ventricular dysplasia present with ventricular arrhythmias.
Endocrine	Hypothyroidism, hyperthyroidism, pheochromocytoma, acromegaly, diabetes	
Metabolic	Hypocalcemia, hypophosphatemia, uremia, carnitine	

TABLE 42-2

Diseases Diagnosed by Endomyocardial Biopsy

1. Myocarditis
     Giant cell arteritis
     Cytomegalovirus infection
     Toxoplasmosis
     Chagas' disease
     Rheumatic fever
     Lyme disease
2. Infiltrative cardiomyopathy
     Amyloid
     Sarcoid
     Hemochromatosis
     Carcinoid
     Hypereosinophilic cardiomyopathy
     Glycogen storage disease
     Cardiac tumors
3. Toxins
     Doxorubicin
     Chloroquine
     Radiation injury
4. Genetic conditions
     Fabry's disease
     Kearns–Sayre syndrome
     Right ventricular dysplasia

The electrocardiogram (ECG) most frequently shows sinus tachycardia. Diffuse ST- and T-wave changes, prolonged QT intervals, conduction delay, low voltage, and even acute infarct patterns can also occur. Echocardiography can reveal LV systolic dysfunction in patients with a normal-sized LV cavity. Segmental wall-motion abnormalities and increased wall thickness secondary to inflammation may be present. Ventricular thrombi are seen in 15% of patients. Tissue alterations associated with myocarditis can be identifiable using MRI. Use of transverse relaxation time (T2)-weighted images may visualize tissue edema with active myocarditis, and gadolinium-enhanced MRI has been used to characterize inflammatory changes *endomyocardial biopsy* can confirm the diagnosis. Because myocarditis can be focal, four to six samples are obtained to reduce sampling error to < 5%. Active myocarditis is defined pathologically as inflammatory infiltrate with myocyte necrosis. As resolution of myocarditis can occur within 4 days of initial biopsy, endomyocardial biopsy should be applied quickly to maximize diagnostic yield. The *Dallas criteria* separate initial biopsies into myocarditis, borderline myocarditis, or no myocarditis. Alternative classification schemes combine histopathologic and clinical criteria, and divide myocarditis into four subgroups—fulminant, acute, chronic active, and chronic persistent. These categories provide prognostic information and suggest which patients can or cannot benefit from immunosuppressive therapy.

Approximately 40% of patients with acute myocarditis will completely recover. One-third will be left with mild myocardial dysfunction to significant heart failure. One-quarter will either die or require cardiac transplantation. For patients with histopathologic confirmation of myocarditis, the 1-year survival is approximately 80%, and 5-year survival is in the range of 50% to 60%. Predictors of recovery include the degree of LV dysfunction at presentation, shorter duration of disease, and less intensive drug therapy. Paradoxically, patients with fulminant myocarditis—defined as rapid onset of symptoms, fever, and severe hemodynamic compromise—have a better survival than patients with acute nonfulminant myocarditis.

Treatment of acute myocarditis is supportive care. Diuretics, angiotensin-converting enzyme inhibitors, blockers, and aldosterone antagonists should be given in the proper clinical context. Digoxin can increase the expression of inflammatory cytokines and should be used cautiously. When acute myocarditis presents with profound hemodynamic collapse, mechanical circulatory support devices can be used to bridge patients either to cardiac transplantation or to recovery. Anti-inflammatory therapy has demonstrated predominantly negative results. The Multicenter Myocarditis Treatment Trial randomized patients with biopsy-proven myocarditis to conventional medical therapy versus steroid/azathioprine or steroid/cyclosporine immunosuppression. Treatment with immunosuppression failed to demonstrate an improvement of ejection fraction, mortality, or attenuate clinical disease. High-dose immunoglobulin (IVIG) showed no benefit over placebo. Thus, the routine use of immunosuppressive therapy in myocarditis is not supported. Although subgroups with ongoing myocarditis and increased HLA expression in biopsy samples may benefit from immunosuppression, no uniform methodology yet exists to identify them.

【 】 CHAGAS' DISEASE

American trypanosomiasis, or Chagas' disease, is the most common cause of CHF in rural South and Central America. The disease results from the bite of the reduviid bug, leading to infection with *Trypanosoma cruzi*. Cardiac injury is thought to be immunologically mediated.

In the acute phase, hematogenous spread of the parasite leads to invasion of various organ systems and an intense inflammatory reaction. Patients experience fever, sweating, myalgias, and myocarditis. The case fatality rate is approximately 5%. Survivors enter an asymptomatic latent phase, but 20% to 30% will develop a chronic form of the disease up to 20 years after the initial infection. The chronic stage is a result of gradual tissue destruction. The gastrointestinal tract and heart are the most common sites of involvement, with the primary cause of death being cardiac failure. Fibrosis of myofibrils and the Purkinje fibers leads to cardiomegaly, CHF, heart block, and arrhythmias.

Diagnosis of the acute disease depends on the discovery of trypomastigotes in the blood of the infected individual. Endomyocardial biopsy can show parasites in one-quarter of individuals. Chronic infection can be confirmed by complement-fixation test and positive serologic tests (such as the indirect immunofluorescent antibody, enzyme-linked immunosorbent assays, and hemagglutination tests) together with symptoms and signs compatible with Chagas' disease. Echocardiography can demonstrate segmental wall-motion abnormalities—specifically apical aneurysms. ECG findings include complete heart block, atrioventricular (AV) block, or right bundle-branch block with or without fascicular block. Treatment of chronic Chagas' disease is symptomatic and includes a pacemaker for complete heart block, an implantable cardioverter-defibrillator for recurrent ventricular arrhythmia, and standard therapy for CHF. Antiparasitic agents, such as nifurtimox and benzimidazole eradicate parasitemia during the acute phase, should be administered for untreated disease, and can be used as prophylaxis in the setting of immunosuppression. The role of immunosuppression therapy for chagasic myocarditis is controversial, and heart transplantation is effective for end-stage refractory cardiac disease.

【 】 LYME CARDITIS

Lyme disease results from infection with the spirochete *Borrelia burgdorferi*, introduced by a tick bite. The initial presenting symptom in patients with the disease who progress to cardiac involvement is frequently complete heart block. LV dysfunction is seen but rare. Endomyocardial biopsy can show active myocarditis; spirochetes are rarely observed. Treatment includes corticosteroids and tetracycline.

【 】 RHEUMATIC CARDITIS

Acute rheumatic fever can occur following group A streptococcal pharyngitis. Clinical diagnosis is made using the *Jones criteria*. The major manifestations are carditis, polyarthritis, chorea, erythema marginatum, subcutaneous nodules, and evidence of preceding streptococcal infection. Minor criteria are nonspecific findings, such as fever, arthralgia, previous rheumatic fever or rheumatic heart disease, elevated erythrocyte sedimentations rate (ESR) or C-reactive protein, and prolonged PR interval. Diagnosis is made by the presence of two major criteria or one major and two minor criteria. Two-thirds of patients present with an antecedent pharyngitis, followed by symptoms of rheumatic fever in 1 to 5 weeks. CHF is observed in only 5% to 10% of cases. Severe carditis is usually mild, and valvular lesions predominate. Physical examination is notable for fever and the Carey Coombs murmur, significant for mitral valvulitis. The mitral valve is involved three times as often as the aortic valve. ECG findings include PR prolongation and nonspecific ST-T–wave changes. Endomyocardial biopsy demonstrates the pathognomonic Aschoff body, a persistent inflammatory lesion. Laboratory tests suggestive of rheumatic fever include antibodies to antistreptolysin O and anti-DNAse B, an elevated ESR, and elevated CRP. Aspirin and penicillin are the mainstays of therapy, although corticosteroids can provide symptomatic relief. Once rheumatic fever is diagnosed, antibiotic prophylaxis is required to prevent recurrent episodes. The most effective method is a single monthly intramuscular injection of 1.2 million U of benzathine penicillin G until the age of 21 years.

NONINFECTIVE MYOCARDITIS

【 】 HYPERSENSITIVITY

Hypersensitivity myocarditis is thought to be caused by an allergic drug reaction and is characterized by peripheral eosinophilia and infiltration into the myocardium by eosinophils, multinucleated giant cells, and leukocytes. Methyldopa, the penicillins, sulfonamides, tetracycline, and the antituberculous drugs are the pharmaceuticals most commonly associated with this entity. Treatment included stopping the offending agent and corticosteroids therapy. Unfortunately, the first manifestation of cardiac involvement is sometimes sudden death caused by arrhythmia.

【 】 GIANT-CELL MYOCARDITIS

Giant-cell myocarditis is an extremely rare but aggressive form of myocarditis, typically progressive and unresponsive to medical therapy. This disease is most prevalent in young adults and an association with other autoimmune disorders is reported in approximately 20% of cases. Diagnosis is made by endomyocardial biopsy. Widespread or multifocal necrosis with a mixed inflammatory infiltrate including lymphocytes and histiocytes is required for histologic diagnosis. Eosinophils are frequently noted, as are multinucleated giant-cells in the absence of granuloma. The clinical course is usually characterized by progressive CHF and is frequently associated with refractory ventricular arrhythmia. It is almost uniformly and rapidly fatal. Case reports and the Giant-Cell Myocarditis Registry suggest that treatment with immunosuppressive regimens, but not steroids alone, can extend transplant-free survival by a few months. Mechanical circulatory support may be required as a bridge to transplant, and rare cases of complete recovery have been described. Cardiac transplantation represents the best treatment option despite the possibility of recurrence in the transplanted heart.

【 】 PERIPARTUM CARDIOMYOPATHY

The incidence of peripartum cardiomyopathy varies from 1 in 3,000 to 1 in 15,000 pregnancies in the United States. A much higher incidence is observed in Africa (1 in 3,000) and Haiti (1 in 350). Predisposing factors include black race, obesity, multiple gestations, preeclampsia, chronic hypertension, and age greater than 30 years. Patients present with heart failure in the last trimester of pregnancy or in the first 5 months postpartum. Absence of a demonstrable cause of heart failure is required to make the diagnosis as the hemodynamic stress of pregnancy can frequently unmask previously unknown cardiac disease. The ECG frequently shows LV hypertrophy. Echocardiographic findings can range from single-chamber LV enlargement to four-chamber dilation. Endomyocardial biopsy can reveal myocarditis in as many as 50% of these women, but generally the findings are nonspecific. Patients with higher ejection fractions and smaller ventricular diastolic dimensions at the time of diagnosis have a better long-term prognosis. Congestive cardiomyopathy persisting for more than 6 months is likely irreversible and associated with a poorer prognosis. Subsequent pregnancies in patients with stable heart failure are subject to recurrence and should be viewed as high risk.

[ ] NEUROMUSCULAR DISEASES

Heritable neuromuscular dystrophies associated with cardiomyopathy include Becker, Duchenne, and X-linked cardioskeletal myopathy, myotonic dystrophy (Steinert disease), congenital myotonic dystrophy, limb-girdle muscular dystrophy (Erb disease), familial centronuclear myopathy, Kugelberg–Welander syndrome, Friedreich ataxia, and Barth syndrome. The myocardial involvement, natural history, and prognosis of each of these disorders are variable. Duchenne dystrophy is an X-linked disease of the dystrophic gene with proximal muscle weakness and cardiomyopathy. Patients with myotonic dystrophy present between age 20 and 50 years, and death usually results from respiratory and/or cardiorespiratory failure. The ECG frequently shows a straight posterior myocardial infarction.

CARDIOMYOPATHY CAUSED BY ENDOCRINE DISORDERS

Thyroid hormone excess or deficiency can lead to reversible cardiomyopathy. Thyroid hormone metabolism is frequently abnormal in patients with CHF. Changes in cardiac function are mediated by triiodothyronine (T_3) regulation of cardiac-specific genes. Hypothyroidism can results in decreased cardiac output, increased peripheral vascular resistance, and impaired exercise performance. Thyroid toxicity can lead to the development of both high- and low-output cardiac failure. A prolonged tachycardia and high-output state caused by thyrotoxicosis is thought eventually to produce LV dilation. A consequent progressive decline in systolic function leads to low-output heart failure.

Pheochromocytoma produces hypertension, swelling, palpitations, and orthostatic hypotension. Although progression to cardiac involvement is unusual, catecholamine-induced myocarditis has been reported. Patients typically die of cardiovascular causes as aggressive disease can lead to CHF or malignant ventricular arrhythmias. Cardiac abnormalities are reversible with tumor resection.

Acromegalic cardiomyopathy appears to be a specific entity that develops in 10% to 20% of patients with excess growth hormone production. The initial increased cardiac output and decreased total peripheral resistance triggered by increased growth hormone levels over time result in myocyte hypertrophy with fibrosis leading to impaired diastolic function and finally systolic dysfunction. CHF that develops in these patients is particularly resistant to conventional therapy owing to higher collagen content in the acromegalic heart. Inflammatory and degenerative damage to the sinoatrial and AV nodes can lead to sudden death. Pituitary surgery and irradiation remain the mainstays of therapy, although the cardiopathic manifestations persist despite a fall in growth hormone levels.

TOXINS

【 】 ALCOHOL

Chronic alcohol abuse is a major risk factor for the development of congestive cardiomyopathy, accounting for up to 45% of all dilated cardiomyopathies. Chronic excessive alcohol use can result in CHF, hypertension, and arrhythmias. Cardiac damage results from direct toxic effects of alcohol and acetaldehyde, a metabolite. Nutritional deficiencies, toxic cofactors, sympathetic stimulation, or coexistent hypertension can also contribute to disease development. The disease is observed most frequently in males age 30 to 55 years with a greater than 10-year history of heavy alcohol use and is extremely rare in premenopausal women. Patients can present with CHF, arrhythmias, or embolic phenomena. Atrial fibrillation is extremely common and sudden death can be the initial presentation. The mainstay of treatment is abstinence from alcohol. The duration and extent of abuse is correlated with outcome. Prognosis is extremely poor in those patients who continue to drink in excess of 100 g of ethanol daily compared with patients who moderate their alcohol consumption. Additionally, patients with structural histologic abnormalities have a poor prognosis.

【 】 COCAINE

Myocardial ischemia, infarction, coronary spasm, cardiac arrhythmias, sudden death, myocarditis, and dilated cardiomyopathy are all reported cardiovascular complications of cocaine abuse. By blocking the reuptake of norepinephrine, cocaine induces tachycardia, vasoconstriction, hypertension, cardiomyopathy, and ventricular arrhythmias. Cardiomyopathy can result from secondary changes in the heart caused by tachycardia or sustained increased ventricular afterload. Endomyocardial biopsy findings are nonspecific and can demonstrate the presence of contraction-band necrosis and a diffuse inflammatory cellular infiltrate. The treatment of cocaine-related myocarditis and cardiomyopathy is aimed at abstinence and treatment of heart failure. Use of beta-blockers is typically avoided as it may potentiate coronary spasm.

【 】 CHEMOTHERAPEUTIC AGENTS

Anthracyclines (doxorubicin) and cyclophosphamide are the most common chemotherapeutic agents associated with heart failure. Doxorubicin cardiotoxicity is suspected to be caused by increased oxidative stress from the generation of free radicals, although the exact cause is questionable. Risk factors for the development of doxorubicin cardiomyopathy include age older than 70 years, combination chemotherapy, mediastinal irradiation, prior cardiac disease, hypertension, and liver disease. The *early or acute cardiotoxicity* manifests as a pericarditis-myocarditis syndrome and is not dose-related. LV dysfunction is rarely seen, but arrhythmias, abnormalities of conduction, decreased QRS voltage, and nonspecific ST-segment and T-wave abnormalities are commonly observed. The prognosis is good, with quick resolution on discontinuation of therapy. *Late or chronic cardiotoxicity* is caused by the development of a dose-dependent degenerative cardiomyopathy. This syndrome generally occurs at cumulative doses above 550 mg/m^2. Serial assessment of nuclear ejection fractions is used clinically to monitor for toxicity. Histopathologic grading delineates best the safety of continued doxorubicin administration. Cardiotoxicity can occur within a year or as late 20 years of the last dose of anthracycline. The best management of anthracycline cardiotoxicity is prevention by limiting dosage. Coadministration of beta-blockers has also been demonstrated to have cardioprotective effects.

In contrast to the anthracyclines, cardiotoxicity associated with cyclophosphamide is not dose-related. Pericarditis, systolic dysfunction, arrhythmias, and myocardial can occur. Prior LV dysfunction is a risk factor for development of significant cardiomyopathy with cyclophosphamide. Although mortality is not trivial, survivors exhibit no residual cardiac abnormalities.

Trastuzumab is a monoclonal antibody directed against the human epidermal growth receptor 2 (HER-2) receptor protein on breast cancer cells that is associated with an increased risk of heart failure. The incidence of heart failure can range from 7% with monotherapy to 28% when trastuzumab is used in association with anthracyclines and cyclophosphamide.

【   】 PSYCHOTROPIC DRUGS

An increased incidence of cardiac complications including myocarditis, pericarditis, and cardiomyopathy has recently been reported with the atypical neuroleptic agent clozapine used in the treatment of schizophrenia. Four-chamber dilation can occur and can be reversible with discontinuation of the drug.

【   】 CHEMICAL TOXINS

A variety of compounds can lead to a spectrum of cardiotoxicity, including cardiomyopathy. They include interferon alpha, IL-2, phenothiazines, emetine, methysergide, chloroquine, lithium, cobalt, hydrocarbons, lead, and carbon monoxide.

CARDIOMYOPATHIES ASSOCIATED WITH NUTRITIONAL DEFICIENCIES

Thiamine deficiency may result in wet beriberi, a clinical syndrome characterized by high-output cardiac failure and severe lactic acidosis. Dramatic hemodynamic improvements are seen after bolus infusion of thiamine. Untreated, beriberi can be fatal. Vitamin D deficiency, or rickets, and vitamin D excess are associated with cardiovascular morbidity and mortality.

Cardiomyopathy associated with inadequate dietary intake of selenium is termed Keshan disease. Low selenium levels have been documented in patients receiving total parenteral nutrition. Whether the cardiomyopathy results from the actual selenium deficiency or the selenium deficiency increases susceptibility to cardiotropic viruses is unclear. Its incidence is dramatically reduced with supplementation of sodium selenite.

L-Carnitine is essential in the transport of long-chain fatty acids into mitochondria, where they undergo beta-oxidation. Normal hearts obtain approximately 60% of total energy production from fatty acid oxidation. Primary carnitine deficiencies result from several genetic disorders and can lead to cardiomyopathy within 3 to 4 years of birth, which responds to carnitine supplementation. Secondary carnitine deficiencies are more common and are associated with liver disease, renal disease, dietary insufficiencies (chronic total parenteral nutrition, malabsorption), diabetes mellitus, and defects in acyl-CoA metabolism.

TAKO-TSUBO CARDIOMYOPATHY

Also termed *broken heart syndrome* or *stress cardiomyopathy*, Tako-Tsubo cardiomyopathy is a reversible cardiomyopathy characterized by apical ballooning observed on left ventriculography. The etiology may be related to adrenergic stimulation. Differences in the density of beta-adrenergic receptors in the apex and base of the heart can account for the apical ballooning. Other potential mechanisms include multivessel spasm, microvascular dysfunction, transient LV outflow obstruction, and/or localized myocarditis. The clinical presentation is generally preceded by a stressful emotional, physical, or psychological event. Symptoms include chest pain, dyspnea, and syncope. Cardiac enzymes are elevated. The most common ECG finding is anterior ST elevations. Echocardiography reveals mild to severe LV dysfunction with anteroapical akinesis or dyskinesis. MRI shows mid to apical LV dyskinesis without delayed gadolinium hyperenhancement consistent with myocardial viability. Coronary angiography is normal and endomyocardial biopsy is nondiagnostic. Recovery of LV function occurs over a period of days to weeks.

NONCOMPACTION CARDIOMYOPATHY

LV noncompaction cardiomyopathy is a genetically heterogenous disorder that may or may not be associated with other congenital abnormalities. In the absence of coexistent congenital defects, this disorder is called *isolated noncompaction of the left ventricle*. The underlying mechanism is postulated to be caused by intrauterine arrest of myocardial development leading to diffuse prominent deep trabeculations in hypertrophied and hypokinetic segments in the left ventricle. Ventricular arrhythmias, embolic events, and heart failure, which can occur in two-thirds of patients, are the most common sequelae. Diastolic dysfunction can occur from both abnormal relaxation and restricted filling from the prominent trabeculae. Diagnosis is made by echocardiography or MRI. Anticoagulation to prevent embolization and close monitoring for arrhythmias with early use of implantable defibrillators are key aspects of patient management.

IDIOPATHIC CARDIOMYOPATHY

Idiopathic cardiomyopathy (IDC) is the term used to describe a group of myocardial diseases of unknown cause. Idiopathic dilated cardiomyopathy is a diagnosis of exclusion and probably represents the end result of a number of disease processes. Surreptitious alcohol use and undiagnosed and untreated hypertension represent other etiologies of cardiomyopathy in many cases. Its prevalence is estimated to be between 7% and 13% of all patients with systolic dysfunction. The prognosis for this condition is better than that for ischemic cardiomyopathy. Mortality for untreated cardiomyopathy approaches 50% at 5 years.

SUGGESTED READING

Cooper LT, Berry GJ, Shabetai R. Idiopathic giant-cell myocarditis—Natural history and treatment. *N Engl J Med.* 1997;336:1860–1866.

Felker GM, Hu W, Hare JM, et al. The spectrum of dilated cardiomyopathy: the Johns Hopkins experience with 1,278 patients. *Medicine.* 1999;78:270–283.

Kawai C. From myocarditis to cardiomyopathy: mechanisms of inflammation and cell death. *Circulation.* 1999;99:1091–1100.

Magnani JW, Dec GW. Myocarditis: current trends in diagnosis and treatment. *Circulation.* 2006;113:876–890.

Mason JW, O'Connell JB, Herskowitz A, et al. A clinical trial of immunosuppressive therapy for myocarditis. *N Engl J Med.* 1995;333:269–275.

McCarthy R, Boehmer J, Hruban R, et al. Long-term outcome of fulminant myocarditis as compared with acute (nonfulminant) myocarditis. *N Engl J Med.* 2000;342:690–695.

McNamara DM, Holubkov R, Starling RC, et al. Controlled trial of intravenous immune globulin in recent-onset dilated cardiomyopathy. *Circulation.* 2001;103:2254–2259.

Pinney SP, Mancini DM. Myocarditis and specific cardiomyopathies. In: Fuster V, O'Rourke RA, Walsh RA, et al., eds. *Hurst's The Heart.* 12th ed. New York, NY: McGraw-Hill; 2008:863–881.

Wu LA, Lapeyre AC III, Cooper LT. Current role of endomyocardial biopsy in the management of dilated cardiomyopathy and myocarditis. *Mayo Clin Proc.* 2001;76:1030–1038.

Yeh ETH, Lenihan DJ, Ewer MS. The diagnosis and management of cardiovascular diseases in cancer patients. In: Fuster V, O'Rourke RA, Walsh RA, et al., eds. *Hurst's The Heart.* 12th ed. New York, NY: McGraw-Hill; 2008:2053–2072.

CHAPTER (43)

The Heart and Noncardiac Drugs, Electricity, Poisons, and Radiation

Andrew L. Smith

NONCARDIAC DRUGS

【 】 CHEMOTHERAPEUTIC AGENTS

Chemotherapeutic agents may cause acute or chronic cardiovascular toxicity. Cardiomyopathy has generally been associated with the anthracyclines (doxorubicin, daunorubicin, epirubicin, idarubicin, and mitoxantrone). Cyclophosphamide has been associated with reversible systolic dysfunction and occasionally hemorrhagic myocarditis. Interleukin-2 and interferon alpha may cause hypotension and rarely cardiomyopathy. 5-Fluorouracil has been associated with coronary vasospasm. Amsacrine and paclitaxel have been associated with cardiac arrhythmias. Herceptin given in combination with doxorubicin may cause systolic dysfunction. Imatinib (Gleevec) has also been associated with heart failure.

Anthracyclines

Doxorubicin (adriamycin) and daunorubicin (cerubidine) cause dose-related cardiotoxicity possibly due to free-radical damage. Most cases of chemotherapy-related heart disease result from these agents. Acute cardiac toxicity may occur after the initial doses, and chronic cardiotoxicity occurs within months of therapy. Additionally, late cardiac systolic dysfunction occurring years later is becoming increasingly recognized. Diffuse left ventricular (LV) dysfunction occurs in up to 7% of patients receiving 550 mg/m^2 of doxorubicin. Toxicity is less with newer dosing schedules, which incorporate prolonged infusions in order to avoid high peak concentrations. Once cardiomyopathy develops, treatment is similar to those with other forms of systolic dysfunction. The clinical course varies from fulminant heart failure to gradually progressive deterioration. In some patients, systolic dysfunction is reversible. Endomyocardial biopsy provides a definitive detection. Dexrazoxane, an iron-chelating agent, is approved as a preventive strategy in women with breast cancer after cumulative doses of doxorubicin of greater than 300 mg/m^2. Trastuzmab (Herceptin), a treatment for metastatic breast cancer, carries as high as a 30% risk of cardiotoxicity when combined with anthracyclines. Use without combined anthracycline therapy carries a much lower risk and is usually reversible.

[ ] PSYCHOTROPIC AGENTS

Tricyclic Antidepressants

Tricyclic antidepressants (TAs) have potentially serious cardiovascular effects, including tachycardia, orthostatic hypotension, electrocardiogram (ECG) changes, and depression of LV function. They have electrophysiologic properties similar to those of the type IA antiarrhythmics and are contraindicated in the recovery phase following myocardial infarction. The threshold for the use of TAs should rise as the severity of heart disease increases or when there is QT prolongation.

TA overdose is lethal in approximately 2% of patients, generally related to cardiac complications. Initial clinical status and initial serum drug levels are not predictive of prognosis. QRS prolongation is a sign of toxicity but is an insensitive finding. Gastric lavage, repeat dosing of activated charcoal, and sodium bicarbonate therapy are appropriate treatment strategies. Type I antiarrhythmics should not be used for cardiac rhythm disturbances. Sodium bicarbonate is the initial therapy for ventricular arrhythmias. Hypotension refractory to volume loading and bicarbonate therapy should be treated with vasopressors such as norepinephrine, or vasopressor doses of dopamine.

Other Psychotropic Agents

The selective serotonin reuptake inhibitors (SSRIs) have rarely been associated with orthostatic hypotension and bradycardia. These drugs may affect the cytochrome P450 system and interfere with other cardiovascular drugs. Case reports of cardiac toxicity are rare. Orthostatic hypotension is common. The major concern with these agents is interaction with tyramine-containing substances, resulting in hypertensive crisis. Lithium may suppress automaticity, particularly of the sinus node. ECG changes may simulate hypokalemia, including T-wave inversion, prominent U waves, and QT prolongation. Overdose with lithium may result in severe bradycardia. Phenothiazine antipsychotic agents, including chlorpromazine and thioridazine, can produce tachycardia, postural hypotension, T-wave changes, QT prolongation, and bundle-branch block. Clozapine has been reported to cause myocarditis.

[ ] NONCARDIAC DRUGS CAUSING TORSADES DE POINTES

Tricyclics, phenothiazine, and other psychotropic agents may prolong the QT interval and induce torsades de points. Other toxic causes of torsades de pointes are haloperidol, terfenadine, astemizole, cisapride, pentamidine, probucol, arsenic, organophosphates, and liquid protein diets.

[ ] DRUG-RELATED VALVULAR HEART DISEASE

Valvular heart disease resembling that seen with carcinoid syndrome has been associated with the antimigraine drugs methysergide and ergotamine, the weight loss medications dexfenfluramine and fenfluramine, and possibly pergolide, used to treat Parkinson's disease (Table 43-1).

[ ] CHLOROQUINE

Chloroquine and hydroxychloroquine can cause skeletal and rarely heart muscle disease. When cardiac involvement occurs, features of restrictive cardiomyopathy are most common. Acute chloroquine poisoning results in hypotension, tachycardia, and prolongation of the QRS; it is often fatal.

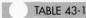
TABLE 43-1

Drug-Related Valvular Disease

Agents
   Methysergide
   Ergotamine
   Dexfenfluramine
   Fenfluramine
   Pergolide mesylate
Pathology
   Fibroendocardial plaque formation on normal valvular architecture
Echocardiographic findings
   Valve thickening and retraction
   Valvular regurgitation

【 】 ANTIMIGRAINE DRUGS

Sumatriptan, in addition to ergotamine and methysergide, is used to treat migraines. It is a selective serotonin type I agonist and may cause *coronary artery vasospasm.* Sumatriptan should not be taken within 24 hours of treatment with ergotamine-like medications because of the risk of prolonged vasoconstriction.

Ergotamine, methysergide, and sumatriptan are generally contraindicated in patients with obstructive coronary artery disease because of vasoconstrictor effects and the possibility of precipitating angina.

【 】 ANABOLIC STEROIDS

Illicit use of androgens is a problem in competitive athletes and body builders. Data on human toxicity are limited. Stanozolol and nandrolone have been associated with marked lipid abnormalities and an increase in coronary atherosclerosis. These agents may also cause LV hypertrophy and hypertension.

【 】 COCAINE

Cocaine is a common drug of abuse and has broad cardiovascular toxicity (Table 43-2). Chest pain is the most common reason for cocaine users to seek medical attention. The evaluation of cocaine-related chest pain is difficult. Approximately 6% of patients presenting to emergency departments with cocaine-related chest pain have myocardial infarction. They are often young men without other risk factors for coronary artery disease except tobacco smoking. The quality or duration of the chest discomfort is often not predictive of infarction. Because young patients often have early repolarization patterns on the ECG, ST-segment elevation in leads V_1 to V_3 may be confused with acute infarction. Patients may require cardiac monitoring for 6 to 12 hours, until enzymes have excluded infarction.

Treatment strategies for cocaine-induced myocardial ischemia have been developed based on the known cardiac and nervous system toxicity of this agent. Patients presenting with anxiety, tachycardia, and/or hypertension may respond well to benzodiazepines. Nitroglycerin may reverse coronary vasoconstriction induced by cocaine. Aspirin may prevent thrombus formation. Patients not responding to these measures may benefit from phentolamine or from calcium-channel blocker therapy with verapamil. Beta-adrenergic antagonists should generally be avoided due to unopposed alpha-mediated vasoconstriction. In documented cocaine-related myocardial infarction, thrombolytic therapy is highly effective. However, emergency coronary angiography may be necessary to distinguish patients with acute infarction from those with ST-segment elevation due to early repolarization.

TABLE 43-2

Cardiovascular Complications of Cocaine

Sudden death
Acute myocardial infarction
Chest pain without myocardial infarction
Accelerated coronary artherosclerosis
Intimal hyperplasia of coronary vessels
Electrocardiographic abnormalities
    Sinus tachycardia
    Premature ventricular complexes
    Ventricular tachycardia
    Torsades de pointes
    Ventricular fibrillation
    Prolongation of QT interval
    Early repolarization (ST-segment changes)
Acute reversible myocarditis
Dilated cardiomyopathy
Acute severe hypertension
Acute aortic dissection, rupture
Pneumopericardium
Stroke
Subarachnoid hemorrhage
Endocarditis (intravenous use)

Cocaine-related cardiac rhythm disturbances are best managed initially with benzodiazepines. Intravenous sodium bicarbonate and magnesium may be beneficial.

【 】 METHAMPHETAMINES

The biological effects of methamphetamines are similar to those of cocaine, but vasoconstriction is less. Cardiovascular toxicity is common and includes tachycardia, hypertension, and arrhythmias. Chest pain and myocardial infarction are less common than with cocaine. Chronic use may result in a catecholamine-mediated dilated cardiomyopathy.

ELECTRICITY

【 】 ENVIRONMENTAL ACCIDENTS

The immediate cardiac effect of injury due to lightning or electrical equipment may be asystole or ventricular fibrillation. Cardiac arrest may also result from apnea and hypoxia. Atrial and ventricular arrhythmias, conduction abnormalities, and LV dysfunction may occur. Cardiac abnormalities occur due to direct myocardial injury or central nervous system injury, with intense catecholamine release. Hypertension and tachycardia may be managed with beta-blocking agents.

Cardiopulmonary resuscitation should be continued for a prolonged period after apparent death from lightning, since late recovery may occur. In lightning strikes involving multiple victims, attention should first be directed to those who are "apparently dead," since lightning victims with vital signs generally survive without immediate medical attention and those without vital signs may recover after prolonged resuscitation.

【 】 ELECTROCONVULSIVE THERAPY

Electroconvulsive therapy (ECT) may produce cardiac arrhythmias and ECG changes during the first few minutes after the shock. ECT produces brief, intense stimulation of the central nervous system. Cardiovascular complications may result from this stimulation or from the drugs used to modify the response. Patients with coronary artery disease should be pretreated with a beta-blocker to blunt tachycardia and hypertension and to reduce the frequency of ventricular ectopic beats. Patients with cardiac pacemakers can safely undergo ECT.

COMPLEMENTARY AND ALTERNATIVE MEDICINES

Complementary and alternative medicines and the heart are discussed in Chapter 62.

POISONS

【 】 SNAKE AND SCORPION VENOMS

Snake venoms affect the coagulation system, cellular components of the blood, endothelium, nervous system, and heart. Cardiac arrhythmias, severe hypotension, and cardiac arrest may occur. Multiple pulmonary emboli may be seen in patients who survive 12 hours or longer. Scorpion venom may cause hypertension, myocardial infarction, arrhythmias, conduction disturbances, and myocarditis.

【 】 MARINE TOXINS

Scorpion fish cause envenomation that may result in rhythm disturbances and heart failure. Ingestion of pufferfish may cause severe bradycardia and cardiovascular collapse. Stingray venom contains phosphodiesterases and rarely may cause cardiac rhythm disturbances.

【 】 HALOGENATED HYDROCARBONS

These substances are used in fire extinguishers, solvents, refrigerants, pesticides, and plastics, paints, and glues. They can suppress myocardial contractility and produce arrhythmias and sudden death.

【 】 CARBON MONOXIDE

Carbon monoxide poisoning produces myocardial ischemia usually manifest by ST-segment and T-wave changes and atrial and ventricular arrhythmias. Extensive myocardial necrosis and cardiomyopathy can occur.

RADIATION

Radiation to the mediastinum can affect the pericardium, myocardium, endocardium, valves, and capillaries of the heart. Radiation may cause acute pericarditis, chronic pericarditis, and pericardial constriction. Pericardial involvement is most frequent 4 to 6 months after radiation therapy.

Clinically important myocardial dysfunction related to radiation generally occurs in combination with pericardial disease. Myocardial fibrosis may result in diastolic dysfunction and, less commonly, systolic dysfunction. Radiation-induced valvular heart disease is rare but usually involves the aortic or mitral valves. Premature coronary artery disease may occur after radiation therapy and often involves the coronary ostia.

Radiation may result in fibrosis of the nodal and infranodal pathways. Right bundle-branch block is especially common; complete heart block is rare.

SUGGESTED READING

Adams MJ, Hardenbergh PH, Constine LS, et al. Radiation-associated cardiovascular disease. *Crit Rev Oncol Hematol.* 2003;45:55–75.

De Smet PAGM. Herbal remedies. *N Engl J Med.* 2002;347:2046–2056.

Jain S, Bandi V. Electrical and lightning injuries. *Crit Care Clin.* 1999;15:319–331.

Kloner RA, Rezkalla SH. Cocaine and the heart. *N Engl J Med.* 2003;348:487–488.

Roden DM. Drug therapy: drug-induced prolongation of the QT interval. *N Engl J Med.* 2004;350:1013–1022.

Smith AL, Book WM. Effect of noncardiac drugs, electricity, poisons, and radiation on the heart. In: Fuster V, O'Rourke RA, Walsh RA, et al., eds. *Hurst's The Heart.* 12th ed. New York, NY: McGraw-Hill; 2008:2132–2142.

Theodoulou MS. Cardiac effects of adjuvant therapy for early breast cancer. *Semin Oncol.* 2003;30:730–739.

Witchel HJ, Hancox JC, Nutt DJ. Psychotropic drugs, cardiac arrhythmia, and sudden death. *J Clin Psychopharmacol.* 2003;23:58–77.

Yeh ETH, Tong AT, Lenihan DJ, et al. Cardiovascular complications of cancer therapy: diagnosis, pathogenesis, and management. *Circulation.* 2004;109:3122–3131.

CHAPTER 44

Diseases of the Pericardium

Sharon L. Roble and Brian D. Hoit

The pericardium consists of an inner visceral and an outer parietal layer, between which is a potential space, the pericardial cavity, which normally contains up to 50 mL of plasma infiltrate. Despite serving many important functions (Table 44-1), the pericardium is not essential for life and no adverse consequences follow either congenital absence or surgical removal of the pericardium. Thus, clinicopathologic processes involving the pericardium are understandably few; indeed, pericardial heart disease comprises only pericarditis and its complications (tamponade and constriction) and congenital lesions. Nevertheless, the pericardium is affected by virtually every category of disease (Table 44-2).

ACUTE PERICARDITIS

Acute fibrinous or dry pericarditis is a syndrome characterized by typical chest pain, a pericardial friction rub, and specific electrocardiographic (ECG) changes. It should be emphasized that the quality, severity, and location of pain vary greatly. The ECG may either confirm the clinical suspicion of pericardial disease or first alert the clinician to the presence of pericarditis. Serial tracings may be needed to distinguish the ST-segment elevations caused by acute pericarditis from those caused by acute myocardial infarction (MI) or normal early repolarization. The ST-T–wave changes in acute pericarditis are diffuse and have characteristic evolutionary changes (Table 44-3).

The chest radiograph is frequently normal, but may reveal an enlarged cardiac silhouette (a moderate or large pericardial effusion) as well as provide evidence of the underlying etiology. When an effusion is present, echocardiography estimates the volume of pericardial fluid, identifies cardiac tamponade, suggests the basis of pericarditis, and documents associated acute myocarditis. Nonspecific blood markers of inflammation usually increase in cases of acute pericarditis, and serum cardiac isoenzymes may increase with extensive epicarditis. Many patients presenting with acute, idiopathic pericarditis have increased serum troponin I levels, often within the range considered diagnostic for acute myocardial infarction.

Hospitalization is warranted for most patients who present with an initial episode of acute pericarditis in order to determine the etiology and to observe for the development of cardiac tamponade. Acute pericarditis usually responds to oral nonsteroidal anti-inflammatory drugs (NSAIDs). Prophylaxis against gastrointestinal bleeding with histamine-2 antagonists or proton-pump inhibitors is warranted, particularly in those at high risk or who require longer durations of treatment. Addition of colchicine to NSAID therapy is effective for the acute episode and may prevent recurrences. Indomethacin reduces coronary blood flow and should be avoided. Chest pain is usually alleviated in 1 to 2 days, and the friction rub and ST-segment elevation resolve shortly thereafter. Most mild cases of idiopathic and viral pericarditis are adequately treated in 1 to 4 days. However, the duration of therapy is variable and patients should be treated

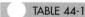

TABLE 44-1

Functions of the Pericardium

Mechanical
    Effects on chambers
        Limits short-term cardiac distention
        Facilitates cardiac chamber coupling and interaction
        Maintains pressure–volume relation of the cardiac chambers and output from
        them
        Maintains geometry of left ventricle
    Effects on whole heart
        Lubricates, minimizes friction
        Equalizes gravitation, inertial, hydrostatic forces
        Mechanical barrier to infection
Immunologic
Vasomotor
Fibrinolytic
Modulation of myocyte structure, function, and gene expression
Vehicle for drug delivery and gene therapy

until an effusion, if present, has resolved. The intensity of therapy is dictated by the distress of the patient; narcotics may be required for severe pain. Cases not responsive to NSAIDs and colchicine may necessitate systemic corticosteroids therapy for a week to control pain, with the dosage tapered rapidly thereafter. Corticosteroids should be avoided unless there is a specific indication, such as uremic pericarditis and connective tissue disease, as they enhance viral multiplication and may produce recurrences when the dosage is tapered.

Painful recurrences of pericarditis may respond to NSAIDs, but commonly require high-dose corticosteroids. Using the lowest possible dose, alternate-day therapy, combinations with nonsteroidal drugs, or colchicine should minimize the risks of long-term steroids. Intrapericardial administration of triamcinolone has been shown to relieve symptoms in patients with recurrent autoreactive myopericarditis and azathioprine has also been used to prevent recurrent episodes Pericardiectomy should be considered only when repeated attempts at medical treatment have clearly failed.

PERICARDIAL EFFUSION

Accumulation of transudate, exudate, or blood in the pericardial sac is a frequent complication of pericardial disease and should be sought in all patients with acute pericarditis. Chronic effusive pericarditis may be associated with large, asymptomatic effusions. Transudative effusions (hydropericardium) occur in heart failure and other states associated with chronic salt and water retention, and exudative effusions occur in a large number of the infectious and inflammatory types of pericarditis. Although frank hemorrhagic effusions suggest recent intrapericardial bleeding, sanguineous and serosanguineous effusions occur in many infectious and inflammatory disorders. Chylous pericarditis implies injury or obstruction to the thoracic duct, and cholesterol pericarditis is either idiopathic or associated with hypothyroidism, rheumatoid arthritis, or tuberculosis.

Echocardiography is the *procedure of choice* for the diagnosis of pericardial effusion. Computed tomography (CT) and magnetic resonance imaging (MRI) may be useful

TABLE 44-2

Causes of Pericardial Heart Disease

Idiopathic
Infectious
    Bacterial
    Viral
    Mycobacterial
    Fungal
    Protozoal
    AIDS-associated
Neoplastic
    Primary
    Secondary (breast, lung, melanoma, lymphoma, leukemia)
Immune/inflammatory
    Connective tissue diseases (rheumatoid arthritis, systemic lupus erythematosus,
        scleroderma, acute rheumatic fever, dermatomyositis, mixed connective tissue
        disease, Wegener's granulomatosis)
    Arteritis (temporal arteritis, polyarteritis nodosa, Takayasu's arteritis)
    Acute myocardial infarction (MI) and post-MI (Dressler's syndrome)
    Postcardiotomy
    Posttraumatic
Metabolic
    Nephrogenic
    Aortic dissection
    Myxedema
    Amyloidosis
Iatrogenic
    Radiation injury
    Instrument/device trauma (implantable defibrillator, pacemakers, catheters)
    Drugs (hydralazine, procainamide, daunorubicin, isoniazid, anticoagulants,
        cyclosporine, methysergide, phenytoin, dantrolene, mesalazine)
    Cardiac resuscitation
Traumatic
    Blunt trauma
    Penetrating trauma
    Surgical trauma
Congenital
    Pericardial cysts
    Congenital absence of pericardium
    Mulibrey nanism

to identify loculated or atypically loculated pericardial effusions and to characterize the nature of the effusion. Epicardial fat may mimic an effusion, but is slightly echogenic and tends to move in concert with the heart, two characteristics that help distinguish it from an effusion, which is generally echolucent and motionless.

The etiology of a pericardial effusion is difficult to determine on historical or clinical grounds. Specific diagnoses are possible using visual, cytologic, and immunologic analysis of the pericardial effusion and pericardioscopic-guided biopsy.

The approach to the management of a moderate-to-large pericardial effusion is shown in Fig. 44-1. Drainage of a pericardial effusion is usually unnecessary unless either purulent pericarditis is suspected or cardiac tamponade supervenes, although on

TABLE 44-3

Electrocardiographic Changes in Acute Pericarditis

Stage	Time Course	ECG Changes
1	ST-segment elevation occurs within hours of onset of chest pain and may persist for days	Upward concave ST-segment elevations usually not exceeding 5 mm; PR-segment depression (except aVR)
2	Hours to days following stage one	ST segments return to baseline; T waves normal or show loss of amplitude
3	T-wave inversions may persist indefinitely (especially when associated with TB, uremia, or neoplasm)	T-wave inversions
4	Usually completed within 2 weeks, but variability common	ECG normalizes

occasion pericardiocentesis is needed to establish the etiology of a hemodynamically insignificant effusion. Persistent or progressive effusion, particularly when the cause is uncertain, also warrants pericardiocentesis.

CARDIAC TAMPONADE

Cardiac tamponade is a hemodynamic condition caused by a pericardial effusion and characterized by equal elevation of atrial, ventricular diastolic, and pericardial pressures; an exaggerated inspiratory decrease in arterial systolic pressure (pulsus paradoxus); and

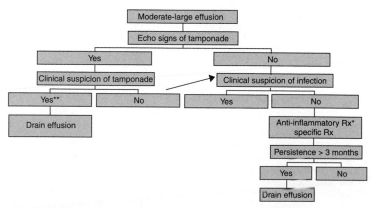

FIGURE 44-1. Algorithm for the management of moderate to large pericardial effusions. (*Anti-inflammatory treatment if there are signs of pericarditis. **Right heart catheterization may be required.)

arterial hypotension. Although the absolute intracardiac pressures are elevated, the transmural pressures are practically zero or even negative. The greatly reduced preload is responsible for the fall in cardiac output, and when compensatory mechanisms are exhausted, arterial pressure decreases.

Cardiac tamponade may be acute or chronic and should be viewed hemodynamically as a continuum, ranging from mild (pericardial pressure less than 10 mm Hg) to severe (pericardial pressure greater than 20 mm Hg). Mild cardiac tamponade is frequently asymptomatic, whereas moderate and especially severe tamponade produces precordial discomfort and dyspnea. Both the severity of cardiac tamponade and the time course of pericardial fluid accumulation dictate symptoms and physical findings. Careful inspection of the jugular venous pulse waveform is essential for the diagnosis; compression of the heart by pericardial fluid results in a characteristic loss of the venous Y descent. An inspiratory decline of systolic arterial pressure exceeding 10 mm Hg defines pulsus paradoxus, a phenomenon with complex and multifactorial origins. However, in the presence of coexisting left ventricular disease, atrial septal defects, or aortic insufficiency, *pulsus paradoxus may not develop*. Low voltage on the ECG and/or electrical alternans should raise the suspicion of cardiac tamponade; unless even a brief delay might prove life threatening, an echocardiogram should be obtained. During inspiration, greater than normal increases in right ventricular dimensions and decreases in left ventricular dimensions occur in many cases of tamponade. These respiratory changes also accompany other conditions associated with pulsus paradoxus, such as chronic obstructive lung disease and pulmonary embolism. Diastolic collapse of the right ventricle and right atrium, which reflects negative transmural pressure, is useful but neither sensitive nor specific as for tamponade. Exaggerated respiratory variation in transvalvular and venous velocities measured by Doppler echocardiography (flow velocity pulsus paradoxus) also helps diagnose cardiac tamponade. It is important to remember that clinically significant tamponade is a clinical diagnosis and *"echocardiographic signs of tamponade"* are not by themselves an indication for pericardiocentesis. Although the absence of any cardiac chamber collapse has a high negative predictive value (92%), the positive predictive value is reduced (58%); and although positive and negative predictive values are high (82% and 88%, respectively) for abnormal right-sided venous flows (i.e., systolic predominance and expiratory diastolic reversal), they could not be evaluated in more than one-third of patients.

The pericardial, right atrial, pulmonary capillary wedge, and pulmonary artery diastolic pressures are elevated and equal; the degree of elevation is related to both the severity of tamponade and the patient's intravascular volume status. The right atrial and wedge pressure tracings reveal an attenuated or absent Y descent. Cardiac output is reduced and systemic vascular resistance is elevated.

Removal of small amounts of pericardial fluid (~50 mL) produces considerable symptomatic and hemodynamic improvement because of the steep pericardial pressure–volume relation. Unless there is concomitant cardiac disease or coexisting constriction, removal of all of the pericardial fluid normalizes pericardial, atrial, ventricular diastolic and arterial pressures, and cardiac output. Drainage of the pericardial fluid using a catheter minimizes trauma, allows measurement of pericardial pressure and instillation of drugs into the pericardium, and helps prevent (but does not guarantee) reaccumulation of pericardial fluid. Extended (3 ± 2 days) catheter drainage is associated with lower recurrence rates over a 4-year follow-up. Generally speaking, drainage should continue until the volume of the aspirated volume is less than 25 mL/d.

Although pericardiocentesis may provide effective relief and has relatively simple logistic and personnel requirements, *surgical drainage* offers several advantages. These include complete drainage, access to pericardial tissue for histopathologic and microbiological diagnoses, the ability to drain loculated effusions, and the avoidance of the risk of traumatic injury due to blind placement of a needle into the pericardial sac. The choice between needle pericardiocentesis, ideally performed under echocardiographic guidance, and surgical drainage depends upon institutional resources and physician experience, the etiology of the effusion, the need for diagnostic tissue samples, and the patient's prognosis. In any case, pericardial fluid should be sent for smear, culture, and cytology. Repeat pericardiocentesis, sclerotherapy with tetracycline, surgical creation of a pericardial window, or pericardiectomy may treat recurrent effusions. A pericardial window is usually placed in patients with malignant effusions, and pericardiectomy may be required for recurrent effusions in dialysis patients. In critically ill patients, a pericardial window may be created percutaneously with a balloon catheter.

CONSTRICTIVE PERICARDITIS

Constrictive pericarditis is a condition in which a thickened, scarred, and often calcified pericardium limits diastolic filling of the ventricles. Although acute pericarditis from most causes may eventuate in constrictive pericarditis, the most common antecedents are idiopathic, cardiac trauma and surgery, tuberculosis and other infectious diseases, neoplasms, radiation therapy, renal failure, and connective tissue diseases.

Constrictive pericarditis resembles the congestive states due to myocardial disease and chronic liver disease. Patients generally complain of fatigue, dyspnea, weight gain, abdominal discomfort, nausea, and increased abdominal girth. Physical findings include ascites, hepatosplenomegaly, edema, and wasting; often these lead to an erroneous diagnosis of hepatic cirrhosis. The venous pressure is elevated and displays deep Y and often deep X descents, and it fails to decrease with inspiration (Kussmaul's sign). Kussmaul's sign lacks specificity, as it is seen also in cases of restrictive cardiomyopathy, right ventricular failure and infarction, and tricuspid stenosis. A pericardial knock, similar in timing to the third heart sound, is pathognomonic but occurs infrequently. Pulsus paradoxus may occur with associated pericardial effusion (effusive-constrictive pericarditis).

Low QRS voltage and nonspecific P- and T-wave changes are common; atrial fibrillation is seen in approximately one-third of cases and atrial flutter less often. The cardiac silhouette may be normal or enlarged, and pericardial calcification is present in less than half of the cases. Pericardial thickening and calcification and abnormal ventricular filling produce characteristic but insensitive and nonspecific changes on the M-mode echocardiogram; these reflect abnormal filling of the ventricles. However, a normal study virtually rules out the diagnosis. Because of the close physiologic similarities of constrictive pericarditis and restrictive cardiomyopathy, increased pericardial thickness detected by CT is the most reliable means of distinguishing between the two disorders. Accurate definition of pericardial thickness and its distribution is also possible with MRI.

Cardiac catheterization is used to confirm the clinical suspicion of pericardial disease, uncover occult constriction, diagnose effusive-constrictive disease, and identify associated coronary, myocardial, and valvular disease. Endomyocardial biopsy is sometimes necessary to exclude restrictive cardiomyopathy.

Pericardiectomy is the definitive treatment for constrictive pericarditis but is unwarranted either in very early constriction or in severe, advanced disease, when the risk of surgery is excessive (30%–40% mortality) and the benefits are diminished. Involvement of the visceral pericardium and evidence for myocardial fibrosis also increases the surgical risk. Symptomatic relief may take several months following pericardiectomy. Postoperative normalization of cardiac pressures may be incomplete in a significant number of patients.

Evidence of transient (acute) constriction may occur in about 15% of patients with acute effusive pericarditis. Therefore, before proceeding with pericardiectomy, the possibility that pericardial constriction may be reversible and amenable to medical therapy should be considered. Constrictive pericarditis may resolve spontaneously or in response to various combinations of nonsteroidal anti-inflammatory agents, steroids, and antibiotics. Diuretics and digoxin are useful in patients who are not candidates for pericardiectomy because of their high surgical risk.

Effusive-constrictive pericarditis is an uncommon entity, which occurs when pericardial fluid accumulates between the thickened layers of pericardium. The hemodynamic picture is consistent with tamponade prior to pericardiocentesis and constrictive pericarditis afterward. Noninvasive testing is not useful in the evaluation of effusive-constrictive pericarditis.

CONGENITAL PERICARDIAL HEART DISEASE

Congenital absence of the pericardium is an uncommon anomaly, usually involving a portion or the whole of the left parietal pericardium. Its presence is usually suspected from the chest radiogram and echocardiogram. Contrast-enhanced CT and MRI reliably establish the anatomy of the defect. Pericardial cysts are rare remnants of defective embryologic development and are benign; their importance lies in differentiation from neoplasm.

SUGGESTED READING

Hoit BD. Diseases of the pericardium. In: Fuster V, O'Rourke RA, Walsh RA, et al., eds. *Hurst's The Heart.* 12th ed. New York, NY: McGraw-Hill; 2008:1951–1974.

Hoit BD. Management of effusive and constrictive pericardial heart disease. *Circulation.* 2002;105:2939–2942.

Maisch B, Seferovic PM, Ristic AD, et al. Guidelines on the diagnosis and management of pericardial diseases executive summary; the task force on the diagnosis and management of pericardial diseases of the European Society of Cardiology. *Eur Heart J.* 2004;25:587–610.

CHAPTER (45)

Cardiovascular Diseases Caused by Genetic Abnormalities

Michael Froeschl and Robert Roberts

Genetic factors play a role in many cardiovascular diseases, from familial disorders such as congenital long QT syndrome to complex, nonfamilial phenotypes, such as atherosclerosis. Molecular genetics, in conjunction with cytogenetics, provides the opportunity to decipher the genetic basis and pathogenesis of cardiovascular diseases. In this chapter, several cardiac genetic disorders are reviewed.

ESSENTIALS OF GENETIC DISORDERS

There are approximately 23,000 genes in the human genome. The gene or genes inherited constitute a person's *genotype*. *Phenotype*, on the other hand, comprises the physical, physiologic, or biochemical features that the individual manifests, which are determined by both genetic makeup and the influence of myriad environmental factors. The percentage of individuals with a genetic mutation who also have one or more features of the genetic disease is referred to as the *penetrance*. Penetrance is an all-or-none phenomenon: any manifestation, however minute, indicates that the gene is penetrant in that individual. *Nonpenetrance* refers to lack of any observable phenotype. This feature is to be distinguished from *expressivity*, which refers to the variable nature of the clinical phenotype, such as severity. Thus, by definition, to have expressivity, the trait must be penetrant.

The most important part of an evaluation for genetic disease is the family history. The individual with the problem who brought the family to medical attention is known as the *proband* or index case. Information should generally be collected on all first-, second-, and third-degree relatives of the proband. A pedigree chart is then generated. Pregnancy and family histories can then be used in conjunction with the findings on physical examination to derive a potential etiologic diagnosis and to plan for further diagnostic studies. Prognosis and recurrence risk are closely tied to an accurate diagnosis and its probable etiology. Genetic counseling should provide information about the diagnosis, possible etiology, and prognosis of a disease. In addition, psychosocial issues, reproductive options, and the availability of prenatal diagnosis should be discussed. Genetic counseling should be nondirective, providing information in a nonjudgmental, unbiased manner. The family should then be able to make decisions based on medical information in the context of their religious, moral, cultural, and social backgrounds and their financial situation. The accelerated pace of progress in gene discovery, molecular medicine, and molecular diagnostics has begun to allow for improved genetic counseling and holds the promise of future genetic therapy. As knowledge about the genetic basis of disease grows, however, so too does the potential for discriminatory health insurance policies to exclude individuals who are at risk for an illness or to charge prohibitively high rates on the basis of predetermined illness.

CARDIOVASCULAR ABNORMALITIES CAUSED BY CHROMOSOMAL DEFECTS

Table 45-1 lists chromosomal defects that cause cardiovascular abnormalities. Two commonly encountered syndromes due to chromosomal defects—Down syndrome and Turner syndrome—are reviewed here.

【 】 DOWN SYNDROME

Down syndrome, or trisomy 21, is a major cause of mental retardation and congenital heart disease. The incidence of Down syndrome is approximately 1 in 700 live births. The risk of having a live-born with Down syndrome increases with maternal age. Clinical manifestations include congenital anomalies of the heart and gastrointestinal tract, epicanthal folds, flattened facial profile, small and rounded ears, upslanted palpebral fissures, excess nuchal skin, and brachycephaly. Cardiac abnormalities are present in approximately half of cases, most commonly atrioventricular canal defects and isolated

TABLE 45-1

Partial List of Chromosomal Abnormalities Associated with Heart Disease

Chromosome Defect	Syndrome	Cardiac Phenotype
45X	Turner syndrome	Coarctation of the aorta, ASD, aortic stenosis
Trisomy 5		Interrupted aortic arch
Trisomy 13	Patau syndrome	CHD, VSD
Trisomy 18	Edwards syndrome	CHD, VSD
Partial trisomy 20q		Dextrocardia
Trisomy 21	Down syndrome	CHD, ASD, VSD, PDA
Trisomy 22		VSD
Partial tetrasomy 22	Schmid–Fraccaro syndrome	CHD Anomalous pulmonary venous return
Deletion 4p	Wolf–Hirschhorn syndrome	CHD
Deletion 7q11.23	Williams syndrome	CHD, supravalvular aortic stenosis, hypertension, MVP
Deletion paternal 15q11	Prader–Willi syndrome	CHD
Deletion 17p	Miller–Dieker syndrome	CHD, ASD
Deletion 22q11	CATCH-22, DiGeorge, and velocardiofacial syndromes	CHD
Rearrangement 5p15.1–3	Cri du chat	CHD
Recombination chromosome 8	San Luis Valley syndrome	Tetralogy of Fallot

ASD, atrial septal defect; CHD, congenital heart disease; MVP, mitral valve prolapse; PDA, patent ductus arteriosus; VSD, ventricular septal defect.

ventricular septal defects (VSDs). Isolated secundum atrial septal defect (ASD) and tetralogy of Fallot are also encountered.

Down syndrome is caused by trisomy 21. It is full trisomy in 95%, chromosomal translocation in 2%, and mosaic in 3%. Most errors in meiosis leading to trisomy 21 are of maternal origin and occur during the first meiosis in two-thirds and during the second meiosis in one-fifth of cases. *DSCR1* (Down syndrome critical region) encodes for calcipressin 1, a calcineurin A inhibitor. It is abundantly expressed in the heart and brain and is a candidate gene for both the cardiac anomalies and the mental retardation.

【　】 TURNER SYNDROME

Turner syndrome is characterized by a constellation of findings that result from partial or complete monosomy of the X chromosome. It is the most common chromosomal abnormality in females, with an incidence of 1 per 2,500 to 3,000 live-born girls. The phenotype is variable and often mild with short stature, low-set ears, broad chest with widely spaced nipples, peripheral lymphedema, and ovarian dysgenesis; intelligence is normal. Cardiac abnormalities are common, with a prevalence estimated between 23% and 40%. The most common are bicuspid aortic valve in 10% to 20% and coarctation of aorta, present in 10% of adult cases. A variety of other cardiac defects may also occur, usually other left heart abnormalities such as aortic stenosis, dilated ascending aorta, and hypoplastic left heart syndrome (HLHS). Women with Turner syndrome are more susceptible to aortic aneurysms and ischemic heart disease.

Turner syndrome is caused by complete or partial absence of an X chromosome. The most common karyotype is monosomy X (45,X). Approximately 5% to 10% of the cases have duplication of the long arm of one X (46,X,i[Xq]) and the rest have mosaicism.

GENETIC BASIS OF SPECIFIC CONGENITAL HEART DISEASES

A number of congenital heart diseases occur in isolation and are not part of complex phenotypes as observed in chromosomal abnormalities. Recently, the causal genes for several congenital heart diseases have been identified. Preliminary studies depict a common theme in the pathogenesis of isolated congenital heart defects that implicates deficiency of several transcriptional factors that regulate cardiac gene expression during embryogenesis.

【　】 SUPRAVALVULAR AORTIC STENOSIS

Supravalvular aortic stenosis is an autosomal dominant disease characterized by discrete narrowing of the ascending aorta above the level of the sinusus of Valsalva. It commonly occurs as a phenotype of Williams syndrome (or Williams–Beuren syndrome) in conjunction with mental retardation in some and exceptional talents in others, hypercalcemia, elfin facies, and stenosis of major arteries. The prevalence of supravalvular aortic stenosis is estimated to be 1 in 25,000 live births.

The gene responsible for supravalvular aortic stenosis was initially mapped to chromosome 7q11.23 and subsequently identified as *ELN,* encoding elastin. Almost all cases of isolated supravalvular aortic stenosis are caused by *ELN* mutations. Mutations result in elastin deficiency, which in the vascular system leads to inelasticity of the vessel wall and subsequent fibrosis as a result of an altered stress–strain relation (elastin arteriopathy).

【　】 FAMILIAL ATRIAL SEPTAL DEFECT

ASD is among the most common congenital heart diseases, with an estimated incidence of 1 in 1,000 live births. ASD is usually sporadic; however, familial ASD with an autosomal dominant mode of inheritance has also been described. The first gene identified for familial ASD was *NKX2–5 (CSX1)*. The gene is located on 5q35 and encodes NKX2.5, a predominantly cardiac-specific transcription factor that regulates expression of several cardiac genes. The spectrum of clinical phenotypes caused by mutations in NKX2.5 extends beyond secundum ASD to include VSDs, tetralogy of Fallot, subvalvular aortic stenosis, and pulmonary atresia.

A second causal gene for familial ASD with an autosomal dominant mode of inheritance is *GATA4* on chromosome 8p22–23. Mutations diminish DNA-binding affinity and transcriptional activity of GATA4 transcription factor and block its physical interaction with TBX5, another transcription factor involved in the pathogenesis of congenital heart disease.

A third causal gene for familial ASD is *MYH6*, which is located in chromosome 14q12 and encodes myosin heavy chain 6. The MYH6 protein is expressed at high levels in atrial tissues and plays an important role in the formation of the interatrial septum.

【 】 HOLT–ORAM SYNDROME

Holt–Oram syndrome is a rare autosomal dominant inherited disorder characterized by anomalies of the heart and upper extremities; hence the name *hand–heart syndrome*. The most common congenital heart defects are ASD and VSD, followed by conduction system abnormalities and atrial fibrillation. Less common cardiac abnormalities include truncus arteriosus, mitral valve defects, patent ductus arteriosus (PDA), and tetralogy of Fallot. Anomalies of the upper limb vary from mild malformation of the carpal bones to phocomelia.

Mutations in *TBX5* on chromosome 12q24, which codes for transcription factor TBX5, are responsible for the cardiac and skeletal abnormalities in Holt–Oram syndrome. A number of mutations have been described resulting in reduced expression of TBX5.

【 】 FAMILIAL MYXOMA SYNDROME

Myxomas are the most common cardiac tumors and are generally sporadic. In approximately 10% of cases, however, myxomas are familial with an autosomal dominant mode of inheritance. Familial myxoma commonly occurs as a part of *Carney complex* with the constellation of cardiac myxoma, endocrine disorders, and skin pigmentation. LAMB (*l*entigines, *a*trial myxoma, *m*ucocutaneous myxoma, *b*lue nevi) and NAME (*n*evi, *a*trial myxoma, *m*yxoid neurofibromata, *e*phelides) syndromes are considered variants of Carney complex. The majority of familial cardiac myxomas (Carney complex) are caused by mutations in the *PRKRA1A* gene on chromosome 17q24, which encodes the alpha-regulatory subunit of cyclic adenosine monophosphate (cAMP)-dependent protein kinase.

GENETIC DISEASES OF CARDIAC MUSCLE

The term *cardiomyopathy* denotes a disorder in which there is a primary defect in the myocardium, affecting cardiac myocyte structure and/or function. Cardiomyopathies are commonly classified into four groups according to their phenotypic characteristics: hypertrophic, dilated, restrictive, and arrhythmogenic right ventricular cardiomyopathy (see also Chapter 39). Each of these groups exhibits important genetic influences.

【 】 HYPERTROPHIC CARDIOMYOPATHY

Hypertrophic cardiomyopathy (HCM) is an autosomal dominant disease diagnosed clinically by the presence of unexplained cardiac hypertrophy (see also Chapter 40). The prevalence of HCM is approximately 1 in 500 in young adults and likely higher in the elderly population because of age-dependent penetrance. The pathologic hallmark of HCM is cardiac *myocyte disarray*. Other pathologic features of HCM include myocyte hypertrophy, interstitial fibrosis, thickening of the media of intramural coronary arteries, and often a malpositioned mitral valve with elongated leaflets. Most patients with HCM are asymptomatic or only mildly symptomatic; symptoms are usually related to heart failure or arrhythmia. HCM is the most common cause of sudden cardiac death (SCD) in young, competitive athletes, accounting for almost half of all cases of SCD in athletes younger than 35 years of age in the United States. However, in the absence of major risk factors for SCD, HCM has a relatively benign course, with an estimated annual mortality of about 1% in the adult population.

HCM is a genetically heterogeneous disease. Approximately two-thirds of patients have a family history of HCM; in the remainder, the disease is sporadic. Both familial and sporadic cases are caused by mutations in sarcomeric proteins. In 1990, an arginine-to-glutamine substitution at codon 403 (R403Q) in the beta-myosin heavy chain (MHC) was identified as the first causal mutation. Since then, more than 300 different mutations in over a dozen genes encoding sarcomeric proteins have been identified (Table 45-2).

TABLE 45-2

Causal Genes for Hypertrophic Cardiomyopathy (Sarcomeric Genes)

Gene	Symbol	Locus	Frequency	Predominant Mutations
β-Myosin heavy chain	MYH7	14q12	~ 30%	Missenses
Myosin binding protein-C	MYBPC3	11p11.2	~ 30%	Splice-junction and insertion/deletion
Cardiac troponin T	TNNT2	1q32	~ 5%	Missenses
Cardiac troponin I	TNNI3	19p13.2	~ 5%	Missense and deletion
α-Tropomyosin	TPM1	15q22.1	~ 5%	Missenses
Essential myosin light chain	MYL3	3p21.3	< 5%	Missenses
Regulatory myosin light chain	MYL2	12q23–24.3	< 5%	Missense and 1 truncation
Cardiac α-actin	ACTC	15q11	< 5%	Missense mutations
Titin	TTN	2q24.1	< 5%	Missense mutations
Telethonin (Tcap)	TCAP	17q2	Rare	Missense mutations
α-Myosin heavy chain	MYH6	14q1	Rare	Missense and rearrangement mutations (association)
Cardiac troponin C	TNNC1	3p21.3– 3p14.3	Rare	Missense mutations (association)
Cardiac myosin light peptide kinase	MYLK2	20q13.3	Rare	Point mutations (association)
Caveolin 3	CAV3	3p25	Rare	Point mutations (association)
Phospholamban	PLN	6p22.1	Rare	Point mutations (association)
Myozenin 2	MYOZ2	4q26–q27	Rare	Missenses

Systematic screening of sarcomeric genes suggests that mutations in *MYH7* and *MYBPC3,* which encode beta-MHC and myosin-binding protein C (MBP-C), respectively, are the most common causes of human HCM, accounting for approximately one-half of all cases. Mutations in *TNNT2* and *TNNI3,* encoding cardiac troponin T and I, respectively, are less common, each accounting for approximately 5% of HCM cases. Overall, the causal genes and mutations for over two-thirds of HCM cases have been identified. The genes accounting for the remainder are yet to be identified or are a result of genes inducing a phenocopy (described later).

A remarkable feature of HCM is the broad spectrum of its phenotypic expression, with respect to both the degree of cardiac hypertrophy and the risk of SCD. This variability is multifactorial. Causal genes and specific mutations are the major determinants of the expressivity of cardiac phenotype. Mutations in *MYH7* are generally associated with early-onset HCM with extensive hypertrophy and a high incidence of SCD, yet there is variability among different *MYH7* mutations. On the other hand, the phenotype in the majority of patients with *MYBPC3* mutations is relatively mild. The age of onset of clinical symptoms tends to be late, the degree of cardiac hypertrophy less severe, and the incidence of SCD low. However, "malignant" mutations have been described that are associated with severe hypertrophy and a high incidence of SCD. The risk of SCD in HCM caused by mutations in *MYH7* and *MYBPC3* is partially reflective of the severity of hypertrophy: mutations associated with mild hypertrophy generally carry a relatively benign prognosis and those with severe hypertrophy indicate a high incidence of SCD. This is in contrast to HCM caused by mutations in *TNNT2,* which is characterized by mild cardiac hypertrophy but extensive myocyte disarray and a high incidence of SCD.

Genes other than the causal genes also affect the phenotype in HCM. They are termed *modifier genes.* Unlike the causal genes, modifier genes are neither necessary nor sufficient to cause HCM. However, they can influence the severity of cardiac hypertrophy and the risk of SCD. *ACE*, encoding angiotensin-I-converting enzyme 1 (ACE-1), was the first gene implicated as a modifier of cardiac phenotype in human HCM. Since then, variants of endothelin-1 (*EDN1*), tumor necrosis factor-alpha (*TNF-α*), angiotensinogen (*AGT*), angiotensin II receptor 1 (*AGTR1*), and platelet-activating factor acetylhydrolase (*PLA2G7*) have also been associated with the severity of the cardiac hypertrophy. Finally, the environment contributes to the phenotypic expression of HCM. The not-uncommon finding of HCM in young competitive athletes who succumb to SCD suggests intense physical exertion may worsen the cardiac phenotype. Moreover, the absence of hypertrophy early on in life, the fact that hypertrophy often spares the low-pressure right ventricle, despite equal expression of mutant sarcomeric protein in both ventricles, and the attenuation of hypertrophy through pharmacologic intervention (at least in animal models) all serve to support the important contribution of the environment to the development of hypertrophy in HCM.

Unexplained cardiac hypertrophy, which clinically denotes HCM, also occurs in other settings, including metabolic disorders, mitochondrial diseases, and triplet repeat syndromes. Although the gross phenotype is similar, the pathogenesis and prognosis of hypertrophy caused by different classes of mutant proteins differ. Therefore, such conditions are considered *phenocopy* (diseases mimicking HCM). The prevalence of HCM phenocopy is not precisely known. Given the prevalence of each particular HCM phenocopy, it is expected that phenocopy accounts for approximately 5% to 10% of cases with the clinical diagnosis of HCM. The distinction between true HCM and HCM phenocopy is important as there may be specific treatments available for some phenocopies. A prototypic example of HCM phenocopy is Fabry's disease, an X-linked lysosomal storage disease. Fabry's disease is present in 1% to 3% of cases with the clinical diagnosis of HCM in the adult population. The phenotype results from deficiency of alpha-galactosidase A (α-Gal A). The deficiency of the enzyme results in deposits of glycosphingolipids in multiple organs, including the heart. Cardiac hypertrophy, which is often indistinguishable from true HCM, is associated with high QRS voltage, conduction defects, and cardiac arrhythmias. Fabry's disease is treatable by enzyme replacement.

【 】 DILATED CARDIOMYOPATHY

Dilated cardiomyopathy (DCM) is a primary disease of the myocardium manifested (see also Chap. 39) by dilatation of the left (and often right) ventricle and a decline in its contractility. It has a prevalence of 40 cases per 100,000 individuals and an incidence of 5 to 8 cases per 100,000 persons. Patients with DCM are often asymptomatic in the early stages but eventually develop symptoms and signs of heart failure and arrhythmia. A family history of DCM is present in approximately half of all index cases with idiopathic DCM; in the remainder, DCM is considered sporadic. Familial DCM is commonly inherited as an autosomal dominant disease, which clinically manifests during the third and fourth decades of life. Multiple causal genes for autosomal dominant DCM have been identified, including several that encode sarcomeric proteins, which are also implicated in HCM (see the previous section). Thus, despite the contrasting phenotypes of HCM and DCM, mutations in sarcomeric genes can cause either phenotype. Several other of the known causal genes for DCM encode myocyte cytoskeleton proteins (Table 45-3). The phenotype of DCM is determined not only by many heterogeneous causal mutations but also by modifier genes and environmental factors. Genetic studies to identify modifier genes for DCM are largely restricted to SNP-association studies (see Chapter 39).

Finally, DCM is often a feature of various genetic multiorgan disorders. Examples include X-linked muscular dystrophies (Duchenne and Becker muscular dystrophies, Emery–Dreifuss syndrome, and Barth syndrome); certain trinucleotide repeat syndromes (myotonic dystrophy, Friedreich ataxia); metabolic disorders (Pompe disease, Refsum disease); and mitochondrial diseases (Kearns–Sayre syndrome, primary L-carnitine deficiency).

【 】 RESTRICTIVE CARDIOMYOPATHY

Restrictive cardiomyopathy (RCM) is a heart-muscle disease characterized by severely enlarged atria as a result of elevated right and left ventricular filling pressures, normal or reduced ventricular volumes, and, usually, preserved global systolic function. The clinical manifestations are those of heart failure, often with predominance of right-sided signs and symptoms. The age of onset of the disease is variable, and the prognosis is relatively poor. RCM can occur because of systemic infiltrative disorders, such as amyloidosis and sarcoidosis, as well as storage diseases, such as Fabry's disease. Although such disorders are also genetic in etiology, RCM in such disorders is an indirect consequence, and not a primary myocardial abnormality.

Familial RCM with an autosomal dominant form of inheritance in conjunction with skeletal myopathy and atrioventricular conduction defects has been described. Two causal genes for RCM—*DES* encoding desmin and *TNNI3* encoding cardiac troponin I—have been identified. Desmin is an intermediary filament that is also involved in desminopathies involving skeletal muscles as well as the heart. Mutations in *TNNI3,* which are known to cause HCM and DCM, also cause RCM. RCM also occurs in patients with Noonan syndrome, which is caused by mutations in the protein tyrosine phosphatase, nonreceptor type II. The pathogenesis of RCM remains largely unknown.

【 】 ARRHYTHMOGENIC RIGHT VENTRICULAR
   CARDIOMYOPATHY

Arrhythmogenic right ventricular cardiomyopathy (ARVC) is an uncommon cardiomyopathy with characteristic pathologic and clinical features. The pathologic phenotype is characterized by gradual replacement of cardiac myocytes by adipocytes and fibrosis. The clinical phenotype comprises ventricular arrhythmias, primarily originating from the right ventricle, SCD and heart failure. ARVC is an important cause of SCD in apparently healthy individuals. In the U.S. population, it accounts for 3% to 4% of

TABLE 45-3

Causal Genes for Dilated Cardiomyopathy (DCM)

Gene	Symbol	Locus	Inheritance	Mutations/Frequency/Context
Sarcomeric/Cytoskeletal				
Cardiac α-actin	ACTC	15q11–14	AD	Missense/uncommon; also causes HCM
β-Myosin heavy chain	MYH7	14q11–13	AD	Missense/~5%; also causes HCM
Cardiac troponin T	TNNT2	1q32	AD	Missense/uncommon; also causes HCM
α-Tropomyosin	TPM1	15q22.1	AD	Missense/rare; also causes HCM
Cypher/ZASP: LIM domain binding 3	LDB3	10q22.3–q23.2	Sporadic and familial	
Titin	TTN	2q24.1	AD	Missense/uncommon; also causes HCM
Telethonin (T-cap)	TCAP	17q12		
Cytoskeletal				
α-Sarcoglycan	SGCA	17q21	AD	Limb–girdle muscular dystrophy
β-Sarcoglycan	SGCB	4q12	AD	
δ-Sarcoglycan	SGCD	5q33–34	AD AR	
Dystrophin	DMD	Xp21	X-linked	Duchenne and Becker Muscular dystrophy
Muscle LIM protein	MLP (CSRP3)	11q15.1	AD	Rare, founder effect in families described
Intermediary Filaments				
Desmin	DES	2q35	AD	Also causes RCM and desminopathies
αB-crystallin	CRYAB	11q35		Desminopathy
Nuclear Proteins				
Lamin A/C	LMNA	1q21.2	AD	DCM, conduction defect, muscular dystrophy, lipodystrophy, insulin resistance
Emerin	EMD	Xq28	X-linked	Emery–Dreifuss syndrome
Vinculin	VCL	10q22.1–q23	Sporadic	Metavincluin isoform
Cell Junction Molecules				
Desmoplakin	DSP	6p23–25 10q21–23	AR AD	Also causes ARVC

TABLE 45-3

Causal Genes for Dilated Cardiomyopathy (DCM) *(Continued)*

Gene	Symbol	Locus	Inheritance	Mutations/Frequency/Context
Unknown				
Taffazin (G4.5)	*TAZ*	Xq28	X-linked	Barth syndrome
		1q32		
		2q14–22		
		2q31		
		3p22–25		
		6q23–24		
		9q13–22		
		10q21–23	AD	
		7p12.1–		
		7q21		

ARVC, arrhythmogenic right ventricular cardiomyopathy; AD, autosomal dominant; AR, autosomal recessive; DCM, dilated cardiomyopathy; HCM, hypertrophic cardiomyopathy; RCM, restrictive cardiomyopathy.

SCD associated with physical activity in young athletes. In some reports, ARVC was found in up to 25% of the cases of nontraumatic SCD.

ARVC is a genetic disease that is estimated to be familial in approximately 30% to 50% of the cases. The most common mode of inheritance is autosomal dominant. Recessive forms in conjunction with keratoderma and woolly hair (Naxos disease) or with predominant involvement of the left ventricle (Carvajal syndrome) also have been described and referred to as *cardiocutaneous syndrome*. The genetic basis of ARVC is partially known. Chromosomal loci have been mapped (Table 45-4). Mutations in *PKP2*, which encodes for plakophilin 2, appear to be the most common causes of ARVC, accounting for approximately 20% of the cases. Mutations in *DSG2* and *DSP*, which encode for desmoglein 2 and desmoplakin, respectively, each account for approximately 10% to 15% of the cases of ARVC. The molecular pathogenesis of ARVC is unknown.

GENETIC DISEASES OF CARDIAC RHYTHM AND CONDUCTION

Cardiac rhythm and conduction abnormalities can occur as the primary phenotypes of genetic disorders that affect ion channels and their regulators (see Table 45-5). Several of these are reviewed below.

【 】 BRUGADA SYNDROME AND ITS VARIANTS

Brugada syndrome is characterized by syncope or SCD in the setting of a structurally normal heart and a distinctive ECG pattern consisting of *ST-segment elevation in V_1 to V_3, usually with a right bundle-branch block*. Episodes of syncope and sudden death are caused by fast polymorphic ventricular tachycardia or ventricular fibrillation. Brugada

TABLE 45-4

Chromosomal Loci and Causal Genes for Arrhythmogenic Right Ventricular Dysplasia

	Chromosome	Symbol	Protein	Function
ARVC1	14q24.3	TGFβ3	Transforming growth factor-beta-3	Mitotic and trophic factor
ARVC2[a]	14q42.2–q43	RYR2	Ryanodine receptor 2	Calcium channel
ARVC3	1q12-q22			
ARVC4	2q32.1			
ARVD5	3p23			
ARVD6	10p12–p14			
ARVD7	10q22			
ARVC8	6p24	DSP	Desmoplakin	Desmosomes
ARVC9	12p11	PKP2	Plakophilin 2	Desmosomes
	18q12.1	DSG2	Desmoglein 2	Desmosomes
Naxos disease	17q21	JUP	Plakoglobin	Desmosomes

[a]Phenocopy. RYR2 mutations cause catecholaminergic polymorphic ventricular tachycardia and not true arrhythmogenic right ventricular cardiomyopathy.

syndrome often manifests in subjects in the third or fourth decades of life, and occasionally in infants as SIDS. Recent studies suggest sudden unexpected death syndrome (SUDS), which is prevalent in Southeast Asia, is a form of Brugada syndrome. Death often occurs at night and more commonly in male subjects (male-to-female ratio is 10:1). Electrocardiographically, the disease is identical to Brugada syndrome.

In 1998, SCN5A, the cardiac sodium channel gene, was identified as the first, and thus far the only, causal gene for Brugada syndrome. More than 60 different mutations in SCN5A have been identified that collectively account for approximately 25% of all cases with Brugada syndrome. As in many other genetic disorders, Brugada syndrome also exhibits locus heterogeneity, and a second locus on chromosome 3 has been mapped; however, the causal gene has not yet been identified. Biophysical characterization of mutations in SCN5A suggests that mutations decrease the sodium current availability by two main mechanisms: decreased expression of the mutant channel or acceleration of inactivation of the channel.

Mutations of SCN5A can lead to a large spectrum of phenotypes, including Brugada syndrome, LQT3, isolated progressive cardiac conduction defect, idiopathic ventricular fibrillation, atrial standstill, and SUDS. The phenotypes are all considered allelic variants.

【 】 LONG QT SYNDROME

Long QT syndrome (LQTS) is a disease of ventricular repolarization identified by the prolongation of the QT interval on ECG. Clinical manifestations include syncopal episodes and SCD due to polymorphic ventricular tachycardia (torsades de pointes) and ventricular fibrillation. LQTS is either acquired or congenital. Two patterns of inheritance have been described in the congenital LQT syndrome: (1) autosomal dominant disease, described by Romano and Ward, which is more common; and (2) autosomal recessive disease, described by Jervell and Lange Nielsen, which is associated with deafness.

TABLE 45-5

Genetic Disorders Causing Cardiac Arrhythmias in the Absence of Structural Heart Disease (Primary Rhythm Disorders)

	Rhythm	Inheritance	Locus	Gene
Supraventricular				
Atrial fibrillation	AF	AD	10q22	—
		AD	11p15	*KCNQ1*
		AD	21q22	KCNE2
		AD	11q13	KCNE3
		AD	17q23	KCNJ2
		AD	12p13	KCNA5
		AD	1q21	*GJA5*
		AD	6q14–16	—
		AR	5p13	—
Atrial standstill	SND, AF	AD	3p21	*SCN5A*
Sick sinus syndrome	SND	AD	15q24	*HCN4*
		AR	3p21	*SCN5A*
Absent sinus rhythm	SND, AF	AD	—	—
WPW	AVRT	AD	—	—
Familial PJRT	AVRT	AD	—	—
Conduction Disorders				
PCCD	AVB	AD	19q13	—
			3p21	*SCN5A*
Ventricular				
LQT syndrome (RW)	TdP	AD		
LQT1			11p15	*KCNQ1*
LQT2			7q35	*HERG*
LQT3			3p21	*SCN5A*
LQT4			4q25	*ANKB*
LQT5			21q22	*minK*
LQT6			21q22	*MiRP1*
LQT7			17q23	*KCNJ2*
LQT8			12p13	*CACNA1C*
LQT syndrome (JLN)	TdP	AR	11p15	*KCNQ1*
			21q22	*minK*
SQT syndrome	VF	AD		
SQT1			7q35	*HERG*
SQT2			11p15	*KCNQ1*
SQT3			17q23	*KCNJ2*
Catecholaminergic PVT	VT	AD	1q42	*RYR2*
		AR	1p13–p11	*CASQ2*
Brugada syndrome	VT/VF	AD	3p21	*SCN5A*

AD, autosomal dominant; AF, atrial fibrillation; AR, autosomal recessive; AVB, atrioventricular block; AVRT, atrioventricular reentrant tachycardia; JLN, Jervell and Lange–Nielsen; LQT, long QT; PCCD, progressive cardiac conduction defect; PJRT, paroxysmal junctional reentrant tachycardia; RW, Romano–Ward; SND, sinus node dysfunction; TdP, torsade de pointes; VF, ventricular fibrillation; VT, ventricular tachycardia; WPW, Wolff–Parkinson–White syndrome.

Autosomal Dominant LQT Syndrome (Romano–Ward Syndrome)

The first locus for the autosomal dominant disease was mapped to chromosome 11 in 1991. Since then seven other loci have been mapped (see Table 45-5). Most genes identified encode proteins that make up potassium channels. *KCNQ1* and *mink* encode for the alpha- and beta-subunits of the slow-activating delayed rectifier potassium channel (I_{Ks}) and are mutated in LQT1 and 5, respectively. *HERG* and *MiRP1* encode for the alpha- and beta-subunits of the rapid-activating delayed rectifier potassium channel (I_{Kr}) and are mutated in LQT2 and 6, respectively. And *KCNJ2* encodes the inward rectifier potassium channel Kir2.1, defective in LQT7 (also known as Andersen syndrome). Mutations in all five of these genes cause decreased function in the corresponding potassium channels and consequently a prolongation in the action potential and in the QT interval. On the other hand, two forms of LQTS involve channels other than potassium. LQT3 is the result of mutations in *SCN5A*, the gene that encodes the cardiac sodium channel, and the same one implicated in Brugada syndrome (see previous section). However here, a gain-of-function mutation is at play resulting in delayed inactivation of the channel, as opposed to Brugada syndrome, in which inactivation is accelerated. Similarly, in LQT8, also known as Timothy syndrome, gain of function mutations in *CACNA1C*, the gene that encodes the (subunit of the L-type calcium channel, increase the inward calcium current and prolong action potential duration. Finally, one form of congenital LQTS is not caused by a mutation in a gene encoding a channel protein at all. LQT4 appears to be caused by a defect in *ANKB*, which encodes for ankyrin-B, a cell membrane anchoring protein.

Several genotype-phenotype correlation studies have been performed to identify the genetic determinants of triggering events, ECG phenotype, and response to therapy. These studies have predominantly focused on the three most common forms of LQT syndrome: LQT1, LQT2, and LQT3. In general, individuals with LQT1 exhibit symptoms during physical activity, such as swimming, and have a T wave of long duration on ECG. Individuals with LQT2 usually develop symptoms related to auditory stimuli and the T wave is small or notched. In contrast, subjects with LQT3 are symptomatic during sleep and the ECG shows a very late T wave with a prolonged ST segment. Mutations also carry prognostic significance, and in all three groups (LQT1, 2, and 3), there is a correlation between cardiac events and the QT interval. Although beta-blockers are considered the first line of therapy in patients with LQT1, they have not been shown to be beneficial in patients with LQT3, who have a slower heart rate. Preliminary data suggest LQT3 patients might benefit from Na^{1+} channel blockers, such as mexiletine, but long-term evidence is not yet available.

Autosomal Recessive LQT Syndrome (Jervell and Lange–Nielsen Syndrome)

The autosomal recessive forms of the LQT syndrome, which are also associated with sensorineuronal deafness, have been linked to mutations in the genes encoding I_{Ks} current, namely *KVLQT1* and *mink*. For the LQT phenotype to express, the patients must inherit a mutation from both parents. Consequently, it is less common than the Romano–Ward syndrome but is associated with a longer QT interval and a more malignant course. The phenotype could also arise in recessive forms when different mutations in the same gene are inherited from the parents (compound heterozygote).

【 】 SHORT QT SYNDROME

The short QT syndrome is a newly described disease characterized by the presence of shortening of the QT interval on ECG and clinically by episodes of syncope, paroxysmal atrial fibrillation and/or life-threatening cardiac arrhythmias. Short QT syndrome usually affects young individuals with no structural heart disease. It may be present in sporadic cases as well as in families. It was originally described in 2000. In 2003, a link was established between the short QT syndrome and familial sudden death with the first clinical report of two families with short QT syndrome and a high incidence of SCD. Three genes, all encoding for potassium channels, have thus far been discovered: *KCNH2, KCNQ1* and *KCNJ2* (see Table 45-5). Biophysical analyses have demonstrated that mutations in each of these genes that cause short QT syndrome result in channel "gain of function" and consequently shortening of the action potential.

【 】 PROGRESSIVE FAMILIAL HEART BLOCK

Familial heart block is an autosomal dominant disease of the cardiac conduction system characterized by development of bundle-branch block and gradual progression to complete heart block. Two forms have been recognized: in type I, the onset is early and the disease is rapidly progressive; in type II, the onset is later in life and the QRS complex is often narrow and AV nodal block predominates. Clinical features of the disease include syncope, SCD, and Stokes–Adams attacks. A locus has been identified in chromosome 19q13, but the gene has not yet been identified. Mutations in *SCN5A* have been identified in some families with familial heart block. In addition, AV block in conjunction with congenital heart disease such as ASD (NKX2.5 mutations) as well as DCM (lamin A/C mutations) have been described.

【 】 CATECHOLAMINERGIC POLYMORPHIC VENTRICULAR TACHYCARDIA

Catecholaminergic polymorphic ventricular tachycardia (CPVT) is an autosomal-dominant inherited disease with a mortality rate of approximately 30% by the age of 30 years. Phenotypically, it is characterized by runs of bidirectional and polymorphic ventricular tachycardia in response to vigorous exercise in the absence of evidence of structural myocardial disease. CPVT is caused by mutations in ryanodine receptors (*RYR2* on 1q42), calcium-activated calcium channels responsible for the release of this ion from the sarcoplasmic reticulum. A recessive form of familial polymorphic ventricular tachycardia has also been described and mapped to 1p13.3-p11. Mutation screening identified a missense mutation in calsequestrin 2 (*CASQ2*) as responsible for the disease. CASQ2 is involved in the same pathway as RYR2 to control calcium release from the sarcoplasmic reticulum.

【 】 SICK SINUS SYNDROME

Sick sinus syndrome (SSS) is characterized by the occurrence of sinus bradycardia, sinus arrest and chronotropic incompetence. Sinus node dysfunction has been linked to loss of function mutations in *HCN4* and, in recessive form, to *SCN5A*. *HCN4* contributes to native f-channels in the sinoatrial node, the natural cardiac pacemaker region. In 2006, a loss of function defect in *HCN4* was also linked to familial sinus bradycardia. *SCN5A* encodes the cardiac sodium channel implicated in Brugada syndrome and LQT3 (see above).

【 】 FAMILIAL ATRIAL FIBRILLATION

Atria fibrillation (AF) in the absence of known causes of secondary AF may be a familial disorder. The mode of inheritance appears autosomal dominant. The first causal gene for familial AF was identified as the *KCNQ1*, also responsible for LQT1. The mutation for AF is a gain of function mutation, in contrast to the loss of function mutations observed in patients with LQT1. Links between *KCNE2, KCNE3, KCNJ2*, and *KCNA5* and AF have confirmed the role of mutations in channels responsible for potassium currents in the development of AF.

【 】 FAMILIAL WOLFF–PARKINSON–WHITE SYNDROME

Familial Wolff–Parkinson–White (WPW) syndrome is a rare syndrome with autosomal dominant mode of inheritance. It occurs in isolation or in conjunction with other disorders, such as HCM and Pompe disease. It is characterized by palpitations, syncope as a result of supraventricular arrhythmias and evidence of preexcitation on the resting ECG. The phenotype of WPW in conjunction with HCM and conduction defects was found in patients with mutations in *PRKAG2*, which encodes AMP-activated protein kinase.

GENETIC BASIS OF CARDIAC DISEASE IN CONNECTIVE TISSUE DISORDERS

Several connective tissue disorders have cardiovascular manifestations. Marfan's and Ehlers–Danlos syndromes are reviewed below (see also Chapters 50 and 54).

【 】 MARFAN'S SYNDROME

Marfan's syndrome is a primary disorder of connective tissue with an estimated incidence of 1 per 5,000 population. It is characterized by increased height, disproportionately long limbs and digits, increased joint laxity, and lens dislocation or subluxation. Cardiovascular manifestations include progressive dilatation of the aortic root, aortic aneurysm and dissection, and aortic and mitral valve prolapse. The age of onset of the clinical manifestations of Marfan's syndrome is variable, but cardiac phenotypes commonly occur in the third or fourth decades. Aortic dissection is the leading cause of premature death in patients with Marfan's syndrome.

Marfan's syndrome is an autosomal dominant disease. The first causal gene to be identified is the *FBN1*, which is located on 15q15.23 and encodes fibrillin. Fibrillin is the major component of extracellular microfibrils in both elastic and nonelastic connective tissues. More than 600 nonrecurring unique mutations in *FBN1* have been described. Mutations are spread throughout most of the gene, and the frequency of each particular mutation is relatively low, thus making screening for mutations tedious. There is significant variability in the phenotypic expression of Marfan's syndrome, partly attributable to locus and allelic heterogeneity and partly to the effect of modifier genes and perhaps environmental factors. A phenocopy of Marfan's syndrome is congenital contractural arachnodactyly (CCA), characterized by severe kyphoscoliosis, generalized osteopenia, flexion contractures of the fingers, abnormally shaped ears, and, less frequently, mitral regurgitation and congenital heart disease. Recently, point mutations in the *FBN2* gene have been described as causes of contractural arachnodactyly.

The pathogenesis of Marfan's syndrome entails decreased expression levels of the fibrillin protein and reduced deposition of fibrillin in vascular adventitia, resulting in weakening of the adventitia and consequent aneurysm formation.

【 】 EHLERS–DANLOS SYNDROME

Ehlers–Danlos syndrome (EDS) is a relatively uncommon group of hereditary connective tissue disorders. There are six primary subtypes and several rarer variants; most are the result of defective collagen synthesis. Cardiovascular abnormalities are most common in EDS classic type (formerly EDS I and II) and EDS vascular type (formerly EDS IV). EDS classic type is caused by deficient types V and I collagen and is characterized by hyperextensible skin, joint hypermobility, mitral valve prolapse, and aortic dilatation. The disorder is transmitted in an autosomal dominant fashion through genes *COL5A1* on 9q34.2-q34.3, *COL5A2* on 2q31, and *COL1A1* on 17q21.3-22.1. Ehlers–Danlos type IV is considered the most malignant form of the disease because of proneness to spontaneous rupture of the bowel and large arteries (including coronary arteries and the aorta) and a high incidence of pregnancy-related complications. It is caused by mutations in *COL3A1*, which is located on 2q31 and encodes type III pro-collagen.

SUGGESTED READING

Farwell D, Gollob M. Electrical heart disease: genetic and molecular basis of cardiac arrhythmias in normal structural hearts. *Can J Cardiol.* 2007;23(suppl A):16A–22A.

Keren A, Syrris P, McKenna WJ. Hypertrophic cardiomyopathy: the genetic determinants of clinical disease expression. *Nat Clin Pract Cardiovasc Med.* 2008;5:158–168.

Marian AJ, Brugada R, Roberts R. Cardiovascular disease caused by genetic abnormalities. In: Fuster V, Walsh RA, O'Rourke RA, et al., eds. *Hurst's The Heart.* 12th ed. New York, NY: McGraw-Hill; 2008:1811–1854.

Roberts R. Principles of molecular cardiology. In: Fuster V, Walsh RA, O'Rourke RA, et al., eds. *Hurst's The Heart.* 12th ed. New York, NY: McGraw-Hill; 2008:110–122.

Roberts R, McNally E. Genetic basis for cardiovascular disease. In: Fuster V, Walsh RA, O'Rourke RA, et al., eds. *Hurst's The Heart.* 12th ed. New York, NY: McGraw-Hill; 2008:177–189.

CHAPTER (46)

Congenital Heart Disease in Adults

Jamil A. Aboulhosn and John S. Child

The incidence of moderate and severe forms of congenital heart disease (CHD) is 6 per 1,000 live births. Without early medical or surgical treatment, the majority of patients with complex CHD would not survive to adulthood. Surgical and medical advances have dramatically improved prognosis; more than 85% of patients with CHD survive to reach adulthood. Many adults with CHD may never require surgical intervention. The most common defects incidentally encountered in adulthood are:

1. Small ventricular septal defect (VSD)
2. Secundum atrial septal defect (ASD)
3. Mild/moderate pulmonary stenosis
4. Bicuspid aortic valve
5. Mitral valve prolapse

Adults with CHD usually present in one of three ways: (1) with a history of prior surgery (palliative or reparative) during childhood, (2) with a known cardiac lesion without prior intervention, or (3) with an unrecognized defect that is diagnosed in adulthood (Table 46-1). With the exception of simple ligation of a small patent ductus arteriosus early in life, there are generally no surgical/interventional cures, and all have certain potential sequelae and complications (Table 46-1). Cyanotic adults require special care and consideration. Cyanosis results from shunting of deoxygenated blood to the systemic circulation, either because of pulmonary stenosis (as in repaired tetralogy of Fallot) or as a result of suprasystemic pulmonary vascular resistance (Eisenmenger syndrome) (Table 46-2). All adults with unrepaired, palliated, or repaired CHD contend with certain medical considerations (Table 46-3). As the patient with CHD makes the transition from adolescence to adulthood it is imperative that the patient understand the nature and implications of his or her heart problem and what interventions have or need to be performed. Appropriate advice and guidance should be available regarding employment, insurance, socialization, contraception, and exercise (Table 46-4).

SELECTED LESIONS

【 】 ATRIAL SEPTAL DEFECT

Seventy-five percent of ASDs are ostium secundum defects; these are among the most common anomalies in adulthood. Twenty percent are ostium primum defects, and five percent are sinus venosus defects.

TABLE 46-1

Surgical Considerations in the Care of the Adult with Congenital Heart Disease

Type of procedure	May be palliative (e.g., systemic-to-pulmonary artery shunt) or reparative. Rarely curative.
Procedural sequelae	Certain procedures have known sequelae (e.g., transannular patch repair of tetralogy of Fallot with resultant severe pulmonary regurgitation) that over time may lead to heart failure or arrhythmias (RV failure, VT, SVT).
Durability of materials used in surgical repair	Valves/conduits have limited durability and may require multiple replacements throughout life. Close follow-up needed.
Sternal/thoracic reentry	Reoperation poses a higher risk than first operations. They are more risky when an extracardiac conduit or high-pressure ventricular chamber lies beneath the sternum.
Transplantation	Ultimate therapeutic option; however, stringent criteria for transplant listing may exclude some CHD patients (e.g. failing Fontan's patients with congestive hepatopathy). Higher rate of organ rejection in CHD patients who have had multiple blood transfusions during previous surgeries. Higher risk of perioperative bleeding in patients with previous sternotomies/thoracotomies.
Noncardiac surgery	Frequent cause of morbidity and mortality in the adult with congenital heart disease. High-risk patients benefit from special expertise, particularly with cardiac anesthesia.

RV, right ventricular; VT, ventricular tachycardia; SVT, supraventricular tachycardia.

Associated lesions must be ruled out (cleft mitral valve and inlet VSD in primum defect, anomalous pulmonary venous return in venosus defect) (Fig. 46-1).

Patients are frequently asymptomatic in early adulthood, presenting because of a murmur or abnormal electrocardiogram (ECG) or chest x-ray (CXR). Auscultation reveals fixed splitting of the second heart sound. Most eventually become symptomatic later in life related to chronic right ventricular (RV) volume overload, pulmonary hypertension, atrial arrhythmias, and rarely paradoxical embolization. Left ventricular (LV) diastolic dysfunction related to age and systemic hypertension may increase left to right shunt with age.

Typical ECG findings in secundum ASD include right axis deviation and incomplete right bundle-branch block (RBBB). Primum ASD presents with left axis deviation.

Management

Closure should be considered in symptomatic patients or asymptomatic patients with a shunt of any significance (Qp/Qs ≥ 1.5, where Qp is pulmonary blood flow and Qs is systemic blood flow) or with RV volume overload. Most have symptomatic improvement.

Transcatheter device closure is commonly used for secundum ASD. There is a very low risk of mortality with device or surgical closure. There is a shorter hospital stay and less morbidity with device closure compared to surgery.

TABLE 46-2

Issues in the Care of the Patient with Cyanotic Heart Disease

Erythrocytosis	This is a physiologic response to chronic hypoxia. Hyperviscosity symptoms may occur if Hgb $\geq$ 20 g/dL (headache, dizziness, fatigue), usually caused by dehydration. Hydration is the preferred initial treatment. Phlebotomy is rarely required.
Phlebotomy	Perform only if Hgb greater than 20 g/dL and there are symptoms of hyperviscosity. Remove 500 mL of whole blood at a time, and always replace with an equal amount of dextrose or saline.
Iron deficiency	Common and may be secondary to injudicious phlebotomies. Iron deficient microcytic red blood cells are less deformable, have decreased oxygen carrying capacity and increase blood viscosity, as well as increased risk of stroke.
Bleeding	Secondary to coagulation factor deficiency, thrombocytopenia and platelet dysfunction, and increased vascular permeability. Hemoptysis is common in those with severe pulmonary hypertension. Anticoagulants and antiplatelet agents are generally avoided unless definitely required for another indication (e.g., indwelling catheters or pacemaker leads in a patient with a right-to-left shunt and risk of thromboembolism).
Cardiovascular	Supraventricular arrhythmias in 50%. Ventricular arrhythmias in 15%. Right ventricular dysfunction and right heart failure may occur. Elevated left ventricular filling pressures are common and may be related to abnormal septal motion in those with right ventricular pressure overload. Systemic arterial atherosclerosis is generally absent but pulmonary arterial atherosclerosis is common. In situ pulmonary artery thrombi are common.
Other	Hyperuricemia with occasional gout, renal dysfunction, paradoxical embolization (use filters in all IV lines), cerebral abscesses, hemoptysis, kyphoscoliosis, infective endocarditis (high risk—all patients should be given prophylaxis for bacteremic procedures). Pregnancy ill-advised because of fetal risk and maternal risk (especially if severe pulmonary hypertension is present).

Surgery is needed in patients with other forms of ASD or those with anomalous pulmonary veins.

Closure of the ASD in adult life does not prevent atrial fibrillation.

【 】 VENTRICULAR SEPTAL DEFECT

There are four types of VSDs: perimembranous (most common), muscular (most common in infancy and childhood but the majority will spontaneously close), inlet (associated with primum ASD and cleft mitral valve), and outlet (Fig. 46-1).

Clinical Presentation

The spectrum of isolated VSDs encountered in the adult patient usually consists of:

1. Small restrictive defects or defects that have closed partially. The pulmonary vascular resistance is not significantly elevated and the left-to-right shunt magnitude is mild

TABLE 46-3

Medical Considerations in Adults with Congenital Heart Disease

Ventricular function	Certain CHD subtypes are at increased risk of progressive ventricular dysfunction (e.g., single ventricle physiology systemic RV or RV with pressure and/or volume overload). Benefits of established heart failure regimens in other cardiomyopathic diseases often guide medical treatment of CHD patients with ventricular dysfunction; however, there are limited prospective or randomized data to support the efficacy in CHD.
Arrhythmias	Arrhythmias are common and are the primary reason most well-repaired and stable adults with CHD seek emergent or urgent medical attention. Underlying hemodynamic problems should always be sought. Atrial arrhythmias are frequently not well tolerated and need to be aggressively treated. VT may be secondary to fibrosis, ventricular dilation, or reentry adjacent to a surgical scar. Sudden cardiac death risk is high in certain subgroups and AICDs may be needed; however, inappropriate shocks are a common problem.
Conduction disease	Intrinsic or postoperative sinus node disease and AV node dysfunction common. Pacing may require epicardial lead placement in certain situations. Multisite ventricular pacing is preferable in patients with low ejection fraction, dyssynchrony, or those requiring ventricular pacing secondary to heart block.
Endocarditis	Both operated and unoperated patients are at risk. Patients need meticulous dental, skin, and nail care. Antibiotic prophylaxis is important. American Heart Association guidelines from 2007 recommend antibiotic prophylaxis for bacteremic procedures in a small subset of patients (cyanotic CHD, prosthetic valve, recently implanted prosthetic material).
Pregnancy	As a rule, stenotic lesions, severe pulmonary hypertension and right-to-left shunts are tolerated poorly, whereas regurgitant lesions and left-to-right shunts do better. Patients need very close follow-up and should deliver in centers with appropriate expertise. Vaginal delivery with epidural anesthesia is usually preferable. Infective endocarditis prophylaxis in certain subsets. Discussion of CHD transmission risk to the fetus, genetic considerations, fetal echocardiography in most patients at 20–22 weeks gestation.
Contraception	Estrogen-containing regimens increase thromboembolic risk. Progesterone based regimens are preferable in patients at increased risk (Fontan's patients, right-to-left shunts).
Exercise	Exercise testing is a useful tool to assess fitness level, determine hemodynamic response to exercise, rule out exertion-induced tachyarrhythmias, evaluate chronotropic competence, and provide an exercise prescription. As a rule, heavy isometric exercise is contraindicated.

AICD, automatic implantable cardiac defibrillator; AV, atrioventricular; CHD, congenital heart disease; RV, right ventricle; VT, ventricular tachycardia.

TABLE 46-4

Nonmedical Considerations in Adults with Congenital Heart Disease

Employment	Most adults with CHD are and can be gainfully employed. Employers may discriminate against patients with known CHD due to misconceptions regarding health status, performance ability, and amount of sick leave required. The CHD specialist may need to be an advocate for the patient. Restrictions for employment do exist for certain jobs in which the safety of others is the direct responsibility of the patient with CHD. CHD specialist may need to estimate the risk of acute disability or sudden cardiac death in such patients.
Insurability	Adults with CHD have difficulty obtaining life insurance. In general, insurance policies are restrictive and patients with CHD are frequently insured at higher rates or not at all. Transition from adolescence to adulthood is difficult with cessation of health insurance under a parent's policy.
Psychosocial development	Psychosocial problems can occur in patients with CHD, manifesting in excessive psychological stress that is not related to the clinical severity of the original cardiac defect. Most patients are well adjusted but many may suffer from fear of isolation and low self-esteem; feelings that are compounded by exercise limitation, surgical scars, and parental overprotection. Psychosocial support is beneficial. Intellectual development may be impacted in complex forms of CHD.

$(Q_p/Q_s \geq 1.5:1)$. The intensity of the precordial holosystolic murmur is inversely related to the size of the defect; therefore a loud and harsh holosystolic murmur is present.

2. Large nonrestrictive defects in cyanotic patients who have developed the Eisenmenger complex, with systemic pulmonary vascular resistance and shunt reversal (right to left).

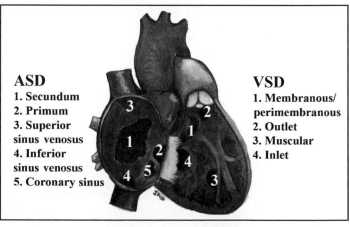

ASD
1. Secundum
2. Primum
3. Superior sinus venosus
4. Inferior sinus venosus
5. Coronary sinus

VSD
1. Membranous/perimembranous
2. Outlet
3. Muscular
4. Inlet

FIGURE 46-1. Types of atrial septal defects (ASDs) and ventricular septal defects (VSDs) in order of prevalence in adults with CHD.

3. Patients with moderately restrictive defects ($Q_p/Q_s \geq 1.6:1$ and $\leq 2:1$) who have not undergone closure. These patients often have mild to moderate pulmonary hypertension.

4. Patients who have had their defects closed in childhood. These patients may have VSD patch leaks.

Perimembranous or outlet defects may be associated with aortic regurgitation due to cusp prolapse.

Management

A small restrictive defect does not require surgical repair unless it is causing hemodynamically significant aortic regurgitation. Patients have a significant risk of endocarditis.

Larger defects may be repaired in the absence of severe pulmonary hypertension and severely elevated pulmonary vascular resistance (>10 Wood U/m^2), which incurs a high perioperative risk.

Transcatheter device occlusion of muscular and perimembranous VSD is feasible, and early trials demonstrate a good safety and efficacy profile.

Patients with pulmonary hypertension may derive symptomatic and functional benefits from pulmonary vasodilators—endothelin blockade (bosentan), phosphodiesterase 5 inhibition (sildenafil or tadalafil), and prostacyclin analogues.

【　】 ATRIOVENTRICULAR SEPTAL DEFECT

Atrioventricular septal defect (ASD) is an umbrella term for endocardial cushion defects representing a spectrum of lesions involving the atrial and ventricular septum, atrioventricular valves, and the LV outflow tract. Defects are classified into "partial" or "complete" forms. The "partial" form may be a primum ASD but no VSD. The "complete" form includes both a primum ASD and an inlet VSD. Deficiency of the inlet ventricular septum plus abnormalities of the atrioventricular valves (overriding, straddling, and/or cleft) commonly occur. Subaortic stenosis is a common association often caused by chordal attachments of the cleft anterior mitral valve to the LV outflow septum; it may also occur de novo following surgical repair. The diagnosis may be missed until adulthood, and patients have a presentation similar to that of secundum ASD, often with coexistent mitral regurgitation.

The typical ECG shows left axis deviation and incomplete RBBB. ASD is the most common cardiac lesion seen in Down syndrome. If a complete and nonrestrictive AVSD is not repaired early in childhood, it results in Eisenmenger physiology.

Management

The complete form requires early surgical repair (age < 6 months) to prevent pulmonary hypertension and pulmonary vascular disease.

Residual mitral regurgitation is common and frequently must be managed surgically.

In the partial form, the need for and timing of repair are dictated by the hemodynamic severity of the dominant lesion. Surgical closure of the defect is usually indicated, with repair of the mitral cleft if necessary.

【　】 TETRALOGY OF FALLOT

Tetralogy of Fallot is the most common cyanotic congenital heart malformation and one of the first complex lesions to be successfully repaired; it occurs in 7% to 10% of children with CHD. The four characteristic findings are (1) malaligned VSD, (2) RV outflow and/or pulmonary valve/artery stenosis or atresia, (3) dextroposed overriding aorta, and (4) RV hypertrophy.

Pentalogy of Fallot consists of additional ASD or patent foramen ovale.

Clinical Presentation

Most patients will have had palliation and/or intracardiac repair during childhood. Rarely, they present in adulthood without prior surgery (pulmonary outflow tract obstruction is mild in those patients with acyanotic or pink tetralogy of Fallot).

The type of surgical intervention predicts long-term complications. If the repair involved a pulmonary valvectomy or the use of a transannular patch, resultant severe pulmonary regurgitation is the rule. This is usually tolerated for one to two decades but ultimately leads to RV enlargement and dysfunction, tricuspid regurgitation, and supraventricular and ventricular arrhythmias.

Other important issues after repair include recurrent RV outflow tract obstruction, residual VSD, peripheral pulmonary stenosis, and the development of RV outflow tract aneurysm after patch outflow repair. Aortic root dilation is common and aortic valve regurgitation may occur.

There is an increased risk of ventricular arrhythmias and sudden cardiac death, especially in patients with elevated LV filling pressure, known or inducible ventricular tachycardia, prior ventriculotomy incision, severe pulmonary regurgitation, prior palliative shunt, and QRS duration ≥ 180 msec.

Management

Timing of pulmonary valve replacement is controversial but most experts agree that symptomatic patients, those with ventricular arrhythmias, and those with progressive RV enlargement and/or dysfunction, should undergo valve replacement.

Reoperation should be considered for a large residual VSD (Qp/Qs ≥ 1.5:1), significant residual RV outflow tract obstruction, large RV outflow tract aneurysm, or hemodynamically significant aortic regurgitation.

Placement of an implantable cardiac defibrillator is recommended in patients with clinical evidence of sustained or nonsustained ventricular tachycardia and those with inducible sustained ventricular tachycardia.

【 】 ISOLATED PULMONARY STENOSIS

In the adult, this is usually due to a trileaflet pulmonary valve with fused commissures, less commonly due to a dysplastic valve as seen in Noonan's syndrome (webbed neck, hypertelorism, low-set ears, small chin, and deformed auricles). Subpulmonary infundibular stenosis is common. Survival to adulthood is common.

Management

Moderate stenosis is usually well tolerated. Balloon valvuloplasty should be considered if the peak gradient is ≥ 40 mm Hg. Regression of subpulmonary infundibular stenosis is the norm following valvuloplasty.

【 】 LEFT VENTRICULAR OUTFLOW TRACT OBSTRUCTION

Clinical Presentation

Obstruction may be valvular (usually bicuspid valve), subvalvular (discrete membrane, more diffuse tunnel, or mitral chordal attachments), or supravalvular (i.e., William's syndrome). Multilevel obstruction is common. Common associations include parachute mitral valve and aortic coarctation (Shone complex). VSD is also commonly associated. Aortic regurgitation is commonly associated with valvular and subvalvular forms. Medial abnormalities of the ascending aorta commonly result in dilation and may lead to dissection.

Management

The development of symptoms (angina, dyspnea, or syncope) mandates intervention in aortic valve stenosis. In asymptomatic patients, intervention may be considered if the stenosis is severe. Surgical valvotomy and transcatheter balloon valvuloplasty can relieve obstruction in young patients with mobile and minimally calcified valves with a risk of resultant regurgitation. Valve replacement may be necessary for valves unsuitable for valvotomy, and various prostheses are available (mechanical, bioprostheses, and Ross procedure). For subvalvular obstruction, surgical intervention may consist of membrane excision together with myotomy and myectomy. Multilevel obstruction may require a Konno procedure (aortic annulus enlargement, aortic valve replacement, and ventricular septal myotomy with patch enlargement). Supravalvular stenosis requires surgical excision with end-to-end anastomosis, aortoplasty, or graft placement.

【 】 COARCTATION OF THE AORTA

Clinical Presentation

In most unrepaired adults, the lesion consists of a discrete narrowing in the descending aorta just distal to the origin of the left subclavian artery. It is often discovered in asymptomatic patients who are found to have upper limb hypertension. A bicuspid valve occurs in up to 50% of patients. An associated aortopathy predisposes the aorta to aneurysm formation and dissection and to development of cerebral aneurysms. Death occurs from complications of hypertension, including stroke, aortic dissection, congestive heart failure, and premature coronary artery disease.

Management

Assessment of severity includes a combination of measuring upper and lower limb blood pressure, measuring blood pressure response to exercise, and estimating pressure gradients at rest and with exercise using Doppler echocardiography. Cross-sectional imaging modalities (magnetic resonance imaging [MRI] and computed tomography [CT]) are very useful in delineating anatomy and planning interventions.

Intervention may be considered if the peak gradient across the coarctation is ≥ 20 mm Hg. Surgical repair is well established, with a low complication rate. Techniques include end-to-end anastomosis, patch grafting, and the use of a subclavian flap (Fig. 46-2).

Percutaneous balloon angioplasty with stenting for primary and recurrent coarctation is an attractive option in selected patients. Stent implantation is preferable to angioplasty alone.

Patients with successfully treated coarctation often continue to have systemic arterial hypertension despite the absence of significant residual coarctation. Late repair (> 14 years of age) is associated with higher rates of hypertension and decreased survival.

【 】 TRANSPOSITION OF THE GREAT ARTERIES

In complete transposition of the great arteries, or d-TGA, the aorta arises from the RV, and the pulmonary artery arises from the LV (ventriculoarterial discordance). This causes deoxygenated systemic venous flow to be directed to the aorta and pulmonary venous flow directed to the lungs. Survival to adulthood without intervention is rare. Frequent associations include VSD, LV outflow tract obstruction, and coronary anomalies.

Creation or enlargement of an existing ASD by transcatheter balloon septostomy or surgical septectomy in the infant with d-TGA allows enough left-to-right shunting of oxygenated blood to keep the patient alive.

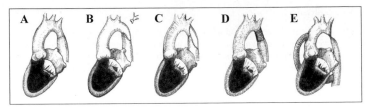

FIGURE 46-2. Types of surgical repair of coarctation of the aorta. **A.** End-to-end anastamosis. **B.** Subclavian flap. **C.** Patch aortoplasty. **D.** Interposition graft. **E.** Bypass graft from ascending to descending aorta.

The early corrective surgical approach consisted of atrial switch, which redirected atrial flow through the creation of a baffle, so that systemic venous blood was diverted to the LV and pulmonary venous flow to the RV (Mustard and Senning operations; Fig. 46-3).

Given all of the above intermediate/long-term complications of the atrial switch operation, since the early 1980s, the surgical approach has consisted of anatomic repair by reconnecting the aorta to the LV and the pulmonary artery to the RV, and coronary artery reimplantation (arterial switch).

Late Results

Mustard and Senning patients need close follow-up. Long-term survival is > 80%; however, over 50% of patients will develop sinus node dysfunction, arrhythmias, baffle-related problems, valve regurgitation, or RV failure.

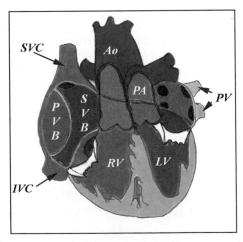

FIGURE 46-3. D-Transposition of the great arteries status-post atrial switch procedure (Senning or Mustard) characterized by "baffling" of deoxygenated blood from the superior vena cava (SVC) and inferior vena cava (IVC) via a systemic venous baffle (SVB) to the left ventricle (LV) and thereafter to the pulmonary artery (PA). Oxygenated blood returns to the heart via pulmonary veins (PV) and is "baffled" via a pulmonary venous baffle (PVB) to the right ventricle (RV), which serves as the systemic ventricle and pumps into an anteriorly dextraposed aorta (Ao).

Long-term results in adults with arterial switch appear promising. Long-term problems include coronary kinking and ischemia, neo-aortic valve regurgitation, and neo-aortic and neo-pulmonary artery aneurysms or stenoses.

【 】 CONGENITALLY CORRECTED TRANSPOSITION OF THE GREAT ARTERIES

In this anomaly (L-TGA), the aorta arises from the RV and the pulmonary artery arises from the LV (ventriculoarterial discordance). In addition, the left atrium enters the RV and the right atrium enters the LV (atrioventricular discordance). From a circulatory oxygenation standpoint, these patients are "congenitally corrected." The pulmonary and systemic circulations run in series, not in parallel as with d-TGA. There is ventricular inversion and the respective atrioventricular valves follow the ventricles. The morphologic RV, however, still functions as a systemic ventricle.

Fewer than 10% of patients are free of associated abnormalities, which include VSD (membranous or muscular) in up to 80%, pulmonic stenosis (valvar or subvalvar) in up to 70%, and tricuspid valve abnormalities (usually Ebstein) in 33%.

Patients are frequently diagnosed in adulthood, when they present with heart block or exercise intolerance secondary to systemic AV valve regurgitation.

Management

The conduction system is intrinsically abnormal in this condition and progressive heart block is common. Patients frequently require pacing. Significant systemic (tricuspid) AV valve regurgitation requires replacement with a prosthesis before ventricular dysfunction occurs. Since the RV is a systemic ventricle and is frequently abnormal, patients may benefit from heart failure therapies but no prospective randomized data support this.

【 】 EBSTEIN'S ANOMALY OF THE TRICUSPID VALVE

Clinical Presentation

The Ebstein anomaly is characterized by apical displacement of the septal leaflet of the tricuspid valve into the RV cavity. The RV is divided into a proximal "atrialized" portion and a distal "functional" portion. The effective volume of the functional RV is often small. The anterior leaflet is usually excessively long and may have attachments to the RV free wall. The "atrialized" portion of the RV is usually thin because of congenital absence of myocardium. The effective right atrium (+ atrialized RV) is invariably large and becomes more so in the presence of tricuspid regurgitation, which is a very common occurrence. An ASD or patent foramen ovale is present in more than one-third of cases. Other associated lesions include pulmonary stenosis, VSD, and patent ductus arteriosus. Twenty-five percent of patients have one or more accessory pathways with ventricular preexcitation (usually right-sided). Patients often present in adulthood with arrhythmias or exercise intolerance.

Management

If functionally mild, TR may not require intervention. Progressive RV dysfunction, impaired functional capacity, right-to-left shunting, and/or paradoxical embolization require surgical intervention.

If a large, mobile anterior leaflet is present, the tricuspid valve may be repaired. Otherwise, a biological prosthesis is usually inserted. The ASD will also be closed, and any accessory pathways can be interrupted at the time of surgical repair.

In patients with severe RV dysfunction, a "one–and-a-half" ventricle repair may be useful. This consists of tricuspid valve repair or replacement along with a "Glenn" shunt (superior vena cava attached to right pulmonary artery) in order to offload the dysfunctional RV.

SUGGESTED READING

Aboulhosn J, Child JA. Congenital heart disease in adults. In: Fuster V, Alexander RW, O'Rourke RA, et al., eds. *Hurst's The Heart.* 12th ed. New York, NY: McGraw-Hill; 2007:1922–1943.

Ammash N, Connolly H, Abel M, et al. Noncardiac surgery in Eisenmenger syndrome. *J Am Coll Cardiol.* 1999;33:222–227.

Brickner ME, Hillis LD, Lange RA. Congenital heart disease in adults. First of two parts. *N Engl J Med.* 2000;342:256–263.

Brickner ME, Hillis LD, Lange RA. Congenital heart disease in adults. Second of two parts. *N Engl J Med.* 2000;342:334–342.

Canadian Cardiovascular Society. Consensus conference on adult congenital heart disease, Montreal, 1996.

CHAPTER (47)

Perioperative Evaluation of Patients with Known or Suspected Cardiovascular Disease Who Undergo Noncardiac Surgery

Michael J. Lim and Kim A. Eagle

Each year 50,000 patients suffer a perioperative myocardial infarction in the United States and more than half of the 40,000 perioperative deaths are caused by cardiac events. Most perioperative cardiac morbidity and mortality is related to myocardial ischemia, congestive heart failure, or arrhythmia. The aims of perioperative evaluation are twofold: first, to identify patients at increased risk of an adverse perioperative cardiac event; and second, to identify patients with a poor long-term prognosis due to cardiovascular disease who come to medical attention only because another noncardiac problem leads to noncardiac surgery.

CLINICAL DETERMINANTS OF PERIOPERATIVE CARDIOVASCULAR RISK

The majority of patients at increased risk of adverse perioperative cardiac events can be identified by performing a careful history, physical examination, and review of the resting 12-lead electrocardiogram (ECG). Current recommendations of the American College of Cardiology (ACC) and the American Heart Association (AHA) designate risk factors as belonging to three groups: major, intermediate, and minor (Table 47-1).

【 】 HISTORY

Risk factors recognized as predictive of increased perioperative risk include advanced age, poor functional capacity, and prior history of coronary artery disease, congestive heart failure, arrhythmia, valvular heart disease, diabetes mellitus, uncontrolled systemic hypertension, renal insufficiency, and stroke. Because most symptoms of cardiac disease are either associated exclusively with or exacerbated by increased physical activity, significant noncardiac limitations in physical capacity are associated with inherent problems in the ability to detect symptoms of underlying cardiac disease and thereby to diagnose it. Impaired conditioning, poor cardiac reserve, poor respiratory reserve, or a combination of these disorders results in a poor functional capacity and in a reduced ability to accommodate the cardiovascular stresses that may accompany noncardiac surgery.

【 】 PHYSICAL EXAMINATION

Systemic hypertension, elevated jugular venous pressure, pulmonary rales, the presence of a third heart sound, murmurs suggestive of significant valvular heart disease, and vascular bruits all may identify a patient as having a higher perioperative risk.

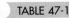

TABLE 47-1

Clinical Predictors of Increased Perioperative Cardiovascular Risk

Major Predictors

Acute or recent myocardial infarction[a] with evidence of ischemia based on symptoms or noninvasive testing
Unstable or severe[b] angina (Canadian class III or IV)
Decompensated heart failure
High-grade atrioventricular block
Symptomatic ventricular arrhythmias with underlying heart disease
Supraventricular arrthythmias with uncontrolled ventricular rate
Severe valvular heart disease

Intermediate Predictors

Mild angina pectoris (1 or 2)
Prior myocardial infarction by history or Q waves on ECG
Compensated or prior heart failure
Diabetes mellitus (particularly insulin-dependent)
Renal insufficiency (creatinine ≥2.0 mg/dL)

Minor Predictors

Advanced age
Abnormal ECG (left ventricular hypertrophy, left bundle-branch block, ST-T abnormalities)
Rhythm other than sinus (e.g., atrial fibrillation)
Low functional capacity (inability to climb one flight of stairs with a bag of groceries)
History of stroke
Uncontrolled systemic hypertension

[a]Recent myocardial infarction is defined as greater than 7 days but less than or equal to 1 month; acute myocardial infraction is within 7 days.
[b]May include stable angina in patients who are usually sedentary.

【 】 COMORBID DISEASES

Patients with diabetes mellitus, restrictive or obstructive pulmonary disease, renal dysfunction, and anemia all have an increased risk of concomitant cardiac complications during the perioperative period. Optimization of management and control of noncardiac conditions may therefore reduce the risk of cardiac morbidity in the perioperative period.

【 】 SURGERY-SPECIFIC RISKS

Emergency procedures are associated with a two- to fivefold increase in perioperative cardiac risk compared with elective procedures. Other types of noncardiac surgery associated with high perioperative risk include aortic and peripheral vascular surgery and prolonged abdominal, thoracic, or head and neck procedures with large fluid shifts. The ACC/AHA task force report on perioperative cardiac evaluation stratifies noncardiac surgical procedures as high, intermediate, and low cardiac risk (Table 47-2). See also Chapter 59.

Perioperative anesthesia technique influences the patient's cardiac physiology and may affect the perioperative cardiac risk. Opioid based anesthesia generally does not affect cardiovascular function, although the commonly employed inhalational agents cause afterload reduction and decreased myocardial contractility. Hemodynamic affects

TABLE 47-2

Cardiac Risk Stratification for Different Types of Surgical Procedures

High Risk (reported cardiac risk[a] > 5%)

Emergency major operations, particularly in the elderly
Aortic, major vascular, and peripheral vascular surgery
Extensive operations with large volume shifts and/or blood loss

Intermediate Risk (reported cardiac risk < 5%)

Intraperitoneal and intrathoracic
Carotid endarterectomy
Head and neck surgery
Orthopedic
Prostate

Low Risk[b] (reported cardiac risk < 1%)

Endoscopic procedures
Superficial biopsy
Cataract
Breast surgery

[a]Combined incidence of cardiac death and nonfatal myocardial infarction.
[b]Does not generally require further preoperative cardiac testing.

are minimal when spinal anesthesia is used for infrainguinal procedures, whereas the higher dermatomal levels of spinal anesthesia required for abdominal procedures may be associated with significant hemodynamic effects, including hypotension and reflex tachycardia.

CLINICAL ASSESSMENT OF PERIOPERATIVE RISK

A general algorithm for use in determining the need for further cardiac testing prior to surgery is shown in Fig. 47-1.

【 】 PREOPERATIVE TESTING

Resting Left Ventricular Function

Unless recently defined, preoperative assessment of left ventricular systolic function should be performed among patients with poorly controlled congestive heart failure and should be considered among patients with prior congestive heart failure and among those with dyspnea of unknown cause.

Functional Testing and Risk of Coronary Artery Disease

Because clinical factors usually serve to identify patients at low or high risk of an adverse cardiac event after noncardiac surgery, preoperative stress testing typically has the greatest utility among patients at intermediate risk. An exercise ECG study allows assessment of functional capacity as well as evaluation for evidence of coronary artery disease based on ST-segment analysis and hemodynamics. Performance of exercise echocardiographic testing or exercise myocardial perfusion imaging should be considered in the presence of

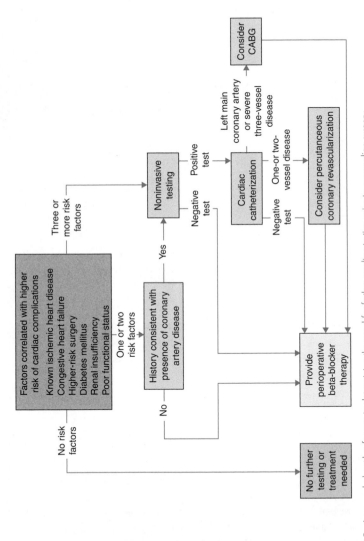

FIGURE 47-1. A general algorithm for use in determining the need for further cardiac testing prior to noncardiac surgery.

significant resting ECG abnormalities that preclude diagnostic testing for coronary artery disease, such as left bundle-branch block, left ventricular hypertrophy with strain, or digitalis effect.

Exercise Testing

Preoperative cardiac stress testing is useful in the objective assessment of functional capacity, to identify patients at risk of perioperative myocardial ischemia or cardiac arrhythmias, and to aid in the assessment of long-term as well as perioperative prognosis. In a general population, the mean sensitivity and specificity of exercise ST-T–wave ECG studies for the detection of coronary artery disease are 68% and 77%, respectively. The mortality rate was 5% per year or more among a high-risk subset, comprising 12% of the total population, who were able to achieve an exercise workload of less than Bruce stage I and had an abnormal exercise ECG. In contrast, mortality was less than 1% per year among a low-risk subset comprising 34% of the total population, who were able to achieve at least Bruce stage III with a normal exercise ECG response.

Nonexercise Stress Testing

Approximately 30% to 50% of patients undergoing noncardiac surgery are unable to achieve an adequate exercise workload for a diagnostic study. In these patients, pharmacologic stress testing for the detection of coronary artery disease can be performed using one of two general methods. Infusion of the adrenergic agonist dobutamine results in increases in heart rate, myocardial contractility, and to a lesser degree, blood pressure, resulting in increased myocardial oxygen demand. In the setting of a limited oxygen supply, increased demand causes myocardial ischemia, which is detected as a regional wall-motion abnormality on echocardiographic imaging. Alternatively, pharmacologic "stress" can be achieved using the coronary vasodilators dipyridamole or adenosine.

Although any abnormality on thallium scintigraphy is suggestive of coronary artery disease and is associated with a higher perioperative cardiac risk compared with patients who have normal scans, perioperative cardiac risk associated with a fixed perfusion defect is substantially lower than that associated with perfusion redistribution. In addition, the size of a perfusion defect is directly related to perioperative cardiac risk.

PREOPERATIVE THERAPY FOR CORONARY ARTERY DISEASE

【 】 CORONARY REVASCULARIZATION

There are no large prospective randomized trials testing the impact of either preoperative coronary artery bypass grafting or percutaneous transluminal coronary angioplasty on perioperative cardiac morbidity and mortality rates. However, several retrospective studies suggest that patients having undergone previous successful surgical coronary revascularization have a low risk of perioperative cardiac events during noncardiac surgery. The risk of death is comparable to that found among patients without clinical indications suggestive of coronary artery disease. The Bypass Angioplasty Revascularization Investigation (BARI) trial investigated 1,049 patients undergoing noncardiac surgery and found a low incidence of myocardial infarction or death among patients having undergone either coronary artery bypass surgery or percutaneous angioplasty. The absence of any evident difference between groups suggests that the previous percutaneous coronary angioplasty confers a protection from perioperative cardiac events that is similar to that conferred by surgical revascularization. However, based on the limited data available, indications for percutaneous coronary angioplasty among patients undergoing preoperative evaluation should be considered the same as for the general population.

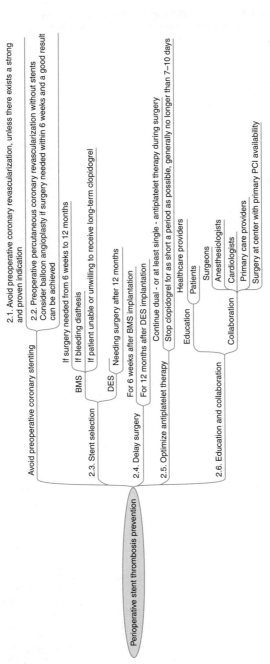

FIGURE 47-2. Perioperative strategy for the minimization of potential stent thrombosis. Reproduced with permission from Brilakis ES, Banerjee S, Berger PB, et al. Perioperative management of patients with coronary stents. *J Am Coll Cardiol.* 2007;49(22):2145-2150.

The optimal timing of noncardiac surgery has not been defined for those patients requiring percutaneous revascularization. Patients who have gone more than 6 months after percutaneous coronary angioplasty with no evidence of recurrent ischemia could be considered to have undergone successful revascularization, presumably with a low perioperative risk. Elective surgery within the first 28 days after the placement of a bare-metal stent has been associated with a high risk of catastrophic events attributed to potential stent thrombosis. The timing for surgery following the placment of a drug-eluting stent also remains unknown. Figure 47-2 represents a proposed strategy for minimization of stent thrombosis in patients undergoing surgical procedures.

【 】 MEDICAL THERAPY FOR CORONARY ARTERY DISEASE

Although data are lacking to support the empiric use of nitroglycerin or calcium-channel blockers, there is increasing evidence that the empiric use of perioperative beta-blockers reduces the risk of an adverse cardiac event in medium- and high-risk patients undergoing vascular surgery. When data from the prospective trials evaluating the use of perioperative beta-blockade are combined, 5 to 30 patients would need to be treated to prevent a single perioperative death. However, beta-blockers should be started preoperatively and carefully titrated upward to achieve a heart rate in the 60s and without hypotension.

MANAGEMENT OF SPECIFIC CONDITIONS

Patients with a variety of medical conditions known to increase cardiovascular risk may require noncardiac surgery. Factors that contribute to increased perioperative risk include interruptions in routine medical therapy as well as physical and mental stresses associated with the surgical procedure and convalescent period. It is important to note that the period of maximum cardiac risk appears to occur in the postoperative period. Because cardiovascular risk is not limited to the intraoperative period, appropriate emphasis should be placed on the treatment of specific conditions throughout all phases of the perioperative period.

SUGGESTED READING

Auerbach AD, Goldman L. Beta-blockers and reduction of cardiac events in noncardiac surgery. *JAMA*. 2002;287:1435–1444.

Boden WE, O'Rourke RA, Teo KK, et al. Optimal medical therapy with or without PCI for stable coronary disease. *N Eng J Med*. 2007;356:1503–1516.

Brilakis ES, Banerjee S, Berger PB. Perioperative management of patients with coronary stents. *J Am Coll Cardiol*. 2007;49:2145–2150.

Eagle KA, Rihal CS, Mickel MC, et al. Cardiac risk of noncardiac surgery: influence of coronary artery disease and type of surgery in 3368 operations. CASS Investigators and University of Michigan Heart Care Program. Coronary Artery Surgery Study. *Circulation*. 1997;96:1882–1887.

Fleisher LA, Beckman JA, Brown KA, et al. ACC/AHA 2007 guidelines on perioperative cardiovascular evaluation and care for noncardiac surgery: a report of the American College of Cardiology/American Heart Association Task Force on Practice Guidelines (Writing Committee to Revise the 2002 Guidelines on Perioperative Cardiovascular Evaluation for Noncardiac Surgery). *J Am Coll Cardiol*. 2007; 50:e159–e241.

Kaluza GL, Joseph J, Lee JR, et al. Catastrophic outcomes of noncardiac surgery soon after coronary stenting. *J Am Coll Cardiol*. 2000;35:1288–1294.

Mukherjee D, Eagle KA. Perioperative evaluation and management of patients with known or suspected cardiovascular disease who undergo noncardiac surgery. In: Fuster V, O' Rourke RA, Walsh RA, et al., eds. *Hurst's The Heart*. 12th ed. New York, NY: McGraw-Hill; 2008.

Poldermans D, Boersma E. Beta-blocker therapy in noncardiac surgery. *N Eng J Med*. 2005;353:412–414.

CHAPTER 48

Metabolic Syndrome, Obesity, and Diet

Stanley S. Wang, Sidney C. Smith, Jr.,
and Scott M. Grundy

Metabolic syndrome (MetS) is a multiplex risk factor for atherosclerotic cardiovascular disease (ASCVD) that involves atherogenic dyslipidemia, elevated blood pressure, dysglycemia, a prothrombotic state, and a proinflammatory state. The syndrome manifests clinically with hyperglycemia, hypertension, hypertriglyceridemia, reduced high-density lipoprotein cholesterol (HDL-C), and increased waist circumference (Table 48-1). The prevalence of MetS continues to increase in the United States owing in large part to an ongoing epidemic of obesity. Among U.S. adults, the mean waist circumference has increased continuously since the late 1980s with over one-half of the adult population having abdominal obesity by 2004. A 2005 population survey from the Centers for Disease Control and Prevention (CDC) found that 60.5% of U.S. adults were overweight (body mass index [BMI] of ≥ 25.0 kg/m²), 23.9% were obese (BMI ≥ 30.0 kg/m²), and 3.0% were extremely obese (BMI ≥ 40 kg/m²). Similar worrisome trends are being reported in U.S. adolescents and children as well. The associated increase in MetS is alarming because individuals with MetS have an approximate doubling of risk for ASCVD and approximately fourfold higher risk for developing type II diabetes mellitus (T2DM) compared to those without the syndrome.

LOW-DENSITY LIPOPROTEIN AND METABOLIC SYNDROME: PARTNERS IN ATHEROGENESIS

Atherosclerosis occurs through injury and response to injury. Low-density lipoprotein cholesterol (LDL-C) is the primary injurious agent. The response to injury is inflammation, a complicated molecular cascade that is exacerbated by various components of MetS. Hypertension enhances deposition of LDL-C and the expression, release, and effect of numerous inflammatory cytokines. Dysglycemia potentiates processes that lead to glycation and further inflammation. Lower HDL-C levels reduce the putatively anti-inflammatory impact of these molecules (although raising HDL-C with currently available pharmaceuticals, such as torcetrapib, has been linked to increased adverse outcomes). Additional evidence suggests that MetS increases circulating cytokines and promotes a prothrombotic state through a series of molecular effects.

OBESITY: THE DRIVING FORCE OF METABOLIC SYNDROME

The prevalence of MetS has risen in parallel with increasing obesity. The underlying process appears to relate to an inflammatory process generated by the release from adipose

TABLE 48-1

Criteria for Clinical Diagnosis of Metabolic Syndrome

Measure (any 3 of 5 Constitute Diagnosis of Metabolic Syndrome)	Categorical Cut Points
Elevated waist circumference[a,b]	≥ 102 cm in males
	≥ 88 cm in females
Elevated triglycerides	≥ 150 mg/dL (1.7 mmol/L)
	or
	Drug treatment for elevated triglyceride
Reduced HDL cholesterol	< 40 mg/dL (0.9 mmol/L) in males
	< 50 mg/dL (1.1 mmol/L) in females
	or
	Drug treatment for reduced HDL-C
Elevated blood pressure	≥ 130 mm Hg systolic blood pressure
	or
	≥ 85 mm Hg diastolic blood pressure
	or
	Antihypertensive drug treatment in a patient with a history of hypertension is an alternate indicator
Elevated fasting glucose	≥ 100 mg/dL
	or
	Drug treatment of elevated glucose

HDL, high-density lipoprotein; HDL-C, HDL cholesterol; in, inches.

[a]To measure waist circumference, locate the top of the right iliac crest. Place a measuring tape in a horizontal plane around the abdomen at the level of the iliac crest. Before reading the tape measure, ensure that the tape is snug, but does not compress the skin, and is parallel to the floor. The measurement is made at the end of a normal expiration.

[b]A lower waist circumference cut point (e.g., ≥ 94 cm [37 in] in men and ≥ 80 cm in women) appears to be appropriate for persons of Asian origin. Moreover, some persons of non-Asian origin with a marginally increased waist circumference (e.g., 94–102 [37–39 in] in men and 80–88 cm [31–35 in] in women) can have a strong genetic contribution to insulin resistance; they should benefit from changes in life habits, similarly to men with categorical increases in waist circumference.

tissue of biologically active products known as adipokines, including nonesterified fatty acids, tumor necrosis factor-alpha, and interleukin 6. The results include increased insulin resistance, a prothrombotic state, elevated cortisol levels, and greater inflammation.

ENDOGENOUS METABOLIC SUSCEPTIBILITY

Although obesity and adiposity are important in the development and propagation of MetS, not all patients with obesity develop MetS; endogenous metabolic susceptibility is required. Dysfunctional adipose tissue, including ectopic distribution of fat in the liver, muscle, and viscera, promotes insulin resistance, abdominal obesity, and MetS. Insulin resistance may also arise from genetic bases. Other potentially relevant endogenous endocrinologic relationships include polycystic ovary syndrome and cortisol dysregulation. Racial/ethnic differences in the expression of the clinical features of MetS also support a role for variable intrinsic susceptibility to MetS.

CLINICAL DIAGNOSIS OF METABOLIC SYNDROME AND PROGNOSTIC IMPLICATIONS

The diagnostic criteria for MetS were updated in 2005 by the American Heart Association (AHA) and the National Heart, Lung, and Blood Institute (NHLBI) (Table 48-1). Although MetS is associated with an almost twofold doubling of the risk of ASCVD, additional prognostication is based on current National Cholesterol Education Panel–Adult Treatment Panel III (ATP III) guidelines using Framingham risk scoring for coronary heart disease (CHD). The ATP III guidelines categorize patients into four levels of risk: high risk (10 year risk for CHD > 20%, including patients with clinically evident ASCVD or diabetes); moderately high risk (two or more risk factors with a 10 year risk of 10%–20%), moderate risk (2 or more risk factors with a 10 year risk of < 10%), and lower risk (0–1 risk factors with a 10 year risk of < 10%). Most patients with MetS can be considered to be at least at moderate risk, and many will have risk > 10%. However, MetS is only one part of overall risk assessment for ASCVD, and patients— including those without established ASCVD or T2DM—should undergo risk assessment under the Framingham risk scoring scheme.

MANAGEMENT OF UNDERLYING CAUSES OF METABOLIC SYNDROME

Overweight and obesity are major driving forces underlying the MetS, and are thus primary targets of therapy. The initial goal for these patients with MetS is to achieve a 10% annual reduction in body weight with an ultimate goal of achieving a BMI < 25 kg/m^2. Clinical guidelines, published by the NHLBI in 1998, recommend behavioral change including exercise and reduced caloric intake as first-line therapies to achieve weight loss.

Recommendations for dietary intervention should include a heart healthy diet, as consumption of foods rich in omega-3 fatty acids and fiber, including fish, fruits, vegetables, nuts, and whole grains; as well as reduction of intake of refined grains and saturated and trans-fats, which may result in reduction in inflammation.

A number of behavioral changes are recommended to promote long-term weight loss. These include the establishment of weight loss and physical activity goals and routines, avoidance of situations conducive to overeating, consuming regular meals and abstaining from snacks and binges, taking smaller portions, eating slowly, self-monitoring (e.g., with a diet diary), and developing a social support structure.

Current AHA/NHLBI recommendations for patients with MetS include 30 minutes daily of moderate intensity physical activity. Examples of recommended activities include brisk walking, jogging, swimming, biking, golfing, team sports, treadmill, exercise bicycling, and substitution of active leisure activities for sedentary ones (such as television and video game use). Longer and more vigorous exercise may confer additional benefit and risk reduction.

MANAGEMENT OF METABOLIC RISK FACTORS

Atherogenic dyslipidemia refers to lipid abnormalities that contribute to ASCVD. These include elevated LDL-C, triglyceride, and non-HDL-C levels, as well as reduced HDL-C levels. Goals for LDL levels are shown in Table 48-2, as well as goals for non-HDL levels (which are 30 mg/dL higher than those for LDL levels). The most established drug treatment for achieving eulipidemia is statin therapy. Numerous trials have shown beneficial effects of statins in subgroups with MetS, including the Air Force Coronary Atherosclerosis Prevention Study/Texas Coronary Atherosclerosis Prevention

Recommended Interventions for Metabolic Syndrome by Framingham Risk Category

Risk Factor 10-yr Risk for Coronary Heart Disease	Lower-to-Moderate Risk (<10%)	Moderately High Risk (10–20%)	High Risk (>20%)[a]
MetS as a whole	Reduce lifetime risk for ASCVD and diabetes	Reduce both lifetime and short-term risk	Reduce short-term risk
Obesity	10% reduction in body weight (preference to lifestyle therapy) → BMI < 25%	10% reduction in body weight (consider weight loss drugs) → BMI < 25%	10% reduction in body weight (consider weight loss drug) → BMI < 25%
Atherogenic diet	Maximal antiatherogenic diet	Maximal antiatherogenic diet	Maximal antiatherogenic diet
Physical inactivity	Exercise 30 min/d → 60 min/d	Exercise 30 min/d → 60 min/d	Exercise 30 min/d → 60 min/d
Atherogenic dyslipidemia: (↑ LDL cholesterol, ↑ non-HDL cholesterol)	LDL cholesterol (non-HDL cholesterol) < 130 (160) mg/dl → <100 (130) mg/dl (with lifestyle)	LDL cholesterol (non-HDL cholesterol) < 130 (160) mg/dl (with drugs if necessary) → <100 (130) mg/dl	LDL cholesterol (non-HDL cholesterol) < 100 (130) mg/dl → < 70 (100) mg/dl (in CHD patients)
Atherogenic dyslipidemia: HDL cholesterol	Raise HDL (lifestyle therapy)	Raise HDL (lifestyle therapy)	Raise HDL (consider drug therapy)
BP	BP < 140/90 mm Hg (with drugs if necessary) → 130/80 (with lifestyle therapies)	BP < 140/90 mm Hg (with drugs if necessary) → 130/80 (with lifestyle therapies)	BP < 140/90 mm Hg (with drugs if necessary) → 130/80 (with drugs in diabetes and chronic renal failure)
Elevated FBG (prediabetes)	FBG < 100 mg/dl (with lifestyle therapy)	FBG < 100 mg/dl (with lifestyle therapy)	FBG < 100 mg/dl (consider insulin sensitizer)
Elevated FBG (diabetes)	HbA1c 6–7%	HbA1c 6–7%	HbA1c 6–7%
Prothrombotic state	No drug	Consider antiplatelet drug[b]	Antiplatelet drug[b]
Proinflammatory state	Complete smoking cessation	Complete smoking cessation	Complete smoking cessation

BP, blood pressure; FBG, fasting blood glucose.

[a]High-risk patients include those ASCVD, diabetes, and those multiple risk factors and 10-yr risk for coronary heart disease greater than 20%.

[b]Antiplatelet drug: typically aspirin (81 mg).

Reproduced with permission from Grundy SM. Metabolic syndrome: a multiplex cardiovascular risk factor. J Clin Endocrinol Metab. 2007;92:399–404.

Study, West of Scotland Coronary Prevention Study, Scandinavian Simvastatin Survival Study, Heart Protection Study, Cholesterol and Recurrent Events Trial, Long-term Intervention with Pravastatin in Ischemic Disease, Anglo-Scandinavian Cardiac Outcomes Trial, and Treating to New Targets.

Alternative (or complementary) drug therapies include nicotinic acid and fibrates to lower triglyceride and raise HDL-C levels, and supportive studies with MetS subgroups (and drugs involved) include the Helsinki Heart Study (gemfibrozil), Veterans Affairs High-Density Lipoprotein Intervention Trial (gemfibrozil), Stockholm Study (clofibrate and nicotinic acid), Bezafibrate Infarction Prevention Study (bezafibrate), Fenofibrate Intervention and Event Lowering in Diabetes study (fenofibrate), and the Coronary Drug Project (nicotinic acid).

In patients at highest risk, including those with established ASCVD, the accepted goal LDL-C is < 100 mg/dL, but numerous trials have suggested that further LDL-C reductions may produce additional risk reduction, prompting the inclusion of an optional goal LDL-C of < 70 mg/dL in the 2006 AHA/American College of Cardiology secondary prevention guidelines. Combination therapy with additional agents may be needed to achieve this lower LDL-C goal as well as to increase HDL-C and reduce triglyceride (TG) levels. When employing combination therapies it is important to consider that although a lipid parameter such as LDL-C, HDL-C, or TG may be favorably altered, evidence of clinical benefit for a particular combination drug strategy should also be established through clinical trials to be certain of the beneficial effects of therapy. For example, an agent designed to raise HDL-C levels, torcetrapib, not only failed to reduce cardiovascular outcomes, but was associated with increased mortality.

Management of hypertension in MetS patients involves nuances that require special attention. Blood pressure levels ≥ 130/85 mm Hg are components of MetS. While the Seventh Report of the Joint National Committee (JNC 7) emphasizes lifestyle intervention as first-line therapy, first-line drug recommendations allow for a wide array of options, including diuretics and beta-blockers. However, because there is some evidence to suggest that high doses of these classes of drugs may increase insulin resistance and raise plasma glucose, many no longer recommend these drugs as first-line agents in patients with T2DM or MetS. Instead, some investigators feel that angiotensin-converting enzyme inhibitors (ACEIs) or angiotensin receptor blockers (ARBs) should be first-line agents in these patients. Regardless, in patients with MetS, the goal is to lower the blood pressure to < 140/90 mm Hg except in patient with renal dysfunction or T2DM, in which case the goal is more ambitious at < 130/80 mm Hg.

Therapy for dysglycemia begins with the lifestyle interventions discussed above, but frequently involves the addition of pharmaceutical agents. Metformin, an insulin sensitizer, has been shown to reduce plasma glucose and reduce progression from prediabetes to diabetes by approximately 40%. Thiazolidinediones (TZD), which are peroxisome proliferator-activated receptor (PPAR) gamma agonists, may provide additional reduction of plasma glucose and diabetes progression. However, troglitazone and rosiglitazone have been associated with liver toxicity and worsened cardiovascular outcomes, respectively, leaving pioglitazone as the only widely accepted TZD on the U.S. market. Target glycosylated hemoglobin (A1C) levels should be lower than 7%; the more intensive goal of 6.5% is controversial in light of preliminary reports from two studies suggesting lack of clinical benefit and possibly increased mortality.

Treatment of the prothrombotic state induced by MetS currently consists of aspirin, with additional antiplatelet therapies being reserved for specific clinical circumstances. Current AHA guidelines recommend primary prevention with aspirin in patients with a Framingham 10 year risk > 10%. Additional anti-inflammatory therapy may be considered in patients with objective evidence of inflammation, such as elevated high-sensitivity C-reactive protein levels, but at this time there is insufficient evidence to support recommendations beyond therapeutic lifestyle changes, although statins have shown promise in this clinical setting.

CONCLUSIONS

MetS encompasses many pathophysiologic processes that contribute to clinically significant ASCVD. Key factors include obesity with adipose tissue dysfunction, dysglycemia, atherogenic dyslipidemia, hypertension, and a prothrombotic and proinflammatory milieu. Although evidence regarding the pathophysiology of and therapeutic interventions for MetS is growing, so is the prevalence of the disease and its risk factors. Given the impending pandemic of MetS, further advances in the understanding and treatment of MetS will be critical in determining the fate of an increasingly large segment of the population.

SUGGESTED READINGS

AHA; ACC; National Heart, Lung, and Blood Institute, Smith SC Jr, Allen J, Blair SN, et al. AHA/ACC guidelines for secondary prevention for patients with coronary and other atherosclerotic vascular disease: 2006 update endorsed by the National Heart, Lung, and Blood Institute. *J Am Coll Cardiol.* 2006;47:2130–2139.

Deedwania P, Barter P, Carmena R, et al; Treating to New Targets Investigators. Reduction of low-density lipoprotein cholesterol in patients with coronary heart disease and metabolic syndrome: analysis of the Treating to New Targets study. *Lancet.* 2006;368:919–928.

Ford ES, Giles WH, Dietz WH. Prevalence of the metabolic syndrome among US adults: findings from the third National Health and Nutrition Examination Survey. *JAMA.* 2002;287:356–359.

Grundy SM. Metabolic syndrome: a multiplex cardiovascular risk factor. *J Clin Endocrinol Metab.* 2007;92:399–404.

Grundy SM. Metabolic syndrome pandemic. *Arterioscler Thromb Vasc Biol.* 2008;28(4):629–636.

Grundy SM, Cleeman JI, Daniels SR, et al. American Heart Association; National Heart, Lung, and Blood Institute. Diagnosis and management of the metabolic syndrome: an American Heart Association/National Heart, Lung, and Blood Institute Scientific Statement. *Circulation.* 2005;112:2735–2752.

Grundy SM, Cleeman JI, Merz CN, et al; Coordinating Committee of the National Cholesterol Education Program. Implications of recent clinical trials for the National Cholesterol Education Program Adult Treatment Panel III Guidelines. *J Am Coll Cardiol.* 2004;44:720–732.

Kong AP, Chan NN, Chan JC. The role of adipocytokines and neurohormonal dysregulation in metabolic syndrome. *Curr Diabetes Rev.* 2006;2:397–407.

Lincoff AM, Wolski K, Nicholls SJ, et al. Pioglitazone and risk of cardiovascular events in patients with type 2 diabetes mellitus: a meta-analysis of randomized trials. *JAMA.* 2007;298:1180–1188.

CHAPTER 49

Diabetes and Cardiovascular Disease

Marc A. Miller, Sammy Elmariah, and
Valentin Fuster

EPIDEMIOLOGY

Diabetes mellitus is a major threat to human health that has reached epidemic proportions. Currently, an estimated 240 million people worldwide are living with diabetes, a figure expected to rise to more than 350 million by the year 2030. Although the prevalence of diabetes is higher in developed countries than in developing countries, low-income and middle-income countries will be hit the hardest by the diabetes epidemic in the future.

The systemic consequences of diabetes are great as it leads to coronary artery disease (CHD), cardiomyopathy, peripheral artery disease, nephropathy, and retinopathy. In regards to atherosclerotic heart disease, diabetes accelerates the natural course of atherosclerosis, involves a greater number of coronary vessels with a more diffuse distribution of atherosclerotic lesions, and increases an affected individual's risk of plaque ulceration and thrombosis (Table 49-1). As such, diabetic patients are at a twofold to fourfold greater risk of cardiovascular disease (CVD) events compared to nondiabetics, and only by understanding the mechanisms underlying each risk will we be more likely to prevent them.

CLINICAL MANIFESTATIONS OF DIABETES

〖 〗 DYSGLYCEMIA

There is a highly significant association between hyperglycemia and adverse cardiovascular events. In the San Antonio Heart study of type 2 diabetics, there was a proportional increase in cardiovascular-related deaths with higher fasting blood glucose levels. Furthermore, for every 1% reduction in mean HbA1c, a measure of glycemia, there is a 14% reduction in the risk of MI and a greater than 20% reduction in the risk of diabetes-related death. Nevertheless, unlike the abundant evidence demonstrating that aggressive glucose lowering reduces microvascular complications, there is less robust data demonstrating a similar effect for reducing macrovascular complications. Postprandial hyperglycemia, in either the absence of fasting hyperglycemia or the presence of normal glucose tolerance, substantially increases an individual's risk for cardiovascular death.

〖 〗 DYSLIPIDEMIA

Lipid disorders constitute the cornerstones in cardiovascular management of diabetic patients. Many factors influence the lipid profile in these patients, including glycemic control, whether the diabetes is type 1 or type 2, and the presence of diabetic nephropathy.

TABLE 49-1

Clinical Evaluation of Risk Factors for the Development of Cardiovascular Disease in Diabetic Patients

Cigarette smoking
   Assess pack-years
Blood pressure
   Duration (if known), current and previous medications, assess presence of orthostatic hypertension
Serum lipids and lipoproteins
   Dietary habits, alcohol intake, amount of exercise and whether aerobic
   Family history of dyslipidemia, eruptive xanthoma, lipemia, retinalis, xanthelasma, thyroid function tests
   LDL, HDL, cholesterol, fasting triglycerides
Spot albumin/creatinine ratio (in micro- and macroalbuminuria)
   Serum creatinine
   Do not rely on dipstick protein, since negative results may reflect lack of sensitivity of test
Glycemic status
   Duration of diabetes; family history of diabetes; vascular, renal, and retinal complications
   Laboratory: FPG, hemoglobin A_1c q 3 months: Dx FPG > 126 × 2: impaired fasting glucose 110–126 × 2; when in doubt, have patient undergo 2-h oral glucose tolerance test

KEY: FPG = fasting blood glucose; HDL = high-density lipoprotein; LDL = low-density lipoprotein.

In type 1 diabetes mellitus, the major determinant of the lipid profile is the level of glycemic control. Low-density lipoprotein (LDL) is moderately increased, triglycerides are markedly increased, and high-density lipoprotein (HDL) is decreased when the level of glycemic control is impaired. For patients with type 2 diabetes, lipid abnormalities are related not only to hyperglycemia but also to the interplay of the insulin-resistant state. Patients with type 2 diabetes may have normal LDL levels, reduced HDL levels, and elevated levels of the very-low-density lipoprotein (VLDL) triglycerides moiety.

Although LDL levels in patients with controlled type 1 or type 2 diabetes may be normal, the atherogenic properties of LDL particles are increased. Glycosylation of the apoprotein B component of LDL, which occurs mainly in the LDL receptor-binding area, impairs LDL receptor-mediated uptake and therefore clearance of LDL. Furthermore, glycosylated LDL is more susceptible to oxidation, and glycoxidized LDL, the combined product of those two processes, is taken up more easily by macrophages and therefore more atherogenic than either glycosylated or oxidized LDL alone. Finally, type 2 diabetic patients have LDL particles that are small and rich with triglycerides but have little cholesterol in them (small, dense LDL), which increases the risk of CHD independent of the total LDL level, probably because of their increased susceptibility to oxidative modification.

Diabetic patients have elevated levels of VLDL as a result of a multiple factors, including increased hepatic de novo fatty acid synthesis, increased free fatty acid mobilization from extrahepatic tissues to the liver, and resistance to the inhibitory effects of insulin on VLDL production. Because the removal of VLDL by lipoprotein lipase is also affected, the level of VLDL triglyceride rises. Although elevated triglyceride levels appear to have a modest association with CHD in nondiabetic patients, there is a stronger association of hypertriglceridemia with increased risk for CHD in diabetic patients.

A low HDL level is a strong risk factor for the development of CHD in the diabetic patient. There is decreased production and increased catabolism of HDL in the diabetic patient. Decreased HDL production is a result of decreased lipoprotein lipase activity and a failure to efficiently catabolize VLDL. These effects culminate in reduced availability of surface components for HDL production. By contrast, increased catabolism of HDL results from the hypertriglyceridemia of diabetes, producing triglyceride-rich HDL_2 that is prone to catabolism by liver enzymes.

【　】 HYPERTENSION

The incidence of hypertension in patients with diabetes is approximately twofold higher than in age-matched subjects without the disease, and this "deadly duo" significantly increases the risk of micro- and macrovascular complications in diabetic patients. It is estimated that more than 10 million Americans have both diabetes and hypertension.

【　】 METABOLIC SYNDROME

The metabolic syndrome is a clustering of cardiovascular risk factors, of which the core components are obesity, insulin resistance, dyslipidemia, and hypertension. Multiple attempts have been made to define the metabolic syndrome, encompassing what each organization deems the relevant clusters (Table 49-2). The most widely used definitions come from the National Cholesterol Education Program Adult Treatment Panel (NCEP-ATP), the World Health Organization (WHO), and the International Diabetes Federation (IDF). The ATP III criteria require any three of the following five: a triglyceride level ≥ 150 mg/dL or receiving a triglyceride-lowering agent; HDL cholesterol < 40 mg/dL in men and < 50 mg/dL in women or receiving an HDL-raising agent; blood pressure ≥ 130/ ≥ 85 mm Hg or receiving antihypertensive therapy; fasting glucose ≥ 100 mg/dL; and a waist circumference in men > 40 in and in women > 35 in, with some variation for different ethnicities. The prevalence of metabolic syndrome, which varies according to which definition is used, is almost 24% in U.S. adult males.

There is a strong relationship between the metabolic syndrome and the development of diabetes, and individuals with the metabolic syndrome are at increased risk of cardiovascular events. The Strong Heart Study of Pima Indians showed that the presence of the metabolic syndrome increased the risk of developing type 2 diabetes 2.1-fold (ATP) and 3.6-fold (WHO). In the WOSCOPS study, which evaluated 5,974 nondiabetics, patients with 4 to 5 metabolic syndrome features had a 24.5-fold increased risk for the development of diabetes. Finally, the Air Force/Texas Coronary Atherosclerosis Prevention Study (AFCAPS/TexCAPS) confirmed a 1.5-fold increase in major adverse cardiovascular events in metabolic syndrome patients, while a meta-analysis of 37 studies, comprising more than 172, 000 individuals, demonstrated a significantly increased risk of cardiovascular events and death (RR 1.78) in people with the metabolic syndrome.

COMPLICATIONS OF DIABETES

【　】 MICROVASCULAR COMPLICATIONS

Renal

Nephropathy occurs in 40% of patients with type 1 and type 2 diabetes, and diabetic nephropathy is the single most common cause of end-stage renal disease in the United States. Risk factors include poor glycemic control and hypertension, while there is disproportionately higher risk in U.S. minority populations compared with whites. The earliest clinical finding of diabetic kidney disease is microalbuminuria, which may occur

TABLE 49-2

Proposed Diagnostic Criteria for the Metabolic Syndrome

Clinical Measure	WHO (1998)	EGIR	ATP III (2001)	AACE (2003)	IDF (2005)
Insulin Resistance	IGT, IFG, T2DM, or lowered insulin sensitivity[a] plus any two of the following	Plasma insulin > 75th percentile plus any two of the following	None, but any three of the following five features	IGT or IFG plus any of the following based on clinical judgment	None
Body Weight	Men: waist-to-hip ratio > 0.90; women: waist-to-hip ratio > 0.85; and/or BMI > 30 kg/m²	WC ≥ 94 cm in men or ≥ 80 cm in women	WC ≥ 102 cm in men or ≥ 88 cm in women[b]	BMI ≥ 25 kg/m²	Increased WC (population specific) plus any two of the following
Lipid	TG ≥ 150 mg/dL and/or HDL-C < 35 mg/dL in men or < 39 mg/dL in women	TG ≥ 150 mg/dL and/or HDL-C < 39 mg/dL in men or women	TG ≥ 150 mg/dL or HDL-C < 40 mg/dL or < 50 mg/dL in women	TG ≥ 150 mg/dL and HDL-C < 40 mg/dL in men or < 50 mg/dL in women	TG ≥ 150 mg/dL or on TG Rx or HDL-C < 40 mg/dL in men or < 50 mg/dL in women or on HDL-C Rx
Blood Pressure	≥ 140/90 mm Hg	≥ 140/90 mm Hg or on hypertensive Rx	≥ 130/85 mm Hg	> 130/85 mm Hg	≥ 130 mm Hg systolic or > 85 mm Hg diastolic or on hypertension Rx

Glucose	IGT, IFG, or T2DM	IGT or IFG (but not diabetes)	> 110 mg/dL (includes diabetes)[c]	IGT or IFG (but not diabetes)	≥ 100 mg/dL (includes diabetes)
Other	Microalbuminuria			Other features of insulin resistance[d]	

T2DM, type 2 diabetes mellitus; WC, waist circumference; BMI, body mass index; and TG, triglycerides. All other abbreviations as in text.

[a]Insulin sensitivity measured under hyperinsulinemic euglycemic conditions, glucose uptake below lowest quartile for background population under investigation.

[b]Some male patients can develop multiple metabolic risk factors when the waist circumference is only marginally increased (e.g., 94–102 cm [37–39 in]). Such patients may have a strong genetic contribution to insulin resistance. They should benefit from changes in lifestyle habits, similar to men with categorical increases in waist circumference.

[c]The 2001 definition identified fasting plasma glucose ≥110 mg/dL (6.1 mmol/L) as elevated. This was modified in 2004 to ≥100 mg/dL (5.6 mmol/L), n accordance with the American Diabetes Association's updated definition of IFG.

[d]Includes family history of type 2 diabetes mellitus, polycystic ovary syndrome, sedentary lifestyle, advancing age, and ethnic groups susceptible to type 2 diabetes mellitus.

Reproduced with permission from Grundy, SM, Cleeman JI, Daniels SR, et al. Dicgnosis and management of the metabolic syndrome: an American Heart Association/National Heart, ung, and Blood Institute Scientific Statement. *Circulation.* 2005;112(17):2735–2752.

at a time when histology is essentially normal. The Diabetes Control and Complications Trial (DCCT) and the UKPDS showed that the development and progression of microalbuminuria can be prevented through strict glycemic control, and while antihypertensive therapy can slow the progression of microalbuminuria to overt nephropathy (secondary prevention) in type 1 and 2 diabetes, there is less convincing evidence that it can prevent the development of microalbuminuria (primary prevention). Nevertheless, blood pressure should be maintained at < 130/80 mm Hg, and anigiotensin-converting enzyme (ACE) inhibitors are the preferred antihypertensive agents. In BENEDICT, a randomized trial of 1,209 patients with type 2 diabetes, hypertension, and normal urinary albumin excretion, trandolapril (either alone or with the addition of verapamil, but not verapamil alone) delayed the development of microalbuminuria. Currently, there is insufficient evidence to recommend ACE inhibitors in normotensive patients without microalbuminuria. Nonetheless, physicians should still recommend screening on at least a yearly basis, since the risk-to-benefit ratio of diagnosing microalbuminuria justifies treatment with an ACE inhibitor, if not for renal disease alone, then for reducing the incidence of myocardial infarction.

Ophthalmologic

Diabetic retinopathy is the most prevalent microvascular complication, affecting nearly 50% of the diabetic population at any given time and eventually occurring in all diabetic patients. Visual loss from diabetes occurs either as a result of proliferative retinopathy or macular edema.

【 】 MACROVASCULAR MANIFESTATIONS

Coronary Heart Disease

Diabetes is so strongly associated with CHD that it is considered a "CHD equivalent." CHD mortality in diabetic subjects without prior evidence of CHD is equal to that in nondiabetic subjects with a prior myocardial infarction. There is a two- to fourfold increase in the relative risk ratio of cardiovascular disease in type 2 diabetes patients compared to the general population, and cardiovascular disease is leading cause of death in patients with diabetes, responsible for more than half of all deaths.

The first detectable sign of a problem in people genetically prone to develop type 2 diabetes is insulin resistance, which can be seen up to 15 to 25 years before the onset of diabetes. Several atherogenic factors are associated with insulin resistance, which can start the atherosclerotic process years before clinical hyperglycemia ensues. Hyperglycemia itself also plays an important role in enhancing the progression of atherosclerosis in type 2 diabetes. The threshold above which hyperglycemia becomes atherogenic is not known, but may be in the range defined as impaired glucose tolerance (i.e., fasting plasma glucose level < 26 mg/dL, or 90-min plasma glucose concentrations > 200 mg/L and a 2-h plasma glucose level of 140 to 200 mg/dL during an oral glucose tolerance test). Population studies show that the degree of hyperglycemia increases the risk for CHD and cardiovascular events.

Acute Coronary Syndromes

Diabetic patients represent a high-risk group for developing and surviving acute myocardial infarction. In particular, diabetic patients treated with insulin have a worse outcome than do non–insulin-treated diabetics. Reperfusion therapy is the cornerstone of the management of acute myocardial infarction. In a meta-analysis of major thrombolytic trials, diabetic patients had a nonsignificant trend toward increased reductions in 35-day mortality rates compared with nondiabetic patients. The potential advantage of angioplasty over thrombolytic therapy has not been addressed in the diabetic population.

The most appropriate method to achieve, and the optimal intensity of, glucose control following myocardial infarction is unclear. The use of insulin and glucose infusion for at least 24 hours after admission, followed by intensive long-term insulin, was compared with usual care in the DIGAMI trial. A total of 620 diabetic patients were randomized, and the trial demonstrated a 30% reduction in mortality at 12 months for the group treated under the intensive program. However, the follow-up DIGAMI-2 trial, which compared three strategies—intensive insulin infusion followed by long-term insulin therapy, intensive insulin infusion followed by long-term standard glucose control, and regular metabolic control—in 1,253 diabetic patients with acute myocardial infarction was unable to show a difference in short- and long-term mortality between any of the arms. A post-hoc analysis of the DIGAMI-2 suggests that insulin therapy may actually be inferior to oral glucose-lowering medications, with the risk of nonfatal myocardial infarction and stroke increased by insulin treatment, whereas treatment with metformin appeared to be protective.

Chronic Coronary Heart Disease

The association between CHD and diabetes has led to screening strategies in diabetic patients even before they are symptomatic. In addition, diabetic patients often are unaware of myocardial ischemic pain, and so silent myocardial infarction and ischemia are markedly increased in this population. In one study of stress, single-photon emission computed tomography (SPECT) in asymptomatic patients with diabetes, abnormal SPECT imaging was present in 60% of patients, including 20% with high-risk features. There is even some evidence to suggest that revascularization, by means of coronary artery bypass surgery, improves survival in those asymptomatic diabetics with high-risk SPECT imaging. Therapeutic modalities in diabetic patients with CHD revolve around standard therapy with aspirin, beta-blockers, calcium-channel blockers, and nitrates.

Diabetic Cardiomyopathy

Diabetic cardiomyopathy is a term used by clinicians to encompass the multiple diabetes-related alterations in left ventricular function, either systolic and/or diastolic, independent of ischemic heart disease and hypertension. The Framingham Heart Study showed that in patients with diabetes who have congestive heart failure, men were twice as likely and women five times as likely as their nondiabetic counterparts to develop congestive heart failure. Furthermore, diabetes has a large adverse impact on survival in heart failure patients, independent of other established variables. Several mechanisms that have been proposed to explain the pathogenesis of diabetic cardiomyopathy include impaired calcium homeostasis, up-regulation of the renin–angiotensin system, increased oxidative stress, altered substrate metabolism, and mitochondrial dysfunction.

In addition to characteristic left ventricular systolic dysfunction of diabetic cardiomyopathy, diastolic abnormalities can occur in patients who have no known diabetic complications, and in fact, diastolic dysfunction frequently precedes the onset systolic dysfunction. The management of heart failure with preserved left ventricular systolic function usually includes beta-blockers and ACE inhibitors, but the evidence supporting these pharmacologic therapies is sparse.

Cerebrovascular Disease

Compared to nondiabetic subjects, the mortality from stroke in diabetic patients is almost threefold higher. The small paramedial penetrating arteries are the most common sites of cerebrovascular disease. In addition, diabetes increases the likelihood of severe carotid atherosclerosis, and diabetic patients are likely to suffer increased brain damage with carotid emboli that would result in transient ischemic attack in a nondiabetic individual.

MANAGEMENT OF DIABETES AND ITS COMPLICATIONS

【 】 THERAPEUTIC LIFESTYLE CHANGES

STENO-2 demonstrated that a comprehensive strategy, which included pharmacologic interventions and behavioral modification, to reduce cardiovascular risk in type 2 diabetic patients with microalbuminuria, was highly effective when compared to usual care. The number needed to treat to prevent a major cardiovascular event was only five patients. The approach—which included targets of HbA1c less than 6.5%, blood pressure of less than 130/80 mm Hg, total cholesterol less than 175 mg/dL, and triglycerides below 150 mg/dL—reduced the risk of cardiovascular and microvascular events by about 50%.

Weight loss is an important therapeutic strategy in all overweight or obese individuals who have type 2 diabetes. In the Finnish Diabetes Prevention Study, intensive lifestyle intervention, which included weight loss, in overweight patients with impaired glucose tolerance, substantially reduced the risk of diabetes by 58%; a beneficial effect that was sustained well after the direct intervention had ended. The primary approach for achieving weight loss, in the vast majority of cases, is therapeutic lifestyle change, which includes a reduction in caloric intake and an increase in physical activity. A moderate decrease in caloric balance (500–1000 kcal/d) will result in a slow but progressive weight loss (1–2 lb/wk). In selected patients, drug therapy to achieve weight loss as an adjunct to lifestyle change may be appropriate. Physical activity is an important component of a comprehensive weight-management program. Regular moderate-intensity physical activity enhances long-term weight maintenance. Initial physical activity recommendations should be based on the patient's willingness and ability, but gradually increases in the duration and frequency of exercise to 30 to 45 minutes of moderate aerobic activity, 3 to 5 days per week, should be recommended when possible.

In patients with severe/morbid obesity, surgical options, such as gastric bypass and gastroplasty, may be appropriate. The Swedish Obese Subjects (SOS) study, a prospective controlled study of 2,010 subjects who underwent bariatric surgery (surgery group) and 2,037 who received conventional treatment (matched control group), demonstrated that bariatric surgery reduced overall mortality and myocardial infarction. Nevertheless, the potential benefits of surgical interventions for weight loss should be weighed against the short- and long-term risks.

【 】 DYSGLYCEMIA MANAGEMENT

The medical community has progressively become more and more aggressive about risk factor modification. Multiple trials in cardiovascular prevention have shown that modification of traditional risk factors show more benefit than glycemic control. Practitioners, however, must realize that because of the importance of glycemic control in preventing microvascular complications, cardiologists have adopted measures to control blood glucose levels.

The American Heart Association (AHA) and the American Diabetes Association (ADA) recommend a HbA1c treatment target of < 7%, based on evidence that lowering A1c to 7% prevents the development and progression of microvascular complications. In both the United Kingdom Prospective Diabetes Study (UKPDS) and the Diabetes Control and Complications Trial (DCCT), intensively treated groups (HbA1c level of 7%) experienced significant reductions in microvascular complications, such as retinopathy and albuminuria, but failed to convincingly demonstrate a reduction in cardiovascular events. In PROactive, a large-scale, prospective, cardiovascular outcomes trial that randomized high-risk type 2 diabetic patients to either pioglitazone or placebo in addition to existing glucose-lowering and cardiovascular medications, there was a 16% risk reduction in favor of pioglitazone in the main secondary end point (the composite of all-cause mortality, nonfatal MI, and nonfatal stroke), but no difference in the primary end point. Nevertheless, in the DCCT/EDIC study of type 1 diabetics, and a meta-analysis of randomized trials of type 1 and 2 diabetics, glycemic control does appear to modestly reduce the incidence of cardiovascular events.

Many type 2 diabetic patients may require more than one antidiabetic agent. Most agents have been studied to measure efficacy as monotherapy and across the board demonstrate a 40% to 60% reduction in the plasma glucose level. The following discussion outlines the mechanisms, advantages, and disadvantages of each of these therapies as individual agents.

Insulin

Insulin is used in the management of type 1 diabetes mellitus (T1DM) or type 2 diabetes mellitus (T2DM) as monotherapy or in combination with oral agents. Insulins currently available differ in their rate of absorption and duration of action; there are also products that are mixtures of rapid short-acting and intermediate-acting insulins. There are three rapid-acting injectable insulins currently available—lispro, aspart, and glulisine—that are used to cover carbohydrates at mealtime to correct for an elevated glucose level, and in insulin pumps. The latest rapid-acting insulin is Exubera, which is inhaled and has an intermediate duration of action (387 minutes); it is faster than lispro and comparable to regular insulin. Neutral pH protamine Hagedorn (NPH) is an intermediate-acting insulin, which can be used to normalize fasting glucose and in combination with rapid-acting insulins during the daytime to provide primarily basal coverage. Insulin glargine and detemir are long-acting insulins that are used once or twice daily to provide broad coverage. The most physiologic way of administering insulin is to give a basal insulin once or twice daily, as well as a bolus of insulin prior to each meal based on carbohydrate counting and a correction factor to bring down the glucose down to premeal levels by 2 h after eating.

Metformin

Metformin decreases hepatic glucose output by inhibiting glucose-6-dehydrogenase activity and stimulating the insulin-induced component of glucose uptake into skeletal muscle and adipocytes. The starting dose for metformin is 500 mg orally with dinner for 1 week then 500 mg orally with breakfast and dinner. A sustained-release preparation is available that allows once-daily dosing. Because of its mechanism of action, there is minimal risk for hypoglycemia. The most common side effects are gastrointestinal—nausea, diarrhea, and abdominal pain—and a metallic taste. Lactic acidosis can also complicate metformin therapy in patients with potential hypoxic states, such as congestive heart failure and severe pulmonary disease, and in those with renal insufficiency. Consequently, caution should be exercised when prescribing metformin to those with impaired renal function (serum creatinine > 1.5 mg/dL in men and > 1.4 mg/dL in women) and the elderly (age > 80 years) unless normal glomerular filtration rate is documented. Regardless, the risk of lactic acidosis is low and is estimated to be 9 per 100,000 person-years. Metformin should be discontinued on the day patients receive an iodinated contrast material for radiographic studies, which can temporarily impair renal function, as well as prior to any surgical procedure. The metformin dose can be resumed 48 hours later if the serum creatinine is in the normal range. Metformin lowers the A1c by 1% to 2%.

Thiazolidinediones

Thiazolidinediones induce peroxisome proliferator-activated receptor (PPAR)-γ binding to nuclear receptors in muscle and adipocytes, allowing insulin-stimulated glucose transport. Three PPARs have been identified to date: PPARα, PPARδ (also known as PPARβ), and PPARγ. PPARα resides mainly in the liver, heart muscle, and vascular endothelium; when it is activated, it controls genes that regulate lipoprotein levels and confers anti-inflammatory effects. PPARδ is located mainly on adipocytes, but is also found in pancreatic cells, vascular endothelium, and macrophages.

Thiazolidinediones (TZDs) lower fasting and postprandial glucose levels, as well as free fatty acid levels, and on average decrease A1c levels by 1% to 1.5%. A first-generation TZD, troglitazone, is no longer available because of its hepatotoxicity. The second-generation TZDs, rosiglitazone and pioglitazone, may be used as monotherapy or in combination with insulin, sulfonylureas, or metformin, and have not been found to be hepatotoxic. TZDs are associated with weight gain caused by fluid retention and proliferation of adipose tissue. However, the TZDs increase fat in the subcutaneous adipose tissue and decrease visceral adipose tissue and fat in the liver. The dose for rosiglitazone is 2 to 8 mg/d; for pioglitazone, it is 15 to 45 mg/d. Two side effects to be noted are peripheral tissue edema and, less frequently, congestive heart failure. TZDs are contraindicated in patients with congestive heart failure and should be used cautiously in at-risk patients.

Sulfonylureas

Sulfonylureas, the oldest class of treatment for type 2 diabetes, act by stimulating beta-cell insulin secretion. The first-generation sulfonylureas have a long half-life and bind ionically to plasma proteins, making them easily displaced. The major concern with these agents is hypoglycemia. The second-generation sulfonylureas have a shorter half-life and bind to plasma proteins nonionically, making them less easily displaced from proteins and available for binding to receptors. Commercially available second-generation sulfonylureas are glyburide (1.25–20 mg/d), glipizide (2.5–40 mg/d), and glimepiride (1–8 mg/d). Sulfonylureas decrease the A1c by 1% to 2%.

Meglitinides

Repaglinide is a member of the meglitinide group of insulin secretagogues with a relatively short half-life of 3.7 h. The binding site on the beta-cell sulfonylurea receptor is distinct from the binding site for sulfonylureas. The drug is taken up to 30 min prior to each meal. Repaglinide is particularly useful in the elderly, patients with chronic renal insufficiency, and patients who are erratic eaters. The dose varies between 0.5 and 4 mg before meals. Repaglinide results in a 1% to 2% decrease in A1c.

Nateglinide, a derivative of phenylalanine, is structurally distinct from both sulfonylureas and repaglinide. It has a quicker onset and shorter duration of action than repaglinide. Nateglinide is available as 60- and 120-mg tablets, taken with each meal. It is effective for lowering postprandial glucose levels. Nateglinide results in a 0.5% to 1.0% decrease in A1c. As with repaglinide, the dose of nateglinide should be omitted if a meal is skipped.

Alpha-Glucosidase Inhibitors

These agents, which are not systemically absorbed, inhibit alpha-glucosidases in the brush border of the small intestine, delaying the absorption of complex carbohydrates. They are most effective in reducing postprandial blood glucose elevations and can be used as adjunctive therapy with other oral agents. The two available agents are acarbose, given 50 to 100 mg with meals, and miglitol, given 50 mg with meals. The side effects are flatulence and gastrointestinal discomfort. One study noted that the prophylactic use of acarbose delayed the development of type 2 diabetes in patients with impaired glucose tolerance. These medications result in a 0.5% to 1.0% decrease in A1c levels and may be useful as an adjunct to other oral hypoglycemic agents with high-carbohydrate meals.

Amylin

Synthetic human amylin, pramlintide, is available as an adjunctive treatment for patients who remain uncontrolled with type 1 or type 2 diabetes despite mealtime insulin use. Amylin is synthesized by pancreatic cells and cosecreted with insulin in response to food intake. Pramlintide has been shown to decrease glucose fluctuations, improve long-term glycemic control, reduce mealtime insulin requirements, and reduce body weight. Empiric reductions in mealtime insulin doses are recommended at the initiation of pramlintide therapy to decrease the risk of hypoglycemia. Pramlintide is available in vials, but not in pen devices thus far.

Incretins

The newest agents available for the treatment of T2DM belong to the class of incretin hormones. The first pharmacologic agent available in this class is the glucagon-like peptide-1 (GLP-1) analogue, exenatide. The two key incretins are GLP-1 and GIP, which are decreased in type 2 diabetes, and when given pharmacologically to animals, these hormones stimulate beta-cell proliferation and can prevent or delay the onset of diabetes. Exenatide (Byetta) is a synthetic peptide that is a GLP-1 agonist (incretin mimetic). It potentiates insulin secretion and decreases glucagons secretion postprandially and is approved as an adjunctive treatment for type 2 diabetics who have not achieved optimal glycemic control on metformin, a sulfonylurea, or both. It can cause nausea, diarrhea, and vomiting, especially when the drug is started and hypoglycemia when added to a sulfonylurea.

See Fig. 49-1 for management of type 2 diabetes.

【 】 DYSLIPIDEMIA MANAGEMENT

Medical therapy for hyperlipidemia is similar in diabetic and nondiabetic patients, but diabetic patients require special consideration.

The hypertriglyceridemia of diabetes can be treated effectively with fibric acid derivatives without an adverse effect on glucose metabolism. These drugs cause a 5% to 15% drop in LDL levels in patients with normal triglyceride levels, but in patients with hypertriglyceridemia, LDL levels go up. This elevation probably is caused by the catabolism of the atherogenic LDL particle, resulting in less atherogenic LDL. Although nicotinic acid lowers both cholesterol and triglyceride levels while raising HDL levels, it generally is not indicated in diabetes. It has an adverse effect on glycemic control, which results from the induction of insulin resistance. Hydroxymethylglutaryl coenzyme A (HMG-CoA) reductase inhibitors—statins—are another group of drugs that are useful in lowering cholesterol levels in type 2 diabetes patients without having an adverse effect on glycemic control. Bile acid resins can decrease the levels of LDL in diabetic patients, but they can cause a significant rise in triglyceride levels, especially if VLDL levels are already high or if diabetes is poorly controlled. In patients with high levels of both LDL and VLDL, bile acid resins can be used in low doses in combination with fibric acid derivatives.

As stated previously, diabetes mellitus is considered a CHD equivalent, and several large-scale clinical trials have assessed the efficacy of statins in both primary and secondary prevention of cardiovascular events in patients with diabetes (Table 49-3). Many of these trials were published after the NCEP-ATP III guidelines, and affirm the notion that diabetics are considered high risk. As such, statin therapy can be considered with LDL levels < 100 mg/dL, with an optional goal of < 70 mg/dL in high-risk diabetic patients. The CARDS trial showed that among 2,838 diabetic subjects with at least one heart disease risk factor, but without elevated cholesterol levels (LDL ≤ 160 mg/dL) and no history of cardiovascular disease, statin therapy was associated with a 37% reduction in the primary composite end point of CHD death, fatal MI, hospitalized unstable angina, resuscitated cardiac arrest, coronary revascularization, and stroke. Based on the subgroup analysis of large statin trials and major primary prevention statin trials that specifically recruited diabetics, there is mounting evidence that type 2 diabetics may be candidates for statin therapy regardless of LDL cholesterol level. The ADA recommends statin therapy, in addition to lifestyle therapy, regardless of baseline lipid levels, for

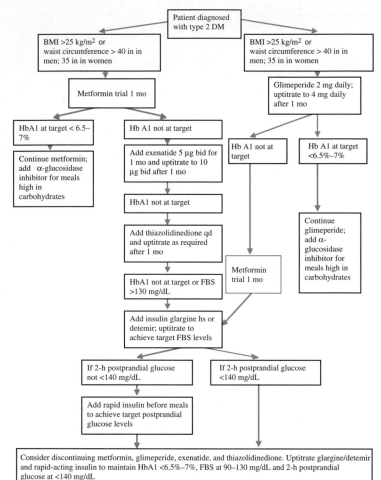

FIGURE 49-1. Algorithm for the management of type 2 diabetes. (BMI, body mass index; DM, diabetes mellitus; FBS, fasting blood sugar; HbA1c, glycosylated hemoglobin.)

diabetic patients without overt CVD who are over the age of 40 and have one or more other CVD risk factors.

【 】 HYPERTENSION MANAGEMENT

Patients with diabetes should be treated to a systolic blood pressure of 130 mm Hg and a diastolic blood pressure of 80 mm Hg. Patients with a blood pressure ≥140/90 should receive drug therapy in addition to lifestyle and behavioral therapy (Table 49-4). All patients with diabetes and hypertension should be treated with a regimen that includes either an ACE inhibitor or an aniogtensin-recepetor blocker (ARB). If one class is not tolerated, the other can be substituted. The HOPE trial evaluated over 9,000 high-risk

○ TABLE 49-3

Studies Evaluating Dyslipidemia Management in Diabetic Patients

Trial	Study Type	Diabetic Sample Size	Type I DM	Type 2 DM	Patient Population and Intervention	Follow-up (Median)	Results	p Value
Cholesterol Treatment Trialists Collaborators	Meta Analysis of 14 major RCT	18,686	1,466	17,220	Statin therapy in diabetics	4.3 yrs (mean)	9% RR reduction in all-cause mortality and 21% RR reduction in major vascular events per mmol/L reduction in LDL	0.02
VA-HIT	RCT	627	–	–	Gemfibrozil vs placebo in diabetic men with low HDL	5.1 yrs	24% RR reduction in death due to CHD, nonfatal MI, and CVA	0.05
FIELD	RCT	9,795	9,795	0	Fenofibrate vs placebo in type 2 DM with total blood cholesterol <6.5 mmol/L	5 yrs	24% RR reduction in nonfatal myocardial infarction; no difference in CHD mortality	0.01

The cholesterol treatment trialists collaborators meta-analysis included the following randomized control trials: 4S, WOSCOPS, CARE, Post-CABG, AFCAPS/TexCAPS, LIPID, GISSH, LIPS, HPS, PROSPER, ALLHAT-LLT, ASCOT-LLA, ALERT, and CARDS.

TABLE 49-4

Studies Evaluating Hypertensive Management Strategies in Diabetic Patients

Trial	Study Type	Diabetic Sample Size	Patient Population and Intervention	Follow-up	Results	p Value
HOT	RCT	1,501	Patients with diastolic hypertension treated with felodipine to a goal DBP vs placebo	3.8 yrs	51% reduction of major cardiovascular event with goal DBP < 80 mmHg vs < 90 mmHg	0.005
Syst-Eur Trial	RCT	492	Nitrendipine vs placebo in hypertensive diabetic patients	2 yrs	62% reduction in all cardiovascular events 41% reduction in all-cause mortality	0.02, 0.09
HOPE	RCT	3,577	Ramipril vs placebo in high-risk patients	5 yrs (mean)	24% RR reduction in composite of myocardial infarction, stroke, or death from cardiovascular cause	0.004
ADVANCE	RCT	11,140	Perindopril/indapamide combination vs placebo in diabetic patients	4.3 yrs (mean)	9% RR reduction of major macrovascular or microvascular event, 18% RR reduction of death from cardiovascular cause	0.04, 0.03
GEMINI	RCT	1,235	Carvedilol vs Metoprolol in diabetic patients with hypertension receiving RAS blockade	35 wks	0.13% difference in HbA1C between two groups in favor of carvedilol	0.004
UKPDS 39	RCT	1,148	Captopril vs atenolol in hypertensive diabetic patients	9 yrs	No advantage of either drug in preventing diabetic complications	NS
SHEP	RCT	583	Chlorthalidone vs placebo and routine care in hypertensive diabetic patients	5 yrs	23% reduction in major cardiovascular events with chlorthalidone	<0.05

DBP, diastolic blood pressure; RCT, randomized control trial; RR, relative risk. All other abbreviations as in text.

patients with evidence of vascular disease or diabetes in a randomized fashion comparing ramipril with placebo over a 5 year period. The MICRO-HOPE substudy, which included the 3,577 patients in the HOPE study with diabetes and at least one cardiovascular risk factor, demonstrated that ramipril lowered the risk of myocardial infarction by 22%, cardiovascular death by 37%, and total mortality by 24%, as compared to placebo. If patients require multiple drug therapy to achieve blood pressure targets, that ALL-HAT (Antihypertensive and Lipid-lowering Treatment to Prevent Heart Attack Trial) results suggest that a thiazide diuretic should then be added as a second-line therapy. The combination of an ACE inhibitor and an ARB is not recommended, since the combination of the two drugs may be associated with more adverse events without an increase in benefit. The use of calcium-channel blockers is not considered front-line therapy in the current recommendations, as they are considered inferior to ACE inhibitors for the treatment of hypertension in diabetic patients.

Beta-blockers have been associated with negative effects on glycemia and new-onset diabetes. In a meta-analysis assessing the effects of antihypertensives on incidence diabetes, the association was lowest for ARBs and ACE inhibitors, and highest for beta-blockers and diuretics. However, whether the metabolic effects of beta-blockers translate into long-term negative outcomes is debatable. Beta-blockers are considered first-line therapy in the management of patients with hypertension and angina and in those post-MI. The GEMINI study demonstrated that use of carvedilol, in the presence of renin–angiotensin blockade, did not affect glycemic control, relative to metoprolol, in diabetic patients with hypertension.

【 】 CORONARY REVASCULARIZATION

Coronary revascularization procedures have become a mainstay of therapy for CHD patients, providing both symptomatic relief and mortality reduction in certain patient subsets. Evidence from well-designed, prospective, randomized clinical trials suggests that surgical revascularization provides a survival advantage compared to medical therapy alone in patients with obstructive left main CHD and in patients with multivessel CHD with decreased left ventricular ejection fraction. Although none of the studies was specifically conducted in diabetic patients, subgroup analyses indicates that diabetic patients (1) are at greater risk for cardiac death and ischemic complications than nondiabetic patients and (2) may derive greater long-term benefit from surgical revascularization than do nondiabetic patients despite greater surgical risk (Table 49-5).

Options for Revascularization in Diabetic Patients: Coronary Artery Bypass Graft Versus Balloon Angioplasty

For the past two decades, the question of preferred revascularization strategies—surgery versus percutaneous intervention (PCI), mostly balloon angioplasty—has led to 13 important randomized clinical trials. There is general consensus that both surgery and percutaneous interventional therapies result in similar death and MI frequency for the overall patient populations observed in these studies. The major departure from this observation was highlighted in the BARI trial substudy, wherein there was a clinically meaningful and statistically significant survival benefit favoring coronary artery bypass grafting (CABG) in diabetic patients. Specifically, in the BARI randomized trial (n = 1,829 patients in total), diabetics on oral agent or insulin (n = 347) undergoing CABG had a 5 year survival rate of 80.6% compared to 65.5% in the balloon angioplasty arm. Notably, at 10 years of follow-up, in the diabetic subgroup, the CABG-assigned group still had a greater survival than the balloon angioplasty group (57.8% vs. PTCA 45.5%, respectively, $p = 0.025$). Although diabetes was not a prespecified subgroup in the original BARI protocol, the 5 year results of the BARI study led to the NIH recommending CABG as the preferred revascularization strategy in diabetics with multivessel coronary artery disease. On the other hand, the BARI registry showed no difference in overall long-term survival between CABG and angioplasty patients.

TABLE 49-5

Studies Comparing Surgical to Percutaneous Revascularization Techniques in Diabetic Patients

Trial	Study Type	Diabetic Sample Size	Patient Population and Intervention	Follow-up	Results	p Value
BARI	RCT	353	PTCA vs CABG in diabetics with severe angina or ischemia and multivessel CAD	10 yrs	Survival was 57.8% with CABG vs 45.5% with PTCA	0.025
BARI-Registry	Observational	339	PTCA vs CABG in diabetics with severe angina or ischemia and multivessel CAD	5 yrs	All-cause mortality was 14.4% with PTCA 14.9% with CABG	0.86
EAST	RCT	59	PTCA vs CABG in patients with multivessel CAD	8 yrs	8-yr survival 75.5% with CABG vs 60.1% with PTCA; no survival difference at 3 yrs	0.23
CABRI	RCT	125	PTCA vs CABG in symptomatic patients with multivessel CAD	4 yrs	4-yr survival was 77.4% with PTCA vs 87.5% with CABG	NS
RITA-1	RCT	62	PTCA vs CABG in patients with CAD	6.5 yrs (median)	Survival was 93% with PTCA vs 78% with CABG	0.09
DUKE	Observational	770	PTCA vs CABG in patients with symptomatic, multivessel CAD	5 yrs	5-yr unadjusted survival was 76% with PTCA vs 74% with CABG; adjusted survival was 86% with PTCA vs 89% with CABG	NS
Mercado et al.	Meta-Analysis of 4 RCT	549	BMS vs CABG in patients with multivessel CAD	1 yr	1-yr survival was 94.4% with BMS vs 96.5% with CABG	NS
New York State Registry	Observational	6,100	All patients undergoing first DES or CABG in New York State from Oct 2003 – Dec 2004	19 mo (mean)	Survival was 93% for DES vs 91.5% for CABG	NS

RCT, randomized control trial; RR, relative risk. All other abbreviations as in text.

Data compiled from Mercado N, Wijn W, Serruys PW, et al. One-year outcomes of coronary artery bypass graft surgery versus percutaneous disease : a meta-analysis of individual patient data from randomized clinical trials. *J Thorac Cardiovasc Surg.* 2005;130:512–519. Included the following randomized control trials: ARTS, SoS, ERACI-2, and MASS-2.

[ ] MODERN PERCUTANEOUS CORONARY INTERVENTION TECHNIQUES

Bare-Metal Stents

Many of the technical limitations of balloon angioplasty have been overcome by coronary stent implantation during PCI. Stenting is more predictable, giving a more reliable angiographic result in a wide variety of lesion types and is associated with lower restenosis in many lesion subsets. The advantage of stent implantation versus percutaneous transluminal coronary angioplasty alone with respect to angiographic restenosis and the need for repeat revascularization is also applicable to diabetic patients, a group that is at significantly higher risk of restenosis.

The introduction and generalized application of stenting with bare-metal stents promised to give PCI parity with CABG as a revascularization strategy. By reducing restenosis and preventing repeat revascularizations, diabetic patients were expected to further benefit from PCI. There have been multiple trials, such as the Arterial Revascularization Therapy Study (ARTS), Stent or Surgery (SOS), the Argentine Randomized Trial of Angioplasty Versus Surgery (ERACI II), and the Medicine, Angioplasty or Surgery Study (MASS-II), which have compared CABG to coronary stenting utilizing bare-metal stents. The ARTS trial, which randomized 1,205 patients with multivessel disease to CABG or stenting, demonstrated no important differences in death, myocardial infarction, or stroke at 1 year. However, the diabetes subset from ARTS revealed that multivessel stenting had a poorer 1 year major adverse cardiac event rate than did CABG, though the results were mainly driven by the higher incidence of repeat revascularization after stenting than after CABG. A quantitative analysis of the 1 year clinical outcomes of patients in ARTS-1, ERACI, SOS, and MASS-II showed that percutaneous intervention with multiple stenting and CABG provided a similar degree of protection against death, myocardial infarction, or stroke.

Drug-Eluting Stents

The advent of drug-eluting stents (DESs) has revolutionized the field of percutaneous interventions, especially in the diabetic patient. Although DESs have not had a major impact on hard cardiovascular end points such as death and MI, they have been successful in reducing angiographic restenosis and the rates of target-vessel revascularizations in both diabetics and nondiabetic populations, especially compared to bare-metal stents. A meta-analysis of DES studies showed that for patients with diabetes the number needed to treat to reduce major cardiac events were four patients for the sirolimus-eluting stents (SES) and six patients for the paclitaxel-eluting stents (PES).

With the superiority of DESs being established in the diabetic population, the next challenge has become the choice of which DES delivers better results—SES or PES. Few studies have compared these major DESs head to head. Although a meta-analysis of 16 randomized DES trials, including both diabetics and nondiabetics, demonstrated that SESs were superior to PESs in terms of a significant reduction of the risk of restenosis and stent thrombosis, other data suggest that SES and PES are associated with similar rates of revascularization, MACE, and stent thrombosis. The question of which DES is superior for the treatment of diabetic patients remains unclear.

[ ] BYPASS OUTCOMES

CABG with the use of an internal mammary artery (IMA) as a bypass conduit has been shown to be more advantageous than CABG with saphenous vein bypass conduits because of greater long-term durability of the arterial conduit. Bilateral IMA grafting provides even further survival advantage than left IMA plus saphenous vein grafts; these data have led to an increased application of CABG with total arterial revascularization.

Nonetheless, the use of bilateral IMA grafting in diabetic patients remains controversial because of the potentially increased risk for sternal wound infection.

Neurologic dysfunction remains a devastating complication of CABG, and diabetes is an important risk factor for stroke during CABG. Additionally, diabetes is the single greatest predictor of mortality during ischemic stroke. If drug-eluting stenting for diabetics with multivessel coronary artery disease proves to be equivalent to coronary bypass surgery in achieving successful revascularization, a significant advantage for stenting may be a reduction in stroke morbidity—the ARTS trial demonstrated no difference in stroke complications between diabetics and nondiabetics.

Inadequate data exists for us to be able to evaluate the definitive impact of DES for diabetic patients on long-term outcomes. Percutaneous coronary intervention using DES is being compared to contemporary CABG in multivessel disease patients with diabetes against the background of aggressive medical therapy in the ongoing NIH-NHLBI-sponsored Future Revascularization Evaluation in Patients with Diabetes Mellitus: Optimal Management of Multivessel Disease (FREEDOM) trial.

EARLY DETECTION OF CARDIOVASCULAR DISEASE IN THE DIABETIC PAIENT

Screening for asymptomatic diabetes in the general population is controversial, because there is a paucity of evidence that the prognosis of such patients will improve with early detection and treatment. The U.S. Preventive Services Task Force (USPSTF) has stated that current evidence is insufficient to recommend for or against routinely screening asymptomatic adults for type 2 diabetes, impaired glucose tolerance, or impaired fasting glucose. Nevertheless, the decision to screen an individual should be based on clinical judgment and patient preference, with special consideration given to those patients with increased cardiovascular risk (e.g., hyperlipidemia, hypertension, increased waist circumference).

More than a fifth of asymptomatic diabetic patients have silent myocardial ischemia and diabetics with inducible ischemia on single-photon emission computed tomography (SPECT) have a significantly worse prognosis than nondiabetic patients; yet routine screening for subclinical atherosclerosis in asymptomatic type 2 diabetic patients remains controversial. Theoretically, identification of silent ischemia, with a modality such as stress SPECT, in an asymptomatic diabetic, would prompt more aggressive treatment of cardiovascular risk factors. In addition, those patients with severe ischemic disease may potentially benefit from revascularization. On the other hand, an unconditional treatment strategy, in which all asymptomatic diabetics are considered high-risk and modifiable cardiovascular risks factors treated accordingly, may cost less and prevent more cardiovascular events. Whether the detection of silent ischemia will result in a reduction in cardiovascular events remains to be seen.

FUTURE DIRECTIONS

On the clinical front, there are still many challenges in the prevention and management of diabetic cardiovascular complications. Glycemic control appears to bet the mainstay of long-term diabetes management. Thus, development of better therapies and devices (e.g., closed-loop pumps, islet and pancreatic transplants) for achieving and maintaining HbA1c < 7% will be a primary goal in the next decade. The advent of drug-eluting stents for percutaneous coronary revascularization has led to a reevaluation of the need for coronary bypass surgery in multivessel disease. Finally, the role of gene therapy in the management of diabetic atherosclerotic disease needs to be addressed in the context of all other advances.

SUGGESTED READINGS

Diabetes Control and Complications Trial Research Group. The effect of intensive treatment of diabetes on the development and progression of long-term complications in insulin-dependent diabetes mellitus. *N Engl J Med*. 1993;329:977–986.

Effects of ramipril on cardiovascular and microvascular outcomes in people with diabetes mellitus: results of the HOPE study and MICRO-HOPE substudy. Heart Outcomes Prevention Evaluation Study Investigators. *Lancet*. 2000;355:253–259.

Executive summary of the third report of the National Cholesterol Education Program (NCEP) Expert Panel on Detection, Evaluation, and Treatment of High Blood Cholesterol in Adults (Adult Treatment Panel III). *JAMA*. 2001;285:2486–2497.

Final 10-year follow-up results from the BARI randomized trial. *J Am Coll Cardiol*. 2007;49:1600–1606.

Grundy SM, Cleeman JI, Daniels SR, et al. Diagnosis and management of the metabolic syndrome: an American Heart Association/National Heart, Lung, and Blood Institute Scientific Statement. *Circulation*. 2005;112:2735–2752.

Grundy SM, Cleeman JI, Merz CN, et al. Implications of recent clinical trials for the National Cholesterol Education Program Adult Treatment Panel III Guidelines. *J Am Coll Cardiol*. 2004;44:720–732.

Juutilainen A, Lehto S, Ronnemaa T, et al. Type 2 diabetes as a "coronary heart disease equivalent": an 18-year prospective population-based study in Finnish subjects. *Diabetes Care*. 2005;28:2901–2907.

Milicevic Z, Raz I, Beattie SD, et al. Natural history of cardiovascular disease in patients with diabetes: role of hyperglycemia. *Diabetes Care*. 2008;31(suppl 2):S155–S160.

Screening for type 2 diabetes mellitus in adults: recommendations and rationale. *Ann Intern Med*. 2003;138:212–214.

Tuomilehto J, Lindstrom J, Eriksson JG, et al. Prevention of type 2 diabetes mellitus by changes in lifestyle among subjects with impaired glucose tolerance. *N Engl J Med*. 2001;344:1343–1350.

CHAPTER (50)

Autoimmune Disorders and the Cardiovascular System

Jose F. Roldan and Robert A. O'Rourke

SYSTEMIC LUPUS ERYTHEMATOSUS

Systemic lupus erythematosus (SLE) is found worldwide and affects all races; it is more common among blacks, Asians, Hispanic-Americans, and females of childbearing age. In the United States, the annual incidence of SLE is about 8 per 100,000 and the prevalence is approximately 1 per 2000 (Table 50-1).

The inflammatory process of SLE involves multiple organ systems, including skin, joints, kidneys, brain, heart, and virtually all serous membranes. Its clinical presentation is varied and depends on the organ systems involved. Fever, arthritis, arthralgias, skin rashes, and pleuritis are common early signs of SLE.

Typical serologic abnormalities include the presence of antinuclear antibodies (ANAs), positive serum anti-DNA antibodies, positive anti-Smith antibodies, positive anti-ribonucleoprotein (anti-RNP) antibodies, and a falsely reactive VDRL. Low C3 and C4 serum complement levels are usually markers of disease activity, especially of renal disease. Careful interpretation of abnormal serologic tests is extremely important. ANA testing is very sensitive for SLE but lacks specificity. About 8% of the *normal population* has a positive ANA test. Although it may have an acute, fulminating course, SLE most often is characterized by a chronic course marked with exacerbations and remissions; the 10 years survival rate exceeds 90%. When patients die of SLE, it is most often in the setting of acute renal failure, central nervous system disease, associated infection, infective endocarditis, or coronary artery disease.

【 】 CARDIAC INVOLVEMENT

About 25% of patients with SLE have cardiac involvement. In addition to the valvular thickening or verrucae, and mitral regurgitation (MR) or aortic regurgitation (AR) (or occasional stenosis), there may be pericardial thickening and/or effusion, left ventricular regional or global systolic or diastolic dysfunction, or evidence of pulmonary hypertension. Either valvular regurgitation or stenosis due to SLE can require valve replacement.

【 】 PERICARDITIS

Pericardial effusions (exudative or transudative) occur at some point in over one-half of the patients with active SLE. In most SLE patients, the pericardial involvement is clinically silent and, when present, has a benign course. Pericardial tamponade is rare. However it should be considered in patients with unexplained signs of venous congestion. Rarely, SLE pericardial disease may lead to pericardial constriction.

TABLE 50-1

Primary Cardiac Manifestations of Nonhereditary Connective Tissue Diseases

Disease	Pericardium	Myocardium	Endocardium (Valves)	Coronary Arteries
Systemic lupus erythematosus	++	+	++	+
Systemic sclerosis	+	++	0	++
Polyarteritis nodosa	±	+	0	++
Ankylosing spondylitis	0	±	++	0
Rheumatoid arthritis	++	+	+	+
Polymyositis/dermatomyositis	++	++	±	±

++, major site of involvement; +, may be involved, but less frequently; ±, rarely involved; 0, not involved.

[ ] ENDOCARDITIS AND VALVE DISEASE

Verrucous endocarditis was first described by Libman and Sacks in 1924. The lesions consist almost entirely of fibrin, and although they may occur on both surfaces of any of the four cardiac valves, they are now most frequently found on the ventricular surface of the posterior mitral leaflet. These *verrucae* are similar histologically to those of nonbacterial thrombotic noninfective endocarditis. Although valvular verrucae in SLE are usually clinically silent, they can be dislodged and embolize and can also become infected, producing infective endocarditis.

[ ] MYOCARDITIS

A severely decreased systolic function similar to what is seen in patients with a septic shock is frequently observed in acutely ill lupus patients. Its cause is not entirely understood but in most cases resolves with the treatment of the primary disease. Several reports have described clinical features consistent with myocarditis, but actual visualization of interstitial myocardial inflammatory cells with associated myofiber necrosis has not been demonstrated histologically. Hemodynamic and echocardiographic studies, however, have shown abnormalities in both systolic and diastolic ventricular function in some SLE patients. T1 spin echo and T2 relaxation time cardiac MRI is being studied extensively in patients with SLE, in its use for the diagnosis of myocarditis. Diagnostic criteria need to be defined.

[ ] CORONARY ARTERY DISEASE

The incidence of myocardial infarction in women with SLE (third and fourth decades of life) is increased by 53-fold in comparison to patients from the Framingham cohort. Two-thirds of the coronary events occurred in women under 55 years of age. Older age at the lupus diagnosis, longer disease duration (>10 years), steroid use, hypercholesterolemia, and postmenopausal status were more common in the patients with coronary events.

Accelerated CAD is increasingly recognized as a leading cause of morbidity and mortality among young women with SLE, who receive long-term glucocorticoids. However, an acute myocardial infarction may occur in the presence of angiographically normal coronary arteries.

Although the causes of this premature CAD are uncertain, glucocorticoid treatment and antiphospholipid (aPL) antibodies have been incriminated. It is speculated that the underlying chronic inflammatory state in SLE may induce an underlying vasculopathy that may facilitate premature atherogenesis.

【 】 PREGNANCY AND THE NEONATAL LUPUS SYNDROME

Neonatal LE is a rare disorder that arises when the so-called anti-Ro, or anti-SSA autoantibodies are formed and circulate in pregnant patients, cross the placenta, and cause a lupus-like syndrome in newborns with the appearance of a skin rash and transient cytopenias from passively acquired maternal autoantibodies. In most cases, the neonatal lupus syndrome is a benign disorder, and most babies of mothers with anti-Ro (SSA), anti-La (SSB), or anti-U1RNP antibodies do not develop neonatal lupus. *A pregnant woman with SLE with positive anti-Ro, anti-La, or anti-RNP antibodies has a less than 3% risk of having a child with neonatal lupus and congenital heart block. The risk that this patient might have an infant with neonatal lupus syndrome but without congenital heart block may be as high as 1 in 3.* Neonatal lupus syndrome with congenital heart block can be diagnosed by the appearance of fetal bradycardia around week 23 of gestation. It is unclear whether aggressive anti-inflammatory therapy to diminish the generalized fetal insult and to lower the titers of circulating anti-Ro (SSA) antibodies makes a difference in fetal cardiac outcome.

【 】 MANAGEMENT

Therapy of cardiovascular SLE is the treatment of the underlying disease and includes nonsteroidal anti-inflammatory drugs (NSAIDs), glucocorticoids, and, in severe cases, immunosuppressive agents such as azathioprine, mycophenolate mophetil, and cyclophosphamide.

Acute Pericarditis

A mild to moderate pericardial effusion can be treated with NSAIDs or prednisone at a dose of 20 to 40 mg/d. A large pericardial effusion may require treatment with a high-dose of steroids (prednisone 1 mg/kg). Pericardiocenthesis or placement of a pericardial window is rarely needed.

Valvular Disease

Valvular disease is clinically silent in most cases. A surgical repair is rarely necessary. There are no studies regarding antimicrobial pophylaxis in patients with lupus and verrucous endocarditis. Therefore, the standard recommendations of the American Heart Association (2007) should be followed (Chapters 32 to 35).

Primary and Secondary Prevention

Since multiple studies have demonstrated a remarkable increased risk of cardiovascular events in patients with SLE and affecting mostly women in the second decade of life, an aggressive control of cardiovascular risk factors is indicated.

The antimalarial agent hydroxychloroquine has a beneficial effect on the lipid profile and is the only disease-modifying antirheumatic agent that has been associated with a decrease of the damage accrual. Every patient with SLE is treated with hydroxychloroquine unless there is a major contraindication for its use.

ANTIPHOSPHOLIPID ANTIBODY SYNDROME

The antiphospholipid syndrome (APS) is defined by the presence of antiphospholipid (aPL) antibodies (any of the following: lupus anticoagulant, moderately elevated titers of IgG or IgM anticardiolipins, and anti-beta-2 glycoprotein IgG or IgM) on two or more occasions 12 weeks apart and less than 5 years prior to a venous or arterial thrombotic event or unexplained recurrent fetal losses after the 10th week of pregnancy.

Livedo reticularis, nonhealing leg ulcers, thrombocytopenia, and Coombs'-positive hemolytic anemia may be also present.

The presence of a prolonged activated partial thromboplastin time should prompt the clinician to rule out the presence of APS.

[ ] MANAGEMENT

Patients with positive aPL antibodies but no evidence of thrombosis or recurrent fetal loss should be given low-dose aspirin only. Patients with APS, who have had thrombotic events or habitual abortions, should be anticoagulated for life. Anticoagulation and antithrombotic therapy in these patients has included unfractionated heparin, low-molecular-weight heparin, or warfarin.

The intensity of the anticoagulation is still controversial. There is no difference in the recurrence of thrombotic events in patients treated with high-level anticoagulation (INR 3.1–4.0) versus low-level anticoagulation (INR 2.0–3.0). The optimal anticoagulation level for these patients is unknown. Whether high- or low-level anticoagulation is used depends on a careful assessment of the risks of anticoagulation, involvement of the arterial site, and history of recurrence of a thrombotic episode on a patient already receiving low-level anticoagulation.

RHEUMATOID ARTHRITIS

The prevalence of rheumatoid arthritis (RA) is 1% to 2%. It is characterized by a symmetric arthritis of large and small joints. Patients with a high-titer rheumatoid factor and severe joint deformities are at the highest risk of suffering the extraarticular manifestations of the disease.

[ ] PERICARDIAL INVOLVEMENT

A diffuse, nonspecific fibrofibrinous pericarditis occurs in about 50% of patients with RA; it is usually clinically silent and is overshadowed by pleuritis or joint pain. The pericardial disease tends to be benign and no treatment is necessary for most cases.

[ ] MYOCARDIAL AND ENDOCARDIAL INVOLVEMENT

A prospective cohort study comparing the incidence of myocardial infarction and cerebrovascular events between RA patients and non-RA patients with known CAD found that patients with RA had a greater incidence of vascular events and mortality. A strong correlation between the presence of inflammatory biochemical markers and carotid atherosclerotic plaques has also been described.

Coronary artery calcification determined by electron-beam computed tomography is significantly higher in patients with RA compared with healthy individuals. The presence of coronary artery calcifications is highly dependent on disease duration. The incidence of valvular infiltration by rheumatoid nodules has been estimated at 1% to 2% in autopsy studies of patients with RA. One echocardiographic study of 39 patients with RA detected left ventricular abnormalities in 25%. A significant excess risk of CHF has been reported in patients with RA.

Management

Methotrexate remains the most important antirheumatic drug for the treatment of rheumatoid arthritis. Longitudinal data supports the addition of an anti-TNF-alpha agent in order to reduce accumulated joint damage over time.

The anti-TNF-alpha agents should not be used in patients with New York Health Association (NYHA) class III or IV heart failure due to the potential risk of decompensation.

【 】 PERICARDIAL INVOLVEMENT

An uncomplicated asymptomatic pericardial effusion does not require any treatment. Moderately severe pericardial effusion with hemodynamic compromise should be treated with corticosteroids (see treatment of pericardial disease in SLE). Pericardiocentesis should be performed only as a lifesaving procedure or when a second disease is suspected such as carcinomatous pericarditis or tuberculosis.

Primary and Secondary Prevention

The accumulated dose of prednisone over time is a major risk factor for atherosclerosis and cardiovascular events. For that reason, its use should be minimized. A steroid-sparing agent must be used or added as soon as possible (methotrexate, anti-TNF-alpha).

It is unknown whether statins have a roll in the primary prevention of cardiovascular events in patients with RA. A randomized doubled-blinded, placebo-control study is currently in progress (Trial of Atorvastatin in the Primary Prevention of Cardiovascular Endpoints in Rheumatoid Arthritis [TRACE RA]).

ANKYLOSING SPONDYLITIS

Ankylosing spondylitis is the prototypical example within the group of the seronegative spondyloarthropathies. It is characterized by a progressive inflammatory lesion of the spine, leading to chronic back pain, deforming dorsal kyphosis, and in its advanced stage, fusion of the costovertebral and sacroiliac joints with immobilization of the spine. This condition is much more frequent in men than it is in women (9:1), generally first occurring early in life but with a chronic progressive course of 20 to 30 years. The HLA-B27 histocompatibility antigen is found in 90% of whites and in 50% of black patients with ankylosing spondylitis.

【 】 CARDIAC INVOLVEMENT

Cardiovascular disease in ankylosing spondylitis is seen typically in patients with severe peripheral joint involvement and long-standing disease. It takes the form of a sclerosing inflammatory lesion that is generally limited to the aortic root area. The inflammatory process extends immediately above and below the aortic valve and typically causes AR (2%–10% of patients).

As the inflammatory process extends below the aortic valve, it can infiltrate the basal portion of the mitral valve, and cause MR. Ventricular diastolic dysfunction may also occur.

【 】 MANAGEMENT

Drug therapy for ankylosing spondylitis used to be directed primarily at relief of the back pain and discomfort. Newer medicines, particularly the anti-TNF-alpha agents, have revolutionized its management.

NSAIDs, methotrexate, and anti-TNF-alpha therapy, in addition to physical therapy, remain the first line of therapy. Glucocorticoids do not have a role except for the treatment of uveitis.

Patients with ankylosing spondylitis also have a high incidence of atlantoaxial instability. For that reason, special caution should be used to avoid a manipulation of the cervical spine, which may result in permanent paralysis.

【 】 VALVE DISEASE

It is not known whether a strict control of the primary disease with anti-TNF-alpha agents will have an impact on the incidence of the valve involvement. Not infrequently, the AR of ankylosing spondylitis may become severe enough to warrant aortic valve replacement.

SYSTEMIC SCLEROSIS (SCLERODERMA)

Scleroderma is characterized by fibrous thickening of the skin and fibrous and degenerative alterations of the fingers and of certain target organs, particularly the esophagus, small and large bowels, kidneys, lung, and heart. Central to this degenerative process are diffuse vascular lesions. Functionally, the vascular disorder is characterized by Raynaud's phenomenon, which is a prominent feature of scleroderma. The underlying pathophysiology of scleroderma that links structure and function is a Raynaud's-type phenomenon of visceral vasculature that leads to focal vascular lesions and parenchymal necrosis and fibrosis. This concept is supported by findings in the heart, the lungs, and the kidneys.

Scleroderma may have a variable clinical expression. Some patients may have skin involvement predominantly; others have minimal skin abnormalities but severe visceral disease that may therefore evade diagnosis. Limited scleroderma (formerly called CREST syndrome) is most of the time a more benign form of scleroderma that presents with relatively mild skin changes limited to the face and fingers, calcinosis, Raynaud's phenomenon, esophageal dysmotility, sclerodactyly, and telangiectasia. Patients with limited scleroderma have a high incidence of pulmonary hypertension.

【 】 CARDIOVASCULAR SYSTEM

Cardiovascular disease in patients with scleroderma can be due to either a primary involvement of the heart by the scalloping disease or a secondary involvement from disease of the kidney or lungs.

Primary Systemic Sclerosis of the Heart

Myocardial involvement is a major determinant of survival in scleroderma. When the heart is involved directly by scleroderma, a myocardial fibrosis occurs. Focal patchy myocardial cell necrosis may be evident, and at autopsy over three-quarters of patients with myocardial scleroderma have foci of necrosis. The type of necrosis is myofibrillar degeneration, or contraction-band necrosis. This lesion is characteristic of myocardium that is subjected to transient occlusion followed by reperfusion. Thus, the morphologic characteristics of the myocardial lesions of primary cardiac scleroderma are very similar to the ones seen in Raynaud's phenomenon.

【 】 CLINICAL MANIFESTATIONS

Autopsy studies have suggested that up to 50% of patients with scleroderma have increased myocardial scar tissue and that up 30% of patients have extensive disease.

The clinical features of myocardial scleroderma include biventricular congestive heart failure, atrial and ventricular arrhythmias, myocardial infarction, angina pectoris, and sudden cardiac death. Idiopathic dilated cardiomyopathy may be simulated.

Pericardial and Endocardial Disease

Pericardial involvement may occur in about 20% of patients with scleroderma. Although the pericardial involvement is due to renal failure in as many as two-thirds of patients, some develop a fibrofibrinous or fibrous pericarditis for which no other cause is evident. *Most cases of pericardial effusion in scleroderma have a benign course.*

Valve Involvement

MR is common in patients with scleroderma. Tricuspid regurgitation occurs in patients with very dilated right ventricular cavities.

Pulmonary Hypertensive Disease

Although the pulmonary fibrosis of scleroderma had been known for years, the recognition of a pulmonary hypertensive lesion independent of parenchymal disease evolved later. Such patients tend to develop rapidly progressive dyspnea and right-sided heart failure in the setting of clear lungs. Morphologically, the pulmonary arterial lesions show the range of advanced alterations as seen in Eisenmenger's syndrome and primary pulmonary hypertension. Pulmonary hypertension portends a poor prognosis.

SECONDARY CARDIOVASCULAR DISEASE

Ventricular hypertrophy and congestive heart failure may be associated with long-standing systemic arterial hypertension and renal disease. Uremic pericarditis may occur. Pulmonary hypertension with marked right ventricular hypertrophy and right-sided heart failure may result from long-standing severe pulmonary scleroderma. Mortality due to scleroderma renal crisis and malignant hypertension has dramatically decreased with the use of angiotensin-converting enzyme (ACE) inhibitors.

【 】 MANAGEMENT

The use of *high-dose glucocorticoids* should be avoided in scleroderma. No uniform therapy is effective for the cardiovascular disease of scleroderma. Treatment consists of standard therapy for congestive heart failure and arrhythmias.

The use of continuous intravenous infusion of epoprostenol, inhaled protacyclin analogue iloprost, or the endothelin-receptor antagonists have improved dramatically the symptoms and mortality due to pulmonary hypertension.

RAYNAUD'S PHENOMENON

Avoiding cool temperatures is of vital importance. Patients should be encouraged not just to use gloves but to wear appropriate clothes to keep a "warm" body temperature. Nifedipine is the first-line agent for the treatment of Raynaud's. Amlodipine has also been shown to be effective; however, in a recent randomized placebo-control trial, patients with scleroderma taking Losartan for the treatment of their Raynaud's had significantly better responses than those treated with nifedipine. Larger trials are needed to determine the true roll of epoprostenol, inhaled protacyclin analogue iloprost, and the endothelin-receptor antagonists for the treatment of severe digital ischemia in order to prevent digital necrosis.

POLYMYOSITIS AND DERMATOMYOSITIS

These idiopathic autoimmune inflammatory myopathies are rare in the United States, with an estimated annual incidence of about 5 to 10 new patients per million. The clinical features include a typical heliotrope rash in dermatomyositis (DM), with periorbital edema and proximal muscle weakness present in both polymyositis (PM) and DM. Typical laboratory findings reflect the presence of muscle breakdown from the inflammatory process. Creatine kinase, myoglobulin, and serum aldolase levels are commonly elevated during acute states. The former is more sensitive in those patients who present with normal, or mildly increased, creatine kinase levels. The so-called anti-Jo-1 antibody, directed against histydil-tRNA synthetase, is detectable in the serum of 20% of patients with PM/DM.

Typical electromyogram (EMG) changes include short-wave potentials, low-amplitude polyphasic units, and increased spontaneous activity with muscle fibrillation (myopathy). Muscle inflammation can be demonstrated on T2-weighted MRI. For that reason it is used nowadays for determining active inflammation and a possible biopsy site. A muscle biopsy remains the gold-standard test for the diagnosis of PM/DM and should be performed on all patients.

【 】 CARDIOVASCULAR INVOLVEMENT

In addition to skeletal muscle involvement, up to 40% of patients may have cardiac abnormalities. A small study of 16 autopsied patients with PM/DM suggests a poor correlation between the degree of skeletal involvement and myocarditis, however, in a study of 55 patients with PM, Behan and associates reported mild diffuse myocarditis, severe inflammation, or fibrosis of the cardiac conduction system in 70% of the patients. Myocarditis leading to congestive heart failure is an uncommon but severe manifestation of PM/DM. The role of gadolinium-DTPA-enhanced MRI appears promising in diagnosing myocarditis in PM/DM. Contrast enhancement and hypokinesia detected by cardiac MRI is reduced after treatment with corticosteroids and immunosuppressive therapy.

【 】 MANAGEMENT

Although coronary arteritis has been reported in few case reports, there are no controlled studies showing evidence of increased incidence of CAD in PM/DM. Glucocorticoids represent the mainstay of therapy. The usual practice is to begin treatment with 40 to 80 mg/d of oral prednisone or its equivalent. Methylprednisolone boluses of 500 to 1000 mg/d for 3 days are reserved for severe and acute cases. Azathioprine (Imuran) and methotrexate are used mostly as steroid-sparing agents. Intravenous immunoglobulin given in monthly boluses is an expensive therapy that is reserved for patients with severe disease (neuromuscular respiratory involvement, dysphagia) and poor response to conventional immunosuppressive therapy. Response can be seen as early as 2 weeks, but typically best effects are seen only after 3 months.

SUGGESTED READING

Behan WM, Behan PO, Gairns J. Cardiac damage in polymyositis associated with antibodies to tissue ribonucleoproteins. *Br Heart J.* 1987;57:176–180.

Crowther MA, Ginsberg JS, Julian J, et al. A comparison of two intensities of warfarin for the prevention of recurrent thrombosis in patients with the antiphospholipid antibody syndrome. *N Engl J Med.* 2003;349:1133–1138.

del Rincon ID, Williams K, Stern MP, et al. High incidence of cardiovascular events in a rheumatoid arthritis cohort not explained by traditional cardiac risk factors. *Arthritis Rheum.* 2001;44:2737–2745.

Manzi S, Meilahn EN, Rairie JE, et al. Age-specific incidence rates of myocardial infarction and angina in women with systemic lupus erythematosus: comparison with the Framingham study. *Am J Epidemiol.* 1997;145:408–415.

Nicola PJ, Maradit-Kremers H, Roger VL, et al. The risk of congestive heart failure in rheumatoid arthritis: a population-based study over 46 years. *Arthritis Rheum.* 2005;52:412–420.

O'Rourke RA. Antiphospholipid antibodies: a marker of lupus carditis? *Circulation.* 1990;82:636–638.

Roldan CA, Shively BK, Crawford MH. An echocardiographic study of valvular heart disease associated with systemic lupus erythematosus. *N Engl J Med.* 1996;335: 1424–1430.

Roldan JF, Escalante A, del Rincon I. Impaired arterial function associated with thinning of cortical bone in rheumatoid artritis. *Arthritis Rheum.* 2008;59:523–530.

Women and Coronary Artery Disease

Pamela Charney

Unfortunately, still there are physicians as well as patients who are not aware that coronary artery disease (CAD) is the most common cause of mortality for women as well as men. Initial CAD research focused on middle-aged populations, among whom men have a dramatically higher rate of CAD than women. As research has expanded to include elderly subjects, less dramatic differences in mortality rates between elderly women and men have been documented. Women develop symptomatic CAD about a decade later then men. Black women are at greater risk of death from CAD and stroke than white women. CAD mortality has been decreasing in women less than in men, probably related to less attention to cardiac risk reduction in women.

PREVENTION OF CAD IN WOMEN

Tobacco exposure and obesity are major modifiable CAD risk factors. Patients requiring aggressive primary prevention include those diagnosed with diabetes, hypertension, lupus, and rheumatoid arthritis, as these diseases are associated with increased rates of CAD events. Postmenopausal hormonal therapy does not protect from CAD mortality and events and increases the rate of stroke and thrombosis. Important risk factors with clinically important gender differences are reviewed in Tables 51-1 and 51-2.

CAD risk factors are additive, and women without traditional cardiovascular risk factors (tobacco, hypertension, old age, high cholesterol, diabetes, physical inactivity, and family history) are at relatively low risk for coronary events. The greatest treatment benefit occurs with aggressive preventive measures in women with multiple risk factors or prior coronary events.

【 】 TOBACCO

Many surveys reveal that physicians can have a powerful effect on smoking cessation, even with minimal effort. Exposure to tobacco is one of the single most important CAD risk factor for both women and men. Cigarette smoking has been associated with an increased risk of CAD, earlier age of first myocardial infarction, and earlier onset of menopause. Women smokers have a higher increase of risk of CAD compared to women nonsmokers, than do men smokers compared to men nonsmokers. Over the last several decades, tobacco use among American women has not decreased as dramatically as it has among men (Fig. 51-1). The prevalence of cigarette use among women reflects both higher initiation and lower successful tobacco cessation rates.

Women contemplating smoking cessation are often concerned about potential weight gain, a common consequence of efforts to stop smoking because tobacco use increases

TABLE 51-1

Sex and Race Considerations in Tobacco Cessation Therapy

Agent	Efficacy	Special Considerations
Nicotine replacement products	Double tobacco cessation compared with tobacco cessation groups alone Can use patch + more rapid release agent	The patch has the highest compliance rate and provides smoother levels than gum, spray, or lozenge. Patch efficacy in women and men similar
Bupropion	Improves tobacco cessation rates in both white and black smokers whether or not depression is present	Increases metabolic rate, so minimizes weight gain while it is used. Can cause seizures, so avoid if history of seizures, prior brain trauma, heavy alcohol use. Avoid with active or history of anorexia and/or bulimia
Varenicline	Try to stop 1 wk after starting drug, with increasing dose if tolerated	Nausea, abnormal dreams, and risk of behavior changes such as agitation, depression, and suicidal thoughts or behavior
Women smokers	Improved cessation with social support— especially children or groups	Surveyed woman smokers unwilling to gain any pounds to stop smoking Accepting weight gain when stopping use leads to greater success in cessation than dieting and stopping tobacco together. Secondary smoke major risk factor for many women
Black smokers	Metabolite level higher, so greater impact with even one cigarette	Fewer cigarettes required to be addicted; therefore initiate pharmacologic therapy sooner. Greater difficulty stopping

one's metabolic rate. Usually weight gain with tobacco cessation is on average 7 to 10 lb, with fewer than 10% gaining >20 lb. However, weight gain tends to be higher among women, blacks, and smokers who inhale more than 25 cigarettes per day. To avoid weight gain with tobacco cessation, realistic expectations may be helpful as well as exercise, careful choice of snacks, and appropriate pharmacotherapy. Increasing physical activity contributes to success in smoking cessation, as does an increased expenditure of calories, even if it does not modify weight gain. Multiple pharmacologic therapies are available (Table 51-1). Second-hand tobacco exposure increases CAD risk by about 20%.

【 】 DIABETES

In the last decade, CAD mortality rates have *increased* by 23% for diabetic women yet decreased by 27% for nondiabetic women. In comparison, men's CAD mortality rates have declined for diabetics (13%) and nondiabetics (36%). Black and Hispanic women have especially high rates of diabetes. Once a woman is diagnosed with diabetes, her "female advantage" in relation to CAD risk is lost. After myocardial infarction, diabetic women have higher risk of congestive heart failure (CHF) and death than do diabetic

TABLE 51-2

Additional Cad Risk Factors with Significant Gender Differences

Risk Factor	Clinically Important Issues for Women
Lipids	Total cholesterol peaks in women age 55–64 (in men at about age 50). LDL is higher with greater age
	HDL in women is greater than in men, remaining similar with aging
	HDL may be most predictive for women, especially low HDL.
	Triglyceride levels may be important in women
	Because women usually develop clinical CAD 10 yrs later than men, many primary prevention trials have inadequate power to assess treatment for women
	There has been adequate power to show that secondary prevention decreases CAD events in women
	Lipid treatment agents are underprescribed after myocardial infarction in women; target treatment levels are often not reached
	Women at high risk, such as women with diabetes, should be aggressively treated. At the time of diabetes diagnosis, women have more adverse lipid abnormalities than nondiabetic age-matched controls
	There is controversy about aggressive treatment in the woman at low risk for vascular disease while results of further primary prevention clinical trials are pending
Obesity	The prevalence of obesity doubled among Americans > age 20 from 1980 to 2002. Racial differences in body-mass index, as well as glycosylated hemoglobin, start in childhood
Hormone replacement therapy	**Not Cardiac Protective.** Women's Health Initiative (WHI): overall no CAD mortality benefit. Increased CAD events with daily estrogen/progesterone, especially in first year
	WHI hysterectomized women treated with estrogen vs. placebo; CAD events rates were similar
	The Heart and Estrogen-Progestin Replacement Study (HERS), the only completed secondary prevention clinical trial of hormonal therapy, revealed no overall reduction in CAD events but substantially more venous thrombotic events and gallbladder disease with hormonal therapy
	HERS subjects at enrollment—low rates of secondary prevention
Aspirin	Aspirin for primary prevention in women > 65 years from the Women's Health Study, a randomized control trial of aspirin (100 mg aspirin on alternating days) or placebo for primary prevention of CVD in women age ≥ 45 with 10 yrs of follow-up with stroke reduction. Overall, an insignificant decrease in CV risk, and no decrease in MI. However, in subgroup analysis, benefit for women > 65 years of age with decreased MI, ischemic stroke, and major CV events
	Aspirin for secondary prevention of CAD and stroke valuable for women
Race and coronary artery disease	Young black women (age < 55) have more than twice the rate of CAD mortality (sudden and nonsudden) than young white women
	Importantly, family income, educational level, and occupational status account for more of this observed difference than traditional coronary risk factors

TABLE 51-2

Additional Cad Risk Factors with Significant Gender Differences (*Continued*)

Risk Factor	Clinically Important Issues for Women
Physical activity and exercise	Obesity is linked to multiple cardiac risk factors Behavioral interventions to decrease weight have been most successful when there is an exercise component Generally, women have smaller hearts, and cardiac output is increased by raising heart rate In national surveys, sedentary lifestyles are reported by as many as 70% of adult women, with higher rates among black and Hispanic women and those with less education or lower income Especially for women, increased activity during daily routines is more helpful than an exercise program Women more likely to exercise regularly with prior weight loss and exercise and if encouraged by their school-age children Both women and men benefit from referral to cardiac rehabilitation programs after MI; fewer women than men are referred for cardiac rehabilitation after CAD events
Menopause	Importance is not fully defined. Historically, women with early surgical menopause have been considered at higher risk for CAD and osteoporosis. However, the Nurse's Health Study found that only women smokers with a younger age of menopause have a greater risk of CAD
Psychocial factors	Depression, an independent risk factor for CAD, is diagnosed twice as often in women than men Depression after myocardial infarction also predicts greater morbidity as well as higher subsequent mortality in women more than men Coronary disease morbidity and mortality is greater among those with lower SES—described as years of formal education, owning a car, income defined by absolute or relative amount, and parental status. More recently, SES has also been defined independent of race. Lower SES has also been related to higher rates of tobacco use and higher inpatient mortality after myocardial infarction
Stress-related cardio-myopathy	*Tako-tsubo* is an acute and reversible severe cardiomyopathy occurring after severe emotional or physical distress seen predominantly in women. Acute symptoms include substernal chest pain or dyspnea (most often associated with ST-segment elevation or T-wave inversion and abnormal cardiac enzymes), with profound systolic dysfunction (ejection fractions often 20%–49%). Low mortality with aggressive supportive care

LDL, low-density lipoprotein; HDL, high-density lipoprotein; CAD, coronary artery disease; SES, socioeconomic status.

men. The mechanisms for these observations are suspected to be at least partially related to lipid abnormalities as well as insulin resistance.

Aggressive management of tobacco exposure, lipoprotein abnormalities, and hypertension, if these are present, are beneficial. Regular exercise can also improve glucose control and insulin resistance. For women at risk of developing diabetes, including those

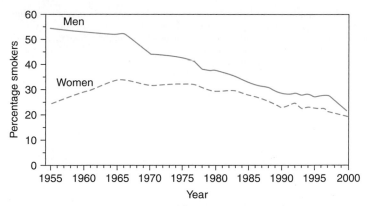

FIGURE 51-1. Prevalence of smoking among men and women age 18 years and under in the United States. Before 1992, current smokers were defined as persons who reported having smoked more than 100 cigarettes and who currently smoked. Since 1992, current smokers have been defined as persons who reported having smoked more than 100 cigarettes during their lifetime and who reported now smoking every day or some days. (1955 Current Population Survey; 1965–1997 National Health Interview Survey.)

who had gestational diabetes, regular physical activity and weight control decrease the risk of subsequently developing diabetes.

[ ] HYPERTENSION

Both systolic and diastolic blood pressures have been found to predict coronary events in women and men. As Kannel states, "Coronary disease is the most common and lethal sequela of hypertension, equaling in incidence all the other cardiovascular outcomes combined." Generally, women are more likely to have controlled blood pressure (BP) than men.

Gender-specific information about pharmacologic therapy is evolving. Thiazide diuretics, a preferred anti-hypertension treatment, are also beneficial for bone health both in epidemiologic studies and clinical trials. Angiotensin-converting enzyme (ACE) inhibitors should be used cautiously in women of reproductive age, as teratogenic effects have been documented in the first as well as second trimester. Infants with only first-trimester ACE inhibitor exposure had increased risk of CV and central nervous system malformations. Therefore, potentially fertile women must understand the potential risk to the fetus before initiating therapy. Cough, a common side effect of first-generation ACE inhibitors, but not the angiotensin receptor blockers (ARBs), occurs substantially more frequently in women than in men.

DIAGNOSIS OF CORONARY ARTERY DISEASE

CAD is often diagnosed clinically by a careful history. Women generally visit physicians more often than men and report more symptoms, including chest pain. Too often, older women ascribe decreased ability to "getting old." Therefore, regular exploration of a patient's exercise tolerance, with CAD in the differential diagnosis, is essential.

Exercise stress testing is a commonly used, noninvasive modality to assess CAD risk. Women have lower sensitivity and specificity with exercise stress testing than men, in part related to lower ECG voltage, as well as more frequent ST-T-wave abnormalities. The maximal exercise capacity and heart rate recovery in women are important prognostically even among asymptomatic women with low-risk Framingham scores. Those with lower exercise capacity and slower heart rate recovery are at increased risk for CV death. A negative exercise stress test with adequate exertion is reassuring and decreases the need to proceed to cardiac catheterization (see also Chapter 5).

Generally, stress imaging techniques are favored in assessing a woman for possible CAD or staging disease severity. Nuclear stress perfusion testing with technetium may be preferred, since thallium can potentially result in soft-tissue attenuation from breast tissue. Stress echocardiography is highly dependent on operator expertise and is technically difficult in obese patients (see also Chapter 5). Many authors prefer stress imaging tests with lower false-positive rates than an exercise stress test for women. Local expertise is an important consideration in deciding whether to use nuclear medicine or echocardiography techniques.

MANAGEMENT OF CLINICAL CORONARY ARTERY DISEASE IN WOMEN

[ ] CHRONIC ANGINA

In the Framingham study, the commonest presenting CAD symptom in women was angina. Women as opposed to men with angina more frequently report anginal symptoms with emotional or mental stress and may more often demonstrate vasospastic responses. Managing angina in women is complicated by the observation that anginal symptoms in women are less predictive of abnormal coronary anatomy than they are in men.

[ ] ACUTE CORONARY ISCHEMIA INCLUDING ACUTE MYOCARDIAL INFARCTION

There are significant gender differences in acute ischemia at the time of presentation and during short-term follow-up. Women tend to delay arrival for medical care longer after symptoms begin; they have less ST-segment elevation on the initial electrocardiogram and are also less likely to receive thrombolytic treatment, aspirin, or beta-blockers. Women more often developed acute pulmonary edema or cardiogenic shock. Both women and black patients receive fewer invasive interventions (catheterization, percutaneous coronary intervention [PCI], and coronary artery bypass grafting [CABG]) for cardiac ischemia. Data analyzed from the National Registry of Myocardial Infarction II noted an interaction of gender and age, with twice the 30-day mortality after myocardial infarction for women aged 30 to 50 than for men of the same age, with a progressive decrease in differences with increasing age until unity was reached at age 75.

In long-term follow-up after myocardial infarction, women have more symptoms than men, although their long-term mortality is similar or better. Specifically, women tend to have more angina and congestive heart failure despite better systolic left ventricular function. Therapies that are efficacious in women as well as men are, in observational studies, often not prescribed for women (i.e., aspirin, beta-blockers, and cholesterol-lowering agents). Furthermore, even when such drugs are prescribed, treatment goals have often not been met. Rehabilitation is also less often recommended for women, although it is equally effective for them. To improve the prognosis of women after myocardial infarction, it is essential to avoid tobacco exposure, to use medications documented to decrease mortality in adequate doses, and to address other risk factors. Ischemic heart disease is the commonest etiology of congestive heart failure (CHF) in women as well as in men.

[ ] INTERVENTIONS FOR CORONARY ARTERY DISEASE: ANGIOPLASTY AND CORONARY ARTERY BYPASS GRAFTING

Both angioplasty and coronary artery bypass grafting are utilized less in women than in men, and there has been controversy as to whether women are undertreated or men overtreated. With the development of smaller coronary artery catheters and stents, angioplasty outcomes and complications have become similar for women and men. The conduit selected in coronary artery bypass grafting (CABG) is less often the internal thoracic artery (ITA) in women than in men, although this graft is associated with the best short- and long-term results. Reasons for avoiding use of the ITA might include higher rates of diabetes in women undergoing CABG and the presence of osteoporosis. Because women compared with men undergoing CABG tend to be older and to have more comorbid conditions, a higher postoperative complication rate—including slower postoperative recovery and higher rates of depression—is not unexpected. With follow-up after several years, gender differences are less apparent.

[ ] ARRHYTHMIAS

Women respond to increasing cardiac demand by increasing heart rate, whereas men increase stroke volume. Women also have a longer QT interval and shorter sinus node recovery time. Palpitations and torsades de pointes are reported more commonly by women than men.

SUGGESTED READING

Charney P. Women and coronary artery disease. In: Fuster V, Alexander RW, O'Rourke RA, et al., eds. *Hurst's The Heart*. 11th ed. New York: McGraw-Hill; 2004:2285–2300.

Cooper WO, Hernandez-Diaz S, Arbogast PG. Major congenital malformations after first-trimester exposure to ACE inhibitors. *N Engl J Med*. 2006;354:2443–2451.

Lerner DS, Kannel W. Patterns of heart disease morbidity and mortality in the sexes: a 26-year follow-up of the Framingham population. *Am Heart J*. 1986;111:383–390.

Mosca L, Banka CL, Benjamin CA, et al. Evidence-based guidelines for cardiovascular disease prevention in women: 2007 update. *J Am Coll Cardiol*. 2007;49:1230–1250.

Ridker PM, Cook NR, Lee IM, et al. A randomized trial of low-dose aspirin in the primary prevention of cardiovascular disease in women. *N Engl J Med*. 2005;352:1293–1304.

Sharkey SW, Lesser JR, Zenovich AG, et al. Acute and reversible cardiomyopathy provoked by stress in women from the United States. *Circulation*. 2005;111:472–479.

Winkleby MA, Robinson TN, Sundquist J, et al. Ethnic variations in cardiovascular disease risk factors among children and young adults: findings from the third national health and nutrition examination survey, 1988–1994. *JAMA*. 1999;281:1006–1013.

CHAPTER (52)

Heart Disease and Pregnancy

Craig S. Broberg and John H. McAnulty

HEART DISEASE ISSUES UNIQUE TO PREGNANCY

Heart disease is the second most common cause of maternal death in Western countries (suicide is first). The health of the developing fetus is predominantly determined by the health of the mother, and thus the safety of the mother should be the highest priority. Some conditions are so risky to mother that pregnancy is contraindicated (Table 52-1). For others, treatment of maternal heart disease can potentially jeopardize the fetus. Certain diagnostic studies, drugs, or interventions may potentially increase fetal loss, result in teratogenicity, or alter fetal growth. Even when labor is successful, the newborn still faces challenges of poor maternal health, with its many implications, or even premature loss of a mother due to heart disease. All these issues are best discussed with a patient well before pregnancy is considered, wherein the risks and expectations are fully discussed by experienced providers so a woman and her partner can make an informed decision about this serious but rewarding personal venture. Each patient deserves a clear plan for labor and delivery laid out in advance by a team of qualified obstetricians, cardiologists, anesthesiologists, and pediatricians.

CLINICAL CONSIDERATIONS

【 】 PRECONCEPTION

Antenatal care should include a discussion of the vulnerability issues explored above. The patient should be told which medications to avoid during pregnancy, and plans made for alternative therapies. Warfarin, angiotensin-converting enzyme (ACE) inhibitors, and angiotensin II receptor blockers (ARBs) should be stopped. Any needed diagnostic tests or interventions should be performed before the risk to the fetus becomes a factor.

【 】 FIRST TRIMESTER

Organ development in the fetus begins at 3 weeks, before some women even know they are pregnant. As soon as pregnancy is confirmed, the patient should be seen by an experienced provider, and coordinated treatment plans made for the entire gestation. Issues to address include warning symptoms, need for scheduled imaging, optimal site for delivery, and plans for delivery. Aspirin should be started in cyanotic patients. Heparin should be used in place of warfarin if necessary.

TABLE 52-1

Cardiovascular Abnormalities Placing a Mother and Infant
at Extremely High Risk

Absolute Contraindications to Pregnancy

Pulmonary hypertension from any cause
Reduced systolic function (LVEF < 35%) with congestive failure
Marfan's syndrome with native aorta > 40 mm

Relative Contraindications/High-Risk Situations

Cyanotic congenital heart disease in the absence of pulmonary hypertension
Prosthetic valve
Unrepaired coarctation of the aorta
Marfan's syndrome with native aorta < 40 mm
Reduced systolic function (LVEF < 35%) in asymptomatic women
Severe obstructive lesions (AS, MS, etc)

LVEF, left ventricular ejection fraction; AS, aortic stenosis; MS, mitral stenosis.

【 】 SECOND AND THIRD TRIMESTER

The expected hemodynamic changes associated with pregnancy reach their peak near the 20th week (Table 52-2). Women should be advised of the likely sensation of dyspnea. An obstetrician should monitor fetal growth and determine the need for fetal echocardiography. Patients needing anticoagulation may be transitioned back to warfarin until labor.

TABLE 52-2

Expected Hemodynamic Alterations During Normal Pregnancy

Variable	Expected Change
Cardiac output	Increases more than 40%. Peaks by midgestation. Can be affected by body position. Goes up further during labor and uterine contraction. Epidural anesthesia will reduce CO
Heart rate	Small increase gradually throughout gestation
Stroke volume	40% increase (main cause of increased cardiac output)
Blood pressure	Falls slightly in early pregnancy, then gradually increases during the remainder of gestation
Hematocrit	Decreases a few percentage points (30% of normal values maximum) because of increased plasma volume
Total body water	Increases by 6–8 liters (mostly extracellular)
Blood volume	Plasma volume increases greater than RBC volume, hence overall reduction in hematocrit
Ejection fraction	No change expected
Ventricular volume	Slight increase (increased cardiac output and stroke volume).
Oxygen consumption	Increases 20% in first 20 weeks. 30% increase by time of delivery

【 】 LABOR AND DELIVERY

Labor and delivery place great demands on the cardiovascular system, and management must be optimized. Warfarin should be stopped in favor of heparin. Vaginal delivery is usually preferred in most patients with heart disease. Caesarean section is not safer hemodynamically. The second stage of labor should not be excessively painful or prolonged, and thus a premeditated plan for epidural anesthesia and assisted delivery (forceps or vacuum suction) to shorten the second stage is best for most patients. In most cases, lumbar epidural anesthesia using low-dose techniques for cardiostability with a pudendal nerve block to minimize pain is effective, least likely to result in hemodynamic compromise, and should be favored over general anesthesia. Induced labor or Caesarean section should be reserved for obstetrical indications or worsening cardiovascular function. Exceptions to this may include patients with extremely high-risk heart disease including Eisenmenger's syndrome and Marfan's syndrome with aortic root dilation. An appropriately planned early delivery may be performed when the fetus is adequately mature, in an effort to shorten gestation and minimize risk. Oxytocin should be avoided or used with caution because of potential hypotension. Antibiotic prophylaxis against bacterial endocarditis is practiced by many experienced centers although not formally recommended.

【 】 POSTPARTUM

Successful delivery does not mean the mother is out of danger. A large proportion of maternal deaths occur more than 1 week postdelivery. Hemodynamic and ECG monitoring should be continued for 48 to 72 hours in those with severe abnormalities (e.g., pulmonary hypertension, cyanotic lesions, severe obstructive lesions, or a severe cardiomyopathy). Sometimes the new mother is reluctant to comply with recommended monitoring. Important changes in clotting factors normally prevent excessive uterine bleeding, but these changes can disrupt the fragile thrombostasis, especially in cyanotic patients.

CARDIOVASCULAR CHANGES DURING PREGNANCY

The added demands on the cardiovascular system during pregnancy require several adaptations (Table 52-2). The presence of cardiovascular abnormalities, therefore, can impair or aggravate these adaptations to the potential detriment of mother or fetus. In general, physiologic changes are better tolerated in patients with volume overload lesions (valvular regurgitation or shunts), than in patients with fixed output (obstructive valves, coarctation, or pulmonary hypertension).

DIAGNOSTIC STUDIES

A number of clinical tools used in cardiovascular assessment are available and safe in the setting of pregnancy (Table 52-3). Interpretation demands an understanding of the normal physiologic changes during pregnancy (Table 52-2), and consideration of the gestational age at the time of the study. Tests involving radiation, particularly CT, are considered unsafe. However, the benefits of diagnostic clarity offered may offset the potential harm from radiation exposure, which can be minimized with shielding.

CARDIOVASCULAR DRUGS AND PREGNANCY

Nearly all cardiac drugs cross the placenta and are secreted in breast milk. Because information about the use of any drug is incomplete, it is best to avoid drug use, but if

TABLE 52-3

Safety Considerations of Cardiovascular Diagnostic Tests During Pregnancy

Study	Safety	Comments
Electrocardiogram	Safe	ST-T wave changes are common and hence interpretation for new ischemic changes is difficult
Chest x-ray	Safe	Radiation exposure is below that expected to cause fetal damage
Transthoracic echocardiogram	Safe	Chamber dimensions and velocity measurements need to be interpreted considering expected hemodynamic changes
Transesophageal echocardiogram	Safe	Some risks from sedation and recumbent position
MRI	Safe	Gadolinium should not be used, however
CT	Unsafe	Radiation exposure increases the risk of abnormal fetal organogenesis or of a subsequent malignancy in the child, particularly leukemia. Standard risks of contrast nephropathy in vulnerable patients
Nuclear	Unsafe	As above, radiation exposure increases risk. Should weigh risks against potential benefit of the diagnostic information

required for maternal safety, drugs should not be withheld. Many common cardiology drugs are listed (Table 52-4) and providers are encouraged to seek additional detail when any drug is used.

MANAGEMENT OF COMPLICATIONS

【 】 VOLUME MANAGEMENT

A low cardiac output is most often caused by intravascular volume depletion. This is particularly dangerous in those with lesions that limit blood flow, such as pulmonary hypertension, aortic or pulmonic valve stenosis, hypertrophic cardiomyopathy, or mitral stenosis. Measures to prevent or treat a fall in central blood volume are outlined (Table 52-5). Hyperemesis gravidarum may aggravate low volume states. If so, intravenous fluids, antiemetics such as *ondansetron*, even in chronic pump infusions, can be required. Conversely, there are conditions where diuretic therapy is necessary, such as mitral stenosis, and aortic stenosis. Diuretics should always be used with care and recognition of the normal need for relative hypervolemia during pregnancy.

【 】 THROMBOEMBOLISM

The risk of venous thromboemboli increases fivefold during and immediately after pregnancy simply as a result of the relative hypercoagulable status and venous stasis. In most patients with heart disease, the risk is even higher. Prophylactic full dose heparin or low-molecular-weight heparin are indicated in those at high risk including (1) thromboemboli during a previous pregnancy and (2) documented hypercoagulable state (antithrombin III deficiency, protein C or S deficiency, factor V *homozygosity*, or anticardiolipin antibody

TABLE 52-4

General Guidelines on Relative Safety of Certain Medications in Pregnancy

Drugs	Safety Profile	Comments
Diuretics	Safe	Avoid hypovolemia
Dopamine/ dobutamine	Unknown	Probably safe, but likely affect uterine blood flow also
Ephedrine	Safe	Presumed safer than other inotropic agents because in animal models ephedrine has no effect on uterine blood flow
Beta-Blockers		
Atenolol/ metoprolol/ bisoprolol	Probably safe	Although warnings report a risk of intrauterine growth retardation, cause/effect relationship is uncertain, and drugs are used widely without reported problems.
Labetolol	Safe	Sometimes used for pregnancy-related hypertension.
Calcium-Channel Blockers		
Dihydropyridines	Safe	No reported problems.
Non-dihydropyridines	Safe	Can cause uterine relaxation.
Antiarrhythmics		
Amiodarone	Unsafe	Fetal thyroid abnormalities, fetal loss and deformity.
Digoxin	Safe	Sometimes used to treat fetal arrhythmia; crosses placenta.
Flecainide	Safe	
Sotalol	Safe	
Lidocaine	Safe	Probably preferred first-line IV agent.
Procainamide	Safe	
Antihypertensives		
ACE inhibitors	Unsafe	Fetal renal abnormalities.
ARBs	Probably unsafe	Presumed risk of fetal renal abnormalities, case reports only.
Nitroprusside	Uncertain	Effective IV antihypertensive and considered safe, though concerns of fetal cyanide poisoning exist from use in late gestation.
Hydralazine	Probably safe	Maternal hypotension reported.
Anticoagulants/Antiplatelet		
Warfarin	Unsafe in first trimester	Warfarin embryopathy from use in first trimester; risk is dose-related (greater if > 5 mg/d). May be safely used in second or third trimester, but should be avoided during labor and delivery.
Heparin	Probably safe	Increased risk of maternal bleeding. Monitoring can be more difficult during pregnancy.

TABLE 52-4

General Guidelines on Relative Safety of Certain Medications in Pregnancy (*Continued*)

Drugs	Safety Profile	Comments
Low-molecular-weight heparin	Probably safe	Needs dose titration with measured factor Xa levels, which can be difficult. Unproven in patients with prosthetic valves, and adverse events have been reported due to improper monitoring.
Aspirin	Probably safe	Associated with fetal growth retardation and loss, but widely used in certain circumstances.
Plavix	Unknown	Anecdotal experience only.

syndrome). For patients with a mechanical prosthetic valve, a careful plan for anticoagulation is mandatory.

 HYPERTENSION

There is no consensus as to what blood pressure should be considered too high. Though 160/105 mm Hg has been cited as a threshold for instigating therapy, many would instigate treatment earlier. Bed rest may not be enough to lower pressure. When associated with proteinuria, pedal edema, CNS irritability, elevation of liver enzymes, and coagulation disturbances, the hypertension syndrome is called *preeclampsia*. If convulsions occur, the diagnosis is *eclampsia*. It is not clear that hypertension alone puts the mother or fetus at risk during pregnancy, but preeclampsia increases maternal risk (1%–2% chance of CNS bleed, convulsions, or other severe systemic illness) and can cause fetal growth retardation (10%–15% chance). Maternal and fetal morbidity and mortality increase still

TABLE 52-5

Measures to Protect Against a Decrease in Central Blood Volume

Acute

Position
- 45–60 degrees left lateral
- 10 degrees Trendelenburg

Volume administration—glucose-free saline

Drugs—ephedrine if unresponsive to fluid replacement

Anesthetics (if required)
- Regional: serial small boluses
- General: emphasis on benzodiazepines and narcotics, low-dose inhalation agents

Chronic

Full leg stockings

Avoid vasodilatation drugs

further with eclampsia. Keeping the systolic blood pressure below 160 mm Hg and the diastolic below 100 mm Hg provides a margin of safety against severe hypertensive episodes. Unless the patient has previously demonstrated salt-sensitive hypertension, sodium restriction is inadvisable. Pharmacotherapy with labetolol or hydralazine is often indicated. Avoid over-aggressive blood pressure lowering. ACE inhibitors and ARBs *should not be used.*

【 】 ARRHYTHMIA

The rules for treatment should be the same as in the nonpregnant patient with the possible exception that a rhythm causing hemodynamic instability should be treated somewhat more rapidly because of concern about diversion of blood flow away from the uterus. As always, if a potentially reversible cause can be identified, it should be corrected.

Atrial or *ventricular premature beats* or *sinus tachycardia* are all very common. In isolation, they do not require specific treatment, but should prompt a search for any potential underlying cause. *Paroxysmal supraventricular tachycardia* is the most common sustained abnormal rhythm occurring with pregnancy. Initial treatment with vagal maneuvers to disrupt the rhythm is warranted. Intravenous adenosine or verapamil are safe, as is electrical cardioversion if required. If recurrent episodes necessitate a daily drug, verapamil or a beta-blocker is often effective. Management of *atrial fibrillation* and *flutter* should be as in the nonpregnant woman, including considerations of anticoagulation. Specifically, mitral stenosis, severe left ventricular (LV) dysfunction, or a previous thromboembolic event requires antithrombotic therapy.

Emergency management of rapid *ventricular tachycardia* or *ventricular fibrillation* should be as recommended for the nonpregnant woman, and prompt a thorough hemodynamic and metabolic review for an underlying cause. During acute management, the woman should be rolled to her left side to enhance blood return from the lower extremities. Situations vary, but a malignant ventricular arrhythmia may justify early Caesarean delivery. Conditions predisposing to ventricular arrhythmia (Brugada syndrome, arrhythmogenic right ventricular dysplaisa, or long QT syndromes) are not well studied during pregnancy. If QT prolongation is present, the presumed cause should be eliminated. Otherwise, management should generally be directed by the clinical situation. Pregnancies have been successful in women with implanted cardioverter/defibrillators; treatment shocks have no demonstrated adverse effects on the baby.

Bradyarrhythmias can occur during pregnancy. Although they are a reason to look for a reversible cause, treatment is generally not required unless the patient has clear hemodynamic compromise. Complete heart block, which in this age group is most likely to be congenital in origin, is consistent with a successful pregnancy. If required, a permanent pacemaker can be inserted.

If a seizure is unlikely or excluded, *syncope* is usually related to volume imbalance or arrhythmia, and treatment should focus on the potential underlying cause.

VALVULAR HEART DISEASE

【 】 MITRAL VALVE DISEASE

Mitral stenosis is typically the most poorly tolerated of any valve lesion during pregnancy. The increased cardiac output, relative tachycardia, and fluid retention of pregnancy can double the resting pressure gradient across a stenotic mitral valve. Symptoms become apparent by the 20th week and can be aggravated still further at the time of labor and delivery. Maternal death is rare when there is careful attention to the management of congestive heart failure. If mitral stenosis is first recognized during pregnancy and symptoms develop, careful fluid management is key. If diuretics do not control symptoms of dyspnea or pulmonary edema, balloon valvuloplasty can be performed. Mitral valve surgical commissurotomy or valve replacement has been performed, but fetal loss exceeds 30%. Atrial fibrillation is common and can be managed with verapamil and/or cardioversion if necessary. In contrast, chronic *mitral regurgitation* is well tolerated during pregnancy. Afterload reduction is an important component of therapy, remembering that ACE inhibitors and ARBs should not be used. Echocardiograms may show trends toward worse valvular regurgitation during gestation, though this likely reflects changes in volume rather than structural worsening. Unless the patient has severe cardiovascular dysfunction, decisions about mitral valve repair or replacement should not be made until several months after pregnancy when hemodynamics has returned to baseline.

【　】 AORTIC VALVE DISEASE

Pregnancy in the presence of *aortic stenosis* can be successful, but if stenosis is severe, maternal deaths have occurred and congestive heart failure is common. Bicuspid aortic valve is the most common cause; thus any coarctation of the aorta and/or an ascending aortic aneurysm should be excluded in all patients. Patients with Turner's syndrome who conceive through artificial means should be especially considered in this regard. If aortic stenosis is severe, measures to avoid hypovolemia are particularly important. If congestive heart failure develops, or if fetal growth retardation becomes an issue, balloon valvuloplasty or aortic valve surgery can be performed with risk of acute aortic regurgitation. Aortic valve surgery can be performed during pregnancy, if the mother is threatened, though with increased fetal loss. *Aortic regurgitation* may be due to an enlarged aorta (including Marfan's syndrome) and/or a bicuspid valve. Like mitral regurgitation, it tends to be better tolerated. If congestive heart failure occurs with pregnancy, treatment should include afterload reduction. *ACE inhibitors and ARBs should be avoided.* If endocarditis should occur and the infection is not rapidly controlled, mortality with medical therapy is high, and surgical therapy is indicated.

【　】 PROSTHETIC VALVE DISEASE

Thromboemboli, maternal or fetal hemorrhage (from anticoagulation), endocarditis, or valve dysfunction may all contribute to substantial morbidity during pregnancy from a prosthetic valve, which is considered a relative contraindication to pregnancy. Mitral prostheses carry the highest risk. Anticoagulation is required. Although debate exists over the optimal means of anticoagulation, current guidelines are shown (Table 52-6). In essence, the guidelines recommend heparin for the first trimester, then warfarin until the 35th week, and then a return to heparin through labor and delivery, with overlap when transitioning from warfarin to heparin. Full-dose subcutaneous heparin should be dose-adjusted to maintain a "high therapeutic level" by following factor Xa levels. Low-molecular-weight heparin is an appealing alternative, but has not been extensively evaluated in patients with prosthetic valves.

SPECIFIC SITUATIONS

【　】 CONGENITAL HEART DISEASE

For the most part, simple shunts such as *atrial septal defects, ventricular septal defects,* or *patent ductus arteriosus,* whether closed or open, are consistent with a successful pregnancy. Arrhythmias are the most common complications. The major exceptions are patients with large shunts who have Eisenmenger's syndrome. Patients with *atrioventricular septal defects* may have left atrioventricular valve (mitral) regurgitation, left ventricular outflow tract obstruction, or conduction abnormalities that can cause

TABLE 52-6

Therapeutic Guidelines for Pregnant Patients with Mechanical Prosthetic Valves[a]

Class I

1. All pregnant patients with mechanical prosthetic valves must receive continuous therapeutic anticoagulation with frequent monitoring. *(Level of Evidence: B)*
2. For women requiring long-term warfarin therapy who are attempting pregnancy, pregnancy tests should be monitored with discussions about subsequent anticoagulation therapy, so that anticoagulation can be continued uninterrupted when pregnancy is achieved. *(Level of Evidence: C)*
3. Pregnant patients with mechanical prosthetic valves who elect to stop warfarin between weeks 6 and 12 of gestation should receive continuous intravenous UFH, dose-adjusted UFH, or dose-adjusted subcutaneous LMWH. *(Level of Evidence: C)*
4. For pregnant patients with mechanical prosthetic valves, up to 36 weeks of gestation, the therapeutic choice of continuous intravenous or dose-adjusted subcutaneous UFH, dose-adjusted LMWH, or warfarin should be discussed fully. If continuous intravenous UFH is used, the fetal risk is lower, but the maternal risks of prosthetic valve thrombosis, systemic embolization, infection, osteoporosis, and heparin-induced thrombocytopenia are relatively higher. *(Level of Evidence: C)*
5. In pregnant patients with mechanical prosthetic valves who receive dose-adjusted LMWH, the LMWH should be administered twice daily subcutaneously to maintain the anti-Xa level between 0.7 and 1.2 U/mL 4 h after administration. *(Level of Evidence: C)*
6. In pregnant patients with mechanical prosthetic valves who receive dose-adjusted UFH, the aPTT should be at least twice control. *(Level of Evidence: C)*
7. In pregnant patients with mechanical prosthetic valves who receive warfarin, the INR goal should be 3.0 (range, 2.5–3.5). *(Level of Evidence: C)*
8. In pregnant patients with mechanical prosthetic valves, warfarin should be discontinued and continuous intravenous UFH given starting 2 to 3 weeks before planned delivery. *(Level of Evidence: C)*

Class IIA

1. In patients with mechanical prosthetic valves, it is reasonable to avoid warfarin between weeks 6 and 12 of gestation, owing to the high risk of fetal defects. *(Level of Evidence: C)*
2. In patients with mechanical prosthetic valves, it is reasonable to resume UFH 4 to 6 h after delivery and begin oral warfarin in the absence of significant bleeding. *(Level of Evidence: C)*
3. In patients with mechanical prosthetic valves, it is reasonable to give low-dose aspirin (75–100 mg/d) in the second and third trimesters of pregnancy in addition to anticoagulation with warfarin or heparin. *(Level of Evidence: C)*

Class III

1. LMWH should not be administered to pregnant patients with mechanical prosthetic valves unless anti-Xa levels are monitored 4 to 6 h after administration. *(Level of Evidence: C)*

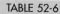

TABLE 52-6

Therapeutic Guidelines for Pregnant Patients with Mechanical Prosthetic Valves (*Continued*)

Class III
1. LMWH should not be administered to pregnant patients with mechanical prosthetic valves unless anti-Xa levels are monitored 4 to 6 h after administration. (*Level of Evidence: C*)
2. Dipyridamole should not be used instead of aspirin as an alternative antiplatelet agent in pregnant patients with mechanical prosthetic valves because of its harmful effects on the fetus. (*Level of Evidence: B*)

PTT, activated partial thromboplastin time; INR, international normalized ratio; LMWH, low-molecular weight heparin; UFH, unfractionated heparin.

*a*See also Chapter 59.

Reproduced with permission from Bonow RO, Carabello BA, Chatterjee K, et al. ACC/AHA 2006 guidelines for the management of patients with valvular heart disease: a report of the American College of Cardiology/American Heart Association Task Force on Practice Guidelines (Writing Committee to Revise the 1998 Guidelines for the Management of Patients with Valvular Heart Disease). Developed in collaboration with the Society of Cardiovascular Anesthesiologists. Endorsed by the Society for Cardiovascular Angiography and Interventions and the Society of Thoracic Surgeons. *J Am Coll Cardiol.* 2006;48:e1–e148.

complications, and pregnancy success depends largely on the presence and severity of these associated lesions.

Generally any obstructive lesion is less well tolerated during pregnancy than a regurgitant lesion. *Subaortic stenosis* from a discrete membrane should be considered similarly to aortic stenosis. *Hypertrophic obstructive cardiomyopathy* (HOCM), with dynamic outflow obstruction, can worsen during pregnancy. The fall in peripheral vascular resistance and peripheral pooling of blood during pregnancy can cause hypotension, and the intermittent high catecholamine state of pregnancy can increase LV outflow tract obstruction. Pregnancy-related deaths have been reported. This is another obstructive lesion where it is important to avoid hypovolemia. Beta-blocker therapy is recommended at the time of labor and delivery.

Safety of pregnancy in *aortic coarctation*, whether or not previously repaired, largely depends on the severity of hypertension, ascending aortic aneurysm, stenosis or restenosis at the coarct site, and the possible presence of intracranial aneurysms. For all of these reasons, blood pressure control is key, typically using beta-blockers (often labetolol). Catheter dilation can be performed if necessary. Patients with *Turner's syndrome* may fall into this category after artificial insemination and should be followed closely.

Tetralogy of Fallot is generally compatible with successful pregnancy. Significant pulmonary valve regurgitation should be excluded and fixed preemptively, particularly if exercise capacity is below 75% of predicted. Many patients are at risk for ventricular tachycardia and should be monitored. *Pulmonary atresia with VSD* is similar.

Maternal *cyanosis* is associated with high fetal loss, prematurity, and reduced infant birthweights. When pulmonary hypertension is not present, maternal mortality is significantly less, but women are at increased risk of heart failure, thromboemboli, and arrhythmias. Aspirin is recommended and early delivery if the situation warrants because of maternal clinical deterioration.

In *Eisenmenger's syndrome*, or cyanosis caused by reversed or bidirectional shunting from elevated pulmonary vascular resistance, pregnancy is strictly contraindicated, and it is advisable to offer interruption of pregnancy early on if conception occurs. A woman who opts to continue should be put on bed rest, heparin, and oxygen for at least the third trimester at an experienced facility, and be monitored closely in the postpartum period.

Most patients with *transposition of the great arteries* (either congenitally corrected TGA or complete TGA with prior atrial redirection surgery) will have a systemic right ventricle, which is prone to dysfunction. Systemic AV valve regurgitation, arrhythmias, and conduction abnormalities are also common. The success of pregnancy in these patients largely depends on attention to these issues. The majority of patients do well if ventricular function is not significantly impaired. Younger women with D-TGA may have been treated with an arterial switch operation and will have a systemic left ventricle, and experience with pregnancy is scarcely reported. Issues here are RVOT obstruction and potential coronary artery problems.

Patients with a *single functional ventricle* will usually have been palliated with some variant of the *Fontan procedure*, where venous blood flows passively to the pulmonary capillary bed. They are complex patients at high risk for venous thromboembolism, atrial arrhythmia, and low-output heart failure, as well as complications related to chronic elevation of central venous pressure including hepatic congestion and protein-losing enteropathy. All should be managed at an appropriate center with experience with such patients. Heart failure or arrhythmia may occur in 10% to 20% of pregnant patients, with a high rate of fetal loss. Still, many do well despite the abnormal circulation. Consideration to anticoagulation should be given especially in late gestation or if circumstances warrant, such as prior atrial arrhythmia or documented atrial thrombus, though routine use of anticoagulation without a clear indication is not necessary.

Women with *Marfan's syndrome* are at risk of death from aortic rupture or dissection especially peripartum. Pregnancy in a woman with a root ≥ 40 mm is contraindicated. Prophylactic use of beta-blockers during pregnancy is generally advised, as well as careful monitoring of the root and valve during gestation.

【 】 PULMONARY HYPERTENSION

Severe *pulmonary arterial hypertension* (PAH) from any cause is a contraindication to pregnancy. Obviously gradations of severity are encountered, and the risk is more substantial in women with near systemic level pressures. If PAH is recognized early enough, interruption of the pregnancy is advised. If this is declined or if the PAH is recognized late in pregnancy, patients should be referred to a tertiary care center with experience with these high-risk patients. Successful use of pulmonary vasodilators has been reported with increasing frequency.

【 】 MYOCARDIAL DYSFUNCTION

Myocardial systolic dysfunction (LV ejection fraction <35%) is considered a contraindication to pregnancy. This includes patients with idiopathic dilated cardiomyopathy, congenital heart disease, or prior *peripartum cardiomyopathy* with persistent systolic dysfunction. If pregnancy is pursued, standard treatment for heart failure, thromboemboli, and arrhythmias is appropriate. Patients should be followed closely and hospital admission late in gestation considered.

【 】 ISCHEMIC HEART DISEASE

Chest discomfort is common during a normal pregnancy and for the most part is caused by abdominal distension or gastroesophageal reflux. Coronary artery disease in pregnancy can result from atherosclerosis, particularly in those with familial hyperlipidemia, diabetes, hypertension, cocaine use, or smoking. Other explanations have been dissection of the coronary artery, spasm, emboli, vasculitis, or anomalous origin of a left coronary artery. Stress imaging without radiation (echocardiography or MRI) is preferred for evaluation if necessary. When demonstrated, significant epicardial CAD should be treated with standard medical therapy. Angioplasty or bypass surgery can be performed at an experienced center.

SUGGESTED READING

Avila WS, Rossi EG, Ramires JA, et al. Pregnancy in patients with heart disease: experience with 1,000 cases. *Clin Cardiol.* 2003;26:135–142.

Capeless EL, Clapp JF. Cardiovascular changes in early phase of pregnancy. *Am J Obstet Gynecol.* 1989;161:1449–1453.

Hameed A, Karaalp IS, Tummala PP, et al. The effect of valvular heart disease on maternal and fetal outcome of pregnancy. *J Am Coll Cardiol.* 2001;37:893–899.

Hung L, Rahimtoola SH. Prosthetic heart valves and pregnancy. *Circulation.* 2003;107: 1240–1246.

Kron J, Conti JB. Arrhythmias in the pregnant patient: current concepts in evaluation and management. *J Interv Card Electrophysiol.* 2007;19:95–107.

Lupton M, Oteng-Ntim E, Ayida G, et al. Cardiac disease in pregnancy. *Curr Opin Obstet Gynecol.* 2002;14:137–143.

Siu SC, Sermer M, Coleman JM, et al. Prospective multicenter study of pregnancy outcomes in women with heart disease. *Circulation.* 2001;104:515–521.

Swan L, Lupton M, Anthony J, et al. Controversies in pregnancy and congenital heart disease. *Congenit Heart Dis.* 2006;1:27–34.

Uebing A, Steer PJ, Yentis SM, et al. Pregnancy and congenital heart disease. *BMJ.* 2006.

Wagner SJ, Barac S, Garovic VD. Hypertensive pregnancy disorders: current concepts. *J Clin Hypertens* (Greenwich). 2007;9:560–566. In press.

CHAPTER 53

The Heart and Obesity

H. Robert Superko and Lakshmana K. Pendyala

Obesity and its associated metabolic syndrome are the most important contributors to premature arterial aging. Obesity, excess accumulation of body fat, is important due to its adverse affect on cardiovascular health, rapidly increasing prevalence, and the future cardiovascular health of the population. This is related to changes in dietary and physical activity patterns that often accompany economic prosperity but, paradoxically, promote increased cardiovascular disease (CVD). Much of this problem is related to the concept of an adverse gene/environment interaction. The rapid and widespread increase in obesity has reached epidemic proportions in the United States (Fig. 53-1). For most individuals, it is chronic, relapsing, and multifactorial in origin. An estimated 122 million (65%) adults in the United States are overweight or obese and 59 million (31%) are obese.

Obesity is an important risk factor for coronary heart disease (CHD), ventricular dysfunction, congestive heart failure, stroke, obstructive sleep apnea, and cardiac arrhythmias. Weight loss in obese patients can be improved or prevented by many of the obesity-related risk factors for CHD (i.e., insulin resistance and type 2 diabetes mellitus, dyslipidemia, hypertension, and inflammation; Fig. 53-2), and can improve diastolic function. Therefore, it is important for health care professionals to understand the clinical effects of weight loss and be able to implement appropriate weight-management strategies in obese patients.

RELEVANT STATISTICS

- 1980: 14.5% of the U.S. population were defined as obese.
- 2003: 32.2% of the U.S. population were defined as obese (110% increase).
- 1980: 46% of the U.S. population had combined overweight (body mass index [BMI] > 25 kg/m^2) + obesity (BMI > 30 kg/m^2).
- 2003: 65% of the U.S. population had combined overweight (BMI > 25 kg/m^2) + obesity (BMI > 30 kg/m^2) (41% increase).
- Disproportionately high in black and Hispanic women as well as Asian and Pacific Islanders, Native Americans, Native Alaskans, and Native Hawaiians.
- Between 1960 and 1980, the percentage of obese adults varied little.
- Between 1980 and 2004, the prevalence of obesity increased (Fig. 53-3).
- Between 1994 and 2000, the percentage of persons with BMI > 25 kg/m^2 increased from 56% to 64%.
- Increase in overweight status in children and adolescents is alarming.
- Degree of obesity is related to years of life lost.
- 20-year-olds to 30-year-olds with a BMI of 30 to 35 have 5 years of life lost.

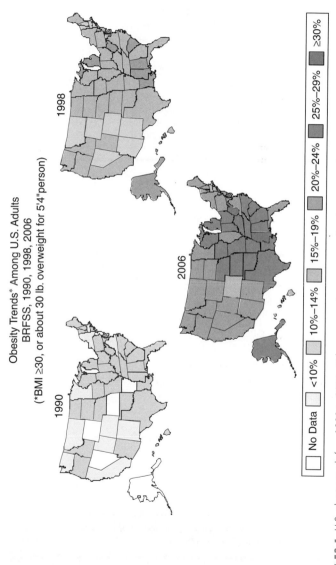

Obesity Trends* Among U.S. Adults
BRFSS, 1990, 1998, 2006
(*BMI ≥30, or about 30 lb. overweight for 5'4"person)

1990

1998

2006

No Data   <10%   10%–14%   15%–19%   20%–24%   25%–29%   ≥30%

FIGURE 53-1. U.S. obesity trends from 1990 to 2006. Colors represent the percentage of each state's population determined to be obese as defined by BMI >30. (http://www.cdc.gov/nccdphp/dnpa/obesity/trend/.)

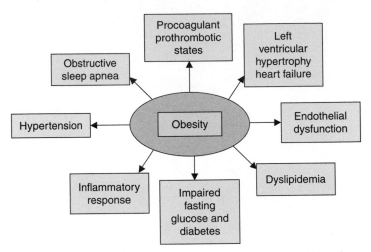

FIGURE 53-2. Interaction of obesity on various other cardiovascular comorbid conditions.

- 20-year-olds to 30-year-olds with a BMI of 35 to 40 have 7 years of life lost.
- Each year an estimated 300,000 American adults die of causes related to obesity.
- $42 billion dollars in direct costs for obesity-related CV disease.
- $30 billion dollars in indirect costs for obesity-related CV disease.
- 17% of all CHD costs related to obesity.

Some specific syndromes are associated with obesity and should be eliminated as treatable causes of obesity in the appropriate patient. These disorders include Cushing's

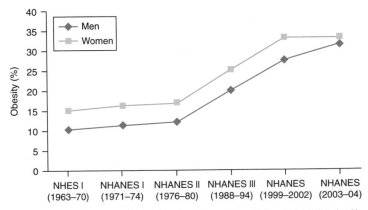

FIGURE 53-3. Percentage of U.S. adults classified as obese (BMI ≥ 30 kg/m²) in health surveys from 1963 to 2004. (NHES, National Health Examination Survey; NHANES, National Health and Nutrition Examination Survey.) (http://www.cdc.gov/nccdphp/dnpa/obesity/trend/.)

> ### TABLE 53-1
>
> Endocrine Diseases Associated with Obesity
>
> Hypothalamic disorders
> Pituitary dysfunction
> Thyroid (hypothyroidism)
> Adrenal (Cushing's syndrome)
> Ovary (polycystic ovarian syndrome)
> Type 2 diabetes

syndrome, hypothyroidism, insulinoma, craniopharyngioma, and other hypothalamus disorders (Table 53-1). Appropriate diagnostic tests should be undertaken to screen for these disorders.

Sleep apnea may contribute to CV complications of obesity and may include:

- Diurnal hypertension
- Nocturnal arrhythmias
- Pulmonary hypertension
- Right and left ventricular failure
- Myocardial infarction
- Stroke
- Increased mortality

DEFINITION

Although not a direct measure of adiposity, body mass index (weight in kilograms/height in meters squared) is a common measure of body fatness used in clinical trials and can be estimated as (weight in pounds/height in inches squared) × 703. Obesity can be defined as a body mass index > 30. CAD risk increases even with mild increases in BMI. In middle-aged women a BMI > 23 but < 25 has a 50% increase in risk for nonfatal or fatal CAD, and in middle-aged men a BMI > 25 but < 29 has a 72% increase in risk (Table 53-2). Use of BMI can be misleading since it does not account for body fat distribution. Likewise, the use of waist circumference to define overweight status can be misleading due to size and anthropomorphic characteristics of individuals. Medically important obesity is an individual excess amount of body fat that contributes to metabolic disturbances, which in turn contribute to increased CVD risk.

【 】 ASSESSMENT OF BODY FAT

Multiple techniques are used to assess the degree of obesity, and each has strengths and weaknesses. Hydrostatic weighing is the "gold standard." However, limitations include the lack of information regarding anatomic fat location, the equipment necessary to accurately conduct a study including an underwater weighing tank, equipment needed to determine pulmonary residual volume by nitrogen dilution, and the ability of the subject to hold their breath underwater for 10 to 15 s on multiple runs. Body mass index (BMI) is used frequently but no indication of actual leanness or fatness can be determined. Skinfold measurements rely on multiple caliper-determined skinfold thicknesses and a mathematical formula that approximates the calculated number to a percent body fat compared to hydrostatic weighing. One measure of the waist-to-hip

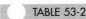

TABLE 53-2

Classification of Overweight Status by BMI and Waist-to-Hip Ratio in Men and Women

			Disease Risk	
Classification	BMI	Obesity Class	Men ≤ 1.0 Women ≤ 0.8	> 1.0 > 0.8
Underweight	≤18.5 kg/m²			
Normal weight	18.5–24.9 kg/m²			
Overweight	25–29.9 kg/m²		Increased	High
Obesity	30–34.9 kg/m²	Class I	High	Very high
Obesity	35–39.9 kg/m²	Class II	Very high	Very high
Extreme obesity	≥40 kg/m²	Class III	Extremely high	Extremely high

ratio (WHR) is the circumference of the waist divided by the circumference of the hips. A WHR > 1.0 in men and > 0.8 in women predicts the complications from obesity independent of BMI.

EFFECTS ON THE HEART

【 】 CARDIAC OUTPUT

Because of the need to move excess body weight, the cardiac workload and output are greater for obese subjects than for nonobese individuals at any given level of activity. The high cardiac output is mostly attributable to increased stroke volume and lower total peripheral resistance because the heart rate increases little if at all. In obesity, left ventricular filling pressure and volume increase, shifting left ventricular function to the left on the Frank–Starling curve and inducing chamber dilatation. The myocardium adapts by increasing contractile elements and myocardial mass, resulting in left ventricular hypertrophy, often of the eccentric type. Diastolic dysfunction from eccentric hypertrophy and systolic dysfunction excessive wall stress results in so-called "obesity cardiomyopathy." Left atrial enlargement is also frequent in normotensive obese individuals and is associated with increased left ventricular mass. Provided that arterial pressure does not change, the increase in cardiac output is associated with a decrease in vascular resistance. When obesity and hypertension are present, obesity increases preload and hypertension postload. The heart of the obese hypertensive individual is now confronted with a double burden, which may result in early left ventricular dysfunction and premature heart failure. Obesity is also associated with persistence of elevated cardiac filling pressures. Loss of excess body fat is associated with beneficial cardiac adaptations (Table 53-3).

【 】 LEFT VENTRICULAR (LV) DYSFUNCTION

Duration of obesity is a strong predictor of heart failure. Components of obesity and the metabolic syndrome are associated with LV changes linked to heart failure. In hypertensive patients, left ventricular wall thickness is related to blood pressure and independently related to insulin sensitivity, which is often present in the obese patient. In young individuals, fasting insulin is an independent predictor of left ventricular mass, reflects an excessive load on the heart relatively early in life, and is associated with obesity and the

TABLE 53-3

Heart Adaptations to Weight Loss

↓	Resting oxygen consumption
↓	Cardiac output (↓ blood volume, ↓ stroke volume)
↓	Left ventricular mass
↓	Systemic arterial pressure
↓	Filling pressures of the right and the left side of the heart
↓	Resting heart rate
↓	QTc interval
↓	or no change in systemic arterial resistance

metabolic syndrome. Mortality rates of heart failure increase as a function of increased BMI. Obesity-related cardiomegaly and impaired function are often are reversible.

【 】 HYPERTENSION

Elevations in blood pressure have long been noted to be associated with an overweight status. A 10-kg higher body weight is associated with 3.0 mm Hg higher systolic and a 2.3 mm Hg higher diastolic blood pressure, and these increments translate into an estimated 12% increased risk for CHD and 24% increased risk for stroke. The link between hypertension and the metabolic syndrome is tightly linked to the central adiposity component of the syndrome. The Olivetti Heart Study reported that waist circumference was the strongest independent predictor of blood pressure, and its association with increased blood pressure was independent of BMI and insulin resistance.

EFFECT ON METABOLISM

Numerous adverse metabolic and hematologic abnormalities are associated with the overweight status (Table 53-4).

【 】 INSULIN RESISTANCE

The term "insulin resistance" is used to describe a metabolic state in which insulin action in the peripheral tissues is less efficient than normal, which results in increased insulin secretion in order to maintain normal blood glucose levels. Insulin resistance, a major component of the metabolic syndrome, is of particular interest to cardiologists because of a link to restenosis following angioplasty and stent placement in patients with elevated post-glucose-load insulin levels. An elevated post-glucose-load insulin value not only marks the insulin-resistant condition but is also linked to the atherogenic small LDL trait and restenosis risk.

Although obesity is related to insulin resistance, the European Group for the Study of Insulin Resistance has concluded that only approximately 25% of obese individuals can be classified as insulin resistant based on insulin-mediated glucose disposal. *Thus, not all overweight individuals are insulin resistant, and not all insulin-resistant individuals are overweight.*

Fasting plasma insulin concentrations, although less accurate than the euglycemic clamp technique, are a reasonable clinical alternative. Values <15 mU/L are considered normal, 15 to 20 mU/L borderline high, and >20 mU/L as high. Fasting glucose between 110 and 126 mg/dL is predictive of insulin resistance but is not a sensitive marker, and most subjects with insulin resistance have a fasting glucose <110 mg/dL.

TABLE 53-4

Metabolic, Hematologic, and Inflammatory Abnormalities Associated with Obesity

↑   Fasting triglycerides
↑   Small, dense LDL
↑   Apolipoprotein B
↑   Fibrinogen
↑   Factor VII activity
↑   Factor VIIIc activity
↑   TPA antigen
↑   PAI-1 antigen and activity
↑   Hs-CRP
↑   Cytokines
↑   TNF-α
↑   HDLC
↑   HDL$_2$ (impaired reverse cholesterol transport)

LDL, low-density lipoprotein; HDL, high-density lipoprotein; TPA, tissue plasminogen activator; PAI-1, plasminogen activator inhibitor; hs-CRP, high-sensitivity C-reactive protein.

Much like insulin resistance, the concept of *leptin resistance* has been proposed. Leptin is a hormone secreted from adipocytes that has an action on the central hypothalamic nuclei that affects consumption of calories and expenditure of body energy. A rich field of research exists in mouse models, but the exact role leptin plays in human obesity and CV risk remains unclear.

【　】 TYPE 2 DIABETES

The development of overt type 2 diabetes mellitus is the eventual conclusion of many obese patients and patients with the metabolic syndrome. Both cross-sectional and longitudinal studies show that abdominal obesity is a major risk factor for type 2 diabetes. The presence of type 2 diabetes is associated with the following:

• 1.5- to 3.0-fold increased CAD risk.

• In type 2 diabetic patients without clinical CAD, 79% of men and 70% of women have a high-grade coronary lesion.

• Type 2 diabetes is a CAD equivalent.

• Repeat revascularization following stent placement is significantly higher in diabetic versus nondiabetic patients.

• Dyslipidemia including the atherogenic lipoprotein profile (ALP).

• Arteriographic severity in type 2 diabetics is significantly related to the presence of intermediate-density and triglyceride-rich lipoproteins characteristic of ALP.

• Four randomized trials have indicated treatment of prediabetics can reduce the development of type 2 diabetes. Either intensive lifestyle or pharmacologic intervention can significantly reduce (25%–58%) the appearance of type 2 diabetes in high-risk individuals.

【　】 LIPID METABOLISM

A major sequel of the overweight status is a dyslipidemia, characterized by:

• Low HDL-C

• Low HDL$_2$

- Elevated fasting triglycerides
- Abundance of small, dense LDL (atherogenic lipoprotein profile [ALP])
- Elevated apolipoprotein B

Obesity is associated with increased free fatty acid (FFA) flux, which inhibits lipolysis *by insulin*. ALP contributes to increased atherosclerosis risk through a variety of associations, reflecting impaired transport.

The term "lipotoxicity" is used to describe toxic effects of an abundance of triglycerides and FFA on normal cell health. High levels of FFA increase oxidative stress, reduce NO synthesis, and contribute to cardiac myocyte apoptosis.

INFLAMMATION

Adipose tissue is a source of inflammatory mediators such as cytokines, tumor necrosis factor-α, and interleukin-6. This pro-inflammatory state is characterized by elevated high-sensitivity C-reactive protein (hs-CRP). Elevated levels of inflammatory markers such as CRP, fibrinogen, and plasminogen activator-1 are components of the obese state, insulin resistance, and the metabolic syndrome. However, the link between overweight status, insulin resistance, and elevated CRP is not consistent or direct.

THROMBOTIC ISSUES

An important component of obesity and the metabolic syndrome is dysfunction within the atherothrombosis system. Fibrinolysis can be suppressed due to elevated plasminogen activator inhibitor (PAI-1) concentrations, increased factor VII, fibrinogen, and von Willebrand factor, all of which have been linked to the development of myocardial infarction.

ENDOTHELIAL DYSFUNCTION

Endothelial dysfunction can be defined as an impaired response to endothelium-dependent vasodilators and has been reported to be present in patients with obesity, type 2 diabetes, and insulin resistance.

NONALCOHOLIC STEATOHEPATITIS

Nonalcoholic steatohepatitis (NASH) is a spectrum of conditions characterized by macrovesicular fatty change in the liver, associated with an absence of alcohol consumption with increasing fibrosis that may proceed to cirrhosis. Insulin resistance is the fundamental operative mechanism as the first step in the development of NASH and oxidative stress as the second. NASH is the second most common chronic liver disease in the United States, with a prevalence of approximately 3%. Treatment is not well established, but includes gradual reduction of excess body fat, control of hyperlipidemia, improvement of insulin sensitivity, and antioxidants.

OBESITY AND CORONARY ARTERY DISEASE

Important early events in the development of atherosclerosis are endothelial cell dysfunction in the epicardial vessels, resistance vessels, or both, and inflammation of the vessel wall. In the setting of the insulin resistance of obesity, coronary endothelial dysfunction is seen at the level of the resistance vessels. Individuals at high risk for CHD can be identified through the measurement of carotid intimal-medial thickness (IMT), a marker of generalized atherosclerosis. Central fat distribution is more important than total fat as a risk factor for atherosclerosis. The preferential deposition of fat centrally after the menopause may explain in part why the risk for CHD events increases 10 to 20 years later in women than men.

GENETICS

Although specific genes have been associated with obesity, the genetics of obesity is complex and involves the concept of gene/environment interaction and the thrifty gene concept. Genetic sites for rare familial obesity syndromes have been identified but none have been identified that are operational in the general population. A few single-gene disorders have obesity as the primary feature (Table 53-5).

PHYSICAL EXAMINATION

The presence of obesity may limit the accuracy of the physical examination and ECG and often underestimates the presence and the extent of heart disease.

- Jugular venous pulse and hepatojugular reflex are often not seen.
- Heart sounds are usually distant.
- Pedal edema may be present (can occur in part as a consequence of elevated ventricular filling pressure, despite elevation in cardiac output).
- Increases in demand for ventilation and breathing workload, especially in the supine position.

TABLE 53-5

Examples of Single-gene Disorders that Have Obesity as a Primary Feature

Gene Product	Gene	Endocrine Abnormalities	Inheritance	Chromosome
Leptin	LEP	Low leptin High insulin High TSH	Autosomal recessive	7q31.3
Leptin receptor	LEPR	High leptin Pituitary dysfunction High insulin	Autosomal recessive	1p31
Pro-opiomelanocortin	POMC1	Red hair pigmentation ACTH deficiency	Autosomal recessive	2p23.3
Prohormone convertase 1	PCI	High POMC Hypogonadism Hypocortisolism	Autosomal recessive	5q1.5–2.1
Melanocortin-4 receptor	MC4R	None	Autosomal dominant	18q22

Data adapted from www.cdc.gov/genomics.

- Blood pressure determination may be inaccurate. Small cuff size may cause considerable increases in blood pressure and could incorrectly classify up to 35% of normotensive obese individuals as hypertensive.

- Evaluate the presence of cor pulmonale.

- Split S_2 heart sound is often best heard at the first left interspace (an increase in the intensity of P_2, suggestive of pulmonary hypertension, may be missed at the bedside).

EFFECT OF OBESITY ON TESTS

【 】 SURFACE ELECTROCARDIOGRAM

Obesity may affect the electrocardiogram (ECG) in several ways: (1) displacement of the heart by elevating the diaphragm in the supine position, (2) increasing the cardiac workload, and (3) increasing the distance between the heart and the recording electrodes. Heart rate, PR interval, QRS interval, QRS voltage, and QTc interval all showed an increase with increasing obesity (Table 53-6).

RADIOLOGY

In obesity, the chest x-ray generally shows an elevated diaphragm with a widened heart in a horizontal direction, with the apex displaced outward to the left. The heart appears enlarged, which is often discordant with the findings on the surface ECG. Apical pericardial fat may obscure the apex or the lower portion of the left border of the heart. Also, many computed tomography (CT) tables have weight restrictions that often prohibit imaging of severely obese patients.

【 】 ECHOCARDIOGRAPHY

Transthoracic echocardiography can be technically difficult in obese patients. This is of importance in evaluating the presence of left ventricular diastolic dysfunction.

Transesophageal echocardiography (TEE) may be of diagnostic use in the evaluation of the presence of CHD in severely obese individuals. Transesophageal dobutamine stress echocardiography combines the advantages of pharmacologic stress testing with superior quality cardiac imaging, has been reported to be safe, and appears to be a good

TABLE 53-6

ECG Changes that May Occur in Obese Individuals

Increase in heart rate
Increase in PR interval
Increase in QRS interval
Increase in QTc interval
Increase in QT dispersion
Increase in late potentials
Increase or decrease in QRS voltage
ST-T abnormalities
Left axis deviation
Flattening of T wave (inferolateral leads)
Left atrial abnormalities
False-positive criteria for inferior myocardial infarction

alternative to cardiac catheterization for assessing the presence of CHD and ischemic threshold in morbidly obese patients. Obese individuals may have limitations because the examination table for nuclear medicine or catheterization usually does not accommodate very obese subjects.

【 】 NUCLEAR MEDICINE

Cardiac function can adequately be assessed in severely obese subjects using nuclear cardiology imaging techniques. Due to exercise limitations, a dipyridamole thallium-201 or technetium-99m perfusion scan may be used instead of exercise testing in very obese patients for the evaluation of the presence of ischemic heart disease.

【 】 CARDIAC CATHETERIZATION

The catheterization laboratory table usually does not accommodate subjects weighing more than 160 kg.

TREATMENT

The initial goal of weight-loss therapy should be to reduce body weight by approximately 10% from baseline. With success, further weight loss can be attempted if indicated through further assessment.

【 】 NUTRITION

A diet that is individually planned and takes into account the patient's overweight status in order to create a deficit of 500 to 1000 cal/d from the patient's current level should be an integral part of any weight-loss program. Specific diet components may assist in weight reduction and include reducing dietary fat and avoidance of simple carbohydrates. Alcohol should be avoided due to the significant amount of calories in relatively small volumes. Key points for nutritional therapy include:

- Decrease daily calories 500 to 1000.
- Avoid simple carbohydrates.
- Reduce dietary fat (saturated).
- Avoid alcohol.
- Include accurate diet assessment tool.
- Include self-monitoring and goal setting.
- Reinforce healthy behaviors.
- Use a continuous care model (obesity is a chronic disease).

【 】 PHYSICAL ACTIVITY

In multiple investigations it has been documented that a key differentiating factor between obese and lean individuals is the amount of routine physical activity or caloric expenditure. In obese individuals, physical activity should be increased gradually to help avoid biomechanical problems associated with excessive weight. Exercise stress tests should be considered prior to high-intensity physical activity.

【 】 MEDICATIONS

When nutrition and physical activity are unable to adequately treat obesity, prescription medications may be used as adjuncts to diet and exercise (Table 53-7). Valvular heart disease was reported to occur in association with the use of some appetite-suppressant

TABLE 53-7

Weight Loss and Physical Activity Benefits for Those Overweight or Obese

Disease/Risk Factor	Weight Loss	Physical Activity
Hypertension	↓↓↓	↓↓↓
Type 2 diabetes mellitus	↓↓↓	↓↓
Lipid profile	Definite improvement	Definite improvement
Coronary heart disease	↓↓	↓↓↓
Stroke	↓	↓↓
Sleep apnea	↓↓	Unknown

↓↓↓, strong decrease in risk; ↓↓, moderate decrease in risk; ↓, slight decrease in risk.

medications and the manufacturer voluntarily withdrew fenfluramine and dexfenfluramine from the market. Primary pulmonary hypertension is a potential complication of fenfluramine or dexfenfluramine taken either alone or in combination. Few studies are available to assess the long-term safety of weight-loss medications, and combination weight-loss drug therapy is even more uncertain.

Orlistat is a medication that works by reducing the body's ability to absorb dietary fat by inhibiting pancreatic lipase and may be complicated by GI distress. Sibutramine is an appetite suppressant that works by decreasing the reuptake of the neurotransmitters norepinephrine, dopamine, and serotonin. It is intended for use in patients with a BMI >30 and on a reduced-calorie diet. Sibutramine and Orlistat are the only weight-loss medications approved for longer-term use in significantly obese patients.

[ ] WEIGHT-LOSS SURGERY

Weight-loss surgery should be reserved for patients in whom efforts at medical therapy have failed and who are suffering from complications of extreme obesity.

SUGGESTED READING

Adams TD, Gress RE, Smith SC, et al. Long-term mortality after gastric bypass surgery. *N Engl J Med.* 2007;357:753–761.

Adams KF, Schatzkin A, Harris TB, et al. Overweight, obesity, and mortality in a large prospective cohort of persons 50 to 71 years old. *N Engl J Med.* 2006;355:763–778.

Bibbins-Domingo K, Coxson P, Pletcher MJ, et al. Adolescent overweight and future adult coronary heart disease. *N Engl J Med.* 2007;357:2371–2379.

Grundy SM. Obesity, metabolic syndrome, and coronary atherosclerosis. *Circulation.* 2002;105:2696–2698.

Krauss RM, Winston M, Fletcher BJ, et al. Obesity. Impact on cardiovascular disease. *Circulation.* 1998;98:1472–1476.

Superko HR. The metabolic syndrome, obesity, and diet. In: Fuster V, O'Rourke R, Alexander RW, et al., eds. *Hurst's The Heart.* 11th ed. New York, NY: McGraw-Hill; 2004:2127–2141.

CHAPTER 54

Diseases of the Aorta

Emily A. Farkas and John A. Elefteriades

DEFINITION

Aortic disease takes the lives of nearly 15,000 patients annually and accounts for more deaths in the United States than human immunodeficiency virus (HIV).

The aorta can be affected by *aneurysm* or *dissection* (Fig. 54-1). *Aneurysm* refers to an undue enlargement of the aorta. In the case of large aneurysms, the aorta has exceeded its normal contours. The criterion for the definition for small aneurysms is less clear. Although the "normal" size of the aorta varies with gender and body size, most agree that no normal aorta should exceed 4 cm in diameter. *Dissection* refers to a splitting of the layers of the aortic wall (within the media), permitting longitudinal propagation of a blood-filled space within the aortic wall. Aortic dissection is the most common cause of death related to the human aorta.

In addition, the aorta can be affected by *atherosclerosis*, which can narrow ostea of the great vessels or produce mobile intra-aortic atheromatous masses capable of embolization to the brain or other organs.

The aorta is an organ in and of itself, with complex intrinsic biological and mechanical properties. In fact, the aorta cooperates with the left ventricle (LV) in a "game of catch" with the stroke volume; that is to say, the intrinsic relaxation and contraction of the aorta augment LV hemodynamic function.

ETIOLOGY

Aneurysm and dissection, previously felt to be "arteriosclerotic" or "idiopathic," are often actually due to genetic and/or metabolic abnormalities affecting the aortic wall. The genetics of the well-known Marfan's syndrome have been fully elucidated. Any of 80 odd specific mutations in the fibrillin gene can produce the phenotypic marfanoid features of excessive height, thin body habitus, aortic aneurysm, valvular regurgitation, ocular lesions, and skeletal abnormalities.

Loeys–Dietz syndrome has been recently defined by mutations in the transforming growth factor-β (TGF-β) receptor, and afflicted individuals develop aneurysms that enlarge rapidly and are prone to rupture. This has a phenotypic overlap with Ehlers–Danlos syndrome, which is another inherited connective tissue disorder associated with aneurysm formation.

Familial aortic aneurysm is now a recognized entity whose existence was heralded by the frequently positive family history noted among patients with non-marfanoid aortic aneurysm. The autosomal dominant inheritance predominates, with other genetic patterns manifest as well (Fig. 54-2). When the proband has a thoracic aortic aneurysm, the chance that a relative has an aortic aneurysm is 1 in 5, or 20%. Of course,

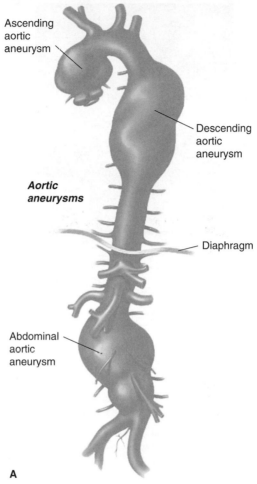

A

FIGURE 54-1. A. Schematic depiction of *aneurysm* of the aorta (ascending, descending, abdominal as indicated by *arrows*). **B.** Schematic depiction of *dissection* of the aorta.

Labels in figure:
Ascending aortic aneurysm
Descending aortic aneurysm
Aortic aneurysms
Diaphragm
Abdominal aortic aneurysm

without a postmortem examination, lethal aortic rupture or dissection of the aorta often masquerades as a myocardial infarction, obscuring the recognition of patterns that exist within families.

Given that a genetic mutation establishes the propensity for the development of an aneurysm, how does this genetic aberration actually bring one about? Evidence is accumulating that the gene substitution sets the stage, but the lytic enzymes known as *matrix metalloproteinases* actually affect the aortic wall. Matrix metalloproteinases (MMPs) degrade the structural proteins of the aortic wall. These enzymes are normally held in check by tissue inhibitor of metalloproteinase (TIMP), which antagonizes the lytic

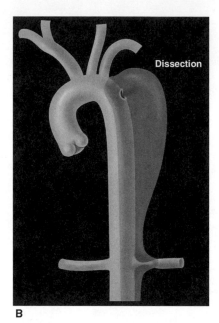

FIGURE 54-1. (Continued)

action of the MMPs. Abdominal aneurysms manifest excess MMP activity, and states of accelerated lysis in ascending aortic aneurysms as well as dissections have recently been confirmed. The authors now believe that aneurysm patients are genetically programmed to manifest excessive MMP activity, leading ultimately to degradation and thinning of the aortic wall.

It is important to recognize the role of a bicuspid aortic valve in aneurysm and dissection disease. *Patients born with a bicuspid aortic valve have structurally inferior aortas, making them vulnerable to aortic aneurysm and dissection.* The fact that aortic dissection in patients with bicuspid aortic valves occurs before the onset of aortic stenosis and its associated symptoms deserves emphasis. Furthermore, because bicuspid valve disease is so common (the most common congenital lesion of the human heart, affecting 1% to 2% of the general population), it actually causes more dissections than the much more commonly appreciated Marfan's syndrome (which occurs in only 1 in 10,000 human beings). In fact, bicuspid aortic valve causes 25 times more acute aortic dissections than Marfan's syndrome (Table 54-1).

What is the immediate event that precipitates the aortic dissection process in a particular individual? Our work suggests that acute hypertension, from a specific severe emotional episode or extreme physical exertion, is commonly the immediate precipitating event. We recently reported catastrophic acute aortic dissections in a series of healthy young athletes engaged in heavy weight training, during which blood pressure can reach a staggering 370 mm Hg.

Older literature refers commonly to the presence of *cystic medial necrosis* as a cause of aortic dissection. This loss of cells and fibers in the aortic wall, producing large spaces or "cysts" within the aortic walls, has proven to be a nonspecific finding that can often be seen in any aged aorta.

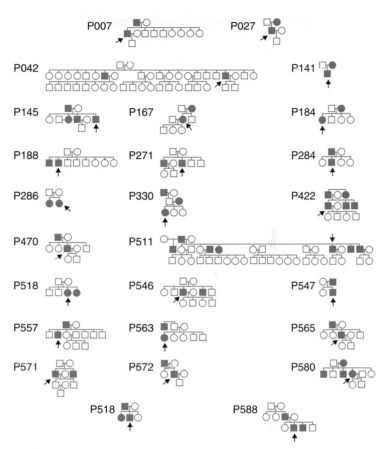

FIGURE 54-2. Thoracic aortic aneurysm (TAA) family pedigrees selected from over 500 family pedigrees. Squares represent men and circles represent women. An arrow indicates the proband with a TAA. Solid blue circles or squares represent affected patients with aortic aneurysms.

TABLE 54-1

Comparison of Epidemiology of Marfan's Syndrome and Bicuspid Aortic valve[a]

	Incidence (%)	AAD Likelihood (Lifetime, %)	AADs Caused (as % of Population)
Marfan's syndrome	1/10,000 (0.01)	40	0.004
Bicuspid aortic valve	2/100 (2)	5	0.1

[a]With special reference to number of cases of aortic dissection brought on by disease.

CLINICAL MANIFESTATIONS

【 　】 ANEURYSM

Unfortunately, the vast majority of thoracic aortic aneurysms are silent, with rupture constituting the very first symptom. Only a fortunate few patients (5%–10%) actually experience symptoms from their aneurysms, permitting earlier detection. Aneurysms of any kind can produce pain, from stretching of the aortic tissue or impingement on adjacent structures. Ascending aneurysms may produce heart failure, with its associated symptoms, by causing aortic regurgitation. As the aortic root enlarges, the aortic valve leaflets are progressively pulled away from each other, permitting backward leakage of blood through the resultant central gap. Ascending aneurysms can distort or even obstruct the trachea, producing respiratory symptoms. Aortic arch aneurysms or descending thoracic aortic aneurysms may produce hoarseness or dysphagia ("dysphagia lusoria") from distortion of the phrenic nerve or direct impingement on the esophagus. Abdominal aortic aneurysms produce back and/or abdominal pain. Rupture of the aorta in any location produces acute symptoms, usually severe pain, followed by a loss of consciousness or death due to internal hemorrhage.

In the present era, thoracic or abdominal aortic aneurysms are most commonly diagnosed incidentally on a computed tomographic scan (or echocardiogram or magnetic resonance imaging study) done for another reason. This provides an unparalleled opportunity to prevent aneurysm-related death by early detection.

【 　】 DISSECTION

Most patients describe the pain of aortic dissection as the most intense pain of their lives. It is often described as tearing or shearing pain, which is quite consistent with the pathophysiology. The pain of ascending dissection is felt in the anterior chest; and that of a descending dissection is felt posteriorly, between the scapulae. It can migrate downward, into the flank or pelvis, as the dissection process propagates distally.

Aortic dissections may be ascending (type A) or descending (type B). The two patterns are determined by the location of the inciting intimal tear. Tears occur in two very specific locations: (1) in the ascending aorta, 2 to 3 cm above the coronary arteries; and (2) in the descending aorta, 1 to 2 cm beyond the left subclavian artery. The first type of tear produces ascending dissection and the second, descending dissection. Note that ascending dissections usually go around the aortic arch to involve the descending and abdominal portions of the aorta.

Aortic dissection can take a patient's life by four mechanisms (Fig. 54-3):

• Intrapericardial rupture (of an ascending dissection).

• Free rupture into the pleural/peritoneal/retroperitoneal cavity (of a descending or abdominal aortic dissection).

• Acute aortic regurgitation (from an ascending aortic dissection).

• Occlusion of *any* branch of the aorta (from an ascending or descending dissection).

Acute aortic regurgitation from the dissection's distortion of the aortic root and impaired leaflet coaptation may be very poorly tolerated, and cardiogenic shock may result. Branch-vessel occlusion comes about by impingement on the true lumen of any branch vessel (coronaries to iliacs) by the distended false lumen with consequent end-organ ischemia.

Approximately 15% to 20% of patients with aortic dissection develop neurologic deficits, with transient cerebral ischemia or stroke in up to 10% of cases resulting from extension of dissection into the carotid or vertebral arteries. When cerebral infarction has occurred, surgery is best avoided for fear of inducing intracerebral bleeding or otherwise extending the zone of injury. When infarction is absent or incomplete, urgent

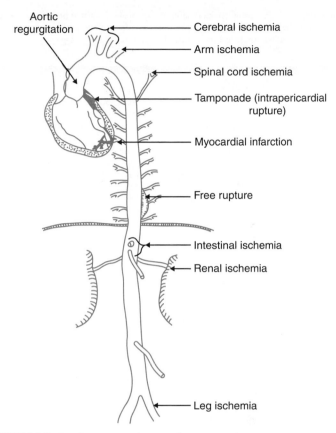

Aortic regurgitation

Cerebral ischemia

Arm ischemia

Spinal cord ischemia

Tamponade (intrapericardial rupture)

Myocardial infarction

Free rupture

Intestinal ischemia

Renal ischemia

Leg ischemia

FIGURE 54-3. Specific major complications of acute aortic dissection.

operation is generally indicated, as repair of the dissection may restore brain perfusion. Similarly, intervention is indicated when interruption of spinal circulation by a dissection of the descending aorta threatens to cause paraplegia.

PHYSICAL EXAMINATION

Ascending aneurysms are not detectable on physical examination unless they produce aortic regurgitation, with its characteristic diastolic blowing murmur heard best to the *right* of the upper sternal border. Descending aneurysms are undetectable on physical examination except with extreme enlargement, when they can occasionally be felt by direct palpation through an attenuated chest wall. The abdominal aorta is easily palpable in most patients. With practice, one can assess the approximate size of the abdominal aorta by palpation between the thumb and index finger.

Aortic dissection produces typical physical signs, including the murmur of aortic regurgitation and decrement or loss of any pulse, most commonly one of the femoral pulses. A substantive difference in blood pressure between the two arms should raise suspicion of aortic dissection. Malperfusion in any involved vascular bed can create correspondent ischemic compromise with neurologic deficits, abdominal tenderness, and threatened extremities as critical indicators of the underlying pathology.

DIAGNOSTIC STUDIES

Plain chest radiography will often suggest thoracic aortic disease, and in the International Registry of Aortic Dissection, chest films were abnormal in 87.6% of patients. It is important to note, however, that a normal study never excludes underlying aortic pathology.

Several types of three-dimensional (3D) imaging are pertinent in aneurysm disease, all with excellent sensitivity and specificity: transesophageal echocardiography (TEE), computed tomography (CT), magnetic resonance imaging (MRI), and abdominal ultrasonography. CT or MRI allows the 3D reconstruction of the entire aorta. The TEE, while blinded to the arch and abdominal aorta, provides information about pericardial effusion/tamponade, valve function, LV function, and images both the ascending and descending aorta well. Abdominal ultrasonography images the abdominal aorta satisfactorily in most cases.

Recent advances in CT technology have made high-resolution noninvasive coronary angiograms possible. New developments permit acquisition of well-opacified images of the coronary arteries, thoracic aorta, and pulmonary arteries from a single CT scan. Utilization of coronary CT angiography (CCTA) as a "triple rule-out" study could potentially exclude fatal causes of chest pain in all three vascular beds (Fig. 54-4).

DIFFERENTIAL DIAGNOSIS

Pertinent blood tests include creatine phosphokinase isoenzyme and troponin levels for evaluation of myocardial infarction. If these enzymes are negative, aortic disease must rise in the differential diagnosis of acute chest pain (this is especially true if the electrocardiogram (ECG) fails to show changes suspicious for ischemia or infarction).

Less well known is the fact that the D-dimer is nearly invariably elevated in acute aortic dissection. The sensitivity of this test is 99%, and if the D-dimer is negative, acute aortic dissection is essentially ruled out.

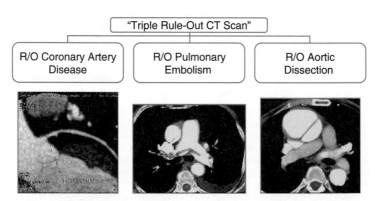

FIGURE 54-4. The "triple rule-out" CT scan that can be used to diagnose or rule out the "big three" conditions that threaten the life of the chest pain patient: coronary artery disease, pulmonary embolism, and aortic dissection. We strongly recommend its use.

Maintaining a high level of suspicion for aneurysmal disease is the primary diagnostic issue. Specifically, all patients admitted with chest and/or abdominal pain *without obvious cause* should have the aorta imaged, and the diagnosis must be considered in any patient with unexplained heart failure, syncope, or neurologic deficit. Patients with an equivocal imaging study and a high pretest probability for an acute aortic event warrant a second complementary imaging examination.

NATURAL HISTORY AND PROGNOSIS

Thoracic aortic aneurysm is a lethal disease, producing an approximated 50% mortality in 5 years with most deaths related to the aneurysm. It is an indolent disease, however, with the aorta growing an average of 0.1 cm/yr. This commonly results in aneurysm development over several decades of adult life.

The ascending thoracic aorta ruptures or dissects at or about 6 cm in diameter. Our in vivo studies in humans have shown that the aorta loses all its normal elasticity at 6 cm; as a consequence, the force of systole can no longer be dissipated in expanding the aorta. Rather, at these large dimensions, the force of systole tends to disrupt the nondistensile, enlarged aorta. At 6 cm, the *yearly* risk of rupture, dissection, or death in patients with ascending aortic aneurysms is a staggering 14.1%. Thus, in patients without overwhelming comorbidities, the *aneurysmal ascending thoracic aorta should be resected before it reaches the critical 6-cm diameter*. Resection is usually done when the aorta reaches 5.5 cm so as to provide a safety margin before rupture or dissection can be expected to occur. For most patients with Marfan's syndrome or a positive family history, a criterion of 5 cm is usually appropriate, as these patients are even more vulnerable to sudden aortic events.

Intervention is generally recommended at larger diameters for patients with aneurysms of the descending aorta, based upon both the different risk of rupture and the greater associated cardiovascular comorbidities that typify these commonly older individuals. Replacement of the descending aorta at about 6.5 cm will preclude most adverse aortic-related events, without prematurely exposing affected patients to the risks of surgical intervention. We apply more stringent criteria for patients with Marfan's syndrome or in those with a family history of aortic disease, intervening prophylactically at 5.0 cm for the ascending aorta and 6.0 cm for the descending aorta (Table 54-2).

  TABLE 54-2

Yale Center for Thoracic Aortic Disease Recommended Surgical Intervention Criteria for Thoracic Aortic Aneurysms

1. Rupture
2. Acute aortic dissection
   a. Ascending requires urgent operation
   b. Descending requires a "complication specific approach"
3. Symptomatic states
   a. Pain consistent with rupture and unexplained by other causes
   b. Compression of adjacent organs, especially trachea, esophagus, or left mainstem bronchus
   c. Significant aortic insufficiency in conjuction with ascending aortic aneurysm
4. Documented enlargement
   a. Growth ≥1 cm/y or substantial growth and aneurysm is rapidly approaching absolute size criteria
5. Absolute size (cm)

	Marfan's	Non-Marfan's
Ascending	5.0	5.5
Descending	6.0	6.5

Abdominal aortic aneurysms between 4.0 and 5.0 cm in diameter are associated with a 1% per year risk of rupture, and decisions regarding surveillance or surgery should be individualized based on age, familial features, and an assessment of surgical risk. Aneurysms of the abdominal aorta greater than 5.5 cm carry a substantial risk of rupture and should be repaired.

Application of these criteria to preemptive extirpation of the aneurysmal human aortic wall prevents most ruptures and dissections. One point deserves emphasis: these criteria apply to asymptomatic aortic aneurysms. *Symptomatic aortic aneurysms should be resected, regardless of size.* The presence of symptoms portends rupture and mandates surgical therapy. At times it may be difficult to determine unequivocally whether symptoms are due to an aneurysm or something else. The authors recommend that pain be considered aneurysm-related unless it can be conclusively demonstrated to be due to another cause.

TREATMENT

Patients with aneurysms are often treated with beta-blocking medications in order to decrease the virulence of the impact of systole on the aortic wall. The effectiveness of this treatment is unproved. Of course, hypertension must be controlled so as to limit the impact of disruptive forces on the aortic wall.

In the setting of acute aortic dissection, the utilization of drugs with anti-impulse properties is well supported. In most cases, the initial agent of choice is an intravenous beta-blocker, which offers the dual advantage of lowering dp/dt max as well as lowering the blood pressure. Vasodilators should only be used as secondary agents alongside anti-impulse medications because of their reflex-mediated positive inotropic and chronotropic effects.

Excellent surgical procedures have been refined over the years for replacement of chronic aneurysms of the ascending, arch, descending, and abdominal or thoracoabdominal aorta. Although surgical dangers exist (bleeding, stroke, paralysis, death), the operations can be performed with considerable safety—especially when done before the aorta ruptures or dissects.

For acute aortic dissection, the following guidelines apply:

- Ascending aortic dissections (type A) require urgent surgery, as death usually occurs in nonoperated patients from intrapericardial rupture, aortic regurgitation, or myocardial infarction due to coronary artery involvement.

- Descending aortic dissections (type B), in the absence of specific vascular complications, do well with medical management (therapy with beta-blockers and afterload-reducing medication). If a specific complication occurs, this is addressed directly by surgery ("complication-specific" approach to descending aortic dissection).

A variety of stent grafts and delivery systems for endovascular repair of aortic aneurysm have been introduced, and analyses of short-term results suggest their value as an alternative therapy for elderly patients and for those with overwhelming comorbid disease. Importantly, however, the mid- to long-term effectiveness of stent therapy in preventing aneurysm growth, rupture, and aneurysm-related mortality (compared to open surgical repair) remains unproved. Although endovascular techniques have not eliminated the reality of stroke and paraplegia that accompanies therapy of complex aortic pathology, they have introduced the technique-specific complication of endoleaks, obliging stringent interval imaging every 6 to 12 months to evaluate the need for reintervention. The psychological impact of "living from scan to scan" is burdensome, and the radiation risks are real.

Although long-term follow-up for endografting of the thoracic aorta is limited, data regarding delayed outcomes following endovascular abdominal aortic aneurysm repair are more robust. One of the largest of such surveys, the EUROSTAR registry, identifies cases of late mortality and rupture even after initially successful intervention. Randomized trials of thoracic endografting versus traditional surgical techniques will be required to conclusively compare stent therapy to open surgical repair, which remains the durable and effective standard of care.

SUGGESTED READING

Achneck HE, Rizzo JA, Tranquilli M, et al. Safety of thoracic aortic surgery in the present era. *Ann Thorac Surg.* 2007;84:1180–1185; discussion 1185.

Albornoz G, Coady MA, Roberts M, et al. Familial thoracic aortic aneurysms and dissections: incidence, modes of inheritance, and phenotypic patterns. *Ann Thorac Surg.* 2006;82:1400–1405.

Davies RR, Kaple RK, Mandapati D, et al. Natural history of ascending aortic aneurysms in the setting of an unreplaced bicuspid aortic valve. *Ann Thorac Surg.* 2007;83:1338–1344.

Elefteriades JA, ed. *Acute Aortic Disease.* New York: Taylor and Francis; 2007.

Elefteriades JA. Beating a sudden killer. *Sci Am.* 2005;293:64–71.

Elefteriades JA. Thoracic aortic aneurysm: reading the enemy's playbook. *Curr Probl Cardiol.* 2008;33:203–277.

Elefteriades JA, Percy A. Endovascular stenting for descending aneurysms: wave of the future or the emperor's new clothes? *J Thorac Cardiovasc Surg.* 2007;133:285–288.

Halperin JL, Olin JW. Diseases of the aorta. In: Fuster V, Alexander RW, O'Rourke RA, et al., eds. *Hurst's the Heart.* 11th ed. New York: McGraw-Hill; 2004:2301–2314.

Laheij RJF, Buth J, Harris PL, et al. Need for secondary interventions after endovascular repair of abdominal aortic aneurysms. Intermediate-term follow-up results of a European collaborative registry (EUROSTAR). *Br J Surg.* 2000;87:1666–1673.

CHAPTER (55)

Cerebrovascular Disease and Neurologic Manifestations of Heart Disease

Megan C. Leary and Louis R. Caplan

CARDIOGENIC BRAIN EMBOLISM

Diagnostic criteria for cardiogenic embolism were formerly very restrictive. Embolism was diagnosed when sudden focal neurologic signs, maximal at onset, developed in patients with peripheral systemic embolism and recent myocardial infarction (MI) or rheumatic mitral stenosis. Using these criteria, cardioembolic infarcts were diagnosed in only 3% to 8% of stroke patients. None of these criteria is definitive. About 20% of patients do *not* have maximal symptoms at onset. Many other cardiac lesions and arrhythmias are also now well-accepted sources of emboli. Lastly, only about 2% of patients with cardiogenic brain embolism have clinically recognized peripheral embolism. Symptoms of peripheral embolism are often so nonspecific that they are seldom diagnosed correctly.

Cardiac sources can be divided into three groups: (1) cardiac wall and chamber abnormalities—for example, cardiomyopathies, hypokinetic and akinetic ventricular regions after MI, atrial septal aneurysms, ventricular aneurysms, atrial myxomas, papillary fibroelastomas and other tumors, septal defects, and patent foramen ovale; (2) valve disorders—for example, rheumatic mitral and aortic disease, prosthetic valves, bacterial endocarditis, fibrous and fibrinous endocardial lesions, mitral valve prolapse, and mitral annulus calcification; and (3) arrhythmias, especially atrial fibrillation and "sick-sinus" syndrome. Some cardiac sources have much higher rates of initial and recurrent embolism. The Stroke Data Bank divided potential sources into high- and medium-risk sources (Table 55-1).

【 】 ATRIAL FIBRILLATION

Persistent and paroxysmal atrial fibrillation (AF) is a potent predictor of first and recurrent stroke, with > 75,000 attributed cases annually. In patients with brain emboli caused by a cardiac source, there is a history of nonvalvular AF in roughly one-half of all cases, of left ventricular (LV) thrombus in almost one-third, and of valvular heart disease in one-fourth. Echocardiographic findings (left atrial diameter, ventricular function and areas of hypokinesis, valve disease, thrombi, spontaneous echo contrast) are helpful in assessing the potential for embolism.

【 】 MITRAL VALVE PROLAPSE

Although MVP is common, the frequency of MVP-related stroke is very low. Morphologic lesions, such as thrombi and fibrous lesions, may clearly suggest embolism; fibrin-platelet depositions on the surfaces of the mitral leaflets and thrombi in the angle

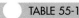

TABLE 55-1

Stroke Data Bank Categorization of Cardiac Risk

High-Risk Categories

Valve surgery
Atrial fibrillation or flutter, sick sinus node with or without valve disease
Left ventricular aneurysm
Left ventricular mural thrombus
Cardiomyopathy or left ventricular hypokinesis
Akinetic region of left ventricle

Medium-Risk Categories

Myocardial infarct within 6 months
Valve disease without atrial fibrillation/flutter or sick sinus node
Congestive heart failure
Decreased left ventricular function
Hypokinetic left ventricular segment
Mitral valve prolapse (by history or echocardiogram)
Mitral annulus calcification

between the posterior mitral valve leaflet and the left atrial wall have been noted. Also, patients may often have atrial fibrillation, syncope, and migraine. The recurrence rate of stroke in MVP alone is very low. Warfarin anticoagulants are ordinarily not indicated in the prophylaxis of patients with MVP, even after an initial stroke. Aspirin prophylaxis (80–325 mg/d) is advisable. Demonstration by echocardiography of an intracardiac thrombus related to MVP changes that recommendation to warfarin.

【 】 MITRAL ANNULUS CALCIFICATION

Mitral annulus calcification (MAC) is an important, often unrecognized cause of embolism. Ulceration and extrusion of calcium through overlapping cusps have been seen at necropsy, thrombi have been found on valves attached to the ulcerative process, and calcific emboli have been seen in surgical embolectomies. Infective endocarditis can also develop on the calcified mitral annulus. Anticoagulation does not prevent calcific emboli. The decision to use antiplatelet agents versus anticoagulants should include consideration of other potential comorbid factors such as AF.

【 】 FIBRINOUS VALVE ABNORMALITIES

Some disorders are associated with fibrous and fibrinous lesions of the heart valves and endocardium. Similar valve lesions occur in patients with systemic lupus erythematosus (Libman–Sacks endocarditis; see Chapter 50), the antiphospholipid antibody syndrome, and cancer and other debilitating diseases (nonbacterial thrombotic endocarditis). Mobile fibrous strands are also often found during echocardiography. Warfarin anticoagulants are *not* effective in the prevention of embolism in these conditions.

【 】 INFECTIVE ENDOCARDITIS

Embolic complications are common in patients who have infective endocarditis. Mycotic aneurysms can cause fatal subarachnoid bleeding. Embolization usually stops when infection is controlled. Warfarin does not prevent embolization and is probably

TABLE 55-2

Types of Embolic Materials

Cardiac	Arterial
Red fibrin-dependent thrombi	Red fibrin-dependent thrombi
White platelet-fibrin nidi	White platelet-fibrin nidi
Material from marantic endocarditis	Combined fibrin-platelet and fibrin-dependent clots
Bacteria from vegetations	Cholesterol crystals
Calcium from valves and mitral annulus calcification	Atheromatous plaque debris
Myxoma cells and debris	Calcium from vascular calcifications
	Air
	Mucin from tumors
	Talc or microcrystalline cellulose from injected drugs

contraindicated unless there are other important lesions, such as prosthetic valves or life-threatening pulmonary embolism. In children and young adults with congenital heart defects, especially those with right-to-left shunts and polycythemia, brain abscess is an important complication.

Emboli often arise from sources other than the heart, such as the aorta, proximal arteries, leg veins (paradoxical emboli), fat in the liver or bones, and materials introduced by the patient or physician (drug particles or air). The types of embolic material also vary.

Atheromatous plaques in the aortic arch and ascending aorta are a very important and previously neglected source of brain embolism. Transesophageal echocardiography (TEE) can show these atheromas. The aorta can also be insonated by B-mode ultrasound probes placed in the supraclavicular fossae on each side. Large (> 4 mm), protruding, mobile aortic atheromas are especially likely to cause embolic strokes and are often recurrent.

ONSET, CLINICAL COURSE, AND DIAGNOSTIC APPROACHES TO BRAIN EMBOLI

Warning signs of stroke can include sudden hemiparesis, hemisensory loss, confusion, trouble speaking or understanding, visual loss, diplopia, ataxia, vertigo, or sudden severe headache with no known cause. Most embolic events occur during activities of daily living. Sudden coughing, sneezing, or rising at night to urinate can precipitate embolism. Although the deficit is most often maximal at outset, 11% of embolic stroke patients in the Harvard Stroke Registry had a stepwise course, whereas 10% had fluctuations or progressive deficits. Later progression, if it occurs, is usually within the first 48 hours. Progression is usually due to distal passage of emboli. Early angiography in embolic stroke patients shows intracranial emboli with high frequency and after 48 hours shows a much lower rate of arterial blockage, presumably due to spontaneous passage or lysis of thrombi. As in all large infarcts, brain edema may develop during the 24 to 72 hours after stroke, causing headache, decreased alertness, and worsening of neurologic signs. The edema is often cytotoxic (inside cells) and *usually does not respond* to corticosteroid treatment.

Emboli usually cause occlusion of distal branches and produce surface infarcts that are roughly triangular, with the apex of the triangle pointing inward. Computed tomography

(CT) and magnetic resonance imaging (MRI) findings can suggest the presence of embolism by the location and shape of the lesion, the presence of superficial wedge-shaped infarcts in multiple different vascular territories, hemorrhagic infarction, and visualization of thrombi within arteries. MRI, particularly with the use of MR diffusion-weighted and MR gradient recall echo (GRE) imaging, is more sensitive for detection of acute brain infarcts than is CT and is also superior in detecting hemorrhagic infarction by imaging hemosiderin. Hemorrhagic infarction has long been considered characteristic of embolism, especially when the artery leading to the infarct is patent. The mechanism of hemorrhagic infarction is reperfusion of ischemic zones, which occurs with spontaneous passage of emboli and after iatrogenic opening of an occluded artery (e.g., endarterectomy, fibrinolytic treatment). At times, it is also possible to image the acute embolus on CT and MRI. Aortic plaques, atrial septal aneurysms, and atrial septal defects, potential sources of emboli, are best seen with transesophageal echocardiography (TEE), but this has limitations. Thromboembolism is a dynamic process. When a clot forms in the heart and embolizes, there may be no residual thrombus in the heart until a clot reforms. Cardiac thrombi are imaged differently on sequential echocardiograms; even large thrombi seen on one echocardiogram can disappear later.

Embolic signals are now detected by monitoring with transcranial Doppler (TCD). Embolic particles passing under TCD probes produce transient, short-duration, high-intensity signals. TCD monitoring of patients with atrial fibrillation, cardiac surgery, prosthetic valves, left ventricular assist devices, carotid artery disease, and carotid endarterectomy have shown a relatively high frequency of embolic signals.

PREVENTION AND TREATMENT

Previously, the intensity of anticoagulation was higher than that currently used, and brain hemorrhages and other bleeding complications were common. Trials now show that lower-intensity warfarin treatment (International Normalized Ratio [INR] 2.0–3.0) is effective in preventing brain emboli in patients with nonrheumatic AF. *Warfarin is about 50% more effective than aspirin* in preventing stroke in patients with atrial fibrillation who do not have valvular disease. Warfarin may not be effective in preventing calcific, myxomatous, bacterial, and fibrin-platelet emboli, and warfarin has been reported to worsen cholesterol crystal embolization. Embolic brain infarcts often become hemorrhagic, and serious brain hemorrhage has occurred after anticoagulation. Large infarcts, hypertension, large bolus doses of heparin, and excessive anticoagulation are associated with hemorrhage. In most patients with hemorrhagic infarction of the brain, the cause is embolic. *Hemorrhagic infarction occurs equally with and without anticoagulation, and development of hemorrhagic infarction is rarely accompanied by clinical worsening.* Patients with hemorrhagic transformation continued on anticoagulants usually do not worsen. The risk of reembolism must be balanced against the small but definite risk of important bleeding. In patients with large brain infarcts, *heparin should be delayed* (but not deferred permanently) and bolus heparin infusions avoided. If the risk for reembolism is high, immediate heparinization without a bolus is advisable; but if the risk seems low, it is prudent to delay anticoagulants for at least 48 hours.

【 】 PARADOXICAL EMBOLISM

Emboli entering the systemic circulation through right-to-left shunting of blood are now more often recognized. By far the *most common potential intracardiac shunt is a patent foramen ovale (PFO).* The high frequency of PFOs in the normal adult population makes it difficult to be certain in an individual stroke patient whether paradoxical embolism through the PFO caused the stroke or was an incidental finding. About 30% of adults have a probe patent PFO at necropsy. The frequency of PFOs declines with age. The average diameter of a PFO is 4.9 mm, and the size tends to increase with age.

There is a high degree of certainty of paradoxical embolism when four or more of five criteria are met: (1) a situation that promotes thrombosis of leg or pelvic veins (e.g., long sitting in one position, recent surgery, etc.); (2) increased coagulability (e.g., the use of oral contraceptives, presence of hypercoagulable state, dehydration); (3) sudden onset of stroke during sexual intercourse, straining at stool, or other activity that includes a Valsalva maneuver; (4) pulmonary embolism shortly before or after the neurologic ischemic event; and (5) the absence of other putative causes of stroke after thorough evaluation. Current treatment options for future stroke prevention in patients with PFO and ischemic stroke include medical therapy, open or minimally invasive cardiac surgical closure, and transcatheter closure. With regard to medical therapies, antiplatelet therapy is reasonable for future stroke prevention in cryptogenic stroke patients with a first ischemic stroke/TIA plus an isolated PFO. Warfarin is considered to be an appropriate treatment option in the subgroup of PFO/ischemic stroke patients with concomitant atrial septal aneurysm, hypercoagulable state, or venous thrombosis.

【 】 BRAIN HYPOPERFUSION DUE TO CARDIAC PUMP FAILURE (CARDIAC ARREST)

Very severe hypoxic-ischemic damage can lead to mortal injury to the cortex and brainstem, irreversible coma, and brain death. When initially examined, such patients have no brainstem reflexes and no response to stimuli except perhaps a decerebration response. These findings do not improve, and respiratory control is absent or lost. When cerebrocortical damage is very severe but brainstem ischemic changes are reversible, brainstem reflexes are preserved but there is no meaningful response to the environment. Automatic facial movements such as blinking, tongue protrusion, and yawning usually persist. The eyes may rest slightly up and move from side to side. When this state does not improve, it is referred to as the persistent vegetative state or "wakefulness without awareness." Laminar cortical necrosis causes seizures. These are often multifocal myoclonic twitches or jerks of the facial and limb muscles, which are difficult to control with anticonvulsants (see also Chapter 18).

With severe border-zone brain injury (watershed infarcts), there is weakness of the arms and proximal lower extremities with preservation of face, leg, and foot movement (the "man in a barrel" syndrome). With less severe ischemia, the symptoms and signs can be predominantly visual. Reading is impossible. Apathy, amnesia, and inertia are also common.

Shortly after arrest, patients with less severe brain injury show reactivity to the environment. Eye opening and restless limb movements develop. The eyes fixate on objects. Noise, a flashlight, or a pinch arouses patients to avoid or react to stimuli. Soon patients awaken and begin to speak. Cognitive and behavioral abnormalities detected after awakening depend on the degree of injury. The initial neurologic findings and course are helpful in predicting outcome. Among patients with meaningful responses to pain at 1 hour, almost all survivors have preserved intellectual function. Patients who do not respond to pain by 24 hours often die or remain in a vegetative state. Coma predicts a poor prognosis. The presence or absence of coma and the response to pain predict neurologic outcome very early.

CT is used to exclude other causes of coma such as brain hemorrhage. Electroencephalography (EEG) may be helpful in studying cortical activity in unresponsive patients and in assessing brain death.

【 】 NEUROLOGIC EFFECTS OF CARDIAC DRUGS AND CARDIAC ENCEPHALOPATHY

Drugs given to patients with cardiac disease often have neurologic side effects. Digitalis can cause visual hallucinations, yellow vision, and confusion. *Digitalis levels need not be excessively elevated; the symptoms disappear with drug cessation.* Quinidine can cause delirium, seizures, coma, vertigo, tinnitus, and visual blurring. Similar toxicity has been seen with lithium. Patients may become acutely comatose while being treated with intravenous lidocaine. *This effect has been associated with the accidental administration of very large doses; more common CNS effects of less extreme toxicity include sedation, irritability, and twitching.* The latter may progress to seizures accompanied by respiratory depression. Amiodarone can cause ataxia, weakness, tremors, paresthesias, visual symptoms, a parkinsonian-like syndrome, and occasionally delirium.

Patients with congestive heart failure often develop an encephalopathy characterized by decreased alertness, sleepiness, decreased intellectual functions, asterixis, and variability of alertness from hour to hour. This cardiac encephalopathy is multifactoral: decreased cardiac output, increased venous pressure, brain edema, increased fluid in the brain ventricles and CSF around the brain, and the effects of drugs and concurrent kidney and liver dysfunction.

NEUROLOGIC AND CEREBROVASCULAR COMPLICATIONS OF CARDIAC SURGERY

Coronary artery bypass graft (CABG) surgery is the most common major cardiovascular operation performed. Abnormalities of intellectual function and behavior are common after heart surgery, and fortunately, most changes are reversed with time. Prospectively, transient complications are noted in 61% of patients. A major concern is that heart surgery will lead to underperfusion of areas supplied by already stenosed or occluded arteries, leading to brain infarcts. This concern underlies neck auscultation for bruits, ultrasound carotid artery testing, and cerebral angiography prior to CABG. However, hemodynamically induced infarction related to preexisting atherosclerotic occlusive cervicocranial arterial disease *is rare*. Embolism arising from cardiac and aortic sources is *much more common*. Patients with carotid bruits have a very low rate of stroke after elective cardiac surgery. In a retrospective study of CABG patients with known carotid disease, ipsilateral strokes occurred in 1.1% of arteries with 50% to 90% stenosis, in 6.2% of arteries with > 90% stenosis, and in only 2% of vessels with carotid occlusion. Embolism arising from cardiac and aortic sources is much more common than atherothrombotic infarcts and of greater concern.

Thromboembolic infarction often occurs in the days following surgery. Strokes occur most often after recovery from anesthesia. If the mechanism of stroke was hemodynamic, the major circulatory stress would be intraoperative and patients would awaken with the deficit. Emboli arise from preexisting cardiac abnormalities (such as hypofunctioning ventricles, dilated atria, and aortic atheromas) or from postoperative arrhythmias. Evidence links operative and postoperative embolism to aortic ulcerative atherosclerotic lesions. Left-body symptoms (right-hemispheric stroke) are twice as common as right-body symptoms. About one-third of embolic signs are detected as the aortic cross-clamps are removed and another 24% as aortic partial occlusion clamps are removed. Necropsy examination of patients dying after cardiac surgery shows severe bilateral, predominantly border-zone infarcts. Patients who are to have elective coronary artery surgery should have preoperative noninvasive assessment of the extent of disease in the carotids and thoracic aorta, and assessment of cardiac function in addition to imaging of their coronary arteries Cardiac, aortic, and intraarterial embolism accounts for the vast majority of cardiac surgery–related focal neurologic deficits.

Drugs are a common cause of encephalopathy in the postoperative period. Particularly important are haloperidol, narcotics, and sedatives. Morphine is sometimes used heavily intraoperatively, and opiate withdrawal with restlessness and hyperactivity can result. Agitation and restlessness are often early signs of organic encephalopathy and may lead to the administration of haloperidol, barbiturates, phenothiazines, or benzodiazepines for calming and sedation. When these drugs wear off and patients begin to awaken, agitation may occur and more sedatives may be given. Haloperidol causes rigidity, restlessness, agitation, hallucinations, and confusion.

CARDIAC EFFECTS OF BRAIN LESIONS

【 】 CARDIAC LESIONS

The most common lesions found in the hearts of patients dying with acute CNS lesions are patchy regions of myocardial necrosis and subendocardial hemorrhage. The abnormalities range from eosinophilic muscle cell staining with preserved striations to transformation of myocardial cells into dense eosinophilic contraction bands. These changes are called *myocytolysis*. Subendocardial petechiae and hemorrhages are also noted. In stroke patients, especially those with subarachnoid hemorrhage, electrocardiograms (ECGs) may show prolonged QT intervals; giant, wide, roller-coaster inverted T waves; and U waves. Patients with stroke who have continuous ECG monitoring have a high incidence of T-wave and ST-segment changes, various arrhythmias, and cardiac enzyme abnormalities. ECG changes also may include a prolonged QT interval, depressed ST segments, flat or inverted T waves, and U waves. Less often, tall, peaked T waves and elevated ST segments are noted. Cardiac and skeletal muscle enzymes, including the MB isoenzyme of creatine kinase (MB-CK), are often abnormal in stroke patients. During the 4 to 7 days after stroke, MB-CK levels show a slow rise and later fall in serum, a pattern different from that found in acute myocardial infarction. Various cardiac arrhythmias have been found in stroke patients, most often sinus bradycardia, tachycardia, and premature ventricular contractions. Some arrhythmias are due to primary cardiac problems, but others are secondary to the brain lesions. Ventricular bigeminy, atrioventricular dissociation and block, ventricular tachycardia, atrial fibrillation, and bundle branch blocks are found less often. Arrhythmias are most common in patients who have brainstem lesions or brainstem compression. Acute pulmonary edema may complicate strokes, especially subarachnoid hemorrhage and posterior circulation ischemia and hemorrhage.

Sudden death associated with stressful situations, including "voodoo death," must involve CNS mechanisms. Ventricular fibrillation can be reliably elicited by stimulation of cardiac sympathetic nerves in both normal and ischemic hearts. Ischemia reduces the threshold for ventricular fibrillation (see also Chapter 18). Stress causes CNS stimulation, which triggers autonomic activation. Patients with lateral medullary and lateral pontine infarcts affecting structures of the reticular formation die unexpectedly; these patients have a high incidence of autonomic dysregulation, such as labile blood pressure, syncope, tachycardia, flushing, and failure of automatic respiration.

SUGGESTED READING

Barbut D, Caplan LR. Brain complications of cardiac surgery. *Curr Probl Cardiol.* 1997;22:455–476.

Barbut D, Hinton RB, Szatrowski TP, et al. Cerebral emboli detected during bypass surgery are associated with clamp removal. *Stroke.* 1994;25:2398–2402.

Caplan LR. *Caplan's Stroke: A Clinical Approach.* 3rd ed. Boston: Butterworth-Heinemann; 2000.

Caplan LR, Hurst JW, Chimowitz MI. *Clinical Neurocardiology.* New York: Marcel Dekker; 1999:186–225.

Caplan LR, Manning WG. *Brain Embolism.* Informa Health Care; London; 2006.

Cohen A, Chauvel C. Transesophageal echocardiography in the management of transient ischemic attack and ischemic stroke. *Cerebrovasc Dis.* 1996;6(suppl 1): 15–25.

French Study of Aortic Plaques in Stroke Group. Atherosclerotic disease of the aortic arch as a risk factor for recurrent ischemic stroke. *N Engl J Med.* 1996;334:1216–1221.

Leary M, Caplan LR. Cerebrovascular disease and neurologic manifestations of heart disease. In: Fuster V, O'Rourke RA, Walsh RA, et al., eds. *Hurst's The Heart*. 12th ed. New York: McGraw-Hill; 2008:2329–2355.

Pessin MS, Estol CJ, Lafranchise F, et al. Safety of anticoagulation after hemorrhagic infarction. *Neurology*. 1993;43:1298–1303.

CHAPTER 56

The Nonsurgical Approach to Carotid Disease

Paul T.L. Chiam, Gary S. Roubin,
Sriram S. Iyer, and Jiri J. Vitek

Carotid stenting (CS) has rapidly evolved over the last decade to become a widely utilized method of carotid artery revascularization. Collective experience with this technique has grown exponentially. Improved peri-procedural outcomes have been achieved through technical and procedural innovations including improved devices, increased operator experience, understanding optimal technique, and understanding the importance of patient selection. It must be noted however, that CS should be viewed as an adjunct to optimal medical therapy; and that to accrue the greatest benefit from CS, concomitant optimal medical therapy is imperative.

For CS to continue to develop, three important issues need to be addressed. These are (1) operator training, (2) application of correct technique, and (3) importance of patient selection.

HISTORICAL PERSPECTIVE

Results of several randomized trials published in the 1990s showed that carotid endarterectomy (CEA) was more effective than medical therapy in reducing the risk of stroke. Based on these data, the American Heart Association (AHA) guidelines recommend CEA for symptomatic carotid stenosis > 50%, and for asymptomatic carotid stenosis > 60% if these asymptomatic patients also have an expected life expectancy of 5 years, provided the peri-procedural complication rates are less than 6% and 3%, respectively. In particular, the asymptomatic corotid surgery trial (ACST) trial reconfirmed that asymptomatic patients derived benefit from CEA with the margin of benefit almost identical to the asymptomatic corotid atherosclerosis study (ACAS) trial. Unlike the ACAS trial, the trial showed that women derived benefit from carotid revascularization. Furthermore, medical management in that trial reflects more contemporary medical therapy in the community with high percentages of patients on antiplatelet therapy, statins, and antihypertensive treatment.

During the evolution of coronary angioplasty in the 1980s, several investigators began to apply the percutaneous approach of angioplasty to carotid revascularization. In 1994, Roubin and coworkers instigated the first rigorous prospective study of CS with independent neurology assessment. Early results by this group and others showed that carotid angioplasty was feasible and had acceptable complication rates despite use of more primitive equipment, lack of distal embolic protection devices (EPDs), and the lack of experience with this novel percutaneous approach. Subsequently, in 2001, the authors published the first long-term follow-up of CS of up to 5 years, which showed that CS could be accomplished with acceptable complication rates and with durable results; and also detection of microembolic signals (MES) with transcranial Doppler during different phases of carotid stenting showed that these signals were reduced with EPDs. More recently, the clinical and anatomic markers of increased risk for CS have been identified and published by our group.

MULTICENTER CLINICAL TRIALS

The stenting angioplasty protection in patients at high risk for endarterectomy (SAPPHIRE) trial showed, in high-surgical risk patients who either were symptomatic with > 50% carotid stenosis or asymptomatic with > 80% carotid stenosis, that Carotid stenting CS was not inferior to Carotid endartesectomy CEA, with MI/stroke/death rates of 12.2% versus 20.1%, respectively, at 1 year, and with clinical equipoise maintained at 3 years.

The carotid revascularization using endarterectomy or stenting systems (CaRESS) trial, a multicenter, nonrandomized, prospective comparative study of symptomatic and asymptomatic patients at high or low surgical risk revealed no significant differences in the stroke or death rates at 30 d and at 1 year between CS and CEA (2.1% vs. 3.6% and 10.0% vs. 13.6%). Although the treatment was decided by the physicians, it imitates true clinical decision-making, suggesting that results of CS are comparable to CEA when appropriate case selection is made.

Recently, however, the endarterectomy versus angioplasty in patients with severe symptomatic carotid stenosis (EVA-3S) and stent- protected percutaneous angioplasty of the carotid versus endarterectomy (SPACE) trials randomizing symptomatic patients showed that CS did not achieve clinical equipoise with CEA. Thirty-day event rates were higher in the CS arm of the EVA-3S study (9.6% vs. 3.9%); in the SPACE trial, although event rates were similar (CS 6.84% vs. CEA 6.34%), CS could not demonstrate noninferiority compared to CEA because of insufficient power as the trial was terminated prematurely due to slow recruitment and lack of funding. Major criticism of the EVA-3S study was that embolic protection was not mandatory early in the trial and the carotid interventionalists were relatively inexperienced compared to the surgeons. Therefore, the results reinforce the important message that distal EPDs must be considered an integral part of the procedure and that rigorous training and credentialing are required.

Multicenter registries of CS that enrolled symptomatic and asymptomatic patients at high surgical-risk provide valuable information regarding outcomes of CS in clinical practice. The stroke or death rates of these registries (ARCHeR, CABERNET, CREATE, CAPTURE, BEACH, CASES-PMS, and ALKK) were between 2.8% and 6.9%. These data show that adverse event rates have decreased even as the procedure has become more widely adopted. The recently reported 1 year results of the BEACH trial (symptomatic and asymptomatic high-surgical-risk patients) showed no difference in event rates between CS (8.9%) and that of CEA as predefined by an FDA-approved objective performance criterion (12.6%).

INDICATIONS AND CONTRAINDICATIONS FOR CAROTID STENTING

The indications of carotid stenting are similar to those for CEA if the procedure can be accomplished with event rates within the AHA guidelines. Certain groups of patients with multiple comorbidities, such as those with severe cardiac or pulmonary disease, which place them at increased surgical risk, are ideal candidates for CS. Several anatomic factors also increase the surgical risk: high lesions (C2 and above), low lesions necessitating thoracic exposure, previous CEA, contralateral ICA occlusion, and prior neck dissection or irradiation are better treated with CS.

With present-day devices and technologies, almost any carotid lesion can be stented. It is not, however, a question of an operator being able to access the stenosis or reduce a lesion stenosis by placing a stent, but is absolutely related to the ability to perform these tasks safely with a low stroke/death rate. Thus, there are several contraindications to CS for

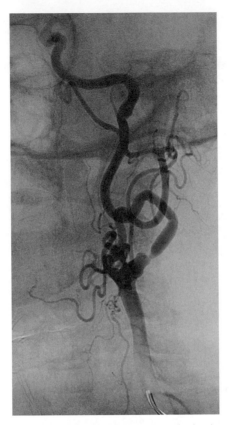

FIGURE 56-1. Angiogram demonstrating severe tortuosity distal to the ICA stenosis, precluding safe deployment of distal filter.

situations that increase the likelihood of adverse events. Two important contraindications are the inability to tolerate dual antiplatelet agents, which are mandatory for at least 1 month post CS; and the inability to advance the EPD distal to the lesion and deployment in a safe "landing" zone (Fig. 56-1). These patients may be more safely treated with CEA. Other contraindications (all relative) include inability to safely access the common carotid artery (CCA), recent (< 14 days) moderate to large cerebral infarction, hostile arch anatomy, severe carotid artery tortuosity, heavy concentric lesion calcification, and the "string sign" (Table 56-1).

ROLE OF CAROTID ANGIOGRAPHY IN PATIENT SELECTION

Many patients with carotid stenosis proceed to CEA based on the findings of severe stenosis on Doppler ultrasound because data from ACAS and North American symptomatic carotid endarterectomy trial (NASCET) revealed a 1% stroke rate associated with diagnostic cerebral angiography. With experienced operators, however, permanent cerebral complications from diagnostic angiography are < 0.3%, and furthermore Doppler ultrasound overestimates stenosis severity in a significant number of patients. Hence diagnostic

TABLE 56-1

Relative Contraindications for Stenting

Inability to tolerate dual antiplatelet therapy
No safe "landing zone" for distal embolic protection device
Inability to safely access the CCA
Recent (< 14 d) moderate to large cerebral infarction
Hostile arch anatomy (type III, severely atheromatous or calcified)
Severe vascular tortuosity
Heavy concentric lesion calcification
"String sign"
Occluded CCA or ICA

cerebral angiography, at least ipsilateral carotid angiography, should be incorporated into the stent procedure as a critical decision-making point.

There have been many instances where the carotid stenosis is found to be less severe during angiography and an unnecessary interventional procedure is avoided. The angiogram provides information on carotid bifurcation level, presence of CCA stenosis, vascular tortuosity, vessel calcification, tandem lesions or intracranial stenoses, lesions characteristics such as presence of ulceration or thrombus, and cerebral collateral flow. We advocate that experienced operators study both carotid arteries, with optional angiographic imaging of a vertebral artery if that can be safely performed. One of the most important points to note is that the final decision to proceed with CS should be made after adequate carotid/cerebral angiograms have been performed. At least two angulated views should be imaged and the view with the most severe tortuosity used in decision-making and to guide the procedure. Often, certain anatomic findings (e.g., vascular tortuosity, heavy concentric lesion calcification) that significantly increase stent risk are first detected during angiography, especially after sheath or guide placement, and depending on findings, the procedure should be terminated and the decision for CS carefully reconsidered.

PATIENT SELECTION

As experience with CS has accumulated, understanding of the entire pathophysiology of the process has deepened. Markers for increased stroke risk during CS (high stent risk) have been identified. These are age, reduced cerebral reserve, excessive vascular tortuosity, and heavy concentric lesion calcification (Table 56-2). Patients with any two or more

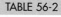

TABLE 56-2

Markers of Increased Risk during Carotid Stenting

	Risk Factor	Features
Clinical	1. Age ≥ 80 y	
	2. Decreased cerebral reserve	Prior (remote) large stroke Multiple lacunar infarcts Intracranial microangiopathy Dementia
Angiographic	3. Excessive tortuosity	≥ 2 90-degree bends within 5 cm of the lesion
	4. Heavy calcification	Concentric calcification; width ≥ 3 mm

of the four risk markers should be excluded from CS, since the risk of peri-procedural stroke will be excessive. Alternative therapies, either medical or surgical, are thus recommended for these patients.

Excessive vascular tortuosity (Fig. 56-2) and heavy concentric lesion calcification (Figs. 56-3 and 56-4B) increase stroke risk due to increased manipulation and procedural time, whereas reduced cerebral reserve decreases brain tolerance to further potential ischemic insult. Age was demonstrated to be a predictor of adverse outcomes before the advent of EPDs and has also been shown to be an adverse predictor even with use of EPDs. The ongoing carotid revascularization endarterectomy versus stenting (CREST) trial (randomizing symptomatic or asymptomatic patients at normal surgical risk) lead-in phase showed that octogenarians had a significantly increased risk of adverse events (12.1% vs. 4.0% in nonoctogenarians) not accounted for by other factors, and recruitment of octogenarians and those of more advanced age was stopped in the lead-in phase of that trial. Possible reasons for these findings are that increased vascular tortuosity and vessel calcification, and reduced cerebral reserve, are more common in elderly patients compared to a younger population.

Several investigators, however, demonstrated that CS can be performed in the octogenarian group with low adverse event rates, raising the question of whether age alone or patient selection and operator experience are the important factors. The authors have recently demonstrated that in the largest single-center series of CS in very elderly patients with independent neurology assessment, CS can be performed in patients selected using the criteria described, with 30-day peri-procedural event rates of 5.1% and 2.6% in the symptomatic and asymptomatic groups, respectively, consistent with the AHA guidelines.

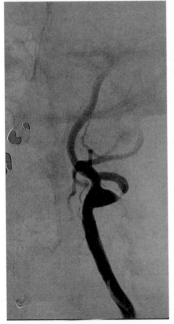 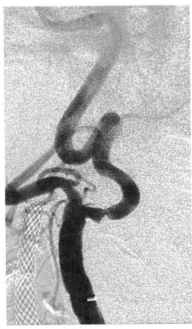

A   **B**

FIGURE 56-2. Angiograms demonstrating excessive vascular tortuotisy (≥ two 90-degree bends within 5 cm of the lesion).

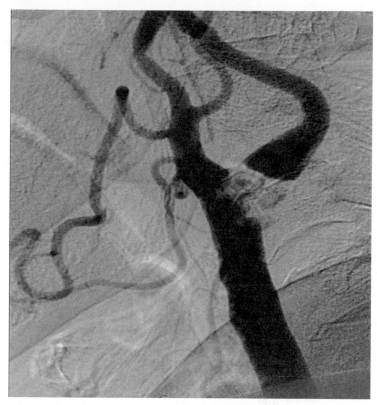

FIGURE 56-3. Angiogram demonstrating heavy concentric lesion calcification.

Therefore, CS and CEA should be view as complementary and not competitive revascularization options There will be patients who are at high surgical risk and more suitable for CS; conversely, there will be patients who are at increased stent risk and will be more suitable for CEA. Thus a new paradigm shift in patient selection is required, and must take into account the stent risk for the individual patient similar to considerations of high surgical risk in patients undergoing CEA. Patients who are at increased risk for both procedures may be better and more safely treated with optimal medical therapy (Fig. 56–5).

TECHNICAL CONSIDERATIONS

Access for the procedure is usually via the femoral artery. Occasionally, in patients with severe peripheral vascular disease, the brachial or radial route can be used. Diagnostic cerebral angiography is routinely performed on all patients to confirm lesion severity and assess vascular tortuosity, vessel calcification, and intracranial collateral circulation. Dedicated neurovascular catheters such as the Vitek catheter (Cook, Bloomington, IN) are used. Arch aortograms are not routinely performed in experienced centers since the

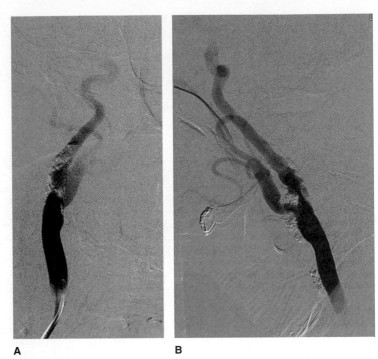

A   **B**

FIGURE 56-4. Angiograms demonstrating heavy concentric lesion calcification.

operators are able to assess arch type based on the configuration of the catheter during diagnostic angiography and also are able to access the CCA even with hostile arches. Thus for these operators, arch angiography does not have significant impact on the choice of equipment or procedure. For operators with lesser experience, arch angiograms are certainly a useful adjunct to help guide decision-making and choice of equipment.

All patients should be on dual antiplatelet therapy with aspirin and clopidogrel. This has been shown to produce superior outcomes compared to aspirin with peri-procedural (24 hour) heparin. Ideally, clopidogrel should be started at least 4 days before the intended procedure, and definitely should not be administered less than 6 hours prior to CS. Strict adherence to this regimen has contributed towards the improved results seen with CS. Control of blood pressure must be meticulous. Antihypertensive medications should be omitted on the morning of the procedure, as mild hypotension and bradycardia usually occur with balloon dilatation and stenting of the carotid bifurcation. Should blood pressure (BP) remain > 160 to 180 systolic after stent implantation, rapidly performing post-dilatation usually reduces BP expeditiously. Less commonly, control of blood pressure is required if it is still > 160 to 180 mm Hg systolic after postdilatation, as it has been shown that strict blood pressure control below 140/90 mm Hg reduces the risk of hyper-perfusion syndrome or cerebral hemorrhage. Intravenous or intra-arterial nitroglycerin or IV labetalol can be used.

Sheaths are preferred over guide catheters as they have a less traumatic tip design, and also require a smaller arteriotomy in the vascular access site. Usually, 6 French (F) sized sheaths are adequate for the vast majority of CS procedures. Occasionally for adverse arch

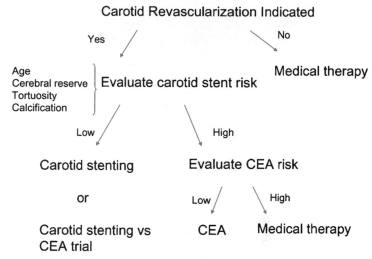

FIGURE 56-5. Clinical decision-making algorithm in the management of carotid artery stenosis.

anatomy or tortuous vessels, a 7F sheath may be required or an 8F guide with the appropriate curve can be utilized. The standard technique of placing the sheath in the common carotid artery (CCA) is most often used. This entails manipulating the diagnostic neurocatheter into the external carotid artery (ECA) over a Glidewire (Terumo, Tokyo) and then exchanging for a sheath over a stiff wire such as the Supracore wire (Abbott Vascular, Santa Clara, CA). Alternatively if the lesion involves the bifurcation of the CCA (Fig. 56-6) or if the ECA is occluded, the "telescopic" technique—where a sheath slides up over a diagnostic neurocatheter and Glidewire/Supracore wire positioned in the CCA—is employed. After sheath or guide placement, vascular tortuosity is reassessed. Occasionally, the vascular tortuosity significantly worsens, and careful reconsideration is required to determine if CS should still proceed as the risk–benefit ratio may have significantly altered.

Anticoagulation is administered once the sheath is in place with either weight-adjusted heparin or bilvalirudin. Bilvalirudin is a direct thrombin inhibitor, and unlike heparin, does not activate platelets. When used in percutaneous coronary intervention, it has been shown to produce the same efficacy as heparin and glycoprotein (GP) IIb/IIIa inhibitors combined but with fewer bleeding complications. Limited data on bivalirudin use in peripheral vascular interventions show that its use appears safe. GP IIb/IIIa inhibitors are no longer used in addition to heparin due to higher risk of cerebral hemorrhage. For these reasons, bivalirudin alone is routinely used during the CS procedure in our institution. Atropine is also administered before balloon predilatation to reduce the incidence of severe bradycardia and hypotension, unless an elevated heart rate is present at the beginning of the procedure or if the lesion is a post CEA restenosis.

After crossing the lesion with a filter wire—the Bare wire system (Abbott Vascular, Santa Clara, CA) where the wire and filter are separate and not fixed, is preferred—the filter is deployed well distal to the lesion in a straight segment of the ICA. In very severe stenotic lesions, where difficulty crossing the stenosis with the filter is anticipated, the "pre-predilatation" technique is used. Any 0.014-in wire, usually a hydrophilic wire such as the PT2 (Boston Scientific, Natick, MA) is first advanced across the severe lesion and "pre-predilatation" is performed with a small 2.0 to 2.5-mm balloon to facilitate

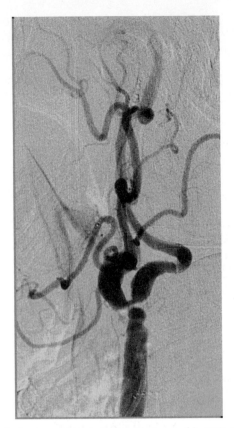

FIGURE 56-6. Angiogram demonstrating severe disease of the CCA. This increases technical difficulty of the procedure, as ECA access for wire support is not possible.

advancement of the filter beyond the stenosis. This unprotected but controlled dilatation with a small balloon is preferable to multiple and prolonged attempts at passing the filter. Once the filter is deployed, predilatation is performed using a small balloon (3.0–3.5 mm) with a single inflation. The intent is to create a track wide enough to facilitate stent placement and yet minimize plaque disruption. Self-expanding nitinol stents are almost exclusively used with stent design falling into two broad groups. The open-cell design (e.g., Acculink, Abbott Vacular, Santa Clara, CA) is more flexible and trackable and conforms better to the vascular anatomy, especially if tortuous. Conversely, the closed-cell design (e.g., Xact stent, Abbott Vascular, Santa Clara, CA) is less flexible but theoretically would entrap atheromatous debris better and also cause less hang-up when retrieving the distal filter with the retrieval catheter. Experience indicates that in only a few cases would placement of a closed-cell stent design be so challenging that an open-cell design is required. Studies examining the superiority of stent cell designs have yielded conflicting results, although it appears that symptomatic patients experience a lower adverse event rate with the use of closed-cell stents. Oversized 9 or 10 mm stents, or 7 to 9 mm or 8 to 10 mm tapered stents, should be used to maximize plaque coverage by metal, and usually include stenting a segment of the 9 to 10 mm CCA.

Postdilatation is performed with a significantly undersized balloon (usually 5.0 mm diameter) with a single inflation. Aggressive postdilatation must be avoided to minimize shearing off plaque fragments that have been squeezed between the stent struts (cheese-grater effect). Contrast injections are kept to a minimum once the wire has passed beyond the stenotic lesion. This reduces risk of injecting microbubbles or microthrombi into the brain, and reduces risk of contrast-induced nephropathy in patients with chronic renal impairment. Balloon dilatation and stent placement can be performed accurately using bony landmarks. Residual stenoses up to 30%, residual ulcers, or mild to moderate distal vessel spasm are best left alone (Fig. 56–7 A and B).

It has been demonstrated using transcranial Doppler that minimal microembolic signals (MES) occur during initial sheath placement, wire crossing, and predilatation; more MES occur during stenting; and the most MES occur during postdilatation. Angioplasty in this setting should be used only to facilitate stent placement and not as a treatment in itself. Therefore, the previous term carotid angioplasty and stenting (CAS) is better termed carotid stenting (CS) in light of this new understanding, emphasizing that stenting is the primary focus, with balloon dilatation only facilitating the process.

CS is performed with EPDs, as previous studies have documented reduction in MES as well as adverse clinical events. Filter dwell time is closely monitored during the procedure to minimize filter deployment time. The CREATE registry showed that filter duration was a predictor for adverse events. Likely reasons are that increased filter duration is a surrogate for case complexity, and that the longer the filter is deployed, the more the accumulation of fibrin and likelihood of embolism. In the vast majority of CS procedures, a distal filter is used. Distal balloon occlusion protection with the Percusurge GuardWire system (Medtronic, Santa Rosa, CA) has the advantage of a lower profile and is more trackable, although it is suitable only in patients with patent intracranial collateral circulation. With all distal protection devices, the initial wiring of the lesion is unprotected and has been shown to cause small amounts of microemboli. Proximal protection devices, such as the Parodi Anti-Emboli System and MOMA, device have been developed to overcome this limitation. Essentially they work using the same principles

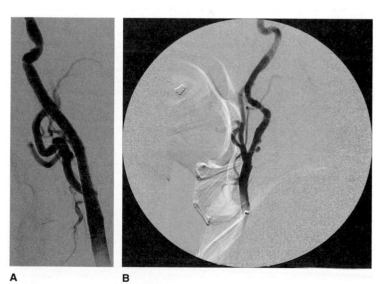

A   **B**

FIGURE 56-7. Post stent angiograms demonstrating residual kinks and ulcer. These should be left alone.

of occluding proximal flow in the common carotid artery and a second balloon occluding flow in the external carotid artery before the lesion is crossed. An added advantage is that any 0.014-in wire can be used. The Parodi system has an extra feature of creating a shunt and reversing blood flow in the ICA. These systems are, however, more cumbersome to use, require a 9F sheath, and like the distal balloon occlusion system, are not suitable for patients with a contralateral ICA occlusion or "isolated hemisphere." To date they have not gained widespread usage.

POSTPROCEDURE MANAGEMENT

Patients are usually monitored closely in a dedicated unit for 4 to 6 hours. Close blood pressure control is essential, as either excessively low or elevated BP may have adverse consequences. Simple hydration should not be overlooked, as this not only reduces risk of contrast-induced nephropathy but also would be beneficial for the relative hypotension that most patients experience postprocedure. Frequent neurologic assessments should be performed during the initial 24 hours, and patients are usually discharged the next day following uncomplicated procedures. Dual antiplatelet therapy is continued for at least 4 weeks, and thereafter aspirin or clopidogrel is maintained indefinitely. A baseline Doppler ultrasound should be performed at the 1-month follow-up as a baseline reference value for future follow-up.

【 】 MANAGEMENT OF HEMODYNAMICS

Hypotension and bradycardia usually occur after stenting and postdilatation due to stretching of the carotid baroreceptors, especially if the procedure involved the carotid bifurcation, and are the commonest complications seen after CS. Usually they are transient and resolve with fluid bolus. More persistent or severe cases can be rapidly reversed with small boluses of IV phenylephrine. Prophylactic atropine administration before balloon dilatation and stenting appears to reduce the occurrence of bradycardia or hypotension. Rarely, hypotension and bradycardia can persist for several days and IV pressors such as dopamine may be required. Early ambulation may reduce the frequency and severity of this phenomenon. In this regard, groin closure devices may provide an advantage in allowing more rapid ambulation.

Hyperperfusion syndrome can occur after relief of a very severe stenosis, especially if peri-procedural BP was elevated. The underlying process is likely to be due to impaired cerebral autoregulation after prolonged and severe ICA stenosis. The classical symptom is headache. Nausea, vomiting, focal neurologic deficits, and seizures may also occur. A high index of suspicion for this complication should be entertained, especially if there was postprocedure hypertension. Velocities in the ipsilateral middle cerebral artery may be normal or increased, and brain CT may be normal or reveal vasogenic edema. Treatment includes BP reduction with intravenous agents, withholding antiplatelet agents until symptom resolution, and close monitoring of neurologic status. Stringent BP control pre- and post-CS has been shown to reduce the hyperperfusion syndrome and the risk of resultant cerebral hemorrhage.

【 】 SPECIAL CONSIDERATIONS

Elderly Patients

The octogenarian group has consistently shown poorer outcomes after CS compared to a younger population. However, more recent studies have demonstrated that with careful patient and lesion selection, CS can be performed in these patients with acceptable outcomes, with results similar to CEA in octogenarians and CS in younger patients. Therefore age itself should not be a high stent-risk criterion provided appropriate patient selection has been made.

Severe Peripheral Vascular Disease

Occasionally, the transfemoral route is precluded due to severe peripheral vascular disease. In these patients, a radial or brachial route can be used. Less commonly, a direct puncture of the CCA could also be performed if the expertise is available.

Challenging Vascular Anatomy

In certain cases with very tortuous vascular anatomy, special measures to maintain stability of the system or to cross the lesion are required. Use of larger-sized sheaths or guides may help provide extra support. An extra 0.014- or 0.018-in wire can also be placed in the ECA as a "buddy wire" to provide extra backup.

Crossing of a lesion in tortuous anatomy may be further aided by simple bedside maneuvers such as removing the patient's head restraint and extending the neck, and getting the patient to turn the head from side to side. Use of separated wire-filter systems such as the Emboshield filter (Abbott Vascular, Santa Clara, CA) or Spider filter (EV3, Plymouth, MN) may be helpful. Other options would include using a hydrophilic 0.014-in wire to cross the lesion to reduce tortuosity (buddy wire) and then pass the filter wire.

In very severely stenotic lesions, "pre-predilatation" with a small balloon may facilitate crossing of the filter wire or filter alone.

Carotid Stent Restenosis

Restenosis post CS is uncommon, with < 5% incidence. Most series reporting restenosis used a cut-off of 80% and 50% for asymptomatic and symptomatic patients, respectively. Frequently, restenosis is detected on Doppler ultrasound, because symptoms are uncommon. Restenosis seems to occur more frequently in those with smaller stent luminal diameter post-stenting, and in patients who undergo CS for post-CEA restenosis and postradiation carotid stenosis.

Patients Undergoing Coronary Artery Bypass Surgery with Severe Carotid Stenosis

The incidence of coexisting carotid and coronary artery disease (CAD) ranges from 2% to 12%. In patients with severe CAD and carotid stenosis, the risk of stroke during CABG is significantly higher than in patients without carotid disease; and conversely, performing CEA before CABG results in higher rates of myocardial infarction and death. The risks of MI/stroke/death in performing CABG and CEA simultaneously are also elevated. An earlier meta-analysis of staged CS followed by CABG revealed a total MI/stroke/death rate of 12.3%; recently, however, it has been shown that with present-day technology and practice, performing CS prior to CABG resulted in a total MI/stroke/death rate of 6.7%. Staged CS in those who are suitable, followed by CABG, may be the safest option in these patients. Ideally, patients are managed medically for 3 to 4 weeks with cessation of antiplatelet therapy at this time. CABG should not be performed immediately if the surgeon will not operate with the patient on aspirin and clopidogrel. In patients with critical aortic stenosis or severe left mainstem CAD, especially if left ventricular ejection fraction is also depressed, CS before cardiac surgery can, in the authors' experience, be performed more safely with intra-aortic balloon pump support.

CONCURRENT MEDICAL THERAPY

Medical therapy should be viewed as an integral part of carotid disease treatment *whether or not* CS is performed. Therefore medical therapy must be optimized to achieve best possible outcomes even if carotid revascularization takes place. Antiplatelet therapy with aspirin or clopidogrel should be universal in patients with carotid disease. Use of dual antiplatelet therapy long term is not recommended, as a previous study showed that this regimen did not significantly reduce stroke rate but increased the rate of major bleeding. Short-term use of dual antiplatelet therapy in symptomatic carotid stenosis, however, appears beneficial. Dual antiplatelet therapy should also be used peri-procedurally if CS is performed.

The usual atherosclerotic risk factors should be assessed and treated. Blood pressure control is probably the most important risk factor in stroke prevention. A lower BP reduces stroke risk, and use of angiotensin-converting enzyme (ACE) inhibitors further reduces stroke risk over and above that attributable to BP lowering alone. Lipid-lowering therapy with statins helps plaque stabilization and may even promote plaque regression. A large randomized trial demonstrated reduction in stroke with aggressive lipid-lowering therapy with statins. Smoking cessation should be advised at every opportunity. Glycemic control in diabetics is also important, although it has been shown that tight glycemic control reduces only microvascular but not macrovascular complications such as stroke. Good glycemic control, however, leads to improved lipid profile, which is important in these patients. Lifestyle changes also should not be forgotten as part of the general measures to reduce the atherosclerotic burden.

FUTURE DIRECTIONS

The optimal timing of CS in symptomatic patients is yet to be well defined. The risk–benefit ratio of revascularization is greatest in the early period after a transient ischemic attack or minor stroke and declines with time as demonstrated in the CEA studies, since the risk of stroke diminishes with time from the initial event. Therefore, performing CS early after an event would theoretically yield the most protective benefit. A recent study showed, however, that CS early (within 2 weeks) after an event resulted in higher adverse event rates than if CS was delayed. For asymptomatic carotid stenoses, future studies will be needed to determine markers that could predict subgroups most at risk of stroke and would hence derive the greatest benefit from CS. In this asymptomatic group, plaque imaging to detect the "vulnerable" plaque more likely to embolize could prove very useful.

Technological advancements will result in decreased profile and increased maneuverability of devices, and better distal protection devices, which may reduce complication rates and improve the safety of the procedure.

Ongoing trials will provide further data on the safety and efficacy of CS compared to CEA. The CREST trial will shed light on both symptomatic and asymptomatic patients with normal surgical risk; ACT1 will provide answers for asymptomatic patients at normal surgical risk.

The most important factor, however, that will further reduce adverse events after CS is that of careful patient selection. Akin to the concept of surgical risk, patients being considered for CS should be selected based on stent risk, and greater efforts must be made to identify additional clinical or anatomic markers that increase the risk of CS.

SUGGESTED READING

Chiam PT, Roubin GS, Iyer SS, et al. Carotid artery stenting in elderly patients: importance of case selection. *Catheter Cardiovasc Interv.* DOI: 10.1002/ccd/21620

Gray WA, Yadav JS, Verta P, et al. The CAPTURE registry: results of carotid stenting with embolic protection in the post approval setting. *Catheter Cardiovasc Interv.* 2007;69:341–348.

Gurm HS, Yadav JS, Fayad P, et al. Long-term results of carotid stenting versus endarterectomy in high-risk patients. *N Engl J Med.* 2008;358:1572–1579.

Halliday A, Mansfield A, Marro J, et al. Prevention of disabling and fatal strokes by successful carotid endarterectomy in patients without recent neurological symptoms: randomised controlled trial. *Lancet.* 2004;363:1491–502.

Mas JL, Chatellier G, Beyssen B, et al. Endarterectomy versus stenting in patients with symptomatic severe carotid stenosis. *N Engl J Med.* 2006;355:1660–1671.

Ringleb PA, Allenberg J, Bruckmann H, et al. 30 day results from the SPACE trial of stent-protected angioplasty versus carotid endarterectomy in symptomatic patients: a randomised non-inferiority trial. *Lancet.* 2006;368:1239–1247.

Roubin GS, Iyer S, Halkin A, et al. Realizing the potential of carotid artery stenting: proposed paradigms for patient selection and procedural technique. *Circulation.* 2006;113:2021–2030.

Roubin GS, New G, Iyer SS, et al. Immediate and late clinical outcomes of carotid artery stenting in patients with symptomatic and asymptomatic carotid artery stenosis: a 5-year prospective analysis. *Circulation.* 2001;103:532–537.

Sacco RL, Adams R, Albers G, et al. Guidelines for prevention of stroke in patients with ischemic stroke or transient ischemic attack: a statement for healthcare professionals from the American Heart Association/American Stroke Association Council on Stroke. Co-sponsored by the Council on Cardiovascular Radiology and Intervention. The American Academy of Neurology affirms the value of this guideline. *Stroke.* 2006;37:577–617.

Yadav JS, Wholey MH, Kuntz RE, et al. Protected carotid-artery stenting versus endarterectomy in high-risk patients. *N Engl J Med.* 2004;351:1493–1501.

CHAPTER 57

Diagnosis and Management of Diseases of the Peripheral Arteries and Veins

Faisal A. Arian and Paul W. Wennberg

ARTERIAL DISEASE

【 】 ATHEROSCLEROTIC ARTERIAL OCCLUSIVE DISEASE

Clinical Presentation

Claudication is reproducible, predictable discomfort in single or multiple muscle groups brought on by sustained exercise and relieved by rest independent of position due to inadequate peripheral arterial blood flow. If a specific position is required for relief, *pseudoclaudication* should be considered (Table 57-1). Advanced peripheral arterial disease (PAD) may present as critical limb ischemia (CLI) characterized by pain at rest with or without tissue loss (ischemic ulcer or gangrene). The presentation of PAD is variable, depending on rate of progression, extent of collateral vessel involvement, comorbidities, and functional status of the patient. Risk factors for PAD are those of coronary artery disease. Diabetes mellitus, tobacco use, age > 65 years, and hyperlipidemia have been linked to progression to CLI. The risk of death (usually due to a cardiovascular event) increases as the ankle–brachial index (ABI) decreases. Classic claudication is present in only 10% of patients, while 40 % remain asymptomatic. The remaining 50% have atypical symptoms.

Examination

Examination includes palpation and auscultation of femoral, iliac, aortic, carotid, and subclavian arteries. Pulse intensity is graded as 0 = absent, 1 = diminished, 2 = normal, and 3 = bounding. Skin temperature, color, and integrity should be compared to that of the proximal and contralateral limbs. A cool, pale extremity with hair loss, pallor on elevation, and rubor (red) with dependent position are signs of advanced disease.

Laboratory Assessment

The ABI is the main test in screening for PAD (Table 57-2). It is calculated by dividing higher of the anterior tibial or posterior tibial artery systolic pressure by the highest brachial artery systolic pressure. Exercise ABI estimates the severity of PAD and also provides excellent prognostic information that may be used to further plan management. Poorly compressible or noncompressible vessels due to arterial calcification (especially in diabetics) limit applicability of the ABI. If the large vessels are noncompressible, the digital vessels in the toes often remain noncalcified and can be used to the estimate

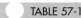 **TABLE 57-1**

Differential Diagnosis of Claudication

Atherosclerosis obliterans	Popliteal entrapment
Arteritis (Takayasu's, giant-cell, etc.)	Venous claudication/varicosities
Embolic disease	Baker's cyst
Arterial spasms (Raynaud's phenomenon)	Degenerative joint disease
Spinal stenosis	Aortic dissection
Myopathy	Aortic coarctation
Thromboangiitis obliterans	Retroperitoneal fibrosis

toe–brachial index. When a pulse is not palpable, *continuous-wave Doppler ultrasound* is used to further define the degree of stenosis. Arterial signals change from a normal triphasic waveform to biphasic, then monophasic, and eventually absent as the severity of stenosis increases. *Transcutaneous partial pressure of oxygen* (TcPO$_2$) may be useful in predicting whether cutaneous perfusion is adequate to heal an ulcer or in planning amputation level.

Angiography is the gold standard for imaging PAD. Computed tomographic angiography (CTA) and *magnetic resonance angiography* (MRA) are noninvasive tests that may be an alternative to catheterization. MRA had historically been a good alternative to CTA in patients with renal failure. However, recent reviews have suggested an association of gadolinium with development of systemic fibrosis and dermopathy in patients with renal failure.

Treatment

Risk-factor modification, especially smoking cessation and a walking program, are the cornerstones of therapy. A *walking program* should be initiated in all patients, with a goal of 30 minutes most days of the week. Diligent foot care and supportive footwear must be emphasized, particularly in diabetics. Control of lipids, hypertension, and diabetes should be optimized. Antiplatelet therapy, with clopidogrel and aspirin (ASA), reduces the risk of adverse cardiovascular outcomes and death in patients with cardiovascular disease by 25% and should be strongly considered. *Cilostazol* is FDA approved to increase the walking distance in patients with claudication. Statins and angiotensin-converting enzyme (ACE) inhibitors have also been shown to improve pain-free walking distance

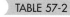 **TABLE 57-2**

Ankle–Brachial Index (ABI) Criteria[a]

	Pre-exercise	Post-exercise	Claudication	Walking Time (min)
Normal	> 0.90[b,c]	> 0.90	None	5
Minimal	> 0.90	< 0.90	None	5
Mild	> 0.80	> 0.50	Present, late	5
Moderate	< 0.80	< 0.50	Present, limiting	< 5
Severe	< 0.50	< 0.15	Early, limiting	< 3

[a]Post-exercise values are taken after walking 5 minutes on a 10% grade at 2 mph. (Speed and distance will vary as tolerated by each patient.)
[b]An ABI > 1.40 (1.30 in some laboratories) is considered noncompressible and an alternative means of investigation should be considered.
[c]Some laboratories use 0.95 as the lower limit for normal.

in patients with claudication. In addition, ACE inhibitors provide protection from adverse cardiovascular events beyond those that can be attributed to blood pressure reduction only. Beta-blockers should *not* be withheld from patients with PAD and concurrent coronary artery disease. Revascularization should be considered in the patients who have failed a trial of conservative therapy or those with rest pain, tissue loss, or lifestyle-limiting claudication. Surgical revascularization is a well established and durable modality. Percutaneous transluminal angioplasty (PTA), with or without stent placement, is beneficial for proximal lesions, such as in the iliac arteries. PTA is less durable when used for distal lesions. However PTA may be a reasonable alternative in patients who are poor surgical candidates and in need of a limb-saving procedure.

【　】 OTHER CAUSES OF CLAUDICATION

Claudication and ischemia may result from numerous disorders (Table 57-1). Some medicines, such as *ergot* compounds, can induce arterial spasm resulting in Raynaud's phenomenon, claudication, acute ischemia, or tissue infarction. With the overall decline in use of ergot for treatment of migraine, this phenomenon is now quite rare. *Fibromuscular dysplasia* (FMD) most commonly affects women in the fourth decade. Renal artery involvement is most common but any artery may be affected. FMD is usually treatable by angioplasty alone. *Microembolism* most often originates from an ulcerated plaque or an aneurysm and less often from the heart. Events may be spontaneous or precipitated by surgery, instrumentation, or anticoagulant therapy. Livedo reticularis (patchy, focal area of bluish discoloration with a lacy pattern) or overt ischemia ("blue-toe syndrome") may be present. Biopsy may be necessary to differentiate microembolization from vasculitis or other etiologies. Antiplatelet agents or systemic anticoagulation may help in preventing recurrence, but the efficacy of these agents is not documented. Solitary plaques may be treated surgically or endovascularly.

【　】 ACUTE ARTERIAL OCCLUSION

Acute arterial occlusion presents with one or more of the following clinical signs: pain, pallor, paresthesia, paralysis, and pulselessness; it may also be cold (polar). Occlusion could be due to trauma, dissection, thrombosis in situ, or embolism. Distal changes caused by microembolization may be present. A search for an embolic source should be undertaken, especially in patients with atrial fibrillation. Attempts to restore blood flow either by pharmacologic (thrombolysis) or mechanical means should begin without delay. Immediate measures include heparinization, limb protection, and pain control. Angiography is often required to plan intervention. If the affected limb is not viable, amputation should be performed as quickly as possible to avoid further complications.

【　】 ARTERIAL DISORDERS OF THE UPPER EXTREMITY

Arterial disease in the upper extremity is less common and more varied in etiology than in the lower extremity. *Thoracic outlet syndrome* (TOS) usually results when the clavicle and the first rib and/or a cervical rib impinge on the subclavian artery. This may predispose the involved arterial segment to develop an aneurysm or a thrombus, which may cause distal embolization. Venous and neurologic complaints may also occur. Imaging for the presence of a functional stenosis with duplex ultrasound or arteriography can document the presence of dynamic obstruction. However, positive thoracic outlet maneuvers are common and the diagnosis of TOS remains a clinical decision. Resection of a cervical rib or first rib should be considered only after physiotherapy has failed or if vascular damage is evident. Improvement of symptoms is variable, particularly for neurogenic complaints. *Hammer hand syndrome* is the result of trauma to the hypothenar area by using the hand as a hammer or by repetitive force with devices. These activities result in aneurysm formation of the ulnar artery, usually at the level of the hamate bone. Ischemia of one or more digits can result from emboli.

TABLE 57-3

Causes of Secondary Raynaud's Phenomenon

Collagen vascular disease	Pulmonary hypertension
Scleroderma	Neurogenic
Mixed connective tissue disease	Thoracic outlet irritation
Rheumatoid arthritis	Carpal tunnel syndrome
Myositis	Neuropathy
Sjögren's syndrome	Medications
Necrotizing vasculitis	Beta-blockers
Hematologic disorders	Ergotamine
Myxedema	Methysergide
Acromegaly	

Takayasu's arteritis and *giant-cell (temporal) arteritis* (GCA) are similar pathologic processes that affect women more than men. Arteries above the diaphragm are usually involved. Generally Takayasu's arteritis affects < 40-year-old and GCA affects > 50-year-old patients. Disease involves arteries bilaterally but the severity is not same on both sides. Both conditions are associated with characteristic clinical and laboratory findings, including an elevated sedimentation rate and classic arteriographic features. These diseases are unique among arteriopathies in that the stenotic lesions improve with steroid therapy.

In *Raynaud's phenomenon*, cold or emotional stimuli induce vasospasm resulting in skin color changes from blue to white to red. The fingers are affected more often than the toes. Many patients describe only the white phase. It may be primary or secondary. *Primary Raynaud's* is defined as bilateral symptoms for 2 consecutive years without evidence of ischemia or other disease processes. Patients without laboratory evidence of digital occlusive disease, thrombophilic disorders, or serologic abnormalities generally have a benign course. These patients do not require any specific therapy and quickly learn to keep not only hands but also the whole body warm. *Secondary Raynaud's phenomenon* has many etiologies (Table 57-3) and the course is generally less benign. Treatment of secondary Raynaud's must be directed at the underlying cause. Calcium-channel blockers and alpha-adrenergic blockers, alone or in combination, can reduce vasospasm severity and frequency but rarely eliminate it.

VENOUS DISEASE

【 】 VARICOSE VEINS

Primary varicose veins are often familial, with onset during young adulthood or pregnancy. Symptoms such as pain, pressure, or burning discomfort over the veins are aggravated by prolonged dependency. Edema and skin changes due to venous stasis are less often present in primary varicosities, and when they are present, a secondary process should be considered. *Secondary varicose veins* are due to a shift in venous return from the deep to the superficial veins. Common causes of secondary varicosities are extrinsic venous compression, prior deep venous thrombosis (DVT), congenital lesions, arteriovenous fistulas, and elevated right heart pressure. Varicosity enlargement and superficial thrombophlebitis may occur over time. Both symptoms and progression can be ameliorated by appropriately fitted graduated compression hose of 20 to 30 mm Hg or more. Ablation of varicose veins should be considered if complications arise or discomfort is present. Sclerotherapy is effective for most small varicosities and cutaneous "spider veins." Surgical or endovascular intervention is indicated for long proximal varicosities, especially if incompetence of perforator veins or the saphenofemoral junction is present.

[ ] DEEP VENOUS THROMBOSIS

The morbidity and mortality of DVT remain high. Risk factors for DVT and pulmonary embolism are listed in Table 57-4. Objective testing to confirm and define the extent of DVT should be obtained whenever DVT is suspected. Venous duplex ultrasound is the most commonly used method. The sensitivity of duplex ultrasonography is operator dependent, especially for small calf vein and pelvic vein DVTs. Duplex ultrasound may be able to differentiate acute from chronic thrombus based on presence of certain features like the presence of distention (acute) and increased echogenicity of the thrombus (chronic). Treatment with heparin (acutely) and warfarin (chronically) is highly effective in preventing clot propagation and pulmonary embolism. Recent literature suggests treatment for a minimum of 3 to 6 months for patients with first spontaneous DVT. Long-term anticoagulation is considered if the patient has an underlying hypercoagulable state or has recurrent venous thrombosis. Low-molecular-weight heparin (LMWH) has been approved for the initial treatment of uncomplicated DVT. Inferior vena cava filters should be considered when anticoagulation is contraindicated or has failed. Thrombolytic therapy has been used in cases of iliofemoral DVT to reduce the incidence and severity of postphlebitic syndrome, but clear indications for thrombolysis in DVT have not yet been established. Once again, use of compression stockings (> 20 mm Hg) reduces the incidence of postphlebitic syndrome, venous stasis, and ulceration. Leg edema should be at a minimum when measurements are taken to get properly fitting stockings.

Isolated calf vein (distal) thrombus is less likely to embolize than a proximal thrombus. However, 20% of calf DVTs will extend proximally, and 10% of these will embolize. Surveillance sonography is required if anticoagulation is not used initially.

[ ] CHRONIC VENOUS INSUFFICIENCY (CVI)

Chronic deep venous incompetence may occur as sequelae of single or multiple episodes of DVT (post-phlebitic syndrome) or may present de novo. It is generally characterized by leg edema and venous dilation progressing to lipodermatosclerosis (intradermal deposition of proteins and hemosiderin) in advanced cases. The postphlebitic syndrome is characterized by symptoms of heavy, congested limbs, venous claudication, pruritus, and ulceration. Cutaneous changes include fibrosis, lichenification, cellulitis, and ulceration. Reduction of the edema is necessary for the ulcers to heal. Indefinite use of 30 to 40 mm Hg compression stockings is indicated. Edema of chronic venous insufficiency usually spares the toes, thus differentiating it from lymphedema.

Phlegmasia cerulea dolens is a rare complication of DVT seen in the setting of extensive iliofemoral thrombosis characterized by rapid onset of massive edema, severe pain, cyanosis, and ischemia due to compartment syndrome. It is seen most commonly with

TABLE 57-4

Risk Factors for Deep Venous Thrombosis

Age	Residency in a health care facility
Immobility	Prior superficial venous thrombosis
Recent surgery	Hospitalization
Progesterone therapy	Malignancy
Prior deep venous thrombosis	Trauma
Underlying coagulopathy	

advanced malignancy or severe infections, but can follow surgery, fractures, or other trauma. One-third of patients die due to pulmonary embolism, and half develop distal gangrene. Urgent treatment—including placement of a caval filter, heparinization, and thrombectomy or thrombolysis—is required to minimize loss of life or limb.

【 】 LYMPHEDEMA

Primary lymphedema may be present at birth as an isolated occurrence or as part of a congenital familial syndrome. *Lymphedema praecox* has its onset in the teens or early twenties and is seen more often in females (usually around menarche). *Lymphedema tarda* has its onset in later years, but is a diagnosis of exclusion since a secondary cause is more likely in this age group. *Secondary lymphedema* may be due to trauma, recurrent infection, obstruction, infiltrative processes, radiation, or other process either directly or indirectly causing damage to the lymphatics. Recurrent cellulitis is common in patients with lymphedema, causing further damage to lymphatic channels. Unlike venous edema and obesity, lymphedema usually involves the toes. The skin is thickened and rough, giving it the characteristic orange-peel *(peau d'orange)* appearance. The cornerstone of treatment for lymphedema is compression. The leg must be reduced in size by elevation, mechanical pumping, or manual massage. Wrapping of the distal-to-proximal portion of the affected limb(s) is required whenever the patient is upright. Once the leg volume has been decreased, a fit-to-measure compression garment at 40 to 50 mm Hg should be worn. Early and aggressive treatment of cellulitis and tinea pedis is recommended.

VASCULAR ULCERS

Vascular ulcers are classified into four categories: arterial, small-vessel, venous, and neurotrophic (Table 57-5). In patients with diabetes or immunosuppression, the ulcers may be multifactorial. Effective treatment must be guided by the etiology. Protection,

TABLE 57-5

Ulcers of Vascular Etiology

Type	Venous	Arterial	Neurotrophic	Small-Vessel
Location	Above medial and lateral malleoli	Shins, toes, sites of injury	Plantar surface, pressure points	Shin, calf
Pain	No, unless infected	Yes	No	Exquisite
Skin	Stasis changes lipodermato-sclerosis	Shiny, pale decreased hair, may see livedo	Callous, normal to changes of ischemia	"Satellite" ulcers in various stages
Edges	Clean	Smooth	Trophic, callused	Serpiginous
Base	Wet, weeping, healthy granulation	Dry, pale with eschar	Healthy to pale depending on ASO	Dry, punched-out, pale thin eschar
Cellulitis	Common	Often	Common	Rare
Treatment	Compression	Revascularize	Relieve pressure	Treat pain, and causal disease

treatment of infection, and establishment of an ulcer base conducive to the formation of granulation tissue are needed. The wound base assists in selection of a dressing. In general, one should choose an absorbent dressing for wet wounds, a hydrating dressing for dry wounds, and a dressing with antibiotic properties for infected wounds. Moisture-neutral dressings are also available. Manual debridement or mechanical debridement using wet-to-dry gauze dressing changes may be necessary.

SUGGESTED READING

Gloviczki P, Yao JST. *Handbook of Venous Disorders: Guidelines of the American Venous Forum.* 2nd ed. Hodder Arnold. London; 2001.

Hirsch AT, Haskal ZJ, Hertzer NR, et al. ACC/AHA 2005 practice guidelines for the management of patients with peripheral arterial disease (lower extremity, renal, mesenteric, and abdominal aortic). *Circulation.* 2006;113:e463–e654.

Creager MA, Dzau VD, Loscalzo J, et al. *Vascular Medicine: A Companion to Braunwald's Heart Disease.* Philadelphia, PA: Saunders; 2006.

Norgren L, Hiatt WR, Dormandy JA, et al. Inter-society consensus for the management of peripheral arterial disease (TASC II). *J Vasc Surg.* 2007;45 (suppl): S5–S67.

Wennberg PW, Rooke TW. Diagnosis and management of diseases of the peripheral arteries and veins. In: Fuster V, O'Rourke RA, Walsh R, et al., eds. *Hurst's The Heart.* 12th ed. New York, NY: McGraw-Hill; 2007:2361–2379.

CHAPTER 58

Endovascular Treatment of Peripheral Vascular Disease

Suhail Allaqaband, Anjan Gupta,
and Tanvir Bajwa

In the past 25 years, significant advances in endovascular treatment for peripheral vascular disease (PVD) have given doctors and their patients minimally invasive alternatives to major surgical procedures that carry significant morbidity and mortality. Dramatic advances in device technology have made it possible to cross difficult lesions and chronic occlusions. The availability of stents has revolutionized endovascular intervention with marked improvement in immediate and long-term results. Endovascular stents are now the standard of care in peripheral vascular intervention. The development of stent grafts now permits minimally invasive treatment of aneurysmal disease of the aorta as well as other major vascular areas. Endovascular intervention is now the first-line therapy in patients who have acute limb ischemia due to thromboembolic disease.

Percutaneous revascularization has revolutionized the treatment of PVD so rapidly within the past decade that it is easy to forget that, not long ago, surgery was the only available treatment for severe PVD and was frequently delayed until rest pain or gangrene forced the issue. The risk of morbidity and death from surgery were simply too high to justify earlier intervention. Not only can we intervene earlier, but we can now offer the benefit of intervention to many categories of patients not previously considered candidates.

With the advent of stents and better device technology, we routinely treat more complex, calcified, occlusive lesions in high-risk patients with excellent short-term as well as long-term results. There are a few instances, for example, in patients with fibromuscular dysplasia, where results with percutaneous balloon angioplasty (PTA) alone are excellent. But for the majority of patients, currently, stents are the destination therapy for most endovascular interventions for PVD.

The future of endovascular intervention looks even more promising with the advent of drug-eluting stents.

OCCLUSIVE DISEASE OF AORTOILIAC ARTERIES

Patients who have atherosclerotic occlusive disease of the distal aortic bifurcation and proximal iliac arteries can present with lifestyle-limiting claudication, limb-threatening ischemia, or impotence. Traditionally, aortoiliac bifurcation disease has been treated with bypass grafting, which yields an excellent long-term outcome but has been associated with a perioperative mortality rate of up to 2% to 4% and a rate of major early complications (including sexual dysfunction, ureteral damage, intestinal ischemia, and spinal cord injury) of 5% to 13%. Endovascular interventions using stents have become the treatment of choice for aortoiliac disease. Our results, and those of others, using kissing stents for the treatment of aortoiliac bifurcation lesions, have been excellent, both immediately post-procedure and long-term. Our rate of procedural success is 100%,

669

TABLE 58-1

PTA Plus Stenting in Iliac Occlusive Disease: Results of Meta-Analysis of 14 Studies

	PTA + Stent	
	Stenosis	Occlusion
Immediate technical success (%)	100	80
Primary patency (%)	77	61
Secondary patency (%)	80	
Major complications (%)	5.2	

with a primary patency rate of 92% over > 18-month follow-up and a secondary patency rate of 100%.

The initial technical success rate for endovascular intervention for iliac artery occlusive disease is (90%, with a 5-year primary patency rate of about 80% and an extremely low mortality and morbidity. In those who have longer, calcified lesions or occluded arteries, the success rate may be lower; in which case, intravascular stents have been employed with excellent results. A meta-analysis of 14 studies (> 2,000 patients) concluded that PTA with stent placement in iliac arteries was associated with high initial procedural success, with long-term patency rates comparable to surgical grafts and significantly lower morbidity (Table 58-1).

Aortoiliac stenting is thus well supported by current data as the initial choice for treatment of patients with occlusive disease because it is less invasive and has an excellent rate of technical success and long-term patency.

We recommend endovascular stenting as the treatment of first choice in patients who have occlusive or stenotic aortoiliac disease and who present with:

- Critical limb-threatening ischemia.
- Lifestyle-limiting claudication.
- Poor inflow prior to distal femoropopliteal bypass.
- Need for vascular access for performing other cardiac interventions.

(See Fig. 58-1).

OCCLUSIVE DISEASE OF FEMOROPOPLITEAL ARTERIES

Atherosclerotic occlusive disease is 2 to 5 times more common in femoropopliteal arteries than in iliac arteries. Patients may vary in their clinical presentation from claudication to rest pain and leg ischemia. Whereas choices for managing iliac artery disease are clear-cut, choices for managing disease in the femoropopliteal arteries are not supported by strong evidence for or against percutaneous intervention (i.e., PTA, atherectomy, laser, stenting, or a combination of these) or peripheral bypass surgery. When pulsatile flow must be restored to prevent limb loss in patients who have rest pain or critical limb-threatening ischemia, some form of intervention is imperative.

Improved techniques and better-designed balloon catheters and wires, especially the introduction of the hydrophilic/glide wire and such devices as the Frontrunner catheter system and the Re-Entry Catheter, have raised the rate of procedural success to 95% to 100% for treating stenotic lesions and 70% to 80% for occluded lesions. Long-term success of endovascular intervention depends upon the lesion type (i.e., stenosis versus occlusion)

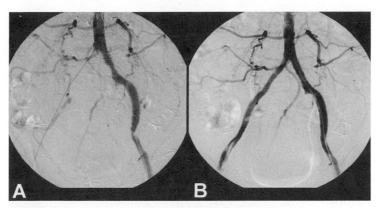

FIGURE 58-1. A 71-year-old male with severe lifestyle-limiting claudication.
A. Angiography showed occluded right common iliac artery and moderate lesion in left common iliac artery and severe lesion in left external iliac artery. **B.** Self-expanding SMART Control stents (Cordis Corp., Minneapolis, MN) deployed with kissing technique followed by postdilatation using kissing balloons.

and the patency of distal runoff vessels. With good distal runoff vessels, the patency rate of PTA in stenotic vessels at 5 years is about 55% to 65%, decreasing to 35% to 45% if the treated vessel is occluded or if runoff is poor. The following indicators adversely affect the degree of patency one can achieve in treating femoropopliteal arteries with PTA:

- Occlusion (especially > 10 cm)
- Calcified vessels
- Multiple-lesion segments
- Rest ischemia (versus claudication)
- Poor distal runoff

Consequently, PTA is increasingly used to treat short, stenotic lesions in the femoropopliteal arteries. Because of poor long-term patency, PTA for occluded femoropopliteal arteries is not recommended unless claudication limits a patient's lifestyle or the patient has progressed to critical limb ischemia.

Although, in treating iliac artery disease, one can expect intravascular stenting to yield excellent long-term patency rates, its long-term benefit for femoropopliteal lesions is unclear. The small number of patients studied and differences in the types of stents used make useful comparison between studies impossible. *In femoropopliteal arteries, use of balloon-expandable stents can no longer be recommended.* At present, only self-expanding stents are used to treat occlusive disease in femoropopliteal arteries; but one must be cautious, because not all self-expanding stents work equally well.

Recently, covered stents (VIABAHN) have been approved by the Food and Drug Administration (FDA) in the treatment of long SFA lesions with a hope of reducing the rate of restenosis and improving long-term patency; however, initial reports have been mixed.

Other devices, like atherectomy cutters, laser catheters, and cryoplasty balloon catheters, have been used with much enthusiasm in femoropopliteal artery repair in the hope of improving long-term patency. However, none of the trials completed so far have shown added benefit for the use of these devices over PTA or stenting.

The BASIL (Bypass versus Angioplasty in Severe Ischemia of the Leg) trial prospectively assigned patients with severe limb ischemia caused by infrainguinal disease to either angioplasty or bypass surgery. At the end of the study, there was no difference seen between the two groups in either mortality rate or rate of survival free of the need for amputation. However, in the angioplasty group, rates for morbidity and length of hospital stay were significantly lower and total cost was significantly less.

Based on the currently available scientific data, we recommend endovascular intervention with PTA ± nitinol self-expandable stent for treatment of femoropopliteal artery lesions in patients with:

- Critical limb-threatening ischemia
- Life-style limiting claudication
- Below-the-knee disease (to improve inflow as well as to serve as a conduit to access the tibioperoneal lesions)

(See Fig. 58-2).

OCCLUSIVE DISEASE OF INFRAPOPLITEAL ARTERIES

Critical limb ischemia is the most severe manifestation of PVD. An estimated 1.5 to 2 million people in the United States and Europe suffer from critical limb ischemia. Mortality rates is high, with 25% dying in 1 year and 60% dying at the end of 3 years. Moreover, about 150,000 patients undergo amputations per year in United States and Europe due to critical limb ischemia. Endovascular therapy has an important and definitive role for patients with infrapopliteal arterial occlusive disease and critical limb ischemia, easily revascularizing outflow lesions with minimal morbidity and mortality.

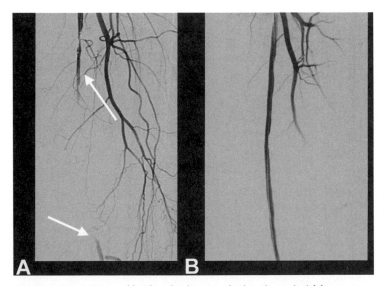

FIGURE 58-2. A 74-year-old male with a history nonhealing ulcer in the left foot.
A. Angiography showed a 15-cm occlusion of the left superficial femoral artery (*arrows*).
B. After percutaneous revascularization with VIABAHN stent-graft (W.L. Gore and Associates, Inc., Flagstaff, AZ).

Tibial artery bypass surgery is seldom used in patients with critical limb ischemia to achieve revascularization in distal to infrapopliteal obstructions because of poor long-term graft patency. This is due to the difficulty of achieving distal anastamoses to small diseased vessels, with diffuse distal arterial occlusive disease producing poor runoff (outflow). A significant majority of these patients have multiple comorbidities, including coronary artery disease and diabetes. This, combined with the increased difficulty of surgery involving grafts crossing a joint, results in an unacceptable level of risk for mortality in these patients. Therefore, endovascular interventions that carry less morbidity and mortality are preferred for limb salvage in these patients.

The immediate and long-term results of PTA for infrapopliteal disease are better in patients who have claudication than in those who have critical limb ischemia. New low-profile balloons and new-generation wires have greatly improved the success rate of infrapopliteal angioplasty for treating occlusions and stenotic lesions. In our published study of 97 patients who had lifestyle-limiting claudication and/or critical limb ischemia, the success rate was 95%, including an 86% rate of successful limb salvage. In another recently published report concerning angioplasty of tibioperoneal vessels for limb salvage, Dorros and associates reported that rest pain was relieved or blood flow to a lower extremity was improved in 95% of the endangered limbs. Clinical 5-year follow-up of the successfully revascularized critical limb ischemia patients documented a limb salvage rate of 91%. These reports demonstrate that patients who have critical limb ischemia due to infrapopliteal disease should be seriously considered for endovascular procedures.

Currently, we recommend endovascular intervention in infrapopliteal arteries only to patients presenting with critical limb ischemia. The goals of intervention are to restore straight-line, pulsatile arterial blood flow to help the wounds heal and relieve ischemic pain.

ENDOVASCULAR TREATMENT OF CLAUDICATION: CURRENT AMERICAN COLLEGE OF CARDIOLOGY/AMERICAN HEART ASSOCIATION PRACTICE GUIDELINES

(See also Chapter 59.)

Class I

1. Endovascular procedures are indicated for individuals with a vocational or lifestyle-limiting disability caused by intermittent claudication when clinical features suggest a reasonable likelihood of symptomatic improvement with endovascular intervention and (a) there has been an inadequate response to exercise or pharmacologic therapy and/or (b) there is a very favorable risk-benefit ratio (e.g., focal aortoiliac occlusive disease).

2. Endovascular intervention is recommended as the preferred revascularization technique for TASC type A iliac and femoropopliteal arterial lesions.

3. Stenting is effective as primary therapy for common and external iliac artery stenoses and occlusions.

Class IIa

1. Stents (and other adjunctive techniques such as lasers, cutting balloons, atherectomy devices, and thermal devices) can be useful in the femoral, popliteal, and tibial arteries as salvage therapy for a suboptimal or failed result from balloon dilation (e.g., persistent translesional gradient, residual diameter stenosis greater than 50%, or flow-limiting dissection)

Class IIb

1. The effectiveness of uncoated/uncovered stents, atherectomy, cutting balloons, thermal devices, and lasers for the treatment of infrapopliteal lesions (except to salvage a suboptimal result from balloon dilation) is not well established.

Class III

1. Endovascular intervention is not indicated if there is no significant pressure gradient across a stenosis despite flow augmentation with vasodilators.

2. Primary stent placement is not recommended in the femoral, popliteal, or tibial arteries.

3. Endovascular intervention is not indicated as prophylactic therapy in an asymptomatic patient with lower-extremity PAD.

ENDOVASCULAR TREATMENT FOR ACUTE LIMB ISCHEMIA

Acute limb ischemia occurs when suddenly decreased blood flow to a limb threatens its viability. The etiology of acute limb ischemia commonly involves an acutely obstructed major artery or bypass graft, obstructed either by an embolus (often from the heart) or by thrombosis in situ. The principal goal of treatment for acute limb ischemia is to rapidly restore blood flow to the ischemic region to forestall irreversible changes. Although surgical intervention was the standard of care for restoring limb perfusion, catheter-directed thrombolysis has proven useful for rapid clot dissolution, unmasking underlying stenoses, and determining the best treatment strategy (surgery or PTA).

Studies have shown that use of catheter-directed thrombolysis in treating limb-threatening ischemia leads to long-term clinical outcomes equal to those of surgical revascularization. The prospective, randomized Surgery Versus Thrombolysis for Ischemia of the Lower Extremity (STILE) trial reported no difference in mortality, amputation, or major morbidity between groups treated surgically and those treated with thrombolysis (urokinase or rt-PA). The rates of limb salvage were also similar (88.2% in the surgical group versus 89.4% in the thrombolysis group). When patients were studied post-hoc on the basis of the duration of their symptoms before enrollment (< 14 days or > 14 days), it was found that those with < 14 days of symptoms had fewer deaths or amputations if they were treated with thrombolysis rather than surgery (15.3% versus 37.5%, $p = 0.01$). The Thrombolysis or Peripheral Arterial Surgery (TOPAS I and II) studies found no difference in rates for mortality and amputation between groups treated with urokinase or with surgery, but the magnitude of surgery was reduced in the thrombolysis group. Accordingly, unless patients present with critical ischemia that demands immediate restoration of pulsatile blood flow by surgical embolectomy (patients with loss of motor and sensory function in a viable limb), catheter-directed thrombolysis should be the initial therapy of choice. Patients who are selected for catheter-directed thrombolysis should be started on aspirin and heparin as soon as possible, followed by angiography and placement of an infusion catheter, with side holes, into the occluded vessel. Thrombolytic agents are introduced through the infusion catheter for a period of 12 to 24 hours, after which angiography is repeated to evaluate results and identify any underlying lesions, which are then usually corrected by PTA, with or without stenting. Urokinase has been studied most extensively in the context of treatment of acute limb ischemia.

In addition to CDT, percutaneous mechanical thrombectomy has also been used to treat acute limb ischemia patients. Of the devices developed to disrupt thrombus formation and remove freshly formed thrombus from the circulation, only the AngioJet Rheolytic Thrombectomy System is currently approved in the United States for use in arterial circulation. Several studies have shown this device to be effective in the treatment of acute limb ischemia, although it is generally used as an adjunct to catheter-directed thrombolysis. Used together, percutaneous mechanical thrombectomy and catheter-directed thrombolysis appear to speed reperfusion and reduce either the duration of thrombolytic infusion, the dose of the agent used, or both.

ENDOVASCULAR TREATMENT FOR CRITICAL LIMB ISCHEMIA (CLI): AMERICAN COLLEGE OF CARDIOLOGY/AMERICAN HEART ASSOCIATION PRACTICE GUIDELINES

(See also Chapter 59.)

Class I

1. For individuals with combined inflow and outflow disease with CLI, inflow lesions should be addressed first.

2. For individuals with combined inflow and outflow disease in whom symptoms of CLI or infection persist after inflow revascularization, an outflow revascularization procedure should be performed.

【 】 THROMBOLYSIS FOR ACUTE AND CHRONIC LIMB ISCHEMIA

Class I

1. Catheter-based thrombolysis is an effective and beneficial therapy and is indicated for patients with acute limb ischemia of < 14 days' duration (Level of evidence: A).

Class IIa

1. Mechanical thrombectomy devices can be used as adjunctive therapy for acute limb ischemia due to peripheral arterial occlusion (Level of evidence: B).

Class IIb

1. Catheter-based thrombolysis or thrombectomy may be considered for patients with acute limb ischemia of > 14 days' duration (Level of evidence: B).

OCCLUSIVE DISEASE OF RENAL ARTERIES

Renal artery stenosis (RAS) is the most common cause of secondary hypertension. Atherosclerosis accounts for 90% of cases of RAS, whereas fibromuscular dysplasia accounts for about 10%. The incidence of atherosclerotic RAS increases with age and is more common in patients who have occlusive disease in other vascular territories. In 18% of 196 unselected patients who presented to our institution with diabetes and hypertension and underwent coronary angiography, renal angiography revealed RAS > 50%.

RAS should be suspected in hypertensive patients if there are any of following conditions:

- Blood pressure that is difficult to control despite trial of multiple pharmacologic therapies.
- Sudden failure of blood pressure control.
- Recurrent pulmonary edema despite a normal left ventricular systolic function.

- Sudden worsening of renal function with the introduction of angiotensin-converting enzyme (ACE) inhibitors.

In most patients, atherosclerotic RAS is progressive, and in a significant number of these patients it results in renal atrophy. Before percutaneous revascularization procedures became widely available, aortorenal bypass surgery was commonly performed to treat patients who had RAS, but rates of perioperative mortality were 2% to 6% with significant morbidity.

Percutaneous revascularization of the renal arteries has been refined and simplified until it has virtually replaced open surgical revascularization of renal arteries for patients who have RAS.

The two major goals of percutaneous revascularization of the renal arteries are

- Control of blood pressure.
- Preservation of renal function.

When RAS is caused by fibromuscular dysplasia, results are excellent for percutaneous transluminal renal angioplasty alone, with a success rate of 82% to 100% and a restenosis rate of about 10%, making PTA the treatment of choice in patients who have uncontrolled hypertension and fibromuscular dysplasia. On the other hand, stand-alone PTA for atherosclerotic RAS has yielded poor results due to high elastic recoil in the *atherosclerotic ostial lesions*. As is the case when used in most other arteries, stents improve both immediate and long-term patency following PTA. As shown in Table 58-2, rates for immediate technical success following renal artery stenting are 97% to 100%, rates for procedure-related major complications are about 2% to 3%, and rates for restenosis are 5% to 21%.

Variations in reporting standards make it hard to judge the efficacy of renal artery stenting in patients who have hypertension and renal function. Nonetheless, renal artery stenting appears to improve control of blood pressure in 70% of patients. Hypertension is cured in only 30% of the patients who have atherosclerotic RAS compared to > 60% of patients with fibromuscular dysplasia. Renal artery stenting improves or stabilizes renal function in approximately 70% of patients. There is evidence that the procedure is more effective if performed in the early stages of RAS, that is, before renal impairment becomes either severe (serum creatinine levels > 4.0 mg/dL) or permanent.

The current consensus is to perform renal artery revascularization in patients who have RAS in order to preserve renal function or to improve control of hypertension. Available data permit no clear-cut recommendations as to the optimal timing of this intervention. However, there is no doubt that PTA should be the procedure of choice in patients who have RAS due to fibromuscular dysplasia, and PTA plus stenting should be the procedure of choice for patients who have atherosclerotic RAS.

Investigations are underway to determine whether devices shown to be effective in preventing distal embolization of atherosclerotic debris in the coronary and carotid arteries are equally as effective during PTA/stenting of the renal arteries (Fig. 58-3).

ENDOVASCULAR TREATMENT FOR RENAL ARTERY STENOSIS (RAS): AMERICAN COLLEGE OF CARDIOLOGY/AMERICAN HEART ASSOCIATION PRACTICE GUIDELINES

(See also Chapter 59.)

Class I

1. Renal stent placement is indicated for ostial atherosclerotic RAS lesions that meet the clinical criteria for intervention (Level of evidence: B).

2. Balloon angioplasty with bailout stent placement, if necessary, is recommended for fibromuscular dysplasia (FMD) lesions (Level of evidence: B)

● TABLE 58-2

Renal Artery Stenting: Results in Recent Studies

Study and Year of Publication	Patients (n)	Arteries (n)	Follow-up (mo)	Technical Success Rate (%)	Hypertension Cured or Control Improved (%)	Renal Function Improved or Stabilized (%)	Restenosis (%)	Major Complications (%)
Lederman (2001)	300	363	16	100	70	73	21	2
Burket (2000)	127	171	15 ± 14	100	71	67	7.8	3
Rodriguez-lopez (1999)	108	125	36	97.6	79	100	5.5	3.2
Rocha-Singh (1999)	150	180	13.1	97.3	91	92	12	1.3
Dorros (1998)	163	202	48	99	49	71	NR	1.8
White (1997)	100	133	8.7 ± 5	99	76	22	18.8	2
Pooled results	948	1174	22.8	98.8	72.6	70.8	13.2	2.2

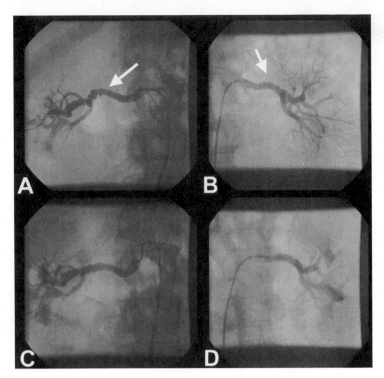

FIGURE 58-3. A 40-year-old male with severe uncontrolled hypertension over the previous year. Selective angiography of right (**A**) and left (**B**) renal arteries showed typical appearance of fibromuscular dysplasia (*arrows*). After balloon, a repeat angioplasty was performed in both renal arteries (**C, D**).

ANEURYSMAL DISEASE OF AORTA AND ILIAC ARTERIES

【 】 DESCENDING THORACIC AORTIC ANEURYSM

The estimated prevalence of thoracic aortic aneurysms is 10 of every 100,000 elderly adults. The incidence of thoracic aortic aneurysms has been increasing in part because of better detection through the wide use of computed tomography (CT). Between 30% and 40% of these aneurysms occur exclusively in the descending thoracic aorta, and with time are likely to expand and rupture. Thoracic aortic aneurysms most often result from cystic medial degeneration that leads to weakening of the aortic wall. Cystic medial degeneration normally occurs with aging and is more extensive in the presence of hypertension. When it occurs in young patients, it is most often caused by Marfan's syndrome or other, less common, connective tissue disorders, such as Ehlers–Danlos syndrome.

The risk of rupture is directly related to the size of the aneurysm. Coady and coworkers found that, in an ascending aorta, an aneurysm with a diameter > 6 cm increased the risk of rupture or dissection by 25%; and in a descending aorta, an aneurysm with a diameter > 7 cm increased the risk by 37%. Davies and coworkers found an annual rate of rupture and dissection of 2% for aneurysms < 5 cm, 3% for aneurysms 5 to 5.9 cm, and 7% for aneurysms > 6 cm in diameter. Therefore, the risk appears to rise abruptly as thoracic aneurysms reach a diameter of 6 cm.

The indications for intervention in patients with thoracic aneurysm include the following:

- Symptoms related to the aneurysm.

- Diameter of 50 mm for an aneurysm in the ascending aorta and 6 mm for an aneurysm in the descending aorta (early in some subgroups, such as Marfan's syndrome patients).

- Growth rate >10 mm/y.

- Complications associated with aneurysm that increase risk of rupture, such as dissection, leak, or ulceration.

The first multicenter nonrandomized trial using Gore Tag thoracic endoprosthesis included 17 sites in the United States. The success rate was 98% in 142 patients. The only reason for failure was inadequate arterial access. The mean diameter size was 64.1 mm and the mean follow-up was 24.0 months. At 2 years, there has been a 97% rate of aneurysm-related survival and an overall survival rate of 75%. Three patients have undergone endovascular revisions for endoleak. No ruptures have been reported. A related trial compared results of implantation using the TAG device with those of surgical therapy and showed that endovascular repair had one-fifth the rate of paraplegia, one-sixth the rate of operative mortality (1% versus 6%), an average of 80% lower procedural blood loss, a lower rate of aneurysm-related death through the first year (3% versus 10%), a shortened average stay in the intensive care unit (1 day versus 3 days), and a shortened average hospital stay (3 days versus 10 days) (Fig. 58-4).

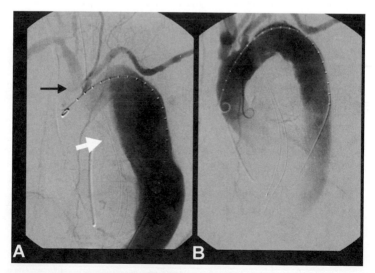

FIGURE 58-4. A 68-year-old female had a 6-cm thoracic aneurysm that surgery failed to repair. **A.** Aortic angiography showed the thoracic aneurysm (*white arrow*) distal to the left subclavian artery (*black arrow*). **B.** After percutaneous intervention with a Gore Tag device (W.L. Gore and Associates, Inc., Flagstaff, AZ).

【 】 ANEURYSMAL DISEASE OF ABDOMINAL AORTA

Abdominal aortic aneurysm (AAA) is defined as focal enlargement of the abdominal aorta (usually involving the infrarenal portion) to a diameter > 3 cm in its largest true transverse dimension. Untreated, the major complication is rupture leading to death. Aneurysmal rupture is directly related to aneurysm size. A recent population-based study from the Mayo Clinic revealed that the estimated risk of rupture was 0% per year for an abdominal aortic aneurysm diameter < 4 cm, with increases to 1% per year for diameters of 4.0 to 4.9 cm, 11% per year for diameters of 5.0 to 5.9 cm, and 25% per year for diameters > 6 cm.

Many of these patients are over age 70 and have other serious comorbidities. Consequently, their operative risk is increased. Even in low-risk patients, open repair of abdominal aortic aneurysm is associated with a mortality rate of up to 5%. In a 36-year population-based study by Mayo Clinic in Olmstead County, Minnesota, the rate of 30-day mortality was 5% in 307 patients who underwent elective open surgical repair of an abdominal aortic aneurysm. The Canadian multicenter study reported a similar rate of 5.4%. In high-risk patients, the mortality rate of open surgical repair of abdominal aortic aneurysm can be as high as 20%.

Implantation of an endoluminal stent graft in a patient with an infrarenal abdominal aortic aneurysm was first described by Parodi. Since then, this technique has evolved to gain widespread acceptance by patients and physicians. Currently, four FDA-approved devices are available for use in the United States.

In the U.S. AneuRx clinical trial (1,192 patients), the rate of implant success was 98%, the rate of procedure-related mortality at 30 days was 1.9%, and the rate of conversion to open repair within the first 30 days was 1.3%. At 4 years, the rate of aneurysm-related mortality was 2.5% (0.5%/y) and the rate of event-free survival was 97.1%. Table 58-3 compares the mortality from endovascular repair to that of open surgical repair in patients who underwent elective abdominal aortic aneurysm repair.

A major limitation of endovascular graft (EVG) repair, however, is that these devices have a large profile that rules out such potential candidates as women who have small iliac arteries and men who have severe PVD. With the currently available devices, only patients who have at least a 10- to 15-mm long infra-renal neck which is less than 28 mm in diameter can be treated with EVG repair. Also bear in mind that the longest follow-up at this time is only 5 to 6 years; without longer follow-up data to go by, the jury is still out regarding lasting benefits.

It is imperative that patients who undergo EVG repair have close follow-up with regular CT or ultrasound scans to detect any late endoleaks (i.e., blood leaking/seeping into

TABLE 58-3

Mortality Related to Open and EVG Repair of AAA

Study	Patients (n)	Follow-up (y)	30-day mortality (%)	Total AAA deaths (%)
Mayo Clinic AAA (open surgical repair)	307	36 (mean, 5.8)	5	7.6
Canadian AAA (open surgical repair)	680	6	5.4	5.8
AneuRx I–III (Endovascular repair)	1192	4	1.9	2.4
Eurostar (Endovascular repair)	2955	4	1.7	2.5

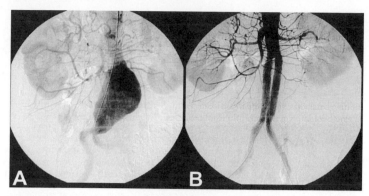

FIGURE 58-5. A 73-year-old male with a history of coronary artery disease, congestive heart failure (ejection fraction 30%), and hypertension was found to have an infrarenal AAA of 8.5 cm. **A.** Angiography showed the large infrarenal AAA. **B.** After successful EVG repair with an AneuRx stent graft (Medtronic, Inc., Minneapolis, MN), there is no evidence of endoleak. (AAA, abdominal aortic aneurysm; EVG, endovascular graft.)

the aneurysmal sac from either around or through the stent graft or via the lumbar vessels). This reported complication of EVG repair could result in continued expansion of the aneurysm and in its rupture if not detected and treated appropriately. Fortunately, most endoleaks can be treated successfully by endovascular procedures, that is, either by deployment of additional cuffs of the stent graft or use of coil or gel foam embolization (Fig. 58-5).

【 】 ANEURYSMAL DISEASE OF ILIAC ARTERIES

Iliac artery aneurysms are most commonly associated with abdominal aortic aneurysms, accounting for up to 50% of all cases. It is rare to find an isolated aneurysm of the iliac artery (an incidence of 0.03%–0.1%). Although most aneurysms in this region are asymptomatic, symptoms may be caused by local compression, thrombosis, or distal embolization of atheromatous debris. Expansive growth and subsequent rupture of iliac artery aneurysms is also well documented.

For patients meeting any of the following criteria, elective repair of iliac artery aneurysm is the treatment of choice:

- Asymptomatic and aneurysm is > 3.5-cm in diameter
- Rapid increase in diameter (> 0.5 cm/y)
- Symptomatic

As with surgical repair of abdominal aortic aneurysms, open surgical repair for iliac artery aneurysms is a major procedure that is associated with high rates of procedure-related morbidity and mortality. Placement of an endovascular stent graft provides a less invasive way to exclude an iliac artery aneurysm.

【 】 POPLITEAL ARTERY ANEURYSM

Popliteal artery aneurysms, defined as localized dilatations of the popliteal artery > 2 cm in diameter, are the most common aneurysms of the peripheral arteries, with a prevalence of 1% in men aged 65 to 80 years. Popliteal aneurysms have a well-documented natural history, tending to occur with significant comorbidity in older men. Popliteal aneurysms are often bilateral (50%) and associated with abdominal aorta aneurysms (40%). Patients usually present with acute limb ischemia caused not by rupture but by either thrombosis or distal embolization. The amputation rate in patients who present with acute limb ischemia due to popliteal artery aneurysms may be as high as 15%.

Surgery has been the procedure of choice for preventing complications. No randomized trials have been conducted to compare results of treatment of popliteal artery aneurysms by medical management with those treated surgically. Dawson and colleagues, reporting on results following elective surgery for popliteal artery aneurysms, found a 90% rate for limb salvage and an 80% rate of graft patency.

Covered stents have been proven safe and feasible for popliteal artery aneurysm repair, with several studies reporting patency rates of 60% to 70% at 18 months. Tellieu and coworkers reported on their prospective study of 28 patients with 23 popliteal artery aneurysms, all of whom underwent endovascular repair with a self-expanding stent graft. Technical success in placing the stent graft and excluding the aneurysm was 100%. During a median follow up of 15 months, 5 of 23 stent grafts became occluded, resulting in a cumulative patency rate of 74%. All occlusions occurred within 6 months after intervention; two occlusions were successfully recanalized.

ENDOVASCULAR TREATMENT FOR ABDOMINAL OR ILIAC ANEURYSMS: AMERICAN COLLEGE OF CARDIOLOGY/ AMERICAN HEART ASSOCIATION PRACTICE GUIDELINES

(See also Chapter 59.)

Class IIa

Endovascular repair of infrarenal aortic and/or iliac aneurysms is reasonable in patients at high risk of complications from open operations.

Class IIb

Endovascular repair of infrarenal aortic and/or iliac aneurysms may be considered in patients at low or average surgical risk.

CONCLUSION

Percutaneous revascularization has revolutionized the treatment of PVD within the last decade. Stents have become the default strategy in the majority of the endovascular interventions because of the excellent immediate results and durable long-term patency. However, when considering treatment options (percutaneous revascularization, conservative medical treatment, or surgical revascularization), it is necessary to judiciously evaluate the scope of the problem in light of the standard question: "Does the benefit of this procedure outweigh the risk?"

At our institution, we triage patients who present with PVD into (1) those who have claudication and (2) those who have rest pain and ischemic ulceration. (Regardless of how they are categorized, all patients are thoroughly evaluated to rule out CAD, by either cardiac angiography or pharmacologic stress testing.)

Considering the high risk for potential loss of limb in patients who have rest pain or ischemic ulcerations, we treat these patients immediately, beginning with angiography and followed by either percutaneous or surgical revascularization, so that pulsatile flow is reestablished. If there is no such significant limitation, we advise our patients that there is no firm basis for the option of percutaneous revascularization, despite their diagnosis of PVD. In such patients we recommend aggressive risk factor modification, smoking cessation, a supervised exercise program, and drug therapy with cilostazol.

In patients suspected of having renal artery stenosis (patients with difficult-to-control blood pressure or worsening renal function on ACE inhibitor therapy), we proceed with renal angiography followed by PTA and stenting.

Endovascular stent grafts have made it possible to treat patients with abdominal aortic aneurysm with minimally invasive intervention. EVG repair is currently the procedure of choice for treatment of abdominal aortic aneurysm, and open surgical repair is reserved only for patients who, for technical reasons, are not suitable candidates for EVG repair. Newer low-profile devices have widened the horizon of EVG repair by allowing physicians to treat patients who have smaller iliac arteries (e.g., women).

In conclusion, by covering familiar ground and mapping out areas of frontier exploration, we hope that we have brought clarity to the challenging task of steering amid the rapidly evolving field of minimally invasive therapies for treatment of PVD and plotting the best course of treatment for each patient.

SUGGESTED READING

Adam DJ, Beard JD, Cleveland T, et al. Bypass versus angioplasty in severe ischaemia of the leg (BASIL): multicentre, randomised controlled trial. *Lancet.* 2005;366: 1925–1934.

Coady MA, Rizzo JA, Elefteriades JA. Developing intervention criteria for thoracic aortic aneurysms. *Cardiaol Clin.* 1999;17:827–839.

Davis RR, Goldstein LJ, Goady MA, et al. Yearly rupture dissection rates for thoracic aortic aneurysms: simple prediction based on size, *Ann Thorac Surg.* 2002:73:17–27.

Dorros G, Jafff MR, Dorros AM, et al. Tibioperoneal (outflow lesion) angioplasty can be used as primary treatment in 235 patients with critical limb ischemia: five-year follow-up. *Circulation.* 2001;104:2057–2062.

Hallett JW Jr. Management of abdominal aortic aneurysms. *Mayo Clin Proc.* 2000;75: 395–399.

Henry M, Amor M, Henry I, et al. Femoropopliteal stenting: results, indications, choice of the stent. *Radiology.* 1999;213:50.

Hirsch AT, Haskal ZJ, Hertzer NR, et al. American College of Cardiology/American Heart Association. ACC/AHA 2005 Guidelines for the Management of Patients with Peripheral Arterial Disease (Lower Extremity, Renal, Mesenteric, and Abdominal Aortic): Executive Summary—A Collaborative Report from the American Association for Vascular Surgery/Society for Vascular Surgery, Society for Cardiovascular Angiography and Interventions, Society for Vascular Medicine and Biology, Society of Interventional Radiology, and the ACC/AHA Task Force on Practice Guidelines (Writing Committee to Develop Guidelines for the Management of Patients with Peripheral Arterial Disease). Endorsed by the American Association of Cardiovascular and Pulmonary Rehabilitation; National Heart, Lung, and Blood Institute; Society for Vascular Nursing; TransAtlantic Inter-Society Consensus; and Vascular Disease Foundation. *J Am Coll Cardiol.* 2006;47:1239–1312. Available at: www.acc.org.

Kidney DD, Deutsch LS. The indications and results of percutaneous transluminal angioplasty and stenting in renal artery stenosis. *Semin Vasc Surg.* 1996;9:188–197.

Mouanotoua M, Maddikunta R, Allaqaband S, et al. Endovascular intervention of aortoiliac occlusive disease in high-risk patients using kissing stents technique: long-term results. *Catheter Cardiovasc Interv.* 2003;60:320–326.

Ouriel K. Surgery versus thrombolytic therapy in the management of peripheral arterial occlusions. *J Vasc Interv Radiol.* 1995;6(suppl):48S–54S.

CHAPTER (59)

Practice Guidelines and Cardiovascular Care

Rajesh Vedanthan and Ira S. Nash

The delivery of medical care in the United States now accounts for approximately 15% of the entire economic activity of the nation. The rapid growth of medical expenditures and the recognition that there are significant deficiencies in the quality of care delivered in the United States and elsewhere have fueled the so-called *quality movement*. This chapter deals with clinical practice guidelines, one of the tools for improving the quality of medical care.

QUALITY OF CARE

【 】 PRACTICE VARIATION

One of the most striking aspects of the delivery of medical care in the United States is its enormous inhomogeneity. Members of ethnic and racial minorities are less likely to be offered intensive cardiac testing and coronary revascularization. Rates of rehospitalization after acute infarction differ markedly among different cities in the absence of clinical differences among the populations. Striking geographic differences exist in the use of effective medications for patients with acute myocardial infarction. Women may be treated less intensively than men.

As the cost, complexity, and potential benefit of medical care have grown, so too has the importance of addressing this variation. Which of the different approaches leads to the greatest benefit for patients? Could similar benefits be achieved at a lower cost? Addressing these and related questions is the essence of evaluating the quality of medical care. Evaluating the quality of care is a necessary prerequisite for improving it.

【 】 DEFINING QUALITY

The Institute of Medicine has defined quality of medical care as "the degree to which health services for individuals and populations increase the likelihood of desired health outcomes and are consistent with current professional knowledge." Simply put, good medical practice is necessarily based on sound medical knowledge, and if done right, benefits patients. Note that even under the best of circumstances, quality medical care improves the *likelihood* of good outcomes but cannot guarantee them. A patient with cardiogenic shock may die even with the best medical care. Many other patients will recover without incident after an infarction even if they do not receive effective therapies, such as thrombolysis or early beta-blockade. It is therefore inappropriate to examine only patient outcomes in judging the quality of care received.

[ ] MEASURING QUALITY: STRUCTURE, PROCESS, AND OUTCOME

A more complete assessment of the quality of care depends on considering three components of medical practice: the structure, process, and outcome of care. The *structure* of care is the environment in which care is delivered. The *process* of care encompasses the myriad steps in the actual delivery of services. Finally, the *outcome* of care is a result that is of interest to patients or providers. Consider, as an example, the assessment of the quality of care provided by a cardiac catheterization laboratory.

The *structure* of care provided by the laboratory includes its physical attributes, such as the modernity of the fluoroscopic equipment and the sophistication of its hemodynamics monitoring. It also encompasses staffing levels, level of training, and maintenance of equipment. The structure of the laboratory also extends beyond its physical boundaries. Is the laboratory a free-standing facility? Is it in a community hospital, where it may be used for general vascular radiology as well as coronary angiography? Is there a cardiac surgical program at the same institution?

The *process* of care addresses what providers do and how they do it. For the catheterization laboratory, this runs the gamut from how patients are scheduled for their procedures through the steps taken to prepare them for the catheterization and all the details of the procedure and postprocedure care. Clearly, this includes an enormous number of potential points of quality assessment. How are patients prepared for the catheterization? Do cardiology trainees perform part (or all) of the procedure under supervision? How are patients monitored after their procedures? Are there dedicated personnel who remove the arterial introducing sheaths? How much heparin is used? How long are patients required to stay in bed? The list goes on.

Finally, an assessment of the laboratory's quality may include an examination of the *outcomes* of the treated patients. This may include complications and mortality but can also be construed more broadly to include "patient-centered outcomes," such as patient satisfaction, functional capacity, or emotional well-being.

[ ] QUALITY ASSESSMENT AND IMPROVEMENT

The assessment and improvement of care require that some component of the structure, process, or outcome of a particular aspect of medical care be selected, defined, and measured. In order for the quality assessment to be meaningful, certain criteria must be met.

First, the focus of the assessment must be something under the control of the providers of care. Particular health outcomes of interest to patients and providers can remain outside the ability of medical care to influence them. Measuring such outcomes would be a waste of resources. A measurable *outcome* of care must therefore be linked with a *controllable* structure or process of care.

A measurable *process* of care can also be the focus of quality assessment and improvement activities as long as it is closely linked to an important health outcome. Since clinical trials have established, for example, the connection between early aspirin administration and improved survival, measuring the extent to which patients actually receive aspirin serves as a measure of the quality of the care delivered.

In clinical circumstances where process and outcome are well linked by clinical evidence, measuring some specific step in the delivery of care instead of the final outcome offers several important advantages. First, it provides an important efficiency. Since every patient is exposed to a system of care but only a small percentage of patients (regardless of the care they receive) is likely to experience a particular outcome such as death, many more patients must be studied if the quality of care they receive is to be judged solely on the outcomes they experience.

In addition, if only the outcomes of care are tracked, any efforts directed at improving an outcome must still ultimately identify and improve those aspects of care delivery that influence it. For example, if hospitals tracked only infarction mortality without measuring the extent to which their patients receive aspirin, the discovery of high mortality rates would necessarily lead to an investigation of care, including such critical steps as the use of aspirin.

Ultimately, improving the quality of care depends on creating the setting, the conditions, and particular processes of care that, if adhered to, maximize the likelihood of good patient outcomes. The summary of these settings, conditions, and processes are practice guidelines.

CLINICAL PRACTICE GUIDELINES

【 】 DEFINITION

In 1990, the Institute of Medicine defined practice guidelines as "systematically developed statements to assist practitioner and patient decisions about appropriate health care for specific clinical circumstances." The intended utility of practice guidelines was expressed in a follow-up report by the Institute of Medicine in 1992:

> Scientific evidence and clinical judgment can be systematically combined to produce clinically valid, operational recommendations for appropriate care that can and will be used to persuade clinicians, patients, and others to change their practices in ways that lead to better health outcomes and lower health care costs.

Although the report acknowledged the existence of substantial barriers to the realization of this ideal, it remains a concise statement of the definition and promise of practice guidelines.

【 】 GUIDELINE DEVELOPMENT

The utility of a practice guideline depends critically on the process by which it was created. Task Force 1 of the 28th Bethesda conference of the American College of Cardiology (ACC) detailed eight phases of successful clinical practice guideline development. Within each of these phases, they outlined specific tasks to be accomplished (Table 59-1). The American Heart Association (AHA) and the ACC have collaborated, often in association with international or subspecialty societies, to produce a series of well-respected clinical practice guidelines for cardiovascular care. They have produced a manual for guideline developers that is consistent with these recommendations.

Perhaps no other step in guideline development is as critical as systematically evaluating the strength of the evidence on which recommendations are based. Some research findings (or other pieces of evidence) reported in the medical literature are more reliable than others. That is, some reported findings are likely to be a true effect, while others may be only an artifact due to a flaw in the study design or a statistical quirk. There is a generally accepted hierarchy of study design. The most reliable research results come from randomized controlled trials (RCTs); among RCTs, those that recruited larger cohorts of patients are generally more reliable than smaller studies. In descending order of reliability (ascending vulnerability to bias), the remaining sources of data are cohort studies, case-control studies, case series and registries, case reports, and expert opinion. The international GRADE (Grades of Recommendations, Assessment, Development, and Evaluation) Working Group also recommended that evidence should be weighed on the basis of consistency and directness. Consistency refers to finding a similar direction and magnitude of treatment effects across different studies. Directness refers to the extent to which the studied population, treatments, and outcomes are similar to those to which the guideline applies. For example, evidence of a greater treatment effect of medication A over placebo compared with the treatment effect of medication B over placebo is only indirect evidence of the superior efficacy of medication A compared with medication B. It is not as reliable as evidence derived from an RCT directly comparing medication A with medication B.

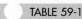

TABLE 59-1

Phases of Guideline Development and Associated Tasks Identified by the 28th Bethesda Conference

---

Phase 1. Administrative Oversight

Task 1. Identify specific goals.
Task 2. Prioritize possible guideline topics.
Task 3. Review the literature to define task, costs, and timeline.

Phase 2. Select Expert Panel

Task 1. Members must bring expertise, diversity, enthusiasm, and commitment.
Task 2. Convene panel electronically (videoconference, e-mail) to begin plans.
Task 3. Confirm outline, map patient-care algorithm.

Phase 3. Literature Search and Evidence Review

Task 1. Computerized literature search.
Task 2. Match literature to guideline outline, rate evidence.
Task 3. Create evidence tables for each topic.
Task 4. Base wording of recommendations on strength of relevant evidence.

Phase 4. Consensus Process

Task 1. Converge on recommendations by an explicit process.

Phase 5. Computerize Guideline Documents in Format for Clinical Use

Task 1. Link recommendations with related evidence.
Task 2. Create preformatted documents to capture data and facilitate care.
Task 3. Create database to store information regarding guideline compliance.

Phase 6. Test and Revise Guideline

Task 1. Expert panel tests computerized guideline in actual patient care.
Task 2. Final revision of guidelines based on testing.

Phase 7. Disseminate Guideline

Task 1. Publish printed version, disseminate computerized version.
Task 2. Encourage local customization.

Phase 8. Revise and Refine Guideline

Task 1. Maintain ongoing literature review.
Task 2. Refine management strategies based on patient outcomes associated with guideline use.

Data adapted from Jones RH, Ritchie JL, Fleming BB, et al. Task Force 1: clinical practice guideline development, dissemination and computerization. *J Am Coll Cardiol.* 1997;29: 1133–1141.

The *2006 Methodology Manual for ACC/AHA Guideline Writing Committees* stipulates that evidence should be characterized as "level" A, B, or C. Level A is defined as "data derived from multiple RCTs or meta-analyses"; Level B as "data derived from a single randomized trial, or nonrandomized studies"; and Level C as "consensus opinion of experts, case studies, or standard of care."

Determining the strength of treatment recommendations rests on making an informed judgment about whether the benefits of a particular intervention outweigh the associated risks, burden, and cost. When this balance is substantially tipped in one direction or the other, and the evidence to support that conclusion is clear, then a strong recommendation about the intervention can be made. When the balance is less clear, then a less definitive recommendation is appropriate. There is no consistent correlation between level of evidence and class of recommendation. If several large RCTs provide conflicting conclusions, then the quality of the available evidence can be high but the recommendation necessarily weak. However, if there is such universal agreement that a particular element of care is so essential that no RCT is ever likely to be done (e.g., the necessity of examining a patient), then a strong recommendation can be appropriate in the absence of rigorous evidence. The classification of recommendations of the ACC and AHA is used throughout this book and is summarized in Fig. 59-1.

All attempts to use evidence from clinical trials to write recommendations for practice must also wrestle with an unavoidable paradox: well-designed clinical trials usually involve highly specified patient populations, while practice guidelines, by their nature, are intended to be broadly applicable. There is no simple or formulaic way to reconcile the nature of the evidence and the need for recommendations.

【 】 GUIDELINE IMPLEMENTATION

Clinical practice guidelines are tools for improving patient care, but their potential can be realized only by influencing physician behavior. Merely making information available to physicians is generally ineffective, so successful implementation of clinical practice guidelines must go beyond making the guidelines accessible.

Lack of physician awareness of or familiarity with specific guidelines has been well documented. Although the large number of practice guidelines makes this virtually inevitable, physicians are often unfamiliar with even the principal recommendations of well-publicized and broadly applicable guidelines.

A negative attitude among clinicians about the value of guidelines is also a significant barrier to implementation. This may be a result of a general mistrust of "cookbook" approaches to clinical practice, a rejection of national (in favor of local) standards of practice, concerns regarding malpractice liability, differences in physician experience, and the paucity of data that adherence to guidelines actually improves care. Many clinicians also believe that guidelines are fundamentally incapable of capturing the nuances and complexity of clinical medicine. Certainly deficiencies in the guidelines themselves, including conflicting recommendations among different guidelines addressing the same conditions, contribute to physician skepticism.

Perhaps the greatest barrier to guideline implementation is the complexity of the health care delivery system itself. Care is provided in a broad range of settings, from private physicians' offices to large academic medical centers; and by a host of practitioners with different levels of interest and expertise in particular clinical conditions. Given the financial pressure present in many medical settings, guideline implementation may be seen as another burden rather than as an aid to clinical practice. Even if guideline adoption is seen as desirable, limitations of physician time and practice resources may hinder efforts to move forward. The inadequacy of many clinical information systems, which under ideal circumstances could identify patients who meet guideline criteria and remind providers of current recommendations, is another important institutional barrier to successful guideline implementation.

There is no single proven strategy for the successful adoption of guidelines. For guideline developers, close attention to the principles of data synthesis and the straightforward presentation of well-documented recommendations are essential. Explicit discussion of potential conflicts with other guidelines and the reasons for different recommendations should be included. Guideline writers should include clear statements regarding the limitations of their own guidelines with respect to the patients or conditions to which they apply.

SIZE of TREATMENT EFFECT

Estimate of Certainty (Precision) of Treatment Effect

	Class I *Benefit >>> Risk*	Class IIa *Benefit >> Risk* *Additional studies with focused objectives needed*	Class IIb *Benefit ≥ Risk* *Additional studies with broad objectives needed; Additional registry data would be helpful*	Class III *Benefit ≥ Risk* *No additional studies needed*
	Procedure/Treatment SHOULD be performed/administered	IT IS REASONABLE to perform procedure/administer treatment	Procedure/Treatment MAY BE CONSIDERED	Procedure/Treatment should NOT be performed/administered SINCE IT IS NOT HELPFUL AND MAY BE HARMFUL
Level A *Multiple (3-5) population risk strata evaluated** *General consistency of direction and magnitude of effect**	• Recommendation that procedure or treatment is useful/effective • Sufficient evidence from multiple randomized trials or meta-analyses	• Recommendation in favor of treatment or procedure being useful/effective • Some conflicting evidence from multiple randomized trials or meta-analyses	• Recommendation's usefulness/efficacy less well established • Greater conflicting evidence from multiple randomized trials or meta-analyses	• Recommendation that procedure or treatment not useful/effective and may be harmful • Sufficient evidence from multiple randomized trials or meta-analyses
Level B *Limited (2-3) population risk strata evaluated**	• Recommendation that procedure or treatment is useful/effective • Limited evidence from single randomized trial or non-randomized studies	• Recommendation in favor of treatment or procedure being useful/effective • Some conflicting evidence from single randomized trial or non-randomized studies	• Recommendation's usefulness/efficacy less well established • Greater conflicting evidence from single randomized trial or non-randomized studies	• Recommendation that procedure or treatment not useful/effective and may be harmful • Limited evidence from single randomized trial or non-randomized studies
Level C *Very limited (1-2) population risk strata evaluated**	• Recommendation that procedure or treatment is useful/effective • Only expert opinion, case studies, or standard-of-care	• Recommendation in favor of treatment or procedure being useful/effective • Only diverging expert opinion, case studies, or standard-of-care	• Recommendation's usefulness/efficacy less well established • Only diverging expert opinion, case studies, or standard-of-care	• Recommendation that procedure or treatment not useful/effective and may be harmful • Only expert opinion, case studies, or standard-of-care
Suggested phrases for writing recommendations	should is recommended is indicated is useful/effective/beneficial	is reasonable can be useful/effective/beneficial is probably recommended or indicated	may/might be considered may/might be reasonable usefulness/effectiveness is unknown/unclear/uncertain or not well established	is not recommended is not indicated should not is not useful/effective/beneficial may be harmful

FIGURE 59-1. Modified with permission from Fuster V, Rydén LE, Cannom DS, et al. ACC/AHA/ESC 2006 guidelines for the management of patients with atrial fibrillation: a report of the American College of Cardiology/American Heart Association Task Force on Practice Guidelines and the European Society of Cardiology Committee for Practice Guidelines (Writing Committee to revise the 2001 guidelines for the management of patients with atrial fibrillation). *Eur Heart J.* 2006;27(16):1979–2030.

Clear demonstration of the value of guideline adoption, through the feedback of local data demonstrating improvements in patient outcomes, is often part of a successful strategy. It is also helpful to modify the incentives for clinicians and invest in clinical information systems.

Recognizing that creating high-quality practice guidelines does not, in itself, improve care, the AHA and the ACC have embarked on their own programs to enhance guideline implementation. The AHA program, called "Get with the Guidelines," is intended to promote the use of a small number of key treatments for patients hospitalized with coronary heart disease, acute coronary syndromes, heart failure, and atrial fibrillation. Hospitals register as program participants and gain access to a Web-based data collection instrument for monitoring guideline adherence, which allows for comparisons of local performance against regional and national data. The program also provides a "toolkit" of educational material, guideline implementation aids, and extensive program support. Similarly, the ACC-sponsored Guidelines Applied in Practice (GAP) program is a rapid-cycle quality improvement initiative that has separate modules for AMI and congestive heart failure. The myocardial infarction tool kit consists of (1) AMI standard admission orders, (2) a clinical pathway, (3) a pocket guide to care, (4) a patient information form, (5) a patient discharge checklist, (6) chart stickers to alert providers, and (7) hospital performance charts.

【 】 GUIDELINE MAINTENANCE

A practice guideline must maintain its scientific currency and relevance to clinical practice. Several different circumstances could necessitate a guideline update:

- Changes in the risks and benefits of current interventions.
- Changes in which outcomes are considered important.
- Changes in the quality of current practice.
- Changes in the value placed on outcomes.
- Changes in available resources.

Establishing the appropriate threshold for any of these criteria is not simple; recognizing when that threshold is achieved is harder still. Some organizations therefore rely on an arbitrary time-based cycle of guideline revision. For example, the National Guideline Clearinghouse deletes guidelines that are more than 5 years old. Such a policy may not be ideal, since it does not allow for a specific update according to the criteria above. Instead, a systematic reassessment of existing guidelines by recognized experts, supplemented by limited searches of the medical literature and operating with prospectively defined criteria for obsolescence, may be the only practical way to assure timely updates. Electronic publication and partial, rather than complete, revisions have been used effectively by the AHA and ACC to reduce the revision cycle time for their guidelines that need updating.

【 】 GUIDELINE QUALITY

Several observers have suggested lists of the attributes that good practice guidelines should have. The Institute of Medicine report lists eight important qualities (Table 59-2). *Validity* implies that the guidelines, if adopted, will actually lead to the anticipated improvements in health outcomes and/or cost of care. *Reliability* or *reproducibility* is achieved if another group of guideline developers would create equivalent guidelines if they relied on the same evidence. Good guidelines should also have clear *clinical applicability*, so that they pertain to a broad, well-defined, explicitly identified population. Guidelines must also allow for some *flexibility* of medical practice and acknowledge the appropriate role of clinical judgment and possible exceptions to broad dictates. *Clarity* of recommendations is another important attribute, and should be promoted through the use of precise definitions of terms, unambiguous recommendations, and a variety of

TABLE 59-2

Desirable Attributes of Clinical Practice Guidelines Identified by the Institute of Medicine

Validity
Reliability
Clinical applicability
Flexibility
Clarity
Multidisciplinary development
Scheduled review
Documentation

Reproduced with permission from Field MJ, Lohr KN, eds. *Clinical Practice Guidelines: Directions for a New Program.* Washington, DC: National Academy Press; 1990.

presentation techniques. Ideally, guidelines should be developed through a *multidisciplinary process*, which elicits the input of a broad range of stakeholders in the field. The report also recommends a provision for *scheduled revision* or an "expiration date," although, as previously discussed, this can be of limited utility. Finally, the Institute report suggests that good guidelines should be *well documented*, so that users will know the "procedures followed in developing guidelines, the participants involved, the evidence used, the assumptions and rationales accepted, and the analytic methods employed."

There are now many practice guidelines put forth by a large number of organizations that deal with a broad array of clinical issues. The National Guideline Clearinghouse lists thousands of practice guidelines on its website. With such a large number of guidelines in the published literature, a number of investigators have attempted to assess how well they fulfill the criteria discussed above.

After examining clinical practice guidelines, some investigators have concluded that most guidelines do not follow established methodologic standards, especially in regard to how the underlying medical evidence is gathered and critically combined. Others have evaluated guidelines in three "dimensions"—rigor of development, context and content, and application—and found that most guidelines did not achieve the majority of criteria in each dimension. Yet another approach has been to describe the type of professionals who developed the guideline, evaluate the sources of information used, and judge whether an explicit method of grading the evidence was described. Such efforts have yielded proposals for uniform reporting of methodology by guideline developers.

More recently, the AGREE (Appraisal of Guidelines, Research, and Evaluation) project has led to the development and validation of a new tool to evaluate guideline quality to judge guidelines across six "domains": scope and purpose, stakeholder involvement, rigor of development, clarity and presentation, applicability, and editorial independence. Each domain is scored independently on the basis of standard criteria. This tool is rapidly becoming the new international standard for the assessment of guideline quality, and is now available through the AGREE website in 14 languages.

【 】 GUIDELINE EFFECTIVENESS

With legitimate questions raised about the quality of guidelines and the challenges associated with their development, implementation, and maintenance, have cardiovascular clinical practice guidelines actually improved the quality of care? The question is difficult to answer. Because the impact of practice guidelines depends on both the quality of the guideline itself and its successful implementation, there is no simple way to allocate observed success or failure between these two. In other words, a failure to demonstrate improvements in cardiovascular care through the use of guidelines may represent deficiencies in the guidelines themselves, operational failure to implement them locally, or some combination of both. Nevertheless, regardless of the frequency with which practice guidelines actually *do* improve care, there is clear and compelling evidence that they *can* improve care.

For example, the Cooperative Cardiovascular Project demonstrated that the feedback on compliance with guidelines for critical process-of-care measures for patients with myocardial infarction was associated with a significant improvement in the quality of care for AMI patients. The success of the guideline implementation programs sponsored by the AHA and ACC also supports the utility of practice guidelines in improving the quality of cardiovascular care. Greater success in implementing practice guidelines depends on the refinement of the guidelines themselves, the more extensive use of clinical information systems to present critical data and guideline recommendations to clinicians at the point of care, and greater sensitivity to the systematic barriers to their adoption.

FINDING PRACTICE GUIDELINES

Most clinical practice guidelines are published in peer-reviewed medical journals. Often, such a journal is the official publication of the parent organization that produced the guideline. Guidelines compiled by the American College of Physicians/American Society of Internal Medicine are published in the *Annals of Internal Medicine*; those of the American College of Chest Physicians appear in *Chest*; and the guidelines of the joint efforts of the ACC/AHA are published in both the *Journal of the American College of Cardiology* and *Circulation*. Guidelines by lesser-known groups are also generally published in mainstream journals. Government agencies often seek to have their guidelines published in journals as well. As a consequence, a computer search of the MEDLINE database of peer-reviewed journals can find many guidelines. This process is far from perfect, however, partially because of the wide variety of key terms used to index guidelines.

Each of these organizations also maintains its own website, where practice guidelines are available. As the pace of medical developments accelerates, guideline updates have become more frequent, and some organizations have adopted a policy of publishing their updated guidelines exclusively in electronic form.

The electronic compendium of guidelines maintained by the National Guideline Clearinghouse is very useful. This searchable website allows the user to specify the subject and/or sponsor of guidelines. The interface is user-friendly, and the list generated by the search contains links to the specified guideline. For example, if one specifies *cardiovascular disease*, more than 850 listed guidelines are presented, along with suggested search terms (*heart disease, vascular disease*, etc.) and the number of guidelines fitting those search criteria. The links allow a user to go directly from the list to a brief summary as well as to the full text of a particular guideline.

CONCLUSION

Assessing and improving the quality of care is a vital component of responsible medical practice. It has taken on increased prominence in recent years because of the widespread evidence of unexplained practice variation, the underutilization of effective therapies, and the increasing pressure for accountability at all levels of health care delivery. Clinical practice guidelines have emerged as an important tool to improve the quality of medical care, and cardiovascular medicine has become a particularly fertile ground for their development. A large number of high-quality clinical practice guidelines are now available that address critical issues in cardiovascular medicine. When they are based on dependable, rigorous evidence, written in clear language, and implemented with sensitivity to the myriad local issues that can thwart their success, clinical practice guidelines can help improve patient care.

SUGGESTED READING

Agree Collaboration. Appraisal of guidelines research and evaluation. http://www
.agreecollaboration.org.

American College of Cardiology. Guidelines applied in practice. http://www.acc.org
/qualityandscience/gap/gap.htm.

American College of Cardiology/American Heart Association. *Methodology Manual for
ACC/AHA Guideline Writing Committees.* http://www.americanheart.org/presenter
.jhtml?identifier=3039684.

American Heart Association. Scientific statements and clinical guidelines. http://my
.americanheart.org/portal/professional/guidelines.

Donabedian A. *Explorations in Quality Assessment and Monitoring.* Vol 1. *The Definition of
Quality and Approaches to Its Assessment.* Ann Arbor: Health Administration Press; 1980.

Field MJ, Lohr KN, eds. *Clinical Practice Guidelines: Directions for a New Program.*
Washington, DC: National Academy Press; 1990.

Field MJ, Lohr KN, eds. *Guidelines for Clinical Practice: From Development to Use.*
Washington, DC: National Academy Press; 1992:4.

GRADE Working Group. Grading quality of evidence and strength of recommendations.
BMJ. 2004;328:1490–1497.

Institute of Medicine. *Medicare: A Strategy for Quality Assurance.* Washington, DC:
National Academy Press; 1990.

Jones RH, Ritchie JL, Fleming BB, et al. Task Force 1: clinical practice guideline development, dissemination and computerization. *J Am Coll Cardiol.* 1997;29:1133–1141.

Marciniak TA, Ellerbeck EF, Radford MJ, et al. Improving the quality of care for
Medicare patients with acute myocardial infarction: results from the Cooperative
Cardiovascular Project. *JAMA.* 1998;279:1351–1357.

CHAPTER 60

Adverse Cardiovascular Drug Interactions and Complications

Julio A. Barcena and Ileana L. Piña

Adverse drug reactions (ADRs) are the fourth leading cause of death in patients hospitalized in the United States. ADRs are responsible for approximately 1 of 16 hospital admissions in Western countries, and occur in as many as 20% of hospitalized patients. The cost of these events, in financial terms, is large, with estimates of $30 billion to more than $130 billion annually.

The World Health Organization defines an ADR as "a response to a drug which is noxious and unintended and occurs at doses normally used in man for the prophylaxis, diagnosis and therapy of disease, or for modification of physiologic function." ADRs are commonly classified as either type A (augmented) or type B (bizarre) reactions. Type A reactions are predictable and based on the pharmacologic characteristics of the drug(s). Type B reactions are unpredictable and idiosyncratic.

Individuals with heart disease are at particular high risk for ADRs. Certain cardiovascular states, such as heart failure, can influence drug metabolism and elimination by altering perfusion of the kidneys, liver, and skeletal muscles. Patients with heart disease are often elderly, and advanced age is associated with higher ADR risk due to age-related alterations in renal and hepatic function, multiple medical comorbidities, and a high prevalence of polypharmacy.

CLINICAL PHARMACOLOGY

Drug interactions are classified as being either *pharmacokinetic* or *pharmacodynamic*. Pharmacokinetic interactions alter the delivery of a drug to its site of action. Pharmacodynamic interactions alter the effect of a drug at its site of action.

【 】 PHARMACOKINETIC INTERACTIONS

The effective delivery of a drug to its biological target depends on its absorption, distribution, metabolism, and elimination. Pharmacokinetic interactions can occur at any of these levels, leading to either magnification or diminution of the drug's primary effect or side effects.

Absorption

Absorption determines drug *bioavailability*. Most orally administered drugs are absorbed by the small intestine, so agents that influence gastrointestinal (GI) metabolism, motility, or pH have the potential to interact with numerous drugs. Drugs that increase GI motility tend to reduce the bioavailability of other drugs, whereas those that decrease motility can increase bioavailability by allowing a longer period of absorption.

Distribution

Once absorbed (or injected), many drugs bind to high-affinity sites on plasma proteins such as albumin and establish some degree of equilibrium between free and protein-bound states. The volume of distribution (Vd) is a theoretical measure that reflects how well a drug is removed from the plasma and distributed in tissue and is related to the serum concentration of a drug. The pharmacologic effect of a drug is proportional to its concentration in the free state.

Metabolism and Elimination

Most drugs undergo hepatic metabolism. Absorbed drugs from the small intestine reach the liver via the portal vein and, through a series of enzymatic reactions, convert these relatively hydrophobic agents into water-soluble compounds that are more readily eliminated. Hepatic metabolism consists of two phases: biotransformation and conjugation. During biotransformation (phase I), drugs are rendered more hydrophilic by oxidation, reduction, or hydrolysis. Phase I is typically followed by conjugation (phase II), during which drugs receive a molecular attachment such as a glucuronate that can facilitate drug transport within the body. Most drug–drug or drug–nutrient interactions involve the induction or inhibition of phase 1 metabolic enzymes. The majority of these interactions involve cytochrome P450 enzyme (CYPs) isozymes. Most drugs are eliminated by the kidneys, either through glomerular filtration, active tubular secretion, or passive tubular reabsorption.

【 】 ADDITIONAL CONTRIBUTORS TO ADVERSE DRUG REACTIONS

Genetic Factors

Human genetic diversity influences the pharmacokinetics and pharmacodynamics of cardiovascular drugs. The frequency of genetic polymorphisms involving CYP isozymes varies by ethnic group, although the clinical relevance of these polymorphisms is not uniform.

Diet

Diet can influence the pharmacokinetics and pharmacodynamics of cardiac drugs. Dietary herbal supplements are commonly used by patients as alternative therapies in the hope of benefiting or preventing cardiac disease. Many of these herbs cause cardiac toxicity or can interact unfavorably with known cardiac drugs. *Hypericum perforatum* (St. John's wort) decreases plasma levels of digoxin, possibly because of P-glycoprotein (Pgp) transport induction. *H. perforatum* also reduces cyclosporine levels and has been implicated as a contributor to acute rejection of a transplanted heart. Black licorice (*Glycyrrhiza glabra*) causes hypertension and competes with aldosterone antagonists for binding at the mineralocorticoid receptor. Feverfew, garlic, and ginger have antiplatelet actions and can pose safety problems in patients taking warfarin.

Age

Drug pharmacokinetics can change with advancing age for several reasons. Body-fat percentage tends to increase with age and can increase the volume of distribution of fat-soluble drugs. Conversely, cachexia can increase serum levels of drugs with a large volume of distribution, such as in the case of digoxin. If an elderly patient is anorectic, certain medications can be more rapidly absorbed in the absence of food ingestion.

Smoking

Cigarette smoking can influence the metabolism of cardiovascular drugs by increasing phase I hepatic enzyme activities. Heavy smoking has been shown to increase the activity of CYP2D6 fourfold when compared to nonsmokers.

DISEASE SPECIFICS AND/OR PATIENT PRESENTATION

【 】 CORONARY ARTERY DISEASE

Fibrinolytic Therapy

Fibrinolysis remains an essential component to STEMI management for many patients. All fibrinolytic drugs work by either directly or indirectly promoting the conversion of plasminogen to plasmin, a nonspecific serum protease that lyses fibrin clot and degrades certain clotting factors. The risk for potentially fatal bleeding complications with the use of any fibrinolytic agent is self evident, and full knowledge of the absolute and relative contraindications of fibrinolytic drugs is mandatory prior to their use.

There are few potential pharmacodynamic interactions to consider when using fibrinolytic drugs. Concomitant use of heparin can increase the potential for serious bleeding in patients treated with fibrinolytic agents. However, in general, this increased risk does not offset the additive benefit of these drugs with respect to maintaining vessel patency. The activated partial thromboplastin time (aPTT) should be frequently monitored when heparin is used in conjunction with a fibrinolytic agent and should be maintained between 1.5 to 2.0 times the upper limit of normal.

Antiplatelet Therapy

Aggressive platelet inhibition is the mainstay in the medical and percutaneous management of coronary artery disease. The success of intracoronary stenting is due largely to the development of potent antiplatelet agents, which prevent catastrophic early and late stent thrombosis and improve long-term stent patency rates.

ASPIRIN   Aspirin plays a broad role in the secondary prevention of coronary artery disease, and its use is essential, along with clopidogrel or ticlopidine, to prevent intracoronary stent thrombosis and maintain stent patency. Like other inhibitors of cyclooxygenase-1, aspirin reduces prostaglandin production, which can attenuate the effects of many antihypertensive drugs, although this phenomenon is more likely to occur at higher (> 100 mg) aspirin doses. Aspirin hypersensitivity, although rare, can result in life-threatening bronchospasm and anaphylaxis. Aspirin use in conjunction with anticoagulants can increase the likelihood for significant bleeding complications.

THIENOPYRIDINES

Ticlopidine   Ticlopidine inhibits platelet function by binding to the surface adenoside diphosphate (ADP) receptors. Its use has been associated with adverse hematologic events including aplastic anemia and thrombotic thrombocytopenic purpura. Although uncommon, these adverse events are potentially dangerous, and the drug should be discontinued if absolute neutrophil and/or platelet counts fall below $1200/m^3$ and $80,000/m^3$, respectively. Ticlopidine is a potent inhibitor of CYP2D6 and CYP2C19 and thus carries a risk for pharmacokinetic interactions with drugs metabolized by these enzymes.

Clopidogrel   Clopidogrel is associated with fewer adverse reactions than ticlopidine and is administered once daily. Hematologic abnormalities associated with clopidogrel use are rare. Clopidogrel is activated by CYP3A4, and its antiplatelet effects can be lessened by concurrent use of CYP3A4 promoters such as amiodarone. Pharmacodynamically, clopidogrel use is associated with an increased risk for significant bleeding when given with anticoagulants or other antiplatelet agents including aspirin.

GLYCOPROTEIN IIB/IIIA ANTAGONISTS   The GP IIb/IIIa antagonists are parenteral drugs that have been shown to reduce ischemic event rates in patients with acute coronary syndromes and in patients receiving intracoronary stents. These molecularly diverse agents are potent inhibitors of the platelet GP IIb/IIIa receptor, and as a group are associated with an increased absolute risk for significant bleeding and thrombocytopenia on the order of approximately 1%.

Abciximab   Abciximab is uniquely suited for use in patients with acute myocardial infarction and thrombosis who require intracoronary stenting. Its benefit in patients with acute coronary syndromes who do not receive a percutaneous coronary intervention has not been clearly demonstrated.

Eptifibatide   Eptifibatide is a small synthetic peptide fashioned after barbourin, a disintegrin found in snake venom. Eptifibatide is efficacious in patients with acute coronary syndromes regardless of the need for percutaneous coronary intervention.

Antithrombotic Therapy

Therapeutic anticoagulation with heparin derivatives and direct thrombin inhibitors has dramatically improved outcomes in patients with coronary artery disease, particularly acute coronary syndromes. The risk for potentially serious bleeding with antithrombin therapy is obvious. However, with appropriate monitoring, the benefit these drugs provide in unstable coronary syndromes far outweighs their collective risk.

UNFRACTIONATED HEPARIN   Heparin potentiates the effect of antithrombin III, which leads to inactivation of thrombin. Heparin also inactivates several clotting factors and prevents the conversion of fibrinogen to fibrin. Heparin has a half-life of approximately 90 minutes and is metabolized by the liver and reticuloendothelial system. Pharmacokinetic drug interactions involving heparin are rare, and most pharmacodynamic interactions involve the concurrent use of drugs with antiplatelet or anticoagulant properties, such as aspirin or warfarin. Life-threatening bleeding complications involving heparin can be usually reverse with protamine sulfate. Early, abrupt cessation of heparin therapy in patients treated for acute coronary syndromes has been associated with rebound ischemia.

One potentially dangerous adverse event associated with heparin use is heparin-induced thrombocytopenia (HIT). HIT occurs in 1% to 5% of heparin-exposed patients and is associated with significant thrombocytopenia (< 100,000/mm³) that typically occurs several days after exposure to any amount of heparin. HIT is caused by autoantibodies directed against the complex of heparin and platelet factor 4 (PF4). HIT management includes discontinuation of heparin and in some cases anticoagulation with direct thrombin inhibitors and warfarin.

LOW-MOLECULAR-WEIGHT HEPARIN   Low-molecular-weight heparin (LMWH) is produced by chemical or enzymatic depolymerization of the unfractionated heparin molecule. This process produces small molecules that maintain activity against factor Xa with less potential to interact with other molecules including PF4. The LMWH enoxaparin has established efficacy in the management of patients with acute coronary syndromes superior to that of heparin, with the advantage of subcutaneous administration and fixed dosing that does not require adjustment or serial monitoring.

WARFARIN   Warfarin is a vitamin K antagonist that binds to several serum clotting factors including factors II, VII, IX, and X. Warfarin has established efficacy in the prevention and treatment of thrombosis in a number of disease states including atrial fibrillation and venous thromboembolic disease, and it is also indicated for thrombosis prevention in patients with mechanical heart valve prostheses. Despite its widespread use, warfarin has a very narrow therapeutic window and carries a substantial risk for bleeding if not closely monitored.

Warfarin Toxicity   The primary manifestation of warfarin overdosage is pathologic bleeding. Patients with an international normalized ratio (INR) > 4 are at increased risk for significant bleeding. One rare complication of warfarin therapy is skin necrosis, which tends to occur more commonly in women treated for deep vein thrombosis. Warfarin has the potential to interact with a wide range of CYP inhibitors and inducers. Closer monitoring of the INR and dose reduction is generally required. Quinolone and macrolide antibiotics potentiate the effects of warfarin by inhibiting CYP1A2 and CYP3A4, respectively. The anticoagulant properties of warfarin can be attenuated by increased dietary vitamin K. Patients on warfarin should be counseled concerning intake of foods that contain high amounts of vitamin K such as kale and spinach, among others.

【 】 RHYTHM DISORDERS

Despite the recent attention given to nonpharmacologic rhythm management options such as device therapy and catheter-based ablation procedures, most patients with rhythm disorders will require antiarrhythmic medication. The potential for significant adverse drug interactions involving antiarrhythmic drugs is large, because antiarrhythmic drugs *in general* function within a narrow therapeutic spectrum; minor alterations in serum levels can result in loss of efficacy or overt toxicity. Many of these agents are dependent on oxidative metabolism by means of subtypes of CYP, thus allowing for possible interactions with inducers and inhibitors of these enzymes.

Class IA Antiarrhythmics

All class IA antiarrhythmic drugs block membrane sodium-channel activity and moderately depress phase 0 of the action potential, slowing conduction and prolonging repolarization. These drugs have utility in treating both atrial and ventricular tachyarrhythmias. QT prolongation increases the risk for potentially fatal arrhythmias such as *torsades de pointes*; therefore the use of QT-prolonging drugs in combination with class IA agents is contraindicated.

QUINIDINE   Quinidine inhibits CYP2D6 and CYP3A4. Coadministration of quinidine with digoxin can result in a rapid, threefold increase in digoxin levels, caused by quinidine-induced reduction in digoxin clearance and displacement of tissue-bound digoxin. Reducing the digoxin dose by one-half is recommended.

PROCAINAMIDE   Procainamide is acetylated by the liver to form the active metabolite *N*-acetylprocainamide (NAPA) and has the distinction of being the only class 1 antiarrhythmic that does not depend on CYP for its metabolism. Procainamide use can result in positive antinuclear antibodies and a drug-induced lupus syndrome in 50% and 30% of patients, respectively. Development of lupus-like syndrome should prompt discontinuation of the drug.

DISOPYRAMIDE   Disopyramide is metabolized by CYP3A4. This drug frequently causes anticholinergic side effects such as dry mouth, urinary retention, and constipation. Disopyramide is also a potent negative inotrope and should be used with extreme caution in patients with left ventricular (LV) dysfunction. Coadministration with beta-blockers can result in profound bradycardia and precipitate heart failure.

Class IB Antiarrhythmics

The class IB antiarrhythmics block membrane sodium channels and have little effect on phase 0 of the action potential in normal cardiac tissue. Class IB agents are useful for the treatment of arrhythmias but also have analgesic properties.

LIDOCAINE   Lidocaine inhibits CYP1A2 and depends on CYP1A2 and CYP3A4 for its oxidative metabolism. Beta-blockers as a class can reduce hepatic blood flow and therefore decrease lidocaine clearance. Some features of lidocaine toxicity include seizure activity, confusion, stroke-like signs and symptoms, respiratory arrest, sinus node inhibition, nausea, and vomiting.

MEXILETENE   Mexiletene, like lidocaine, inhibits CYP1A2 and depends on this enzyme for oxidative metabolism, along with CYP2D6. Mexiletine levels can fall substantially in the presence of P450 inducers such as rifampicin and phenytoin, and patients can require higher mexiletene doses to achieve efficacy.

Class IC Antiarrhythmics

Class IC antiarrhythmic drugs block membrane sodium channels and markedly reduce phase 0 of the action potential, slowing conduction with little effect on repolarization. The Cardiac Arrhythmia Suppression Trial (CAST) documented higher arrhythmic death rates in patients who were treated with certain class IC agents following myocardial infarction, illustrating the pro-arrhythmic potential of these drugs.

FLECAINIDE   Flecainide inhibits the enzyme responsible for its oxidation, CYP2D6, and dose reduction should be considered when flecainide is used in conjunction with CYP2D6 inhibitors such as amiodarone and the selective serotonin reuptake inhibitors. Flecainide is also an AV nodal blocker and negative inotrope with the potential for pharmacologic interactions with agents such as beta-blockers and calcium-channel antagonists. In general, flecainide should not be used in patients with known structural heart disease because of its pro-arrhythmic potential.

PROPAFENONE   Propafenone inhibits CYP2A6 and undergoes oxidative metabolism to variable degrees by means of CYP3A4, CYP1A2, and CYP2A6.

Class II Antiarrhythmic Drugs

The class II agents are beta-adrenergic receptor blockers, ubiquitous in cardiovascular medicine because of their broad clinical utility. Clinical trial data suggest that combining beta-blockers with class III agents in patients with ischemic heart disease can improve outcomes when compared to either class alone; however, such combinations also carry an increased risk for clinically significant bradycardia, especially among the elderly.

Class III Antiarrhythmic Drugs

The class III antiarrhythmic drugs prolong repolarization and alter membrane potassium channel function. Several class III drugs have sodium-channel antagonist properties and some have beta-blocker activity. The class III drugs are used to treat both supraventricular and ventricular rhythm disorders in a diverse population of patients with a broad array of comorbid medical issues. Awareness of the potential for adverse interactions, especially QT prolongation, with the use of these drugs is mandatory, because both hypokalemia and hypomagnesemia can contribute to the development of torsades de pointes.

AMIODARONE   Amiodarone is arguably the most widely used antiarrhythmic agent available, but its propensity to interact with other drugs deserves special attention (see Chapter 9). It interacts with CYP 3A4 and can cause low cardiac output, bradycardia, and hypotension. Other side effects include visual disturbances, hyper- or hypothyroidism, phototoxicity, and pulmonary fibrosis with chronic long-term use. Monitoring is required in a drug with such a high profile of adverse effects. The approach shown in Table 60-1 is highly recommended.

DOFETILIDE   Dofetilide undergoes oxidative metabolism via CYP3A4 and is excreted in the urine by the renal cation transport system. Drugs that inhibit the renal cation transport system are also contraindicated with dofetilide and include ketoconazole, cimetidine, trimethoprim, prochlorperazine, and megestrol.

IBUTILIDE   Ibutilide is used acutely for the conversion of atrial fibrillation or flutter to sinus rhythm. This drug is not metabolized by CYP2D6 or CYP3A4 and does not appear to interact significantly with other drugs.

SOTALOL   Sotalol is a class III antiarrhythmic agent with nonselective beta-adrenergic antagonist properties. Most of the administered dose is excreted unchanged in the urine. Antacids containing magnesium or aluminum salts can decrease the bioavailability of sotalol.

TABLE 60-1

Recommended Approach to Monitoring for Amiodarone Toxicity in Clinical Practice

Baseline
Complete history and physical examination
Ophthalmologic examination
Liver function panel
Thyroid function panel
Renal function panel with electrolytes
ECG
CXR
Pulmonary function tests (including DL_{CO})

Every 6 Months
Liver function panel
Thyroid function panel

Every Year
ECG
CXR

As Clinically Indicated
Any of the above at any time

CXR, chest x-ray; DL_{CO}, carbon monoxide diffusing capacity; ECG, electrocardiogram.
Data adapted from Goldschlager N, et al. *Arch Intern Med.* 2000;160:1741–1748.

Class IV Antiarrhythmic Drugs

The class IV antiarrhythmic drugs block calcium channels and include verapamil and diltiazem. Like the class II drugs (beta-blockers), many of the adverse interaction involving class IV antiarrhythmic drugs are pharmacodynamic.

[ ] HYPERTENSION

Hypertension perhaps more than any other medical diagnosis is associated with an increased risk for ADRs due to the frequent need for multidrug therapy for blood pressure control.

Diuretic Therapy

THIAZIDE DIURETICS   Thiazide-type diuretics are considered first-line agents in hypertension management because of their efficacy and favorable effects on cardiovascular and all-cause mortality. These agents are most effective at lower doses, as higher doses do not result in a substantial increase in antihypertensive effect but have been associated with class-specific adverse events such as hyperlipidemia, insulin resistance, and erectile dysfunction. Thiazide diuretics can cause clinically relevant hypovolemia and electrolyte disturbances such as hypokalemia and hypomagnesemia. Thiazide diuretics can also promote hyperuricemia and precipitate gout.

LOOP DIURETICS   A significant difference between loop and thiazide diuretics is that loop diuretics promote renal calcium *excretion*, which can potentially promote nephrolithiasis. Loop diuretics are also used extensively in patients with heart failure and renal insufficiency. These higher-risk patients are susceptible to diuretic-induced hypovolemia and can experience hypotension and worsening renal function with the administration of drugs such as angiotensin–converting enzyme (ACE) inhibitors and angiotensin receptor blockers (ARBs). Loop diuretic–induced renal insufficiency, hypokalemia, and hypomagnesemia can also precipitate digitalis toxicity.

POTASSIUM-SPARING DIURETICS   Triamterene and amiloride are mild potassium-sparing diuretics that are often coadministered with thiazide diuretics for the treatment of hypertension. This combination substantially reduces the risk of thiazide-induced hypokalemia.

Adrenergic Antagonists

BETA-ADRENERGIC BLOCKERS   Beta-blockers promote peripheral vasodilation, reduce myocardial contractility, and slow electrical conduction through the AV node and thus have the potential for significant pharmacodynamic interactions with drugs of similar design. Synergistic hypotension and bradycardia can also occur when beta-blockers are given in conjunction with antiarrhythmic drugs such as amiodarone. Beta-blocker therapy can result in significant, sometimes life- threatening hypertension through unopposed alpha-adrenergic stimulation in patients who are beginning therapy with clonidine or methyldopa or who abuse stimulant drugs (e.g., cocaine). Previous concerns regarding the risk of beta-blocker therapy in patients with lung diseases such as asthma and chronic obstructive pulmonary disease (COPD) have been largely dismissed, in part because of the introduction of beta-1-specific agents such as metoprolol and the strong benefit of these agents. All beta-blockers can reduce hepatic blood flow and can therefore interfere with hepatic drug metabolism. Many commonly used beta-blockers (carvedilol, metoprolol, propranolol, and labetalol) are metabolized by hepatic CYP2D6 and are therefore susceptible to hepatic pharmacokinetic changes imposed by other drugs.

Once thought to be contraindicated in patients with LV systolic dysfunction, certain beta-blockers have since been shown to dramatically reduce morbidity and mortality in patients with heart failure. The benefits extend from patients with NYHA class II symptoms to those with advanced disease. The administration and dosing of beta-blockers requires some careful attention given the fact that beta-blockers are negative inotropic agents that acutely reduce heart rate and ventricular contractility.

ALPHA-ADRENERGIC RECEPTOR BLOCKERS   The alpha-adrenergic receptor antagonists (alpha-blockers) currently play a limited role in first-line hypertension management. Nonetheless these drugs still play a role as adjunctive agents in refractory hypertension and in the management of patients with symptomatic benign prostatic hyperplasia (BPH). Not unexpectedly, the major pharmacodynamic limitation of alpha-blocker therapy is postural hypotension, and this can be exacerbated by other antihypertensive agents. Volume retention can also occur, particularly in patients with impaired LV function.

CALCIUM-CHANNEL BLOCKERS   Calcium-channel blockers are metabolized by means of hepatic CYP3A4. Therefore as a drug class, calcium-channel blockers are sensitive to pharmacokinetic alterations in CYP3A4 activity. Grapefruit juice, a known CYP3A4 inhibitor, increases plasma concentrations of calcium-channel blockers, which can lead to significant hypotension.

Verapamil   Verapamil is useful for the treatment of hypertension and angina. Verapamil reduces AV nodal conduction, myocardial contractility, and systemic arterial tone and so can act synergistically with beta-blockers to induce hypotension, heart failure, and bradycardia as previously described. Similar pharmacodynamic interactions have been observed between verapamil and antiarrhythmic agents such as amiodarone and flecainide, and the coadministration of verapamil and clonidine can result in serious hypotension and atrioventricular block. Verapamil is oxidized in the liver by CYP3A and inhibits the Pgp-mediated drug transport. This drug also enhances hepatic blood flow and can potentially alter the first-pass metabolism of hepatically-modified drugs. Digoxin levels can increase by as much 50% to 90% in the presence of verapamil, and digoxin dosing should be proportionally reduced if both drugs are required.

Diltiazem   Diltiazem is similar to verapamil in most respects, especially regarding the potential for pharmacodynamic interactions with drugs such as beta-blockers. Diltiazem does not appear to have the same effect on Pgp as verapamil and thus does not influence digoxin levels appreciably. Diltiazem, along with verapamil, does reduce the hepatic clearance of cyclosporine. This interaction can be exploited in hypertensive solid-organ transplant patients where diltiazem therapy permits lower cyclosporine doses. Another potentially significant pharmacokinetic interaction involves hydroxymethylglutaryl coenzyme A (HMG-CoA) reductase inhibitors (statins). Diltiazem increases serum levels of simvastatin, lovastatin, and atorvastatin.

Dihydropyridines   The dihydropyridine-type calcium-channel blockers are potent vasodilators with minimal direct effect on myocardial contractility or conduction, and these agents can be useful in the management of hypertension and angina. As a consequence of vasodilation-induced intercompartment fluid shifts, dihydropyridines produce significant leg edema in up to 20% of users.

Angiotensin-Converting Enzyme Inhibitors

ACE inhibitors have widespread applicability in cardiovascular disease and are commonly used in the management of hypertension, heart failure, and coronary artery disease. ACE inhibitors improve survival and decrease hospitalizations in patients with impaired systolic function.

All ACE inhibitors have the potential to provoke a chronic, nonproductive cough in anywhere from 5% to 35% of patients. The cough associated with ACE inhibitors use can be mediated by bradykinin-induced sensitization of airway sensory nerves (bradykinin in the lung is degraded by ACE), and typically resolves on discontinuation of the drug. Another rare but potentially fatal adverse reaction to ACE inhibitor therapy is angioedema.

ACE inhibitors interfere with the pharmacokinetics of lithium, and concurrent use of both agents results in increased serum lithium levels, occasionally leading to lithium toxicity. ACE inhibitors should be used cautiously with potassium supplements or potassium-sparing diuretic agents to avoid significant hyperkalemia. Similarly, patients with hypovolemia, often a consequence of diuretic therapy, are at increased risk for ACE inhibitor–related acute renal failure; thus appropriate clinical assessment of intravascular volume is mandatory prior to initiation or titration of ACE inhibitor therapy.

Angiotensin Receptor Blockers

ARBs are effective antihypertensive agents that also have benefit in patients with heart failure, particularly in those patients who are ACE-inhibitor intolerant. ARBs are associated with few adverse reactions relative to other antihypertensive drug classes, possibly because of the limited role of the angiotensin receptor outside the cardiovascular system. Unlike with ACE inhibitors, the risk of cough and angioedema with ARB therapy is rare.

Vasodilators

Direct vasodilators such as hydralazine and minoxidil are generally reserved for use in patients with refractory hypertension or in heart-failure patients who do not tolerate ACE inhibitors or ARBs. Hydralazine in combination with long-acting nitrates has been recently shown to improve survival in African Americans with heart failure.

Hydralazine is a direct arteriolar vasodilator that, like the dihydropyridine calcium-channel blockers, can produce peripheral edema in a minority of patients. Hydralazine can also induce a lupus-like syndrome. The syndrome typically resolves several weeks after discontinuation of the drug. Hydralazine is acetylated by the liver and is a weak inhibitor of CYP3A4.

Minoxidil is a potent peripheral arteriolar vasodilator that is pharmacodynamically similar to hydralazine, and thus the same precautions regarding peripheral edema and reflex tachycardia apply. Minoxidil can cause hypertrichosis, a unique side effect that has been exploited for the benefit of those suffering from certain forms of alopecia.

PREVENTIVE CARDIOLOGY

[ ] HMG-CoA REDUCTASE INHIBITORS

Aggressive risk-factor modification plays a crucial role in our ongoing attempt to reduce cardiovascular event rates. The HMG-CoA reductase inhibitors (statins) have revolutionized preventive cardiology since their introduction in the mid-1980s, and the mortality and morbidity benefits of statins have been firmly established in primary and secondary prevention trials.

Hepatotoxicity

All statins have the potential to cause asymptomatic elevation of serum hepatic aminotransferase levels. Significant (> 3 × the upper limit of normal) elevations in serum aminotransferase levels occur in 1% to 3% of statin-treated patients.

Myotoxicity

Statin use is associated with diffuse myalgias in a minority of patients, but clinically significant muscle injury occurs in only 0.5% of statin-treated patients. The mechanism of statin-induced myotoxicity is unknown but can be related to the depletion of metabolic intermediaries such as ubiquinone (coenzyme-Q).

Drug–Drug Interactions with Statins

Most statins are dependent on CYP3A4 for metabolism and are thus subject to pharmacokinetic interactions with agents that inhibit or induce CYP3A4. One notable exception to this rule is pravastatin, which undergoes hepatic metabolism primarily by means of non–CYP-dependent mechanisms. Statin levels can increase substantially in the presence of potent CYP3A4, and the use of grapefruit juice in patients taking statins should be avoided.

【 】 OTHER ANTILIPEMIC AGENTS

Ezetimibe

Ezetimibe is a novel inhibitor of Niemann-Pick C1-like protein, a small-bowel transport protein that facilitates the absorption of dietary and biliary cholesterol. Ezetimibe preferentially blocks the absorption of cholesterol and allows the absorption of triglycerides and fat-soluble vitamins. The drug is metabolized through hepatic glucuronidation and is excreted predominantly in the feces. Ezetimibe does not interact with CYP450 isozymes or Pgp, and so it results in relatively few significant pharmacokinetic interactions. Recent studies have cast doubt on the outcomes benefit of ezetimibe.

Niacin

Nicotinic acid (niacin) has a favorable influence on lipid profiles, but drug tolerance is poor secondary to bothersome cutaneous reactions including flushing and pruritus. These reactions are somewhat common and can be caused by prostaglandin release. Supporting this is the observation that 325 mg of oral aspirin given with niacin greatly attenuates these cutaneous effects. Sustained-release niacin is associated with an increased risk for elevated serum aminotransferases, and fulminant hepatic failure has been described.

Fibrates and Bile-Acid Sequestrants

Use of fibric-acid derivatives is associated with a number of mild complaints including GI upset, headache, and skin reactions such as increased photosensitivity. These drugs can also cause transient elevation of hepatic aminotransferase levels, but overt liver injury is rare. Fibrates can cause myopathy, especially when combined with statins or ezetimibe. Bile-acid sequestrants such as cholestyramine are associated with GI bloating and discomfort and can interfere with the absorption of other drugs, particularly warfarin.

HEART FAILURE AND TRANSPLANTATION

【 】 HEART FAILURE

The impaired cardiac output that is characteristic of advanced heart failure can slow GI transit time, affecting drug absorption and influencing hepatic blood flow. Renal dysfunction is also common in patients with heart failure (~ 30%) and can affect drug elimination. Therefore, heart failure patients should be considered at high risk for ADRs.

Aldosterone Antagonists

The Randomized Aldactone Evaluation Study (RALES) trial showed that the addition of an aldosterone antagonist to standard therapy dramatically improved survival in severe heart failure patients. However, the extension of spironolactone use to patients with less severe heart failure has resulted in an increase in the occurrence of hyperkalemia and its consequences. The addition of spironolactone should be done with close monitoring of renal function and serum potassium levels.

Inotropic Agents

Intravenous inotropic drugs are indicated for short-term in-hospital use in patients with severe decompensated systolic heart failure who do not have mechanical outflow obstruction such as aortic stenosis or hypertrophic cardiomyopathy. Although short-term use of inotropic drugs often improves symptoms and hemodynamics in patients with advanced heart failure, long-term oral or intravenous inotrope therapy has been associated with increased mortality and has no role in chronic outpatient therapy other than for end-of-life care.

DOBUTAMINE   Dobutamine stimulates beta-1-adrenergic receptors on the myocyte surface, resulting in increased contractility and heart rate. The drug has a short elimination half-life (2 minutes) and is metabolized by the liver and in the peripheral circulation. Dobutamine can interact pharmacodynamically with beta-blockers, resulting in hypertension. Dobutamine can also cause reversible eosinophilia.

MILRINONE   Milrinone is a phosphodiesterase inhibitor that undergoes minor hepatic metabolism and is excreted by active tubular secretion. Hypotension and ventricular tachycardia can occur as a result of reduced drug clearance in patients with renal dysfunction, particularly with a loading dose.

Intravenous Vasodilators

NESIRITIDE   Nesiritide is a recombinant human B-type natriuretic peptide (h-BNP) that binds to the guanylate cyclase receptor on vascular endothelial and smooth muscle cells and facilitates vasodilation and venodilation. Nesiritide is used for the short-term inpatient management of acute decompensated NYHA class IV heart failure without hypotension; use in patients with systolic blood pressure (SBP) < 90 mm Hg is contraindicated. Recent concerns have been raised regarding potential adverse effects of nesiritide on kidney function and mortality.

【 】 CARDIAC TRANSPLANTATION

Cardiac transplant recipients are at unique danger of drug–drug interactions because of general unfamiliarity with immunosuppressive drugs by most nontransplant clinicians and because of the narrow therapeutic window that these drugs possess. Interactions with cyclosporine are numerous, and can lead to increased serum levels with subsequent hypertension and renal failure; or conversely, to graft rejection if levels drop significantly.

Cyclosporine and Tacrolimus

Cyclosporine (CSA) and tacrolimus (TAC) belong to the family of calcineurin inhibitors that undergo metabolism by means of hepatic and intestinal CYP3A4. Oral CSA and TAC have incomplete, irregular absorption that varies from patient to patient. It is important to remember that after transplantation, hypertension and hyperlipidemia are common. Careful monitoring of CSA and TAC levels is critical to avoid rejection or alternatively excessive levels and side effects.

Mycophenolate Mofetil

Mycophenolate mofetil (MMF) is an antiproliferative drug that is well absorbed after oral administration and converts to its active metabolite mycophenolic acid (MPA). MPA is metabolized by glucuronyl transferase and excreted in the urine and bile. When CSA and MMF are given in combination, the result can be lower plasma MMF levels secondary to CSA-induced alterations in biliary clearance.

Agents for Post-Transplantation Hypertension

Diltiazem is a commonly used antihypertensive because of a positive effect on transplant arteriopathy. Diltiazem inhibits both CYP3A4 and Pgp and raises CSA levels 1.5- to 6-fold, requiring a reduction in cyclosporine dosing by 20% to 75%.

Lipid-Lowering Agents

Atorvastatin, simvastatin, and lovastatin are all substrates for CYP3A4 that can pharmacokinetically interact with CSA and TAC, resulting in myopathy or even rhabdomyolysis. Fluvastatin is metabolized primarily by CYP2C9 and pravastatin through other pathways, which do not fully involve the CYP system.

SUGGESTED READING

Brunton LL, Parker KL, Lazo JS, eds. *Goodman and Gilman's The Pharmacological Basis of Therapeutics*. 11th ed. New York, NY: McGraw-Hill; 2005.

Faulx M, Piña I, Francis G. Adverse cardiovascular drug interactions and complications. In: Fuster V, O'Rourke RA, Walsh R, et al., eds. *Hurst's The Heart*. 12th ed. New York, NY: McGraw-Hill; Chapter 94.

Opie LH, Gersh BJ. *Drugs for the Heart*. 6th ed. Philadelphia, PA: Saunders; 2005.

CHAPTER (61)

Treatment Consideration in Elderly Patients with Cardiovascular Diseases*

Robert A. O'Rourke

The elderly are the fastest-growing segment of the world's population. In 2035, one in four individuals will be 65 years of age or older. Cardiovascular diseases are the leading causes of morbidity and mortality in the elderly (Fig. 61-1). The manifestations and severity of cardiovascular disease in the elderly may be modified to a certain extent by the cardiovascular changes that occur with normal aging. This chapter reviews the age-associated changes in the cardiovascular system in healthy humans and how they provide the current best evidence for treating the most common cardiovascular diseases of the elderly.

EFFECTS OF AGING ON CARDIOVASCULAR STRUCTURE AND FUNCTION

The age-associated structural changes in the cardiovascular system of healthy humans are listed in Table 61-1. Autopsy studies confirm that older subjects without apparent cardiovascular disease have cardiac myocyte enlargement with a decrease in myocyte number due to apoptosis (programmed cell death). Pacemaker cells in the sinus node also decrease in number with advancing age. At 75 years of age, only 10% of sinus node pacemaker cells remain.

Resting left ventricular (LV) early diastolic filling declines linearly with increasing age (Table 61-2), and by the age of 80 years, the rate may be reduced up to 50%. Despite this slowing of early diastolic filling of the LV, more filling occurs in end-diastole due to increased atrial contraction. This leads to atrial hypertrophy and is manifested as a fourth heart sound. On Doppler echocardiography, there is an age-related decrease in the E:A ratio.

The resting LV ejection fraction (EF) is preserved with aging (Table 61-2). In elderly patients without coronary artery disease, the maximum EF during exercise is decreased. This results from the inability to reduce the end-systolic volume index (ESVI). Even though older persons use the Frank–Starling mechanism during exercise, it cannot appropriately reduce the end-systolic volume (ESV). Therefore, stroke volume (SV) does not increase (Table 61-3).

Exercise tolerance decreases linearly with aging. Despite a greater rise in the plasma concentration of norepinephrine in older persons, there is a reduction in postsynoptic adrenergic responsiveness. Consequently, there is a decreased chronotropic and inotropic

---

*Modified from Shulman S. Cardiovascular aging in health and therapeutic considerations with respect to cardiovascular diseases in older patients. In: Fuster V, Alexander W, O'Rourke RA, et al., eds. *Hurst's the Heart Manual of Cardiology.* New York, NY: McGraw-Hill; 2001.

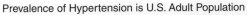

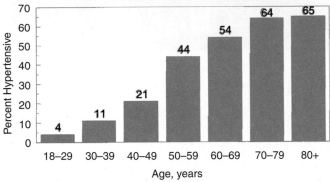

Prevalence of Hypertension is U.S. Adult Population

Based on NHANES III survey: 1988–1991
HTN defined by BP >140/90 mm Hg or treated

A

FIGURE 61-1. A. Prevalence of hypertension, defined as systolic blood pressure ≥ 40 mm Hg or diastolic blood pressure ≥ 90 mm Hg or current use of medication for purposes of treating high blood pressure. Data compiled from National Health and Nutrition Examination Survey III (1988–1991) Burt VL, Whelton P, Roccella EJ, et al. Prevalence of hypertension in the US adult population: results from the Third National Health and Nutrition Examination Survey, 1988–1991. *Hypertension.* 1995;25:305–313.

B. Incidence of atherothrombotic stroke (per 1,000 subjects per year) by age in men (*light bars*) and women (*dark bars*) from the Framingham Heart Study. Data compiled from Wolf PA, Lewis A. Conner lecture: contributions of epidemiology to the prevention of stroke. *Circulation.* 1993;88:2471–2478.

C. Incidence of coronary heart disease by age in men (*light bars*) and women (*dark bars*) from the Framingham Heart Study. Data compiled from Kannel WB, Wolf PA, Garrison RJ, eds. *Framington Study: An Epidemiological Investigation of Cardiovascular Disease.* Sec. 34. NIH Publication No. 87–2703. Bethesda, MD: National Heart, Lung and Blood Institute, 1987.

D. Prevalence of echocardiographic left ventricular hypertrophy in women according to baseline age and systolic blood pressure. Reproduced with permission from Levy D, Anderson KM, Savage DD, et al: Echocardiographically detected left ventricular hypertrophy: prevalence and risk factors. The Framingham Heart Study. *Ann Intern Med.* 1988;108(1):7–13.

E. Prevalence of echocardiographic left ventricular hypertrophy in men according to baseline age and systolic blood pressure. Reproduced with permission from Levy D, Anderson KM, Savage DD, et al: Echocardiographically detected left ventricular hypertrophy: prevalence and risk factors. The Framingham Heart Study. *Ann Intern Med.* 1988;108(1):7–13.

F. Prevalence of heart failure by age in Framingham Heart Study men (*light bars*) and women (*dark bars*). Reproduced with permission from Ho KK, Pinsky JL, Kannel WB, et al: The epidemiology of heart failure: the Framingham Study. *J Am Coll Cardiol.* Oct;22 (4 Suppl A):6A–13A, 1993.

G. Prevalence of atrial fibrillation by age in subjects from the Framingham Heart Study. Reproduced with permission from Lakatta EG, Levy D. Arterial and cardiac aging: major shareholders in cardiovascular disease enterprises. Part 2. The aging heart in health: links to heart disease. *Circulation.* 2003;107:346–354.

Incidence of Atherothrombotic Stroke by Age in Framingham

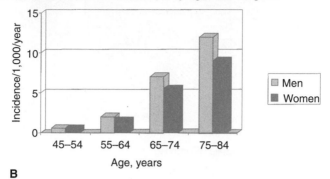

B

Incidence of CHD by Age and Sex

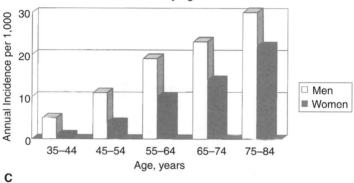

C

Age-Adjusted Prevalence of LVH
Women

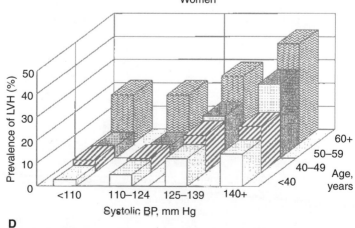

D

FIGURE 61-1. (Continued)

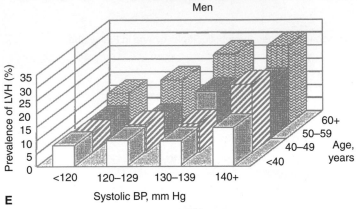

E

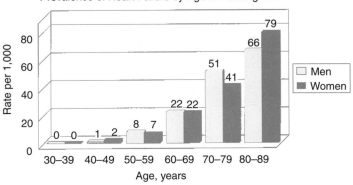

F

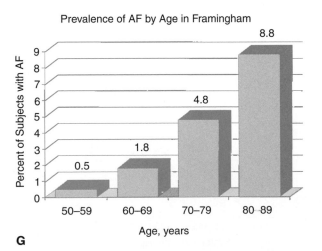

G

FIGURE 61-1. (Continued)

TABLE 61-1

Age-Associated Structural Changes in the Cardiovascular System

Structural	Age-Associated Change	Structural	Age-Associated Change
LV wall thickness	→ Increased	Large arteries	→ Dilate
Myocyte size	→ Increased	Arterial intima	→ Thickened
Myocyte number	→ Decreased	Arterial collagen	→ Increased
Myocardial collagen/elastin	→ Increased	SAN pacemaker cells	→ Decreased

LV, left ventricle; SAN, sinus node.

TABLE 61-2

Age-Associated Changes in Resting Supine Cardiovascular Function

Cardiac Function	Age-Associated Change	Vascular Function	Age-Associated Change
Early diastolic filling	→ Decreased	Arterial compliance	→ Decreased
Atrial contraction	→ Increased	Aortic pulse-wave velocity	→ Increased
Cardiac volumes	→ Unchanged	Reflected waves	→ Early
Heart rate	→ Unchanged	Systemic vascular resistance	→ Increased
Cardiac index	→ Unchanged	Systolic blood pressure	→ Increased
Ejection fraction	→ Unchanged	Pulse pressure	→ Increased
Ventricular-vascular coupling	→ Unchanged	Inertance	→ Increased

TABLE 61-3

Age-Associated Changes in Maximal Exercise Cardiovascular Function

Cardiac Function	Age-Associated Change	Cardiac Function	Age-Associated Change
EDVI	→ Increased	SVI	→ Unchanged
ESVI	→ Increased	Cardiac index	→ Decreased
Heart rate	→ Decreased	Ejection fraction	→ Decreased

EDVI, end-diastolic volume index; ESVI, end-systolic volume index; SVI, stroke volume index.

response of the heart to catecholamines. As noted previously, there is also a decrease in the LVEF with vigorous exercise.

ISCHEMIC HEART DISEASE

Sixty percent of myocardial infarctions (MI) occur in patients above 65 years of age, and one-third of all infarcts occur in those older than 75 years (see also Chapters 22 to 25). Eighty percent of all infarct-related mortality occurs in patients over 65 years, and 60% in those greater than 75 years of age. In unstable angina and non–ST-elevation MI cohorts and in patients suffering an ST-elevation MI, age is the most important demographic predictor of short- and long-term mortality. Table 61-4 shows some of the common features of ST-segment elevation MI in the elderly.

Even in older patients with a first ST-segment elevation MI who are thrombolytic eligible, the in-hospital morbidity and mortality is much greater than in younger patients. This is true despite the fact that indices of infarct size, such as creatinine phosphokinase levels and QRS scores, do not change with age. The incidence of heart failure and cardiogenic shock is three- to fourfold greater among the elderly than among younger infarct patients. Their age-associated decreased LV filling, aortic compliance, and beta-adrenergic responsiveness may contribute to the high incidence of these complications in the elderly.

Thrombolytic therapy decreases mortality in subjects aged 65 to 74 in both randomized and observational trials. There is less agreement about the benefits of thrombolytic therapy given to otherwise eligible patients greater than 75 years of age with ST-segment elevation MI. In high-volume centers, direct percutaneous coronary interventions (PCI) appear to be a reasonable alternative in this age group.

Like younger patients, older patients have large reductions in morbidity and mortality with appropriate postinfarction therapy, including beta-adrenergic receptor blockers, lipid-lowering agents, angiotensin-converting enzyme (ACE) inhibitors, and aspirin. Despite randomized, placebo-controlled trials and observational trials supporting the use of these agents in the older postinfarct patient, these drugs are underutilized in the elderly.

TABLE 61-4

Features and Treatment of ST-Segment Elevation Myocardial Infarction in the Elderly

Feature	Age-Associated Change	Treatment	Result
Complications	→ Shock, CHF, rupture, death	Thrombolytics	Lifesaving for patients 65–75 y; controversial in those > 75 y
Prior symptoms	→ Angina	Direct angioplasty	Lifesaving in high-volume centers
Symptoms	More often atypical	Beta-blockers	Lifesaving
Unrecognized	≈1/2	Aspirin	Lifesaving
Recurrent ischemia	More frequent	ACE inhibitors	Lifesaving
Gender	Female	Lipid lowering	Reduces recurrent events

ACE, angiotensin-converting enzyme inhibitor; CHF, congestive heart failure.

The use of PCI and coronary artery bypass (CAB) surgery in older patients with chronic coronary artery disease has increased over the last 10 to 20 years. Although short- and long-term mortality is greater among the very elderly than in younger subjects, mortality in this group with revascularization procedures has declined and procedural success improved over the last decade. Increasing age is a significant predictor of mortality and stroke during CAB surgery. Lipid-lowering therapy benefits older patients with chronic coronary artery disease.

CONGESTIVE HEART FAILURE

The prevalence of congestive heart failure (CHF) is dramatically increasing. It is the number one discharge diagnosis for older adults. CHF is associated with over 300,000 deaths annually.

Older patients with newly diagnosed heart failure symptoms need careful evaluation, including two-dimensional echocardiography coupled with Doppler flow studies. If left ventricular systolic dysfunction (LVSD) is present in patients with angina and there are no contraindications to coronary revascularization, coronary angiography should be performed.

Older patients with symptomatic LVSD should be treated with an ACE inhibitor, beta-blocker, diuretic if there is evidence of volume overload, and digoxin. Spironolactone is recommended for patients with NYHA class IV symptoms. Nonsteroidal anti-inflammatory drugs (NSAIDs) should be avoided.

HYPERTENSION

The lifetime risk of developing hypertension exceeds 90%. The blood pressure (BP) control rate in the elderly is < 20%, mainly due to poor control of systolic BP (SBP). Weight loss and decreased sodium intake are particularly beneficial in the elderly. A thiazide-type diuretic or a long-acting, dihydropyridine, calcium-channel blocker have been shown in randomized controlled trials to reduce stroke and cardiovascular events. The choice of initial agent may be less important than the degree of SPB reduction achieved.

AORTIC STENOSIS

Calcific aortic stenosis (AS) is by far the most frequent clinically significant valvular abnormality afflicting the elderly (see also Chapter 32). The development of clinically significant AS may be rapid in this age group (months to several years). The predictors of rapid progression to symptoms or death in the elderly with initially asymptomatic calcific AS include a heavily calcified valve and rapid yearly progression of the echocardiographic Doppler gradient across the aortic valve. This noninvasive technique is the most helpful study to detect AS. Asymptomatic older patients require careful follow-up for the development of symptoms, including angina, syncope, and heart failure. Aortic valve replacement often results in marked improvement in symptoms and survival, even in the very elderly. Age itself should not be an exclusion for valve replacement; other surgical risk factors—including low EF, atrial fibrillation, need for coronary artery bypass grafting, and a small-sized aortic root—need be taken into consideration.

For elderly patients requiring valve replacement, the bleeding risk from lifelong anticoagulation with a mechanical valve must be balanced against the risk of structural deterioration and need for repeat surgery with a bioprosthetic valve. Considerations include the age of the patient, anticoagulation risk, and valve position, with mitral bioprosthetic valves deteriorating at a higher rate than bioprosthetic valves in the aortic position (see also Chapters 32 and 37).

ATRIAL FIBRILLATION

The prevalence of atrial fibrillation (AF) is strikingly age dependent. By 80 years of age, nearly 10% will have AF. AF is classified as paroxysmal, persistent, or permanent. AF raises the risk of stroke fivefold. Cardioversion with aggressive rhythm control has not been shown to decrease mortality. Anticoagulation therapy with warfarin can decrease the risk of ischemic stroke with adequate safety. Clinicians should achieve a target international normalized ratio (INR) of 2.5 (range, 2.0–3.0).

SUGGESTED READING

Ahmed A. American College of Cardiology/American Heart Association chronic heart failure evaluation and management guidelines: relevance to the geriatric practice. *J Am Geriatr Soc.* 2003;51:123–126.

Lakatta EG. Cellular and molecular clues to heart and arterial aging. *Circulation.* 2003;107:490–497.

Lakatta EG, Levy D. Arterial and cardiac aging: major shareholders in cardiovascular disease enterprises. Part II. The aging heart in health: links to heart disease. *Circulation.* 2003;107:346–354.

Lakatta EG, Najjar SS, Schulman SP, et al. Aging and cardiovascular disease in the elderly. In: Fuster F, O'Rourke R, Walsh RA, et al., eds. *Hurst's The Heart.* 12th ed. New York, NY: McGraw-Hill; 2008:2247–2274.

White HD, Barbash GI, Califf RM, et al. Age and outcome with contemporary thrombolytic therapy. Results from the GUSTO-I trial. *Circulation.* 1996;94:1826–1833.

CHAPTER (62)

Complementary Medicine in Relation to Cardiovascular Disease

Prashant Kaul, Rebecca B. Costello, Daniel B. Mark, John H. K. Vogel, and Mitchell W. Krucoff

Although complementary and alternative medicine (CAM) therapies have been practiced for thousands of years in culturally based health systems, there is a growing but still very immature literature in most of these areas. With publication of the consensus paper on CAM practices in cardiovascular care, the American College of Cardiology (ACC) has pointed cardiologists to a unique dimension of health care concepts, research, and practice. The introduction to this consensus document observes that "topics chosen for coverage by Expert Consensus Documents are so designed because the evidence base and experience with technology or clinical practice are not considered sufficiently well developed to be evaluated by the formal ACC/AHA Practice Guidelines process."

The National Center for Complementary and Alterative Medicine (NCCAM) at the National Institutes of Health is mandated to explore complementary and alternative healing practices in the context of rigorous science. With even the terms *alternative, complementary, integrative,* and others still in flux, in this chapter the authors have taken selected therapies and references from the general topical framework that NCCAM has developed for CAM therapies with a focus, where possible, specifically on cardiovascular applications across NCCAM's five key treatment areas: biologically based therapies, manipulative and body-based methods, energy therapies, mind–body interventions, and alternative medical systems.

BIOLOGICALLY BASED THERAPIES: SELECTED BOTANICALS AND DIETARY SUPPLEMENTS

[ ] GARLIC (*ALLIUM SAVITUM*)

Garlic has long been touted as a natural product useful for the modulation of immune system activity, in the treatment of hyperlipidemia and hypertension, as well as the primary and secondary prevention of myocardial infarction (MI). Allicin is felt to be the bioactive component responsible for the potential cardiovascular activity of garlic. Allicin content is determined by the nature of the garlic preparation, with raw crushed garlic having the highest concentration. Multiple mechanisms of action have been proposed, including decrease in cholesterol and fatty acid synthesis and cholesterol absorption as well as potent antioxidant properties. Antiplatelet and fibrinolytic activity with garlic has also been reported.

Clinical studies of garlic have yielded contradictory results, with significant design flaws notable in trials of garlic's effectiveness. Short-term studies have shown some benefit in the lipid profiles of patients taking garlic, whereas long-term studies of 6 months or more fail to show a sustained benefit by garlic alone. A well-designed 6-month RCT using highly characterized diet and supplement interventions comparing the effects of raw garlic, powdered garlic supplement, aged garlic supplement, and placebo in 192 moderately hypercholesterolemic patients demonstrated no significant difference in LDC-C by groups. Studies of garlic's effectiveness in hypertension have also suffered from poor methodology, and results show mostly insignificant decreases in blood pressure. Evidence for the supplemental intake of garlic for both the primary and secondary prevention of heart disease is not sufficient to recommend its use for this indication.

The anticoagulant properties of garlic can be problematic in the perioperative period and have been reported to interact with the P450 enzyme system. Garlic will also decrease the effectiveness of some HIV drugs. Side effects are minor other than occasional nausea with excessive raw intake of garlic and the development of an unpleasant odor.

【 】 HAWTHORN (*CRATAEGUS* SPECIES)

Hawthorn species are a group of small trees and shrubs found throughout North America, Asia, and Europe. Purported cardiovascular indications include congestive heart failure, angina, and arrhythmias. Hawthorn's activity is thought to be related to the presence of a number of key constituents, including flavonoids and oligomeric procyanidins.

A review of the literature reveals significant evidence for hawthorn's efficacy in the treatment of mild to moderate heart failure. Animal and in vitro models reveal positive inotropism with a mechanism of action similar to that of digitalis through a cyclic adenosine monophosphate (AMP)-independent effect. There is also evidence of a direct vasodilating effect. Some efficacy has been documented in increasing maximal workload capacity and decreasing symptom severity in patients with heart failure. No published studies have examined mortality effects. The recently completed SPICE (Survival and Prognosis: Investigation of Crataegus Extract WS 1442 in CHF) trial, conducted in 13 European countries in 2,681 patients with NYHA class 2 to 3 heart failure, compared 900 mg of a standardized hawthorn extract with placebo during a 24-month treatment period and noted a reduction in the rate of cardiac deaths after 6 months but not in the primary end point of interest—a composite of cardiac death, death due to progressive heart failure, fatal MI, nonfatal MI, or hospitalization. The number of adverse events and serious events was slightly lower in the hawthorn group compared to placebo. There are very limited human data on relief of anginal symptoms, and antiarrhythmic effects have been studied only in animal models.

The usual dose of hawthorn for heart failure is 300 to 600 mg three times daily of an extract standardized to contain approximately 2% to 3% flavonoids or 18% to 20% procyanidins. Effects can take up to 6 months to equilibrate. Combination with cardiac glycosides and central nervous system depressants should be avoided. Side effects are rare but include gastrointestinal upset, sedation, dizziness, vertigo, headaches, migraines, and palpitations.

【 】 *GINKGO BILOBA*

Ginkgo extracts are derived from the leaf of the ginkgo tree. Ginkgo is the most commonly purchased herbal remedy in the United States, with total sales of over $150 million. Widely used for its purported benefits in treating nondementia-related memory problems, Alzheimer's disease, and vertigo, ginkgo has also been proposed as a treatment for intermittent claudication and peripheral vascular disease. ACC/AHA Practice Guidelines (2005) noted marginal effectiveness of ginkgo to improve walking distance for patients with intermittent claudication.

Ginkgo has been reported to inhibit platelet activation factor, scavenge free radicals, decrease blood viscosity, and decrease vascular resistance, although it is not clear which of these pathways might mechanistically explain ginkgo's effectiveness in peripheral vascular disease. Individual studies have revealed benefit in increasing mean pain-free walking distance. Two meta-analyses have examined the literature and reported a statistically significant increase in walking average distances of 25 m. The clinical significance of this difference is unclear.

The usual dose of ginkgo for the treatment of claudication is 40 to 80 mg three times daily of a 50:1 extract standardized to contain 24% ginkgo-flavone glycosides. Caution must be exercised with its use, because it has been reported to increase both spontaneous and trauma-related bleeding, including bleeding during surgery and other procedures. Caution is also advised when using gingko in conjunction with other anticoagulant or antiplatelet drugs. Ginkgo has been reported to decrease the metabolism of trazodone in at least one case report, perhaps by an inhibition of monoamine oxidase. Side effects are common and include headaches, dizziness, gastrointestinal complaints, and skin reactions.

【　】 HORSE CHESTNUT TREE EXTRACT (*AESCULUS HIPPOCASTANUM*)

The horse chestnut tree is found worldwide. Its seeds contain active compounds known as saponins, which have mild anti-inflammatory properties. Aescin, a combination of triterpene saponins, appears to be the pharmacologically active component. Its mechanism of action is considered to be sensitization to Ca^{2+} ions and a sealing effect on small vessel permeability to water. Traditionally, this botanical has been used for hemorrhoids, rheumatism, swellings, varicose veins, and leg ulcers. Research has focused on horse chestnut tree extract in the treatment of *chronic venous insufficiency*, and multiple studies have reported the superiority of horse chestnut tree extract over placebo. A recent systematic review of 17 RCTs found horse chestnut seed to be efficacious and safe with short-term use (2–16 weeks).

The usual dose of horse chestnut tree extract is 300 mg twice daily, standardized to contain 50 mg aescin per dose, for a total daily dose of 100 mg aescin. Aescin binds to plasma protein and can affect the binding of other drugs. Side effects are rare, including headache, itching, and dizziness. Concerns regarding risk of renal impairment do not appear to be warranted.

【　】 POLICOSANOL

Policosanol is a combination of aliphatic alcohols derived most commonly from sugar cane wax, although octacosanol, the predominant active ingredient, is also present in wheat germ oil and other vegetable oils. Policosanol *inhibits cholesterol biosynthesis* in a step located between acetate and mevalonate as well as by an increase in low-density lipoprotein (LDL) receptor–dependent processing. There is no evidence for a direct inhibition of hydroxymethylglutaryl coenzyme A (HMG-CoA) reductase. Policosanol has been extensively used clinically and researched in Cuba. These studies suggest a lipid-lowering effect of approximately 15% for total cholesterol and 20% for LDL cholesterol, which can be increased to 30% with higher doses. Maximal effects are seen after 6 to 8 weeks of use, and benefits have been demonstrated in studies lasting longer than 1 year. In a head-to-head comparison of 10 mg policosanol with 20 mg fluvastatin in women with elevated cholesterol, the lipid-lowering effects of policosanol were slightly superior to those of fluvastatin, and policosanol alone significantly inhibited the susceptibility of LDL to lipid peroxidation. A recent review has noted the efficacy of policosanol and suggested a unique role for this natural compound, in particular for patients desiring a natural alternative to synthetically derived drugs for cholesterol management. However, efficacy data from newer studies outside of Cuba have failed to report any benefits. There are no studies of clinical outcomes in patients treated with policosanol.

The typical starting dose of policosanol is 5 mg/d, which can be increased to a maximal dose of 20 mg/d. Side effects are infrequent, with weight loss, polyuria, and headache most commonly reported. There is concern that policosanol can potentiate anticoagulant activity and it should therefore be used with caution with other known agents that increase the risk of bleeding.

【 　】 RED RICE YEAST (MONASCUS PURPUREUS)

Red rice yeast, derived from yeast that grows on rice, has been a food staple and folk remedy for thousands of years in Asia. It was noted in the 1970s that a product of the yeast, monacolin K (lovastatin), was an *inhibitor of HMG-CoA reductase*. The concentration of lovastatin varies in red rice yeast but averages near 0.4% by weight.

In a multicenter study of 187 subjects, red rice yeast lowered total cholesterol by 16.4%, LDL cholesterol by 21.0%, triglycerides by 24.5%, and the ratio of total cholesterol to high-density lipoprotein (HDL) cholesterol by 17.7%; it increased HDL cholesterol by 14.6%. Although the reported side effects of red rice yeast are few—including mainly gastrointestinal upset, headaches, and dizziness—red rice yeast must theoretically be considered a typical HMG-CoA reductase inhibitor, and caution is advised with regard to potential side effects, including rhabdomyolysis.

【 　】 DIETARY SUPPLEMENTS

A number of dietary supplements have been postulated to have beneficial effects on cardiovascular disease. These include antioxidant vitamins, B vitamins, omega-3 fatty acids, plant sterols, soluble fiber, soy, nuts, alcohol, and teas.

Omega-3 Fatty Acids

Omega-3 polyunsaturated fatty acids (FAs) can be derived from either plant or marine sources. The principal plant-based omega-3 FA, alpha linolenic acid (ALA), is found in soy and its derivative tofu as well as in canola oil, flax seeds, and nuts. Omega-3 FAs derived from the tissues of marine animals (*fish oil*) include docosahexaenoic acid (DHA) and eicosapentaenoic acid (EPA). Typical dietary sources include mackerel, salmon, herring, sardines, anchovies, and albacore tuna. Three epidemiologic studies in the 1980s found that persons who ate fish every week had a lower mortality from CAD. Proposed mechanisms of benefit for omega-3 FAs include a direct antiarrhythmic effect, reduction in serum triglyceride concentrations and a small drop in blood pressure as well as decreased platelet aggregation. Other suggested mechanisms include an anti-inflammatory effect and enhanced production of vascular nitric oxide.

More than 40 cohort studies have now examined the effects of fish consumption on CAD outcomes. The most robust of these suggest a protective effect. Additional reports suggest that atherosclerotic progression in native coronaries and vein grafts may be slowed in males taking fish oil.

A systematic review of randomized trials of omega-3 FAs published 1966 to 2003 involving more than 33,000 patients found a small but nonsignificant reduction in all-cause mortality with a strategy of high omega-3 intake relative to low omega-3 intake (RR 0.87, 95% confidence interval 0.73–1.03). Overall, studies suggesting the largest apparent benefit for high omega-3 intake were those with the smallest cohorts. The largest of these was the GISSI-Prevenzione study, which randomized 5,666 post-MI patients to 1 g/d or usual therapy. The primary analysis showed a 20% reduction in all-cause mortality ($p = 0.01$) and a 45% reduction in sudden death ($p < 0.01$). The Japan EPA Lipid Intervention Study (JELIS) is the largest primary prevention trial to date randomizing over 18,000 hyperlipidemic patients to 1,800 mg/d of eicosapentaenoic acid (EPA) in addition to a statin or a statin alone. After 4.6 years the primary end point of major coronary events was significantly reduced by 19% in the EPA treated patients.

Currently, the American Heart Association recommends two servings of fish (especially fatty fish) per week as part of a heart-healthy diet for the general public. In Europe, use of fish oil for secondary prevention after MI is generally considered standard of care. Nonetheless, the value of supplemental fish oil for primary or secondary prevention will need significant new studies to clarify current uncertainties. One important ongoing trial is GISSI-Heart Failure, which is testing omega-3 FAs versus placebo in more than 7,000 class II to IV heart failure patients over 3 years. Results are expected in 2008.

Antioxidants and Antioxidant Vitamins

Despite a large body of epidemiologic evidence suggesting a favorable association between a diet high in antioxidants and reduced risk of coronary heart disease (CHD), *no clinical trial has confirmed such benefits.* Most of the observational studies examined the consumption of foods and estimated the likely vitamin content, whereas a few studies have examined the supplemental consumption of vitamins.

Vitamin E refers to a group of molecules that includes four tocopherols and four tocotrienols. Alpha tocopherol is the most prevalent and most potent lipid-soluble antioxidant in plasma. Several large epidemiologic studies involving more than 170,000 subjects have assessed the association between dietary and supplement-based vitamin E and CHD outcomes. Three of these found supplement-based vitamin E to be associated with a significant reduction in hard cardiac events, especially in doses >100 international unit (IU) for > 2 years.

The Cambridge Heart Antioxidant Study (CHAOS) demonstrated that 400 to 800 IU of vitamin E given as secondary prevention reduced the combined end point of death or nonfatal MI by 47%. However, larger and more recent trials including the Heart Outcomes Prevention Evaluation (HOPE) trial, HOPE—The Ongoing Outcomes (TOO) trial, the GISSI-Prevenzione trial, and the Primary Prevention Project (PPP), found *no therapeutic benefit* on a variety of outcome measures including disease progression as assessed by carotid ultrasound. The Women's Heath Study of 39,876 apparently healthy women age 45 and older found that vitamin E (600 IU on alternate days) reduced cardiovascular death (RR 0.76, $p = 0.03$) but had no effect on total cardiovascular events, MI, or stroke. In further analysis of the same data those women randomized to vitamin E demonstrated an overall 21% reduced risk of venous thromboembolism (VTE). The observed risk reduction was 44% among those with prothrombotic mutations or a personal history of VTE. The authors also noted that overall, vitamin E was associated with lower bleeding risk than those observed for low-dose aspirin. At present, however, the preponderance of the evidence *does not support a role for vitamin E* supplements in either primary or secondary prevention of CHD.

Vitamin C (ascorbic acid) is a strong water-soluble antioxidant. Several randomized trials have tested vitamin C supplements in varying doses for CHD prevention. In the Heart Protection Study, 20,536 patients with CAD or diabetes were randomized to antioxidant vitamins (600 mg of vitamin E, 250 mg of vitamin C, and 20 mg of beta-carotene) versus placebo. Although the vitamin regimen was found to be safe, there was *no evidence for a therapeutic effect* after 5 years of treatment. In contrast, in the Antioxidant Supplementation in Atherosclerosis Prevention (ASAP) study, hypercholesterolemic patients were randomized to twice-daily supplements of 136 IU of vitamin E, 250 mg of slow-release vitamin C, both, or placebo only. At 6 years among the 440 subjects completing the study, vitamin supplementation slowed common carotid intimal-medial thickness by 25%.

B Vitamins

Moderate elevations of plasma homocysteine levels have been associated with an enhanced risk for atherosclerotic disease. The metabolism of homocysteine requires several B vitamins as cofactors, specifically vitamins B_6, B_{12}, and folate. *Homocysteine* levels can be decreased by the administration of supplemental folate, with or without vitamins B_6 and B_{12}. Although epidemiologic studies suggested potential cardiovascular benefit with B-vitamin supplementation, either through this or other undefined mechanisms, most trial results have shown no such benefit. A meta-analysis of four randomized, controlled trials of B-vitamin therapy found *no evidence that B vitamin supplements slowed the progression of atherosclerosis.* However, folic acid may affect the early stages of CVD through moderating endothelial dysfunction, as substantiated in a meta-analysis of 14 intervention trials where high doses of folic acid were administered for 4 months or more and flow-mediated dilatation was evaluated. A randomized, placebo-controlled trial with 636 patients suggests that combined folate, B_6, and B_{12} therapy may actually increase the risk of restenosis and revascularization after coronary stenting with bare-metal stents. The AHA notes that available evidence is *inadequate to recommend folic acid and other B-vitamin supplements* as a means to reduce CVD risk at this time.

Chelation Therapy

The intravenous infusion of ethylenediamine-tetraacetic acid (EDTA) is a form of alternative medicine commonly used for the treatment of atherosclerotic vascular disease. The original rationale behind this therapy was that EDTA chelation would remove calcium from atheromatous arterial lesions. However, there is little empiric support for this putative mechanism, and other possible benefits such as an antioxidant effect have been proposed. *The bulk of the evidence base on chelation is from case reports and case series involving a total of more than 4,600 patients, largely describing the beneficial effects of EDTA chelation.*

There have been *four small randomized trials of chelation therapy*. The most recent is the Program to Assess Alternative Treatment Strategies to Achieve Cardiac Health (PATCH), which randomized 84 stable angina patients and followed them for 6 months. Event rates in this trial were low, and there were *no differences* between the *chelation* and the *placebo* arms. The investigators concluded that a much larger trial would be required.

The National Institutes of Health has funded a major randomized trial of chelation, the Trial to Assess Chelation Therapy (TACT). This study, which started enrollment in 2003, will randomize 1,950 patients ≥ 50 years of age with a prior MI to either chelation therapy or placebo. Results are expected by 2010.

Soluble Fiber

Dietary fiber supplements have been shown to produce desirable changes in LDL cholesterol and blood sugar levels. Epidemiologic findings suggest a possible impact on coronary disease and outcome. However, there are *no prospective trials* of the effect of these dietary supplements on cardiac outcomes.

Soy Protein and Isoflavones

Substitution of soy protein for animal protein can produce significant reductions in LDL cholesterol and triglycerides. Whether this reflects a unique benefit of soy or isoflavones in particular or merely a reduction in dietary animal protein and fat is unclear. Much of the most favorable evidence on this intervention is observational and suggests an inverse association between vegetable protein intake and blood pressure. A review of the benefits of soy protein and isoflavones has been published by the AHA Nutrition Committee. A total of 22 randomized trials tested the effects of soy protein and 19 studies tested soy isoflavones and found a small decrease in LDL cholesterol with no effects on other lipid fractions or blood pressure. Therefore, the AHA believes there is no meaningful benefit to soy protein consumption with regard to HDL cholesterol, triglycerides, or lipoprotein(a), but consumption of soy-protein rich foods may indirectly reduce CVD risk by replacing animal and dairy products that may be higher in saturated fats.

Plant Sterols

Plant sterols and stanols have been persuasively shown to lower cholesterol and are now commercially available in margarine products. To sustain the LDL cholesterol reductions of up to 15% noted in the literature with these products, individuals need to consume them daily.

[ ] ALCOHOL

Mild to moderate alcohol consumption has been associated in a variety of reports with reduction in stroke and rates of MI, functional improvement with claudication, and improved cardiovascular survival. Vasodilating and central nervous system effects, as well as antioxidant compounds in alcohol preparations such as red wine, have all been proposed as potential mechanisms of these benefits. At higher dose in susceptible individuals, alcohol is a well-known myocardial toxin, with equally deleterious potential in other end organs such as the liver, gastrointestinal tract, and central nervous system.

MANIPULATIVE AND BODY-BASED METHODS

Acupuncture, acupressure, and an array of massage techniques represent manipulative and body-based therapies. Of these, the most robust scientific information is available on acupuncture.

[ ] ACUPUNCTURE

Worldwide, more than 40% of physicians recommend acupuncture to their patients, and more than 50% of physicians want to add this modality to their therapeutic armamentarium. More than 35 state boards in the United States regulate the practice of acupuncture, although specific certification is not required for licensed physicians. Furthermore, the FDA regulates the use of disposable stainless steel and acupuncture needles as medical devices. The National Institutes of Health has published a consensus statement indicating that many issues related to acupuncture—including efficacy, sham effects, adverse reactions, acupuncture points, training, credentialing, and mechanism of action—need further definition.

Clinically, acupuncture is most accepted for the treatment of pain. In cardiovascular care, there are three areas for which acupuncture has been explored: anginal pain from ischemia, hypertension, and arrhythmias. The rationale for using acupuncture to treat these conditions can stem from its ability to inhibit autonomic sympathetic outflow. Acupuncture techniques can release endorphins in a number of regions in the hypothalamus, midbrain, and medulla concerned with processing information that influences sympathetic neuroactivity. Other neurotransmitters that can also be associated with the cardiovascular effects of acupuncture include gamma-aminobutyric acid, serotonin, and acetylcholine. Because placebo effects can occur in as many as 40% of patients, and because acupuncture seems to be efficacious in only approximately 70% of patients, the actual therapeutic window of benefit may be narrow.

Mechanistic studies suggest that catecholamine reduction with acupuncture can affect myocardial ischemia and stress-induced hypertension. These studies indicate that acupuncture probably limits myocardial ischemia by reducing myocardial oxygen demand rather than by increasing coronary blood flow. There are currently no trials showing reduction in mortality or other clinical outcomes with acupuncture in ischemic heart disease.

General vascular reactivity can be affected by acupuncture. Improvement in primary Raynaud cold-induced vasoconstriction by acupuncture compared to sham treatment has been reported. Hypertension can also be improved by acupuncture, although the absolute effects on blood pressure reported are small. These findings can be more profound in selected hypertensive syndromes responsive to central nervous system modulation.

Most authorities agree that the risk of an adverse event resulting from acupuncture is small, generally below 10% when performed by physicians. Pneumothorax, spinal cord lesions, hepatitis HIV infections, endocarditis, arthritis, and osteomyelitis have been reported but are rare, with an overall rate of less than 2%. The risk of an adverse event for nonphysician acupuncturists is higher, although the risk of serious events is low.

ENERGY THERAPIES

Bioenergetics or energy therapies are a series of healing *disciplines* that claim to harness intangible natural forces to influence physiologic, emotional, and spiritual healing. Although termed "energy" therapies, no electromagnetically defined field effects have actually been characterized. Examples of bioenergy disciplines include therapeutic and healing touch, Qigong, Johrei, Reiki, crystal therapy, and magnet therapy. Energy therapies are generally administered by an active practitioner who conducts both diagnostic and therapeutic functions by *sensing* or *reading* energy patterns and then manipulating or adding to those energy patterns, with the patient in a more passive role. It is quite conceivable that placebo effects, hypnosis, and other trance states can be included in this largely metaphorically defined practice area.

Practitioners of the ancient Chinese healing tradition of Qigong use deep breathing, meditation, and body movement to capture and focus the vital life energy, Qi. In cardiovascular application, Qigong has been claimed to influence hypertension in patients with heart disease as well as sudden death by accentuating vagal tone, as demonstrated by changes in heart-rate variability.

Healing touch and Reiki therapies conceptually involve concentration and transmission of bioenergy from healer to patient, with restoration and realignment of energy fields in the patient, either by touching the patient directly or by touching the energy fields around the body. The Vedic paradigm of energy concentrated in and through anatomically related chakras along the spine and central nervous system, with the energy flow between and around the chakras determined by paths or meridians both within the somatic body and in a field around the body, is frequently included in the conceptual constructs of these practices.

In hospitalized patients, therapeutic touch has been reported to palliate anxiety, with a potential effect on serum catecholamines prior to invasive procedures. *In a small pilot study of healing touch prior to urgent percutaneous coronary intervention, this modality was associated with a suggestive trend toward improved short-term outcomes.*

MIND–BODY INTERVENTIONS

A remarkably large and consistent observational literature provides evidence that the presence or absence of acute and chronic stress; emotional states such as obsessive behavior, depression, and hostility; spiritual attitudes such as faith and hope; and interactive support systems such as companionship and community *connectedness*; have significant correlations to cardiovascular outcomes such as hypertension, MI, stroke, and cardiac death. It is possible that these observations result from genetically driven physiologic responses to stress, with measurable impact on catecholamine levels, cortisol levels, glucose metabolism, autonomic tone, vascular tone, coagulability, pain perception, and immune reactivity. Furthermore, these states of mind and spirit are frequently paired with behaviors such smoking, eating disorders, obesity, diabetes, hypercholesterolemia, a sedentary lifestyle, and hypertension. Coping strategies and therapies that address this mind–body axis may have the potential to improve cardiovascular outcome, although the actual impact of these interventions is unclear. Examples of such therapies include yoga, meditation, mindfulness, relaxation therapy, guided imagery, music, mirthful laughter, and prayer.

One area of mind–body therapy that has been reported in application to cardiovascular disorders is relaxation therapy, where triggering of relative bradycardia, vasodilatation, and changes in the electroencephalogram have been described as the "relaxation response." Relaxation therapies generally involve some combination of relaxed abdominal breathing, quieting of the mind with meditation or related techniques, and somatic relaxation of the body. Relaxation therapies are frequently applied for stress reduction, including prior to invasive procedures.

Other mind–body techniques with published experience in cardiology include music and imagery. Anxiety reduction has been observed with music in coronary care units and MI populations, although an outcomes benefit has not been established. Imagery has been reported to reduce pain or the need for sedation in patients undergoing catheterization and to shorten hospital stay after bypass surgery.

Yoga, meditation, and mindfulness constitute a very broad range of disciplines providing tools that, with practice, cultivate personal access to calming of the body and quieting of the mind, with a variety of potential healing effects including reduction of angina and improved quality of life. One common aspect across these therapies is the use of relaxed abdominal breathing as the focus of concentration.

Many forms of meditation, including prayer, metaphorically extend beyond the mind–body complex into the dimension of mind–body–spirit. Patients suffering from heart disease are confronted by issues of personal mortality, and many turn to prayer both for comfort and to influence outcome. Such spiritual practices have been documented in almost 90% of patients undergoing elective coronary interventions. Beyond anecdote, little is actually known about the role of the human spirit in response to therapy, tolerance of procedures, or as an influence on outcomes.

To date, a total of six prospective, randomized clinical trials of distant intercessory prayer in cardiovascular populations have been published, but data on therapeutic benefit are inconclusive.

The Monitoring and Actualization of Noetic Trainings (MANTRA) Study Project from Duke University published the first multicenter randomized study of noetic therapies in cardiovascular care, in which both double-blinded distant prayer and open-label bedside music-imagery-touch (MIT) therapy were applied in 750 patients undergoing elective percutaneous coronary intervention (PCI) in the MANTRA II study. The 6-month composite primary clinical end point was negative, but the bedside MIT group had lower 6-month mortality ($p < 0.02$), and there was a trend toward outcome differences with different prayer methods. Most recently, Harvard University reported the Study of Therapeutic Effects of Intercessory Prayer (STEP) in 1,802 cardiac bypass surgery patients randomized in six centers to double-blinded placebo, double-blinded off-site prayer, and open label off-site prayer. Patients in the group who received distant prayer and knew about it had a significantly higher incidence of adverse outcomes, in particular postoperative atrial fibrillation, than patients in the double-blinded standard care group.

The MANTRA II and STEP studies in particular represent applications of noetic therapies in more robust multicenter, randomized, blinded study designs, and data from these studies raise key questions on the effects of patient participation as well as potential safety issues related to the use of noetic therapies in human subjects with heart disease.

ALTERNATIVE MEDICAL SYSTEMS

Alternative medical systems broadly constitute approaches to diagnostic and therapeutic applications that are based on paradigms conceptually distinct from the allopathic structure of modern medical practices in the Western world. By and large, alternative medical systems are culturally based and in many cases ancient in their history. Perhaps the most notable hallmark of these systems is their holistic character.

In traditional Chinese medicine, cardiovascular disorders are simply one feature of symptom complexes characterized across four relative states of yin deficiency or excess combined with yang deficiency or excess, where both yin and yang energies are associated with a broad range of emotional states, symbolic imagery, as well as specific body organs. In Ayurvedic medical systems, the body is essentially referenced across five inorganic elements constituting the material universe—earth, water, fire, air, and ether. The body itself is envisioned as coarse material, or *maya*, that is structurally configured by vibrational energy conveyed from a collective or cosmic source, or Atma. In both of these paradigms, wellness and illness exist in the individual human being, but they are also structurally shared across populations and beyond.

Although alternative medical systems appear radical in their departure from the rigorously articulate Western scientific medical model, current directions in wellness-oriented lifestyle modification strategies for both the primary and secondary prevention of cardiovascular disease represent a movement with a distinctively holistic character in the mainstream of modern practice.

SUGGESTED READING

Benson H. The relaxation response: therapeutic effect. *Science.* 1997;278:1694–1695.

De Smet PA. Herbal remedies. *N Engl J Med.* 2002;347:2046–2056.

Eisenberg DM, Davis R, Ettner S, et al. Trends in alternative medicine use in the United States 1990–1997: results of a follow-up national survey. *JAMA.* 1998;280:1569–1575.

Jonas WB, Crawford CC. Science and spiritual healing: a critical review of spiritual healing, "energy" medicine and intentionality. *Alt Ther Health Med.* 2003;9:56–61.

Krucoff MW, Costello R, Mark D, et al. Complementary and alternative medical therapy in cardiovascular care. In: Fuster V, Walsh RA, O'Rourke RA, et al., eds. *Hurst's The Heart.* 12th ed. New York, NY: McGraw-Hill; 2008:2462–2469.

Krucoff MW, Crater SW, Gallup D, et al. Music, imagery, touch and prayer as adjuncts to interventional cardiac care: the Monitoring and Actualization of Noetic Trainings (MANTRA) II randomized study. *Lancet.* 2005;366:211–217.

National Institutes of Health. National Center for Complementary and Alternative Medicine (NCCAM). http://nccam.nih.gov.

Vogel JHK, Bolling SF, Costello RB, et al. Integrating complementary medicine into cardiovascular medicine: a report of the American College of Cardiology Foundation Task Force on Clinical Expert Consensus Documents (Writing Committee to Develop an Expert Consensus Document on Complementary and Integrative Medicine). *J Am Coll Cardiol.* 2005;46:184–221.

Vogel JHK, Krucoff MW, eds. *Integrative Cardiology: Complementary and Alternative Medicine for the Heart.* New York, NY: McGraw-Hill; 2007.

Yager JEE, Crater SW, Krucoff MW. Prayer and cardiovascular disease. In: Stein R, Oz M, eds. *Complementary and Alternative Medicine in Cardiovascular Disease.* Totowa, NJ: Humana Press; 2004.

INDEX

Note: Page numbers followed by *f* or *t* indicate figures or tables, respectively.